MULTIDETECTOR CT

MULTIDETECTOR CT

Principles, Techniques,
and
Clinical Applications

Editors

Elliot K. Fishman, M.D.
Professor
Departments of Radiology and Oncology
The Johns Hopkins University School of Medicine
Baltimore, Maryland

R. Brooke Jeffrey, Jr., M.D.
Professor
Department of Radiology
Stanford University School of Medicine
Stanford, California

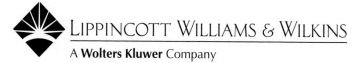

LIPPINCOTT WILLIAMS & WILKINS
A **Wolters Kluwer** Company
Philadelphia · Baltimore · New York · London
Buenos Aires · Hong Kong · Sydney · Tokyo

Acquisitions Editor: Lisa McAllister
Development Editor: Jenny Kim
Manufacturing Manager: Ben Rivera
Supervising Editor: Mary Ann McLaughlin
Production Editor: Kathy Cleghorn, Chernow Editorial Services, Inc.
Cover Designer: Christine Jenny
Compositor: Maryland Composition, Inc.
Printer: Edwards Brothers

© 2004 by LIPPINCOTT WILLIAMS & WILKINS
530 Walnut Street
Philadelphia, PA 19106 USA
LWW.com

Printed in the USA

Library of Congress Cataloging-in-Publication Data

Multidetector CT: principles, techniques, and clinical applications / editors, Elliot K.
    Fishman, R. Brooke Jeffrey Jr.
        p.; cm.
    Includes bibliographical references and index.
    ISBN 0–7817–4087–8
    1. Tomography. I. Fishman, Elliot K. II. Jeffrey, R. Brooke
    [DNLM: 1. Tomography, X-Ray Computed—methods. 2. Tomography Scanners, X-Ray
    Computed. WN 206 M9603 2003]
    RC78.7.T62M85 2003
    616.07′572—dc22
    2003060191

Care has been taken to confirm the accuracy of the information presented and to describe generally accepted
practices. However, the authors, editors, and publisher are not responsible for errors or omissions or for any
consequences from application of the information in this book and make no warranty, expressed or implied,
with respect to the currency, completeness, or accuracy of the contents of the publication. Application of this
information in a particular situation remains the professional responsibility of the practitioner.

The authors, editors, and publisher have exerted every effort to ensure that drug selection and dosage set
forth in this text are in accordance with current recommendations and practice at the time of publication.
However, in view of ongoing research, changes in government regulations, and the constant flow of
information relating to drug therapy and drug reactions, the reader is urged to check the package insert for
each drug for any change in indications and dosage and for added warnings and precautions. This is
particularly important when the recommended agent is a new or infrequently employed drug.

Some drugs and medical devices presented in this publication have Food and Drug Administration (FDA)
clearance for limited use in restricted research settings. It is the responsibility of the health care provider to
ascertain the FDA status of each drug or device planned for use in their clinical practice.

10 9 8 7 6 5 4 3 2 1

Contents

Contributing Authors

Norman J. Beauchamp, Jr., M.D. M.H.S. *Professor and Chair, Department of Radiology, University of Washington, Seattle, Washington*

Christopher F. Beaulieu, M.D., Ph.D. *Associate Professor, Department of Radiology, Chief of Musculoskeletal Imaging, Stanford University School of Medicine, Stanford, California*

Paul D. Campbell, Jr., M.D. *Department of Radiology, The Johns Hopkins University School of Medicine, Baltimore, Maryland*

Frandics P. Chan, M.D. *Assistant Professor, Department of Radiology, Stanford University School of Medicine, Stanford, California*

Lawrence C. Chow, M.D. *Assistant Professor, Department of Radiology, Stanford University School of Medicine, Stanford, California*

Marta Davila, M.D. *Department of Medicine, Division of Gastroenterology, Stanford University School of Medicine, Stanford, California*

Elliot K. Fishman, M.D. *Professor, Departments of Radiology and Oncology, The Johns Hopkins University School of Medicine, Baltimore, Maryland*

Karen M. Horton, M.D. *Associate Professor, Department of Radiology, The Johns Hopkins Medical Institutions, Baltimore, Maryland*

R. Brooke Jeffrey, Jr., M.D. *Professor, Department of Radiology, Stanford University School of Medicine, Stanford, California*

Ihab R. Kamel, M.D., Ph.D. *Assistant Professor, Department of Radiology, The Johns Hopkins Outpatient Center, Baltimore, Maryland*

Satomi Kawamoto, M.D. *Assistant Professor, Department of Radiology, The Johns Hopkins Outpatient Center, Baltimore, Maryland*

Ella A. Kazerooni, M.D. *Assistant Professor, Department of Radiology, University of Michigan Medical Center, Ann Arbor, Michigan*

Leo P. Lawler, M.D., F.R.C.R. *Assistant Professor, Department of Radiology and Radiological Sciences, The Johns Hopkins University, Baltimore, Maryland*

Ann N. Leung, M.D. *Associate Chair of Clinical Affairs, Section Chief, Thoracic Imaging, Associate Professor, Stanford University School of Medicine, Stanford, California*

Sandy Napel, Ph.D. *Associate Professor, Department of Radiology, Stanford University School of Medicine, Stanford, California*

Harpreet K. Pannu, M.D. *Assistant Profesor, Department of Radiology, The Johns Hopkins Outpatient Center, Baltimore, Maryland*

Geoffrey D. Rubin, M.D. *Chief of Cardiovascular Imaging, Associate Professor, Department of Radiology, Stanford University School of Medicine, Stanford, California*

John Paul Schreiber, II *Resident, Department of Radiology, Stanford University School of Medicine, Stanford, California*

Marilyn J. Siegel, M.D. *Professor, Departments of Radiology and Pediatrics, Mallinckrodt Institute of Radiology, St. Louis, Missouri*

F. Graham Sommer, M.D. *Professor, Department of Radiology, Stanford University School of Medicine, Stanford, California*

Preface

In the five years since the publication of the second edition of Spiral CT: Principles Techniques, and Clinical Applications, the imaging world has once again changed dramatically, with the introduction and rapid clinical dissemination of multidetector CT. A new era of "volumetric" imaging has been made possible through the development of 16-slice scanners and the ability to generate near-isotropic datasets. With single slice spiral scanners, we could only peer over the horizon and anticipate this future, which has now been rendered commonplace with the clinical implementation of multidetector CT. What was once thought to be an exciting possibility has become the clinical reality, as workstations closely integrated into the clinical environment enable 3D volumetric imaging, CT angiography, and cardiac imaging to be performed with a degree of anatomic resolution that is truly breathtaking. What is remarkable is that CT has not only proven to be a vital field for technological innovation, but has also maintained its crucial role for routine imaging studies, particularly in acutely ill and traumatized patients.

There are challenges posed by this technological revolution, such as an explosion in data and the greater complexity of managing image acquisition and transfer throughout a clinical enterprise. The clinical utility of using CT to screen asymptomatic patients in high-risk categories for such diseases as lung cancer or colon cancer will no doubt be debated for years to come, until there are definitive prospective studies documenting improved survival. The entire new field of computer-assisted diagnosis is poised to become a clinical reality for many of these applications, as there is a parallel revolution in the CT software in conjunction with the hardware revolution of the multidetector CT scanner.

The challenge in writing a book like this is that there is an ever increasing and expanding array of clinical applications for CT. A typical example is the fact that, within the past few years, CT has become the technique of choice to evaluate patients with suspected pulmonary embolism, replacing nuclear medicine studies and pulmonary angiography. The whole realm of cardiac CT is poised for rapid development as scan acquisition times get faster and faster, and there is no doubt that this will be a critical area for technological development to rival that of cardiac MRI. As the clinical applications and use of CT expand, we must be ever mindful of the need to reduce radiation, particularly in pediatric patients and in young adults. This has not received sufficient attention in years past, but it is clearly becoming a priority. Thus, far greater emphasis will be placed on reducing radiation dosage than has been in the past.

In summary, while it may be difficult to predict the future, one thing is certain: there will be continued hardware and software innovations that will further this technology and will lead to earlier diagnosis and better patient outcomes. This book strives to review the current state of our knowledge of multidetector CT, but that knowledge is moving so rapidly that we, as diagnostic radiologists, must accept the challenge of assimilating this new technological revolution and apply it to improve the care of our patients.

Elliot K. Fishman, M.D.
R. Brooke Jeffrey, Jr., M.D.

Acknowledgments

I would like to acknowledge the Body CT technologists at Johns Hopkins. Their commitment to excellence and dedication to patient care have always been a beacon of light, even in the most trying of moments.

E.K.F.

I would like to acknowledge the hard work and dedication of our technologists, residents and fellows working in Body CT at Stanford. Their commitment to imaging excellence has been the key to superior patient care.

R.B.J.

SECTION I

Basic Principles

CHAPTER 1

Basic Principles of MDCT

Sandy Napel

INTRODUCTION

Since its introduction in 1972, X-ray computed tomography (CT) has evolved into an essential diagnostic imaging tool for a continually increasing variety of clinical applications. The technology has made two major evolutionary leaps during the past decade. The first of these occurred in the early 1990s with the introduction of CT scanners with simultaneous patient translation and data acquisition (1–3). The main technological advances that led to these developments were slip-ring gantry designs, very-high-power X-ray tubes, and interpolation algorithms to handle the non-coplanar projection data. Two terms arose to describe this technology: *spiral* and *helical* CT. Initially, there was some controversy as to which was the more correct and/or precise term, and individual vendors took different stands on the issue. In 1994, Kalender's eloquent letter to the editor of *Radiology*, and the editor's reply, ended the controversy; thereafter, both terms would be equally acceptable (4). For the sake of consistency, this methodology for CT scanning will be referred to as *spiral CT*. These scanners revolutionized the use of CT, creating new applications that could not have been attempted before, such as CT angiography (5,6) and virtual endoscopy (7,8).

The second leap occurred mid-decade, with one vendor's introduction of a dual-detector row spiral CT scanner (9). By late 1998, all major CT manufacturers were shipping multidetector CT (MDCT) scanners capable of acquiring four slices per X-ray tube rotation. Currently, 8- and 16-slice scanners are available, with a capacity for 32 and higher numbers being anticipated. The major advantages of MDCT scanners are improved volume coverage speed and/or longitudinal spatial resolution (10,11). In addition, several new applications are being studied and performed that have been facilitated by the increased volume scanning speed (12–17).

The arrival of MDCT scanners has brought with it many new terms and concepts that must be understood for routine clinical and advanced research operation. To complicate the matter, different vendors have chosen different implementations for several of the key components and user controls. The purpose of this chapter is to provide a general understanding that hopefully can be applied with a little thought to any of these implementations. While vendor-specific examples will be shown, an attempt will be made to focus on the points of similarity, rather than on the differences, among the specific implementations. Obviously, the understanding of MDCT is based on many of the same concepts as prior generations of scanners. In this chapter, there will be no attempt to describe the basic physics of conventional or spiral CT, as these have been well described in many articles and books (18–20). Instead, this chapter will concentrate only on the technology unique to MDCT. It begins with a discussion of the detector, collimation, and data-acquisition systems. A description of the two primary modes of MDCT operation—axial multislice and spiral modes—and a discussion of the various tradeoffs involved when selecting operational parameters follows. The chapter concludes with a brief summary and references to advanced topics that are likely to affect image quality and clinical capabilities in the not-too-distant future.

DETECTOR AND DATA-ACQUISITION SYSTEM

Unless otherwise indicated, note that all detector and X-ray-source-collimation dimensions given in this chapter refer to the their projection at the scanner isocenter. Physical dimensions may be larger or smaller due to magnification caused by the relative sizes and locations of the devices.

The MDCT detector differs from that of a single detector CT (SDCT) in that in addition to being divided in the transaxial plane, it is divided further into rows in the longitudinal (or slice) direction. Figure 1-1 shows an example comparing a SDCT scanner with a 10-mm maximum-slice thickness to an MDCT scanner with 16 equally sized detector rows of height d. The increased length of the MDCT detector array in the slice direction permits a thicker maximum band of radiation to be detected compared to a SDCT

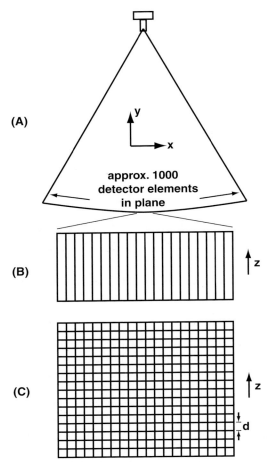

the potential to acquire 16 slices simultaneously, the cost and size of the DAS required to sample all rows simultaneously might be prohibitive. That is, the number of simultaneously acquired scanner *slices* may be limited by the DAS, independent of the number of *rows* offered by a given design. We define a *DAS channel* as the electronics required to sample one slice from the MDCT detector. Thus, an *M*-slice MDCT scanner is one that contains *M* DAS channels and therefore can sample simultaneously a maximum of *M* slices.

The first true MDCT scanners delivered in 1998 had four DAS channels and a larger number of detector rows. One might question whether there was any use for a source collimation other than that shown in Figure 1-2A; that is, why illuminate more than the central four rows if it was not possible to sample more than four? The following discussion explains how scanners with fewer DAS channels than rows operate. While advances in DAS design may be closing the gap between the maximum number of rows and the maximum number of DAS channels available, it is instructive to understand this design as its principles are still in use, and may continue to be for years to come.

In order to handle the disparity between the number of rows in the longitudinal direction and the number of DAS channels, the detector is integrated with an array of computer-controlled electronic switches and adders that can combine the analog outputs from several rows into one ana-

FIG. 1–1. SDCT and MDCT detector geometries. **A:** In-plane (*x,y*) fan of X-rays originates at tube **(top)** and is measured by detector elements along arc **(bottom)**. **B:** Small section of 1000-element detector showing 20 elements with through-plane (longitudinal or *z*-axis) dimension of 10 mm. Collimation at tube controls slice thickness (i.e., *z* width of detector illumination). **C:** MDCT detector is sectioned into rows along the *z*-axis and is generally longer in this dimension, as well. Note: illustration shows equi-spaced sectioning (height *d*) along the *z*-axis; variable width designs also are in use (Figure 1–4).

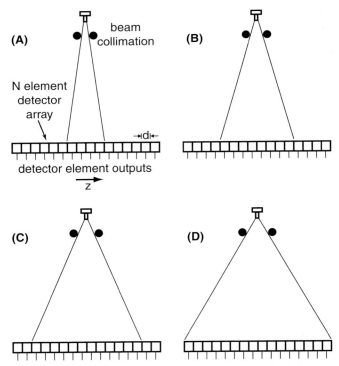

FIG. 1–2. Relationship of longitudinal beam collimation to illumination of detector rows. Figures **(A)** through **(D)** progress from narrow to wider collimation illuminating 8, 12, and 16 rows, respectively. Detector rows outside of direct illumination generally are not sampled.

scanner, and the sectioning of the detector into rows in the slice direction allows better localization (in the slice direction) of the attenuation within the band. This key change to detector design allows multiple thin slices to be acquired simultaneously with greater volume coverage per unit time.

As with SDCT scanners, an X-ray source collimator controls the longitudinal width of X-ray exposure. Figure 1-2 shows the relationship between the adjustment of the collimator opening and the number of detector rows illuminated.

In all CT scanners, the signals from the detector array are sampled (i.e., converted from analog to digital form) by a data-acquisition system (DAS) before they travel from the gantry to the computer system for image reconstruction. While the particular detector illustrated in Figure 1-1 has

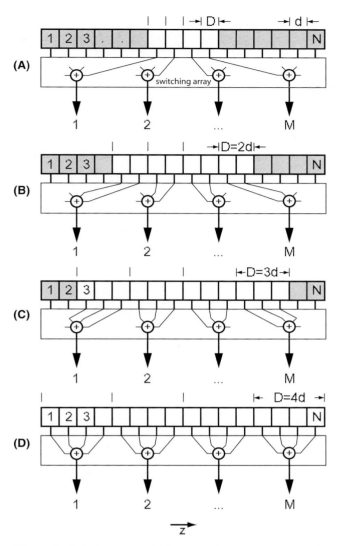

the ratio *M/N* towards unity by more modern designs, as this allows greater longitudinal coverage per rotation with thinner slices. Also note that while there is no satisfactory way of converting thick slices to thin ones (for relatively small *M/N*), there are several ways of converting thin slices to thicker ones (for relatively large *M/N*) if so desired, as will be explained in the "Axial Multislice Mode" and "Spiral Multislice Mode" sections of this chapter.

In addition to the equally sized detector designs discussed thus far and illustrated in Figures 1–1 to 1–3, it is possible to divide the detector longitudinally in other ways. Figure 1-4 shows an example of a so-called adaptive array, that is, an array with variable row width, implemented by one manufacturer. Hybrid designs that combine equally sized elements in one portion with other-sized elements in other portions also exist. One advantage of the adaptive design is that it contains a smaller number of dividers, or *septa*, between the elements than does an equally sized array of the

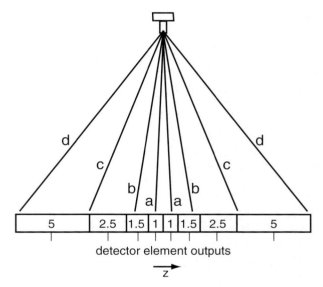

FIG. 1–4. Example of an adaptive (i.e., variable element width) detector array for a 4-slice MDCT scanner. Switching array (not shown) performs a similar function as one used for equally sized detector elements (Figure 1-3), adding outputs of detector elements to produce slice outputs of various thicknesses. Beam collimation between lines *(a)* illuminates only the inner half of the 1-mm elements, producing two 0.5-mm-thick slice outputs. Beam collimation between lines *(b)* illuminates the inner 1-mm elements and the inner ⅔ of the 1.5-mm elements. The inner four detector outputs then are passed straight through the switching array, producing four 1-mm-thick slice outputs. Beam collimation between lines *(c)* illuminates the inner six elements. The 2.5-mm outputs are passed straight through the array, and each 1-mm element is summed with its neighboring 1.5-mm element, thereby producing four 2.5-mm-thick slice outputs. Beam collimation between lines *(d)* illuminates all detector elements. The 5-mm elements are passed straight through the array, and each 1-mm element is summed with its neighboring 1.5-mm element and its neighboring 2.5-mm element, thereby producing four 5-mm-thick slice outputs.

FIG. 1–3. Relationship of *N* detector element outputs to the *M* slice outputs of the DAS. In this design (*N* = 16; *M* = 4), the outputs from equi-sized detector elements are channeled into slice outputs by a switching array. Detector rows not directly illuminated (and therefore not sampled) are shaded gray. **A:** With the narrowest collimation, only four rows are illuminated and each passes through the array as a separate slice output. In **(B)**, **(C)**, and **(D)**, there are more illuminated detector rows than slice outputs, and each of the slice outputs is comprised of the sum of pairs, triples, and quadruples of rows, respectively. The effective slice width, *D* (i.e., the longitudinal distance sampled by each slice output), is then **(A)** *D* = *d*, **(B)** *D* = 2*d*, **(C)** *D* = 3*d*, and **(D)** *D* = 4*d*.

log signal. Figure 1-3 illustrates this for a 16-row detector array and a 4-channel DAS, although the concepts are generalized easily to other implementations. Note in general that as the collimation widens to illuminate a larger longitudinal extent and, therefore, more detector rows, the number of rows summed into each DAS channel increases. Consequently, the effective slice width, *D*, increases as well. From this example, we can see easily the advantages of increasing

same longitudinal extent (e.g., 7 vs. 15 for Figs. 1–4 and 1–3, respectively). These septa reduce the active area of the detector in proportion to their number, and therefore degrade dose efficiency in the same proportion. Alternatively, adaptive arrays do not permit the acquisition of thin slices away from the longitudinal center. When listening to the debate between manufacturers, one must remember that the various performance measures of any scanner design may trade off each other, and each is affected by a multitude of design choices, components, and reconstruction algorithms and not just the design of any single component.

Also note that even in the adaptive design, subsequent to summation by the switching array, the M DAS channels produce projections of slices of equal width. The choice of detector design will not be important in the discussions to follow.

OPERATIONAL MODES

As with most SDCT scanners in use today, MDCT scanners can acquire data with the patient stationary (axial or "step-and-shoot" mode), or with simultaneous patient translation (spiral mode). Figure 1-5 illustrates these modes for a 4-slice MDCT scanner. The following sections describe the practical concepts necessary for understanding the use of each of these modes.

Axial Multislice Mode

In this mode, the MDCT scanner acquires M slices during a single gantry rotation and then translates the patient with the X-rays off before acquiring additional M slices. Consequently, the axial multislice mode has approximately an M-times volume coverage speed relative to SDCT. The detector configuration, that is, the mapping between the N detector elements and the M DAS channels imposed by the setting of the switching array, sets the menu of possible choices for slice thickness and, therefore, volume coverage per unit time.

Figure 1-6 shows an example of a detector array with 16 equally sized rows and a 4-slice scanner. As one compares the rows in the figure, two effects are evident. First, at the end of a given gantry rotation, the distance the patient can be translated increases at the expense of increased individual slice thickness. More specifically, the detector configurations shown in rows 1 through 4 allow 5-mm translation (for four 1.25-mm slices), 10-mm translation (for four 2.5-mm slices), 15-mm translation (for four 3.75-mm slices), and 20-mm translation (for four 5-mm slices), respectively, between rotations.

Second, Figure 1-6 shows multiple slice thicknesses available for each detector configuration. For example, the configuration shown in the first row can produce four 1.25-mm slices, two 2.5-mm slices, or one 5-mm slice by summing neighboring DAS channels (or slice outputs). [This is different than the summation that occurs within the switch-

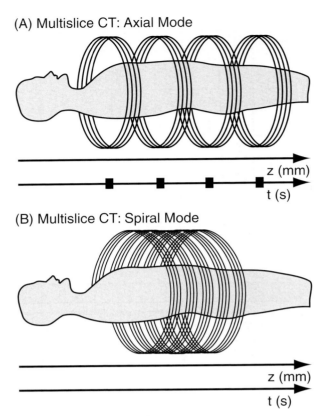

(A) Multislice CT: Axial Mode

(B) Multislice CT: Spiral Mode

FIG. 1–5. Operational modes of MDCT using a 4-slice scanner as an example. **A:** In axial multislice mode, 4 slices are acquired per rotation. Note that the four groups of slices shown are separated along the z-axis for clarity only; in clinical operation, there normally would not be gaps along the z-axis. Each group of four slices is acquired during the block of time shown on the *t*-axis, followed by a delay to reposition the patient to acquire the subsequent group. **B:** In spiral multislice mode, data from each slice output are acquired continuously in time as the patient is translated along the z-axis. The distance between groups acquired during each active rotation depends on the pitch setting, and may be positive (pitch > 1) as shown, or negative (pitch < 1).

ing array for a given detector configuration (Figure 1-3) as, once summed in the array, the data for the thinner sections seen by the elemental outputs can never be recovered.] Thus, axial multislice mode can present several slice-thickness options for a given detector configuration. Depending on the specific manufacturer's implementation and operator choice, the data may be reconstructed first as thick slices and retrospectively as thinner ones, or vice versa.

Another thing to notice is that there may be several configurations that may result in slices of a given thickness. For example, there are three ways to make 5-mm slices (rows 1, 2, and 4) and two ways to make 2.5-mm slices (rows 1 and 2). The choice must be made on the basis of volume coverage speed desired, which increases as one moves from row 1 to 4, and/or the ability to review retrospectively thinner slices, which decreases as one moves from row 1 to 4. A

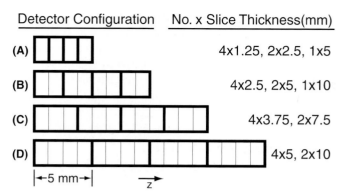

Detector Configuration	No. x Slice Thickness(mm)
(A)	4x1.25, 2x2.5, 1x5
(B)	4x2.5, 2x5, 1x10
(C)	4x3.75, 2x7.5
(D)	4x5, 2x10

|←5 mm→| →z

FIG. 1–6. Slice-thickness options for axial multislice mode as a function of detector configuration. In this design, there are 16 detector rows of height $d = 1.25$ mm and $M = 4$ slice outputs. **A:** Basic configuration, where the inner four 1.25-mm detector rows each produces its own slice output. Figures **(B)**, **(C)**, and **(D)** show configurations where pairs, triples, and quadruples of neighboring detector rows are summed to produce four 2.5-mm-, 3.75-mm-, and 5-mm-thick slice outputs, respectively. The first listed slice thickness in each row of the figure matches the detector configuration. Successive entries list slice thicknesses made available by averaging neighboring pairs **(A–D)** and quadruples **(A,B)** of slice outputs.

more subtle effect that may be of interest in certain clinical situations is that image quality for a given reconstructed slice thickness may be better by configurations shown in the upper rows of the figure. This is because they are made up of thinner sub-slices, each of which is subject to less non-linear partial volume artifact and, therefore, less streaking than slices made using longitudinally wider outputs (21,22). For example, when acquiring 5-mm slices in the brain, where the posterior fossa are known to generate streaks caused by this effect, it may be advantageous to use the configuration given by row 1 or row 2 rather than the one shown in row 4. While the latter permits the fastest volume coverage speed (4 times that of SDCT), row 2 permits a speed of twice that of SDCT, but has reduced artifact because each 5-mm slice is the result of the summation of two 2.5-mm slices. Row 1 produces a 5-mm slice by summing four 1.25-mm slices and thus presents the least artifact, but its volume coverage speed is equal only to that of SDCT (23).

Note that while the preceding discussion revolved around a specific example using an equally sized detector element array of the given dimensions, the concepts are generalized easily to adaptive detector arrays and different dimensions because ultimately only the longitudinal width of the equally sized slice outputs is important.

Spiral Multislice Mode

In this mode, the MDCT scanner acquires multiple slices simultaneously with patient translation through the gantry. This is directly analogous to spiral scanning on a SDCT scanner. However, whereas in SDCT, projections for a single slice are interpolated from data from the single DAS channel, data from all DAS channels contribute to each reconstructed slice in MDCT. Before understanding how this is done, the concept of spiral pitch as it relates to MDCT must be understood.

Spiral Pitch

Pitch is a function of slice width and table speed. For SDCT scanners, the definition of pitch, p, is unambiguous:

$$p = \frac{z_1 - z_0}{D} \qquad (1)$$

where z_0 and z_1 are the locations of the center of rotation at the start and end, respectively, of one gantry rotation, and D is the slice width at the isocenter. For SDCT, the slice width is controlled entirely by the source collimator, which additionally controls the radiation profile. Relationships between pitch, image quality, and dose are generally well understood and consistent from manufacturer to manufacturer. However, pitch in MDCT is complicated because the detector configuration has the ultimate control of slice width. If Eq. 1 were used for MDCT, these relationships would not hold when comparing scanners with different numbers of DAS channels, M. For example, consider a 4-slice scanner ($M = 4$) and an 8-slice scanner ($M = 8$), each covering the same distance ($z_1 - z_0 = 4D$) per gantry rotation with the same slice width (D). Equation 1 computes pitch, $p = 4$, in both cases. However, the width of the X-ray beam at the isocenter is $4D$ for the 4-slice scanner, indicating that the X-ray beam at the start of one rotation does not overlap with its position at the end of it. Alternatively, the width of the X-ray beam of the 8-slice scanner is $8D$, indicating that there is 50% overlap between the beam at the start and end of a single rotation. Thus, if Eq. 1 were used as the definition of pitch, one could have two scanners operating at the same pitch with very different dose implications. Generally, as in the preceding example, the X-ray-beam width at the isocenter is equal to $M \times D$; thus, for MDCT, the accepted (24) definition for pitch is:

$$p = \frac{z_1 - z_0}{M\,D} \qquad (2)$$

With this definition, the above example results in the 8-slice scanner operating at half the pitch of the 4-slice scanner and thereby gives the correct impression of the relative dose relationships.

Figure 1-7 shows an example of a 4-slice scanner operating at two different pitches. Recall that for MDCT, D is the longitudinal width sampled by a single DAS channel, not the size of any particular detector element in the detector array. Thus, the preceding example comparing a 4-slice and an 8-slice scanner, as well as the example shown by Figure 1-7, are independent of the design of the detector array.

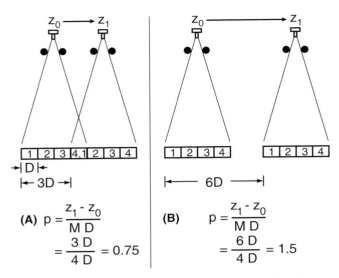

(A) $p = \dfrac{z_1 - z_0}{M \, D}$

$\qquad = \dfrac{3\,D}{4\,D} = 0.75$

(B) $p = \dfrac{z_1 - z_0}{M \, D}$

$\qquad = \dfrac{6\,D}{4\,D} = 1.5$

FIG. 1–7. Two examples of pitch setting for a 4-slice (i.e., M = 4) MDCT scanner in spiral mode. In both cases, patient is translated $z_1 - z_0$ mm to the left during one gantry rotation period, equivalent to X-ray tube tube/detector translation in the opposite direction as shown. **A:** Speed = $3D$ per rotation (pitch = 0.75) results in a 25% overlap, equivalent to the width D of one slice output; slice 1 at the start of a given rotation exactly overlaps slice 4 at the start of the previous one. **B:** Speed = $6D$ per rotation (pitch = 1.5).

Image Reconstruction

As has been the case for spiral SDCT, slices for spiral MDCT may be reconstructed at arbitrary positions along the longitudinal axis. However, whereas in SDCT the projection data used for reconstructing a single slice are interpolated from readings from the single detector array (1,2,19), the projection data in MDCT are interpolated from readings from all M detector rows (20,25,26). In addition, MDCT makes practical the creation of slices of various thicknesses from a single acquisition through a process known as z-filtering (27). Most manufacturers' algorithms create the projection data for a given slice location via these two processes, and then use standard filtered back-projection algorithms (28,29) for slice reconstruction. The following sections discuss interpolation and z-filtering for MDCT; slice reconstruction will not be covered as, barring exceptions (''cone-beam''), this process is unchanged relative to the traditional methods referenced above.

Interpolation

The relationship between sampling density along the longitudinal axis and pitch, or table speed, for SDCT is reviewed first. Consider a line drawn between the X-ray source at a given point in time through the isocenter towards the center of the detector array. Figure 1-8 plots the angle of this line as a function of location along the longitudinal axis for spiral SDCT with a slice width D and pitch = 1 (i.e.,

table speed = D/rotation). Notice that in these examples, one, and only one, projection angle is exactly available at the desired slice location. All of the other required angles (spanning a range of somewhere between 180 degrees and 360 degrees, depending on the reconstruction algorithm) must be interpolated from the available proejctions. Suppose

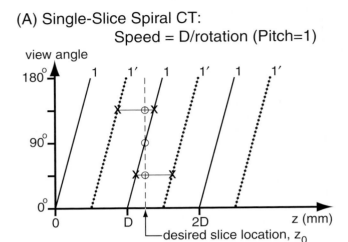

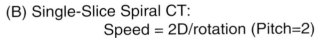

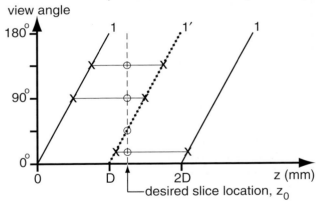

FIG. 1–8. Sampling pattern and interpolation in single-slice spiral CT. Plots show X-ray tube/detector angle versus position (relative to patient landmark) for **(A)** pitch = 1 and **(B)** pitch = 2. Solid lines (labeled "*1*") show angles of rays connecting the X-ray tube to the central detector channel on one side of the gantry (0 degrees–180 degrees), whereas dotted lines (labeled "*1′*") show complementary lines (i.e., at same angle, but originating from X-ray tube on the opposite side), as a function of position. Commonly used 180 degree linear interpolation methods synthesize co-planar rays by weighted summation of the nearest (along z) samples for each tube angle. Circles show examples of desired samples interpolated by weighted summation of the samples at the *x*s on either side of them. While some rays may be acquired incidentally without need for interpolation (e.g., in these examples **(A)** at 90 degrees at pitch = 1 and **(B)** 45 degrees at pitch = 2), rays at other angles are interpolated from a ray on one side of the desired slice and its complement on the other side.

the desired slice location is z_0. A slice of width D integrates attenuation from $z_0 - D/2$ to $z_0 + D/2$; thus, at pitch $= 1$ (Figure 1-8A), there is considerable overlap in anatomy, as seen by the detector from either of two locations (xs) used to interpolate a given angle. However, at pitch $= 2$ (Figure 1-8B), the overlap is marginal. Thus, it can be seen that the sampling density (the distance between the slanted lines along the z axis) relative to the slice width varies as a function of pitch in SDCT. As this density decreases, image artifacts increase due to the relative inconsistency between the samples used to interpolate each required angle.

Figure 1-9 extends the discussion above to faster table speeds and MDCT. Figure 1-9A shows the longitudinal sampling density for a SDCT scanner operating at pitch $= 3$. Note that with a slice width of D, there is no overlap between what the detector "sees" at the beginning and end of a given rotation; this condition leads to severe artifacts under most conditions, and therefore is not in general use today [although there are exceptions (30)]. Figure 1-9B shows what happens to the sampling pattern and density at the same table speed, but with a 4-slice MDCT scanner with slice width D. First, note that although the table speed is unchanged relative to Figure 1-9A, the pitch for 4-slice MDCT is $\frac{1}{4}$ of that for the SDCT according to the accepted definition for pitch (Eq. 2). Furthermore, note that the density of lines along z has improved considerably relative to SDCT (Figure 1-9A) and, in fact, is identical to that of spiral SDCT at pitch $= 1$ (Figure 1-8A). Thus, reduced artifacts at this table speed and slice width relative to SDCT would be expected, which is consistent with the reported literature (31).

Figure 1-9C illustrates what happens in 4-slice MDCT when the table speed, or pitch, is doubled (to $p = 1.5$) relative to that shown in Figure 1-9B ($p = 0.75$). Note the sampling density along z for $p = 1.5$ is half that of $p = 0.75$ and, in fact, is identical to that of spiral SDCT at pitch $= 2$ (Figure 1-8B). Moreover, the table speed of $6D$/rotation exemplified here would represent pitch $= 6$ for SDCT, a condition that has never resulted in clinically acceptable images. However, even the earliest MDCT scanners ($M = 4$) generate excellent images for many applications at this volume coverage speed (31).

z-Filtering

It is well known that the choice of image-reconstruction kernel (sometimes called *filter* or *algorithm*) trades off image noise versus spatial resolution to satisfy clinical requirements. MDCT, through a process known as "z-filtering," additionally allows the operator to generate slices of arbitrary thickness from a single acquisition, allowing the choice of thin slices where high resolution is required and high contrast is available, or thick slices for low-contrast situations requiring low noise.

Figure 1-10 illustrates the creation of three different reconstructed slice widths, w, at two different pitches for a 4-slice MDCT scanner with the detector configured to create

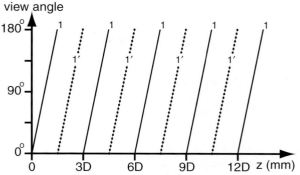

(A) Single-Slice Spiral CT:
Speed = 3D/rotation (Pitch=3)

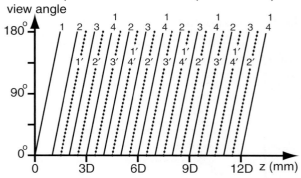

(B) Four-Slice Spiral CT:
Speed = 3D/rotation (Pitch=0.75)

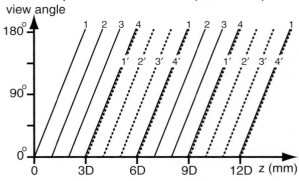

(C) Four-Slice Spiral CT:
Speed = 6D/rotation (Pitch=1.5)

FIG. 1–9. Sampling pattern of **(A)** single slice spiral CT at table translation of $3D$ (3 times the slice width) per rotation, or, pitch $= 3$, compared to a 4-slice (i.e., $M = 4$) MDCT scanner in spiral mode at a table translation of **(B)** $3D$/rotation (pitch $= 0.75$) and **(C)** $6D$/rotation (pitch $= 1.5$). As in Figure 1-8, solid lines show X-ray-tube angle versus location of ray connecting the X-ray tube to the central detector channel for one half of a rotation, and dotted lines show the other half (i.e., complementary rays). Note also that the horizontal (z-axis) scale is compressed compared to Figure 1–8. At **(B)** pitch $= 0.75$, slice output 4 covers the same coordinates as does slice output 1, as shown also by Figure 1-7. At **(C)** pitch $= 1.5$, slice output 4 covers the same coordinates as does slice output 1', and slice output 4' covers the same coordinates as does slice output 1.

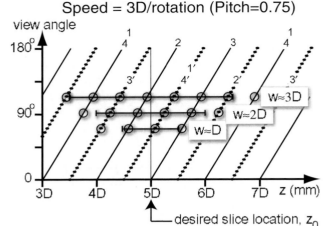

(A) Four-Slice Spiral CT:
Speed = 3D/rotation (Pitch=0.75)

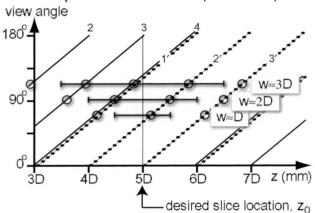

(B) Four-Slice Spiral CT:
Speed = 6D/rotation (Pitch=1.5)

FIG. 1–10. Multiple-slice width options by use of z-filtering. Note the z-axis is identical in scale to Figure 1-8 (expanded compared to Figure 1-9). Sampling patterns are identical to those shown in Figure 1-9. On each plot, horizontal lines with vertical end bars represent desired interpolated slice width (D, $2D$, $3D$) at location $z = z_0$. Circles represent samples that are recruited for interpolation. **A:** At pitch = 0.75, 4, 6, and 8, samples are used to interpolate rays for reconstructed slice widths $w = D$, $w = 2D$, and $w = 3D$, respectively. **B:** At pitch = 1.5, 3, 4, and 5, samples are used to interpolate rays for reconstructed slice widths of D, $2D$, and $3D$, respectively, for the ray angles (same as for pitch = 0.75) shown. Note that, in general, the number of samples used to interpolate a given slice width varies inversely with pitch.

ples) and reduced longitudinal spatial resolution (because samples cover increased longitudinal distance). This tradeoff is directly analogous to tradeoffs that may be made in plane by choice of reconstruction kernel.

Figure 1-10 also implies that for a given desired slice width, the number of samples available for interpolation increases with decreasing pitch. For example, reconstructing a slice of width $2D$ at pitch 0.75 combines six samples, whereas reconstructing the same slice width at pitch = 1.5 combines only four. Combining more samples lowers noise; thus, it can be seen that at constant exposure, noise in MDCT is a function of pitch, a fact that is not true for SDCT (1). Note, however, that some manufacturers provide automatic adjustment of X-ray-tube current (mA) to compensate for this effect. For example, to maintain image noise at higher pitch, the scanner operating software automatically may increase the X-ray-tube current. This means that the traditional notion of reducing dose by increasing pitch may not hold for particular MDCT implementations; therefore, great care must be exercised in this regard.

Tradeoffs in Spiral Multislice Mode

A number of observations may be made from the discussions above on image reconstruction and z-filtering. First, there are three adjustable parameters that affect image quality and the final reconstructed slice width, w: (i) detector configuration, D (i.e., the width of the slice outputs from the detector-switching array; (ii) pitch, p (i.e., the ratio of the table travel per gantry rotation to D; and (iii) the amount of z-filtering used. Figure 1-11 gives an example of available slice widths, w, for a hypothetical 4-slice scanner operated

Available Slice Widths

	speed (mm/rot)	D	nominal slice width (w)					
			1.25	2.5	3.75	5	7.5	10
PITCH = 0.75	3.75	1.25	*	†				
	7.5	2.5		*	†	†		
	11.25	3.75			*	†	†	
	15	5				*	†	†
PITCH = 1.5	7.5	1.25	*	†				
	15	2.5		*	†	†		
	22.5	3.75			*	†	†	
	30	5				*	†	†

FIG. 1–11. Table of available reconstructed slice widths, w, for a hypothetical 4-slice scanner with detector output widths of $D = \{1.25, 2.5, 3.75, 5 \text{ mm}\}$, operated at pitches $p = \{0.75, 1.5\}$. Asterisks (*) indicate smallest possible reconstructed slice widths for a given choice of D and p. Crosses (†) indicate other available slice widths. At fixed D and p, increasing amounts of z-filtering are used to create thicker slices as one moves to the right away from the asterisk.

slice outputs of width D. In all cases, projection data for a given angle at the desired slice location are produced by interpolation, that is, weighted summation of neighboring (along z) samples with the weights selected to produce the desired slice profile. Note that more samples (along z) are required for producing thick slices than thin ones; hence, thick slices have lower noise (due to averaging of more samat two different pitch settings. First, note that because D, p, and speed (i.e., distance traveled per rotation) are related through Eq. 2 at each pitch shown, choosing speed defines detector configuration, D, or vice versa. Second, note that in any row of the table, several slice thicknesses are available from the thinnest (limited by D) to thicker ones created by z-filtering. There is no theoretical reason why there are only two or three thicknesses available in each row, as thick slices can always be created from thin ones; however, manufacturers may limit the choices to simplify use. Third, and perhaps the most disconcerting to a new user, is that there are several settings that result in slices of the same width. For example, Figure 1-11 shows six ways to make a 5-mm slice! Final choices will be a direct function of clinical need. For example, if a large longitudinal extent needs to be covered in a short time (as, e.g., in a CT angiography study), higher pitches may be favored. The remainder of the chapters in this book will provide examples of how these choices should be made in given situations. However, the following "rules of thumb" may be useful in understanding why certain choices are advantageous:

- Creating thicker slices from thinner detector configurations (i.e., $w \gg D$) using z-filtering allows for the retrospective reconstruction of slices as thin as D. That is, if the parameter settings *land* at a cross (†) in the table, thinner slices may be reconstructed [crosses or the asterisk (*) to the left of where the parameter settings land]. Conversely, when $w = D$, the minimum amount of z-filtering is applied and thinner slices may not be reconstructed.
- Because pitch is defined as a ratio (Eq. 2), increasing table speed at constant pitch requires an increase in detector-slice output width, D, and thereby moves one down through the rows in the table. Of course, this permits greater volume coverage speed and requires less X-ray-tube output (because the total scan time decreases), but results in thicker minimum slice widths, and perhaps fewer choices for retrospective thin-slice reconstruction, because less z-filtering is used as D approaches w. Dose at constant mA decreases but, as mentioned above, manufacturers may increase mA automatically as the table speed increases to maintain noise levels.
- Increasing pitch while maintaining detector-slice-output width, D, and reconstructed slice width, w (i.e., moving from a given row in the top half of the table to the same row in the bottom half) may result in increased artifacts (31). Because D and w do not change, the number of choices for retrospective thin-slice reconstruction is not affected, theoretically (although, again, manufacturers may limit choices for other reasons). In addition, note that, at constant mA, dose decreases. However, as mentioned above, manufacturers automatically may increase mA with increased pitch to maintain noise levels.

ADVANCED TOPICS

This chapter was written following the first three years of clinical use of MDCT. During this time, in which 4-slice scanners dominated the scene, MDCT scanner technology has evolved considerably. At the time of this writing, 8- and 16-slice scanners have just appeared, and discussions of even larger numbers of simultaneous slices in the future have excited researchers and clinicians alike. As the technology evolved, new opportunities have arisen, as well as new problems begging for solutions. This section briefly covers some advanced topics, with pointers to the current literature, that are likely to influence the MDCT's continued evolution.

Cone-beam

Figure 1-2 makes it very clear that lines drawn in MDCT from the X-ray source to detector do not pass through the scanner isocenter. Thus, the projections acquired during one complete rotation do not lie on a plane, a condition required by standard methods of CT image reconstruction (28). Instead, they lie on the surface of a cone, hence the term cone-beam. This effect increases as the angle between lines drawn from the X-ray source to the center of the detector element, and to the scanner isocenter, becomes larger compared to the slice width, w. For a 4-slice scanner, the effect is small; only the innermost elements are used for the smallest slice widths and, as the outer elements are recruited, detector elements are summed to create larger widths (Figure 1-3). However, as the number of simultaneous slices, M, increases, thinner slices may be reconstructed from detector elements further from the central ones. This increases the ratio of the cone angle to the slice thickness; consequently, cone-beam artifacts increase.

There is no doubt, then, that as the number of simultaneous slices increases with the evolution of MDCT technology, more attention will be paid to the cone-beam problem. Direct cone-beam reconstructions (32–35) are impractical due to prohibitively long reconstruction times. Approximations such as the Feldkamp algorithm (36) are more practical, but artifacts increase as a function of the cone angle (37). More recently, other approaches have been published that are promising and very likely to be the basis of solutions to the cone-beam problem for future MDCT implementations (38–46).

Cardiac

Until the advent of MDCT, volumetric imaging of the heart most often was accomplished on electron-beam CT scanners, which had 50- or 100-ms acquisition times and therefore could image the heart with minimal motion blur and/or artifact (47). With the patient stationary, the electrocardiogram triggered the acquisition of single or multiple slices. Subsequent slices were acquired following translation of the patient to the next contiguous location.

Multidetector spiral CT scanners offered a new possibility for cardiac imaging because multiple detector rings acquire projections through a given portion of the heart at different times (11,15,48–52). If the rotation rate is asynchronous to the cardiac cycle, each projection of a particular section is acquired at a different cardiac phase. Projections then can be binned into different portions of the cardiac cycle; provided each bin contains projections over a sufficient and sufficiently dense angular range, those projections can be reconstructed into an image representative of that particular range of phases. Typically, one scans at low pitch to allow multiple angles to be captured by each detector ring for a given cardiac phase, a situation that can increase the dose relative to more usual head and body scanning at larger pitch. Faster gantry rotations permit higher temporal resolution and larger pitch. Minimum gantry rotation periods have decreased from 1 s to less than 0.5 s in the past 5 years; further reductions in rotation period, as well as expected increases in the number of simultaneously acquired slices, will lead to fewer artifacts and lower dose.

SUMMARY

The emergence of MDCT scanners has presented new opportunities for improved patient imaging and throughput. However, these scanners bring with them new concepts that have to be understood and new tradeoffs that have to be made. This chapter covered current concepts in detector design and schemes for dealing with limited capability for sampling the entire number of detector elements that can be fabricated. It also covered two modes of operation, axial and spiral multislice, and explored the tradeoffs that can be made when designing protocols for their use. Finally, it touched on several advanced topics that are likely to change further the face and use of MDCT scanners in the near future. The remaining chapters in this book will give examples and results of using the capabilities of current MDCT scanners. Hopefully, the topics covered in this chapter will have helped the reader understand the tradeoffs made in specific clinical applications.

ACKNOWLEDGMENTS

I offer sincere thanks to my physician collaborators, including Christopher F. Beaulieu, R. Brooke Jeffrey, Jr., and Geoffrey D. Rubin, for exciting collaborations using this new technology. In addition, I am grateful to Dr. Stanley Fox and Sholom Ackelsberg for providing introductory materials in the early days of MDCT, and to Christopher F. Beaulieu and Padma Sundaram for careful reading of the text and figures. I gratefully acknowledge support from the National Institutes of Health, General Electric Medical Systems, Siemens Medical Solutions, and the Lucas Foundation. Finally, thanks to my wife, Lyn Furness, my son, Walt, and my daughter, Madeline, who offer continued support and encouragement, and put up with my frequent absences to get things like this done.

REFERENCES

1. Kalender WA, Polacin A. Physical performance characteristics of spiral CT scanning. *Med Phys* 1991;18:910–915.

2. Crawford CR, King KF. Computed tomography scanning with simultaneous patient translation. *Med Phys* 1990;17:967–982.

3. Napel S. Principles and techniques of 3D spiral CT angiography. In: Fishman EK, Jeffrey RB Jr, eds. *Spiral CT.* 2 ed. New York: Lippincott–Raven Press, 1998:339–360.

4. Kalender WA. Spiral or helical CT: right or wrong? [Letter]. *Radiology* 1994;193:583.

5. Napel S, Marks MP, Rubin GD, et al. CT angiography with spiral CT and maximum intensity projection. *Radiology* 1992;185:607–610.

6. Rubin GD, Shiau MC, Schmidt AJ, et al. Computed tomographic angiography: historical perspective and new state-of-the-art using multi-detector-row helical computed tomography. *J Comput Assist Tomogr* 1999;23[Suppl 1]:S83–S90.

7. Rubin GD, Beaulieu CF, Argiro V, et al. Perspective volume rendering of CT and MR images: applications for endoscopic viewing. *Radiology* 1996;199:321–330.

8. Vining DJ. Virtual endoscopy: is it reality? [Editorial; comment]. *Radiology* 1996;200:30–31.

9. Liang Y, Kruger RA. Dual-slice spiral versus single-slice spiral scanning: comparison of the physical performance of two computed tomography scanners. *Med Phys*1996;23:205–220.

10. Hu H, He HD, Foley WD, et al. Four multidetector-row helical CT: image quality and volume coverage speed. *Radiology* 2000;215:55–62.

11. Flohr T, Prokop M, Becker C, et al. A retrospectively ECG-gated multislice spiral CT scan and reconstruction technique with suppression of heart pulsation artifacts for cardio-thoracic imaging with extended volume coverage. *Eur Radiol* 2002;12:1497–1503.

12. Becker CR, Ohnesorge BM, Schoepf UJ, et al. Current development of cardiac imaging with multidetector-row CT. *Eur J Radiol* 2000;36:97–103.

13. Chow LC, Sommer FG. Multidetector CT urography with abdominal compression and three-dimensional reconstruction. *AJR Am J Roentgenol* 2001;177:849–855.

14. Giesler T, Baum U, Ropers D, et al. Noninvasive visualization of coronary arteries using contrast-enhanced multidetector CT: influence of heart rate on image quality and stenosis detection. *AJR Am J Roentgenol* 2002;179:911–916.

15. Horiguchi J, Nakanishi T, Ito K. Quantification of coronary artery calcium using multidetector CT and a retrospective ECG-gating reconstruction algorithm. *AJR Am J Roentgenol* 2001;177:1429–1435.

16. Kopp AF, Kuttner A, Heuschmid M, et al. Multidetector-row CT cardiac imaging with 4 and 16 slices for coronary CTA and imaging of atherosclerotic plaques. *Eur Radiol* 2002;12[Suppl 2]:S17–S24.

17. Nino-Murcia M, Jeffrey RB Jr, Beaulieu CF, et al. Multidetector CT of the pancreas and bile duct system: value of curved planar reformations. *AJR Am J Roentgenol* 2001;176:689–693.

18. Newton TH, Potts DG, eds. *Radiology of the skull and brain: technical aspects of computed tomography.* St. Louis: C.V. Mosby, 1981.

19. Napel S. Basic principles of spiral CT. In: Fishman EK, Jeffrey RB Jr, eds. *Spiral CT.* 2 ed. New York: Lippincott-Raven Press, 1998:3–15.

20. Kalender WA. *Computed tomography: fundamentals, system technology, image quality, applications.* Munich: Publicis MCD Verlag, 2000.

21. Joseph P. Artifacts in computed tomography. In: Newton TH, Potts DG, eds. *Radiology of the skull and brain: technical aspects of computed tomography.* St. Louis: C.V. Mosby, 1981;3956–3992.

22. Levy JM, Hupke R. Composite addition technique: a new method in CT scanning of the posterior fossa. *AJNR* 1991;12:686–688.

23. Jones TR, Kaplan RT, Lane B, et al. Single- versus multi-detector row CT of the brain: quality assessment. *Radiology* 2001;219:750–755.

24. IEC: International Electrotechnical Commission: Medical Electrical Equipment—60601 Part 2-44. Particular requirements for the safety of X-ray equipment for computed tomography. Geneva, Switzerland, 1999.

25. Taguchi K, Aradate H. Algorithm for image reconstruction in multi-slice helical CT. *Med Phys* 1998;25:550–561.

26. Hu H. Multi-slice helical CT: scan and reconstruction. *Med Phys* 1999;26:5–18.

27. Hu H, Shen Y. Helical CT reconstruction with longitudinal filtration. *Med Phys* 1998;25:2130–2138.

28. Herman GT. *Image reconstruction from projections: the fundamentals of computerized tomography.* New York: Academic Press, 1980.

29. Macovski A, Herman GT. Principles of reconstruction algorithms. In: Newton TH, Potts DG, eds. *Radiology of the skull and brain: technical*

aspects of computed tomography. St. Louis: C.V. Mosby, 1981; 3877–3903.

30. Diel J, Perlmutter S, Venkataramanan N, et al. Unenhanced helical CT using increased pitch for suspected renal colic: an effective technique for radiation dose reduction? *J Comput Assist Tomogr* 2000; 24:795–801.

31. Fleischmann D, Rubin GD, Paik DS, et al. Stair-step artifacts with single versus multiple detector-row helical CT. *Radiology* 2000; 216:185–196.

32. Grangeat P. Mathematical framework for of cone-beam 3D-reconstruction algorithm for non-planar orbits. In: *Mathematical models in tomography. Lecture notes in mathematics.* Berlin, 1991;66–97.

33. Defrise M, Clack R. A cone-beam reconstruction algorithm using shift variant filtering and cone-beam backprojection. *IEEE Trans Med Imaging* 1994;13:186–195.

34. Kudo H, Saito T. Derivation and implementation of a cone-beam reconstruction algorithm for circular orbits. *IEEE Trans Med Imaging* 1994; 13:186–195.

35. Lauritsch G, Tam K, Sourbelle K, et al. Exact local regions-of-interest in spiral cone-beam filtered backprojection CT: numerical implementation and first image results. In: Hanson KM, ed. *Medical Imaging 2000—Image Processing.* Bellingham, WA: SPIE—International Society for Optical Engineering, 2000;3979:520–532.

36. Feldcamp L, Davis L, Kress J. Practical cone-beam algorithm. *J Opt Soc Am* 1984;1:612–619.

37. Kohler T, Proksa R, Bontus C, et al.. Artifact analysis of approximate helical cone-beam CT reconstruction algorithms. *Med Phys* 2002; 29:51–64.

38. Mueller K, Yagel R, Wheller JJ. Fast implementations of algebraic methods for three-dimensional reconstruction from cone-beam data. *IEEE Trans Med Imaging* 1999;18:538–548.

39. Wang G, Crawford CR, Kalender WA. Multirow detector and cone-beam spiral/helical CT. *IEEE Trans Med Imaging* 2000;19:817–821.

40. Schaller S, Sauer F, Tam KC, et al. Exact radon rebinning algorithm for the long object problem in helical cone-beam CT. *IEEE Trans Med Imaging* 2000;19:361–375.

41. Kachelriess M, Schaller S, Kalender WA. Advanced single-slice rebinning in cone-beam spiral CT. *Med Phys* 2000;27:754–772.

42. Kachelriess M, Fuchs T, Schaller S, Kalender WA. Advanced single-slice rebinning for tilted spiral cone-beam CT. *Med Phys* 2001; 28:1033–1041.

43. Kachelriess M, Watzke O, Kalender WA. Generalized multi-dimensional adaptive filtering for conventional and spiral single-slice, multi-slice, and cone-beam CT. *Med Phys* 2001;28:475–490.

44. Taguchi K, Zeng GL, Gullberg GT. Cone-beam image reconstruction using spherical harmonics. *Phys Med Biol* 2001;46:N127–N138.

45. Kohler T, Proksa R, Grass M. A fast and efficient method for sequential cone-beam tomography. *Med Phys* 2001;28:2318–2327.

46. Wang G, Zhao S, Heuscher D. A knowledge-based cone-beam x-ray CT algorithm for dynamic volumetric cardiac imaging. *Med Phys* 2002; 29:1807–1822.

47. Moshage WE, Achenbach S, Seese B, et al. Coronary artery stenoses: three-dimensional imaging with electrocardiographically triggered, contrast agent-enhanced, electron-beam CT. *Radiology* 1995; 196:707–714.

48. Kachelriess M, Sennst DA, Maxlmoser W, et al. Kymogram detection and kymogram-correlated image reconstruction from subsecond spiral computed tomography scans of the heart. *Med Phys* 2002; 29:1489–1503.

49. Kachelriess M, Ulzheimer S, Kalender WA. ECG-correlated image reconstruction from subsecond multi-slice spiral CT scans of the heart. *Med Phys* 2000;27:1881–1902.

50. Kachelriess M, Ulzheimer S, Kalender WA. ECG-correlated imaging of the heart with subsecond multislice spiral CT. *IEEE Trans Med Imaging* 2000;19:888–901.

51. Becker CR, Ohnesorge BM, Schoepf UJ, et al. Current development of cardiac imaging with multidetector-row CT. *Eur J Radiol* 2000; 36:97–103.

52. Achenbach S, Ulzheimer S, Baum U, et al. Noninvasive coronary angiography by retrospectively ECG-gated multislice spiral CT. *Circulation* 2000;102:2823–2828.

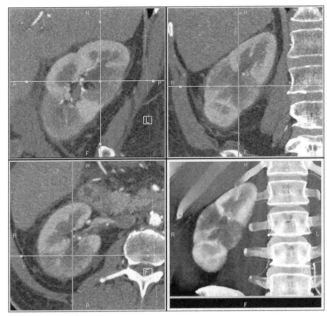

FIG. 2–1. Composite display of acute renal infarction. Computer-screen capture demonstrates the ability to integrate multiple displays for user interface. Renal infarct is displayed interactively in axial, coronal, sagittal, and 3D volume-rendered image. There is no need to jump from screen to screen with this display.

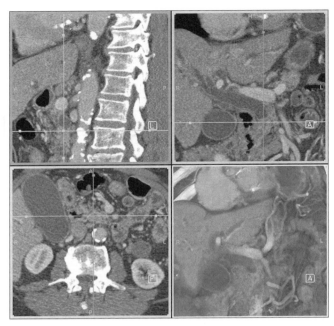

FIG. 2–2. Composite image of ampullary carcinoma. Dilated common bile duct caused by an ampullary tumor is displayed interactively in axial, coronal, sagittal, and 3D volume-rendered image. Information provided in this manner is ideal for transfer to the referring physician.

ume rendering, maximum-intensity projection (MIP), or minimum-intensity projection (MinIP) evaluation (Figures 2–1, 2–2, and 2–3) High-quality mapping of any tissue type is possible. The interactive software moves the process from a secondary interpretation mode to a primary display and interpretation mode. Of course there are a number of other workstations available, but a comparison of various workstations, hardware, and software solutions is beyond the scope of this chapter. However, a current state of the art workstation is required to perform many of the techniques discussed in this chapter.

The clinical role of 3D imaging has been a controversial topic in the past. Many radiologists felt that 3D images were of little value to them, but that they did have some value to referring physicians, citing the relative lack of image quality compared to the initial source CT data. In many cases, this was true, however, it was due to poor quality of initial datasets for 3D rendering, poor quality of 3D workstations and/ or their algorithms, or lack of user experience. In addition, 3D imaging was performed almost exclusively by technologists with little, if any, radiologist input. Although some centers have designed 3D imaging labs with dedicated technologists, this has been the exception, and in most cases, the 3D images were generated in a less-than-ideal scenario. Although dedicated technologists may excel at creating 3D images, it is believed that, in order for 3D imaging to reach the mainstream, radiologists will have to take primary responsibility for the entire process. In addition, a paradigm

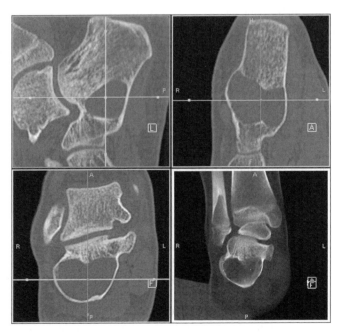

FIG. 2–3. Composite image of unicameral bone cyst. A cystic bone lesion is displayed interactively in axial, sagittal, and 3D volume-rendered image. The user can integrate quickly information from all views for final diagnosis.

shift to 3D mapping as part of the radiologist's initial interpretation of the CT dataset will be necessary. This change will not be a simple one, as it will require changes in practice delivery and workflow. However, it is possible that within 3 years to 5 years, this will become the technique of choice for CT service delivery. Several important barriers must be overcome first, such as the limited number and location of workstations in most institutions. Although some of the newer 16-slice multidetector CT (MDCT) scanners come with sophisticated 3D postprocessing software, these are limited in number and location. Picture archival and communications systems (PACs) workstations were designed to read axial-CT scans, but they were not designed for analysis of volume datasets. These systems were designed classically as mouse-driven soft-copy systems. It is both expensive and cumbersome to duplicate the functions of 3D CT workstation with the functions of classic PACs-system workstations. Merging these two systems into a truly integrated single workstation will both lower costs and accelerate implementation of volume visualization into the mainstream.

DATA ACQUISITION

The quality of a 3D image is dependent on the quality of the initial CT dataset. Unless a quality CT dataset is obtained, it is impossible to get good 3D images, regardless of the technique used. Specific protocols for applications are addressed in detail in the various chapters of this book; however, several general themes cannot be overemphasized. There are several key parameters that need to be optimized in order to obtain superior 3D images. These factors include scanning parameters (i.e., slice thickness, interscan spacing), timing of contrast injection and data acquisition in contrast-enhanced studies, and several other core-study design factors.

The key to high-quality 3D imaging is the use of thin-section reconstruction with narrow interscan spacing. For clinical studies, the prespiral CT protocol was 4-mm slice collimation reconstructed at 3-mm intervals; while a typical protocol for 4-slice MDCT is 1-mm collimation, 1.25-mm slice thickness, and reconstruction at 1-mm intervals. With 16-slice MDCT, .75-mm collimation, .75-mm slice thickness, and reconstruction at .5-mm intervals is used. Specific scan protocols for kilovolts peak (kVp) and milliamperes (mAs) will vary among scanners, but parameter selection must balance image quality and minimizing patient dose from the study. An up-to-date listing of protocols can be found on our website, http://www.ctisus.com. In cases where intravenous (IV) contrast is used (i.e., CT angiography), timing and delivery of contrast material relative to scan acquisition is critical. Optimal timing of arterial- or venous-phase imaging is dependent upon proper acquisition parameters. The use of preset defined-timing delays (i.e., 25 seconds for arterial phase, 55 seconds for venous phase), timing based on test-bolus injections, or computer-triggered imaging delays [i.e., preset value of 150 Hounsfield units (H.U.) in aorta to

trigger abdominal scan] all have been advocated by different authors. Finally, it is critical to understand the impact of reconstruction algorithms on the ability to create quality 3D images. For example, when studying bone pathology, images with a high spatial-frequency reconstruction algorithm are ideal for bone definition when axial slices alone are considered. However, when 3D imaging is performed, especially with volume rendering, the use of a high spatial-frequency reconstruction algorithm may result in images with excessive noise. In select cases, images may need to be reconstructed twice to provide optimal datasets for the entire case. Once the dataset is acquired, it is necessary to analyze the data using 3D rendering algorithms.

RENDERING TECHNIQUES FOR 3D IMAGE PROCESSING

Once a quality dataset has been acquired, the rendering technique is the most important technical determinant of 3D image quality in most circumstances (8–10). The rendering technique is the computer algorithm used to transform conventional serial transaxial-CT imaging data into simulated 3D images. There are a number of different volume-rendering methods, which can be divided into two classes: thresholding, or surface-based (binary), techniques, and percentage, or semitransparent (continuum) volume-based, techniques. This initial selection of rendering technique has great impact on the quality of final images in any given 3D application (11–16) (Figure 2-4).

Either technique consists of three steps: volume formation, classification, and image projection. Volume formation consists of the actual acquisition of imaging data, the stacking of resultant data to form a volume, and preprocessing

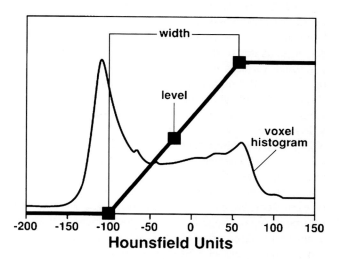

FIG. 2–4. Diagram illustrating the effect of adjustment in window width and level with respect to the voxel histogram of a CT dataset. Such adjustments alter attenuation of structures displayed in the 3D image. Changing the width (slope) alters image contrast, whereas changing level (shift on the *x*-axis) alters data inclusion and voxel attenuation in the resulting image.

that varies according to the specific technique. Typical pre-processing includes resizing (by interpolation or resampling) of each volume element (voxel), image smoothing, and data editing (e.g., removing the CT table on which the patient lies). The classification step consists of determining the types of tissue present in each voxel and determining whether it is binary or continuous in nature. In CT, most voxels can be classified into four basic tissue types: fat, soft tissue, bone, and contrast-enhanced tissue. Other imaging modalities may yield different categories of classification. The final step consists of projecting the classified volume data as a 3D volume viewed from a specific vantage point.

Most early 3D imaging involved the use of thresholding in order to produce a model of object surfaces within the volume. For thresholding classification, each type of tissue to be classified is assigned two numbers: the low and high thresholds. For a voxel to be considered a particular tissue, its signal must fall within the range defined by the low and high thresholds. Bone usually is assigned a low threshold of 100 H.U. and a high threshold of more than 3000 H.U. (essentially the top of the scale for most CT datasets) (17,18).

To classify the volume, the value or signal intensity at each voxel is analyzed and compared with the low and high thresholds for each tissue. If the signal intensity falls between the high and low thresholds defined for a tissue, the voxel is considered to contain that type of tissue. If the signal intensity lies outside the defined thresholds, it is not considered to be that tissue type. The defined ranges of thresholds for various tissue types should not overlap. This classification is binary; that is, it defines each voxel as containing either 100% or 0% of a given tissue type, but nothing in between. Each tissue type is assigned a color (and possibly a level of transparency). Once the volume has been classified, most thresholding-based algorithms will extract surfaces from the classified data. A surface is defined as a boundary between two different voxel types. An image then can be generated by defining a viewing orientation, calculating which surfaces would be visible from such an orientation, and projecting the information into a two-dimensional (2D) viewing plane. The display may be reflective, with a simulated light source, or self-luminous, both of which provide perspective and depth cues.

The thresholding technique has a number of limitations, the most significant being that voxels representing volume averaging (mixed tissue interfaces) cannot be classified correctly. Volume averaging is produced when two or more types of tissue are present in one voxel. Thus, in CT, a voxel encompassing the boundary of muscle and bone will contain a volume average of attenuation values for bone and soft tissue. All imaging modalities will produce voxels with volume averaging because voxels have a finite size. With the thresholding classification, it is expected that each volume element contains only one type of tissue. Thus, it is incompatible with volume averaging and incorrectly classifies voxels that contain volume averaging. The effects of volume averaging appear greatest at tissue–surface interfaces. For instance, of the voxels along the periosteal surface of bone, many average both bone and apposed soft tissue. This geometric reality makes the accurate imaging of surfaces by means of thresholding classification difficult. Ubiquitous volume averaging makes it difficult to define a set of thresholds representing a particular surface as it is modified by anatomic variation and pathologic conditions. This severely constrains the technique. The threshold that would approximate bone in a healthy patient, for instance, exceeds the attenuation values for markedly osteopenic bone, creating artificial *holes* in the data and final image. The thresholding technique also is susceptible to noise introduced in the scan. A small amount of noise can modify attenuation values, creating a soft-tissue voxel out of one that actually is mostly bone.

All of these disadvantages adversely affect the quality of the final image: artificial holes in structures, artificial contours representing voxel boundaries rather than true tissue interfaces, artificial fragments of structures floating in space, and artificial absence or exaggeration of detail, such as bone fractures or fragments. The main advantage of thresholding-based imaging is its speed, since a comparatively small amount of computational power is needed to generate images in a reasonable amount of time.

From a clinical perspective, the limitations of thresholding techniques are underscored when one recognizes that less than 10% of the actual image data is represented in the final image. Although most clinical applications with thresholding-based techniques had been with skeletal applications, the technique also was used with variable success in CT angiography for display of the aorta and branch vessels. The thresholding technique is not used at John Hopkins University School of Medicine, and discussion of this technique soon may be merely historical note.

Volume rendering is another technique for 3D reconstruction and display that originated in the late 1980s. Unlike thresholding techniques, volume rendering has the advantage of displaying data without classifying it into rigid categories. Volume rendering is combined most often with a method of classification termed *percentage classification* (Figure 2-5). The key difference between thresholding classification and percentage classification is that thresholding assumes that each voxel contains either all or none of a particular tissue type, and no mixture of tissues. Percentage classification assumes that a voxel can contain one or more tissue types, and the amount of each tissue is a continuum between 0% and 100%. This allows percentage classification to approximate more closely true voxel content in voxels containing tissue mixtures, or volume averaging. Percentage classification involves examination of each voxel to determine the amount (percentage) of each tissue type present in the voxel. The resultant volume data consist of voxels representing the percentage of each identified tissue type.

The most common method used to determine the content percentage is a probabilistic classification involving a trapezoidal approximation. This method for determining tis-

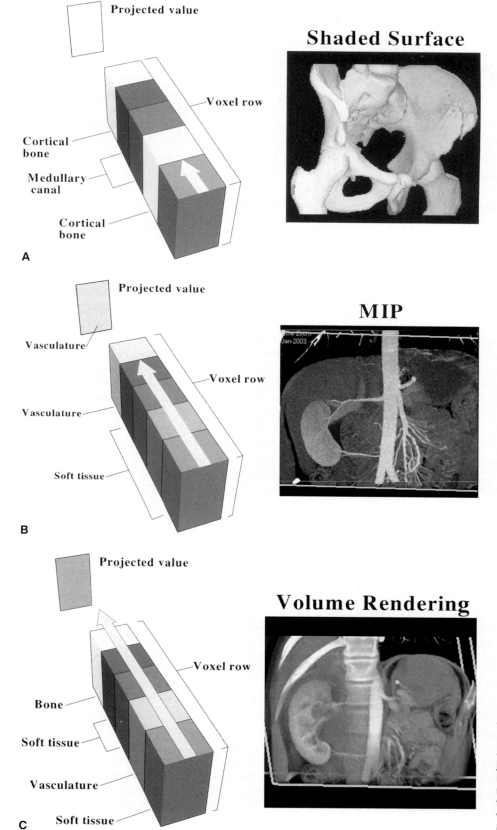

Shaded Surface

MIP

Volume Rendering

FIG. 2–5. Schematic diagrams illustrating how various rendering techniques handle a CT volume dataset. **A:** Shaded-surface technique projects surface of the volume only. **B:** Maximum-intensity-projection technique projects the brightest voxels in the dataset. **C:** Volume rendering visualizes the entire volume, including a range of different tissue types.

sue-type percentages works well for CT data. For trapezoidal classification, each tissue type is assigned a nominal value range that, in theory, exactly represents the tissue type. A voxel with a signal within the nominal value range is considered to contain 100% of that tissue. Around this ideal nominal value range, another range is defined by choosing high and low points representing attenuation values at which a voxel would contain none of the designated tissue. Voxels with signal intensities between the 0% point and the corresponding 100% point are assigned a corresponding percentage between 0% and 100%. Thus, a voxel with signal intensity precisely halfway between the 0% and 100% points would be assigned 50% of that tissue. A voxel with signal intensity three-fourths of the way toward the 100% point would be assigned 75% of that tissue. All values between the 0% and 100% points represent voxels in which volume averaging is present (i.e., more than one tissue is present). This trapezoidal classification models closely the actual volume averaging in CT voxels.

Once the data have been assigned percentages, they must be processed further to form a final image. Each tissue is assigned a color and transparency, and each voxel is assigned a color and transparency. This is accomplished by taking a weighted sum of the percentage of each tissue present in the voxel and the color and transparency assigned to those tissues. A final image is produced by casting simulated rays of light through a volume containing classified and colored voxels. As the simulated rays pass through the voxel, the color and transparency of the voxel modulates the color of the ray. The result is an image that can be displayed on a computer screen or film. Volume rendering requires more computer power than surface-based techniques because each voxel in the dataset must be projected into an image, whereas with a surface-based technique, only the surfaces need to be processed. The final generated images using volume rendering do not have many of the significant computer-generated artifacts found in surface-based or thresholded images. At best, computer-generated artifacts tend to engender distrust of 3D images and, at worst, could lead to diagnostic or therapeutic errors.

One of the principle clinical advantages of volume rendering is its ability to vary opacity values, allowing selection of specific tissue types in a rendered image (Figure 2-6). Opacity refers to the degree with which structures that appear close to the user obscure structures that seem farther away. Opacity can vary from 0% to 100%. High-opacity values can create images that accentuate the surface detail and look similar to surface-rendered images. A low-opacity value allows the user to see through structures, and it is especially useful in viewing bone and soft tissue and their relationship to vascular structures. One potential pitfall with varying opacity is that it may change object size, which may be important when grading stenoses. For example, higher opacity values make objects appear larger, whereas lower opacity values make objects appear smaller. Caution is critical when using volume rendering for quantitative measurements.

Over the last few years, the medical-imaging community has embraced volume rendering for a variety of 3D-imaging applications including CT angiography, oncologic imaging, virtual imaging, and orthopedic applications (Figures 2–7 through 2–13). The increasing power of computer hardware (and its reduction in cost) makes volume rendering the technique of choice for 3D medical imaging.

Another technique routinely used for CT angiography to supplement volume rendering is MIP technique (19,20). This technique is much simpler in principle than volume rendering, as it looks at the entire dataset and projects the brightest objects (highest H.U.) present. That is, pixels are displayed with gray scale relative to voxel attenuation. Maximum-intensity projection provides no depth cues, and because the brightest structures in the image seem closest to you, the technique cannot be used to define 3D relationships. Maximum-intensity-projection technique cannot define soft tissue in detail, limiting the ability to view organs such as the pancreas or liver. However, MIP is ideal for viewing vessels, and it may be valuable especially in organs where vessel mapping is needed but organ enhancement may be significant. Two examples are defining the hepatic arterial or venous anatomy and defining the renal arteries as they travel into the renal cortex (Figures 2–14, 2–15, and 2–16). Maximum-intensity projection does have select limitations, including a "string-of-beads" artifact in small vessels coursing obliquely through the dataset, and potential overestimation of the degree of vessel stenosis, especially when calcium is present. Calcified plaque may obscure regions of stenosis and result in either an overestimation of the extent of stenosis or a suggestion of vessel occlusion.

Maximum-intensity projection typically requires editing the dataset to remove overlying bone in order to avoid obscuring vascular structures. Fortunately, with newer workstations, editing is fairly rapid. Another modification of these techniques uses slabs of data rather than whole volume to display MIP images, often eliminating the need for any significant editing. Prior experience has shown that slabs of 20 mm to 50 mm usually work well in the chest or abdomen (Figures 2–17 and 2–18).

One potential practical advantage of MIP over volume-rendering techniques (VRT) is that implementation of volume-rendering algorithms may differ significantly between vendors, to the point that one may have difficulty determining whether an image is in fact volume rendered. Maximum-intensity-projection images are more likely to look similar, regardless of the workstation or end user. Recent changes in MIP algorithms have improved substantially MIP quality. Classically, because of the flexibility of VRT, it traditionally has been more difficult to train radiologists and technologists to become expert in this technique. The flexibility of VRT also can result in errors, especially when VRT is used for quantification (i.e., measure percent stenosis). Therefore, training is critical before implementing VRT in practice. However, on the newer workstations, the learning curve is no longer a barrier to training and implementation.

(Text continues on page 29)

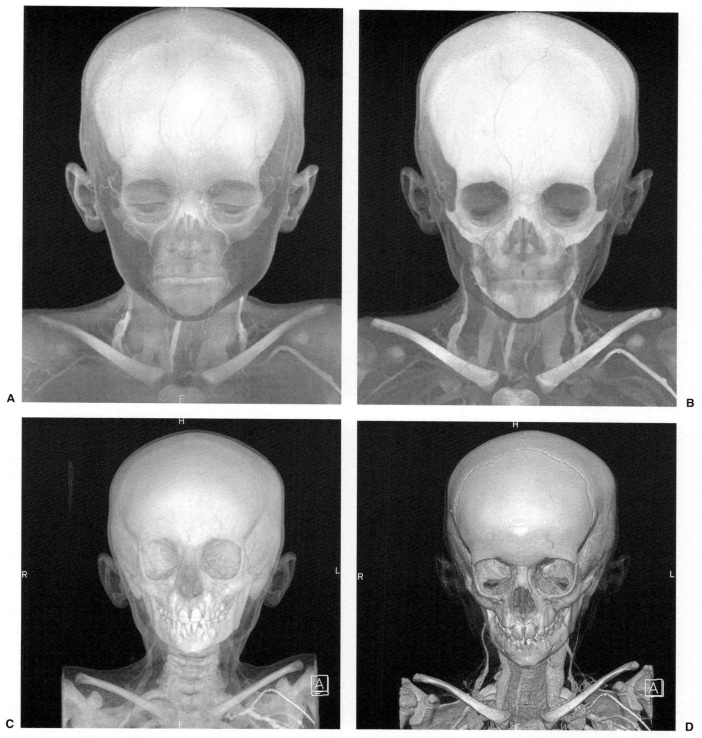

FIG. 2–6. Sequence of images showing advantages of varying opacity in volume-rendering technique. **A–D:** Four images of pediatric skull, where opacity is the only parameter adjusted. Note significant difference in bone detail with changes in opacity values.

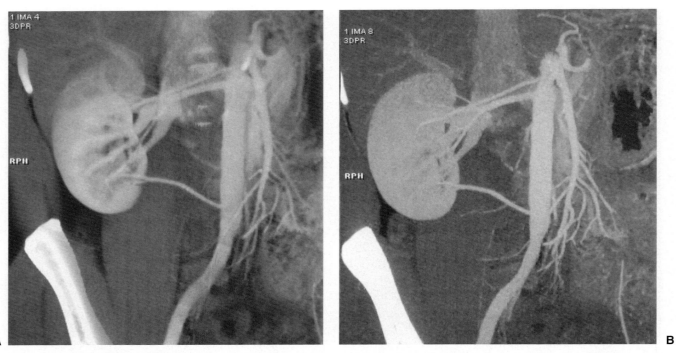

FIG. 2-7. Volume rendering versus MIP in display of kidneys. **A,B:** Although both reconstructions define the presence of three right renal arteries, the volume-rendered image **(A)** defines details of renal parenchyma, which is not seen in the MIP image **(B)**.

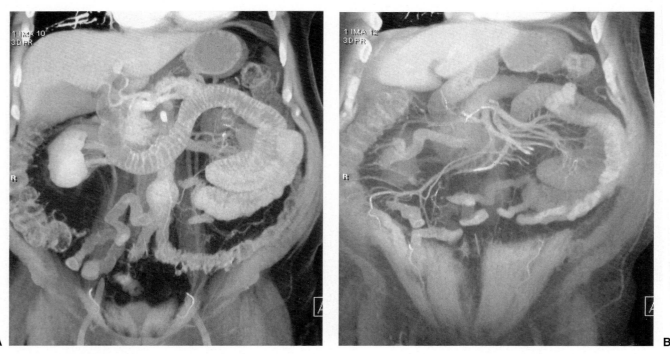

FIG. 2-8. Variable displays with volume rendering allow accentuation of specific details within the volume. This provides unique capabilities for real-time rendering. **A,B:** Volume-rendered image accentuates details of the small bowel **(A)** and mesenteric vasculature **(B)**.

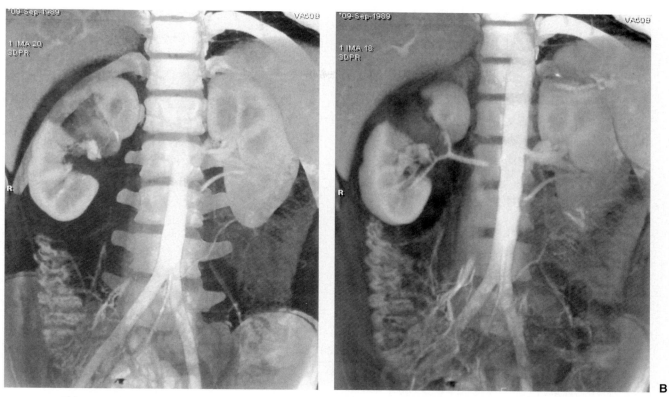

FIG. 2–9. A,B: Volume-rendered image of renal laceration with active-contrast extravasation. Note the ability to define cortical medullary interface, as well as renal artery and area-of-contrast extravasation, depending on the selection of rendering parameters.

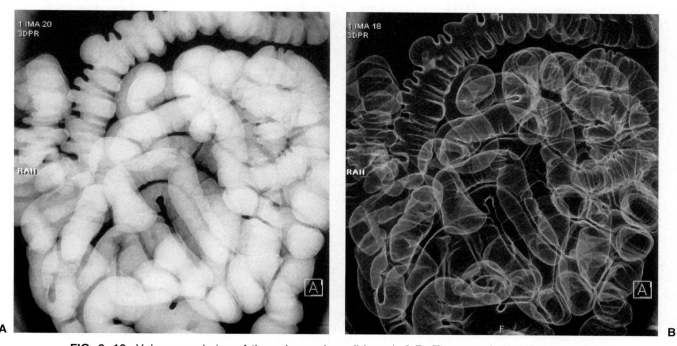

FIG. 2–10. Volume rendering of the colon and small bowel. **A,B:** The use of changes in rendering parameters allows bowel to be displayed as classic barium-study appearance **(A)** or double-contrast appearance **(B)**.

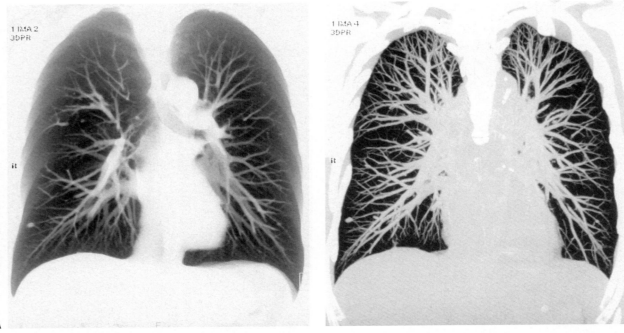

FIG. 2–11. Volume-rendering techniques versus MIP of the lung. **A,B:** Comparison of VRT **(A)** versus MIP **(B)** in display of the lung. Note that ribs and spine are edited from the MIP image, while this is not necessary in the VRT image.

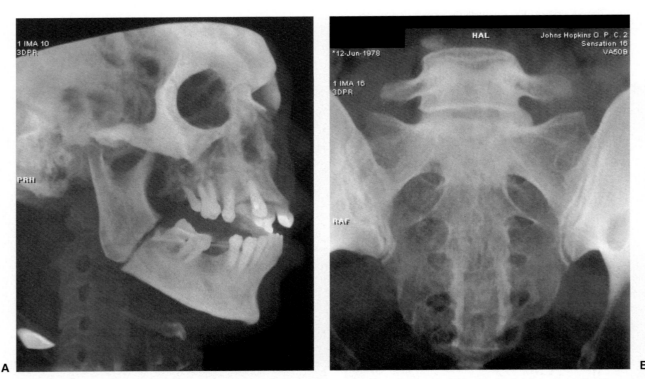

FIG. 2–12. Volume-rendered images of bone using variable opacity. **A:** Mandibular fracture is defined clearly. Note detail of bony orbit, zygomatic arch, and temporal bone. **B:** Detailed imaging of sacrum clearly defines SI joints and sacral foramina. Detail is possible only with correct implementation of volume-rendering algorithm.

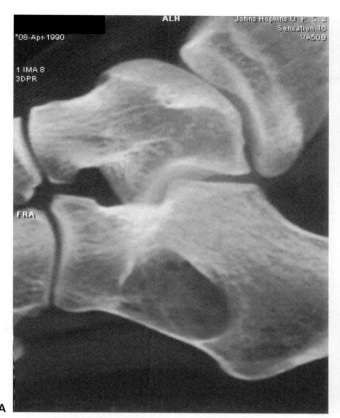

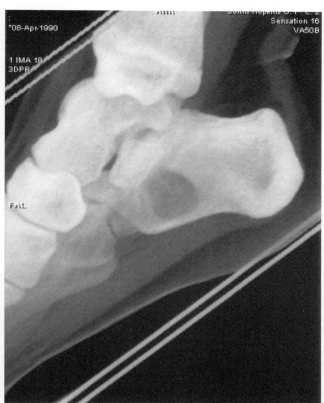

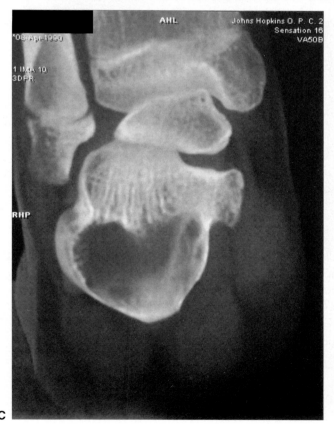

FIG. 2–13. Volume-rendered images of unicameral bone cyst. **A,B:** Sagittal 3D images with varying opacities show the ability to define both lytic bone lesion and normal bone texture. **C:** Coronal image defines in detail extent of the bone cyst and articular joint surfaces.

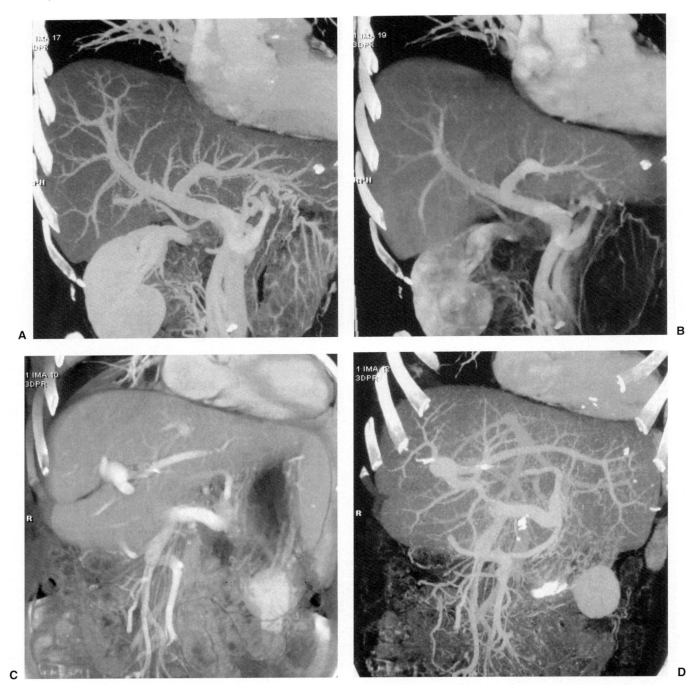

FIG. 2–14. Volume-rendered techniques versus MIP in display of liver parenchyma and venous map showing potential synergy between the two techniques. **A,B:** Although both images use the same dataset, MIP image **(A)** shows more vascular branching than VRT image **(B)**, as it projects the entire vascular map from the entire volume, whereas VRT image projects only a select portion of the volume. Volume-rendered techniques better define the liver texture. **C,D:** Another example shows better liver-texture details with VRT **(C)**, but more vascular mapping with MIP **(D)**. Note that VRT can show all of these vessels, but adjustment of rendering parameters would be needed.

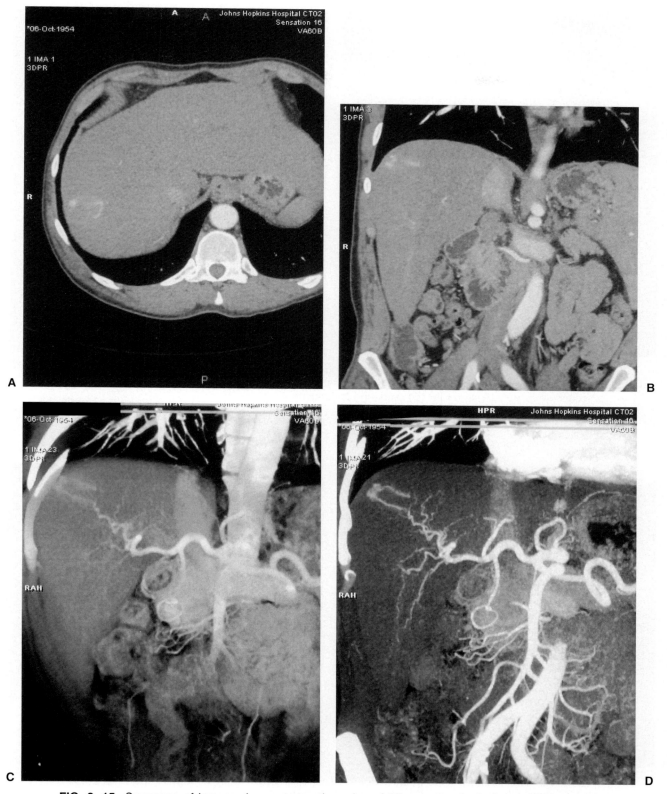

FIG. 2–15. Sequence of images demonstrates the value of 3D mapping for lesion detection by CT angiography to enhance subtle findings. **A,B:** Axial and coronal images define subtle area of hypervascularity in dome of the liver. Volume-rendered techniques **(C)** and MIP **(D)** images show 1-cm tumor with neovascularity. Three-dimensional displays may detect subtle tumors and provide additional information for lesion discrimination.

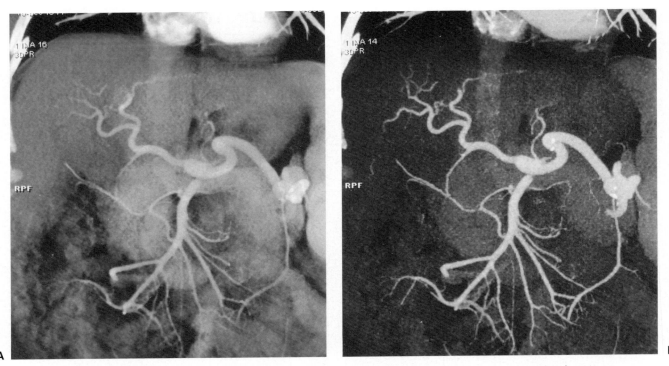

FIG. 2–16. Computed tomography angiographic map of celiac axis and superior mesenteric artery (SMA). **A,B:** Sixteen-slice MDCT with isotropic datasets provides true angiographic details of mesenteric vasculature in VRT **(A)** and MIP **(B)** rendering techniques.

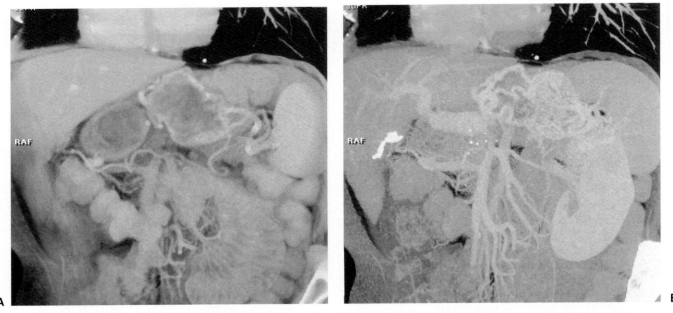

FIG. 2–17. Gastric varices due to splenic vein occlusion. **A,B:** Images generated with VRT **(A)** and MIP **(B)** show differences between the ability of VRT to show true soft-tissue detail and vessels, whereas MIP displays only the brightest structures (vasculature and kidneys) projected through the dataset.

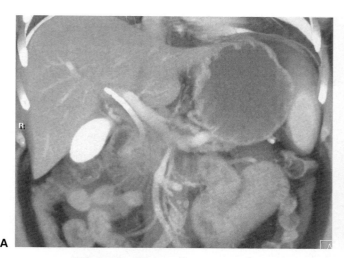
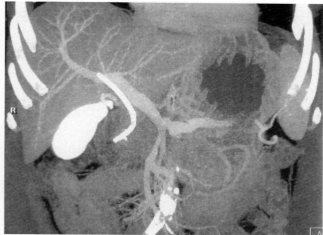

FIG. 2–18. Pancreatic cancer with early invasion of portal vein or superior mesenteric vein using volume-rendering technique and MIP. **A,B:** Volume-rendered image **(A)** shows clear 3D relationships between pancreatic mass, biliary stent, gallbladder, liver, and stomach. Maximum-intensity-projection image **(B)** details the vascular map, but other 3D relationships are lost due to nature of MIP algorithm.

DISPLAY TECHNIQUES

In addition to rendering technique, another important aspect of any 3D system is the system functionality with regard to image display and analysis. Yet another important aspect is the use of real-time interactivity in viewing the datasets. Classic 3D imaging usually presented the radiologist and referring physician with a preset selection of views around one or more axes. Interactive real-time rendering at a minimum of 8 to 10 frames per second, but ideally at 20 or more frames per second, allows the user to choose an infinite number of displays and projections in real time. The single best view then can be selected for any given application. In addition, display of data in stereo, as well as capabilities for fly throughs and fly arounds, can prove very useful. Stereo displays especially are valuable for defining vessel relationships, including orientation, displacement, and vessel encasement (21–23). This is especially useful with volume rendering. Stereo display conveys perspective and depth cues by presenting two separate renderings from slightly different points of view to the left and right eye. This results in an immediate perception of depth due to the inherent integrating capability of the brain (stereopsis). Image separation on a single computer display is achieved with left and right shutter devices incorporated into eyewear that open and close to alternate frames. Although the process requires specialized hardware and software, the cost of these systems is decreasing.

Fly throughs are useful in applications such as virtual colonoscopy for polyp detection and virtual bronchoscopy for determining extent of tumor, stent design or placement, or planning surgical reconstruction or radiation therapy (24,25). This technology also is being applied to endoluminal evaluation of the bladder (26). On a practical note, fly throughs are becoming more popular with virtual colonoscopy as the user interface becomes more intuitive and easier

to use. One potential limitation may be the time required to review the study (10 minutes to 30 minutes). Further discussion of the principles and use fly throughs is provided in Chapter 19 on virtual colonoscopy. We currently use the fly-through technology in many vascular cases, but its value has not yet been scientifically documented.

USE OF COLOR IN 3D RENDERING

The ability to use color in 3D imaging has been available for a number of years and has been used with mixed success. Color initially was used more as a marketing tool, and colors often were chosen more for effect than for clinical utility. The coloring of organs (i.e., spleen in green, liver in red, kidney in blue, etc.) may seem interesting to a lay audience, but it usually was done to mask the lack of fidelity in 3D rendering.

Today, color is used with more impact and may have important implications. Color for fly throughs with virtual colonoscopy enhances realism of the dataset and now is becoming standard. Fly throughs of the airway or bladder also have increased value when appropriate color schemes are used. Color also can be used with vascular imaging to enhance 3D detail and spatial relationships, particularly when images are stored on film or slides. Careful use of color can accentuate pathology and detail when used correctly (Figures 2–19 through 2–22), and may enhance the 3D effect on a dataset by the use of shadowing and changes in the lighting model.

Another application of color is to image patients with orthopedic hardware. Using blue to color the metal implant allows display of 3D images with minimal artifact or noise. Applications range from postacetabular fracture repair to spinal screws to total hip replacement for this clinical technique (Figure 2-23).

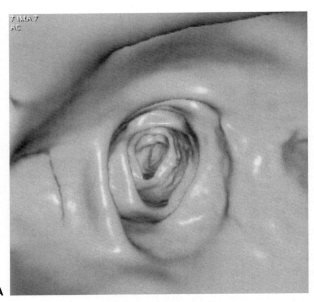
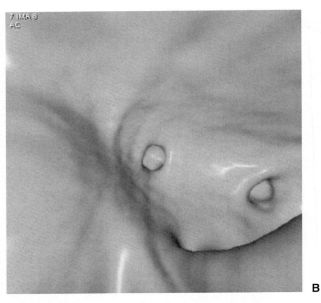

FIG. 2–19. Virtual colonoscopy with color mapping. **A,B:** Use of color allows realistic imaging in endoscopic projection. **A:** Normal haustral folds of the ascending colon are shown; **(B)** shows diverticula in sigmoid colon. (See Color Fig. 2–19)

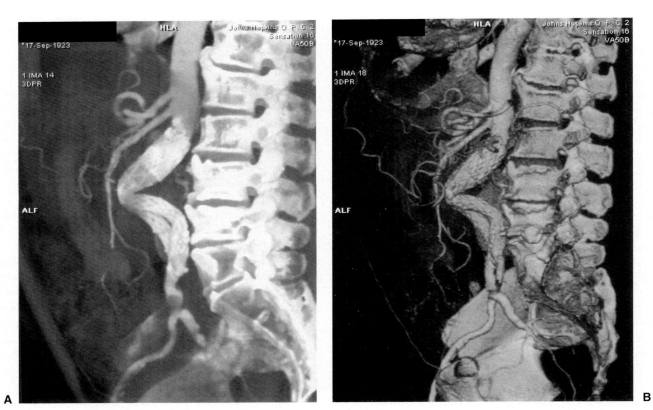

FIG. 2–20. Failing endovascular stent used for repair of abdominal aortic aneurysm. **A,B:** Stress-related failure of endovascular stent is defined in gray scale **(A)** and color **(B)**. The color image gives a more realistic 3D effect. (See Color Fig. 2–20B)

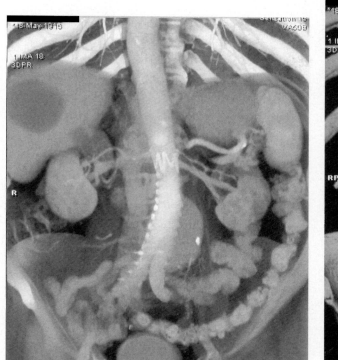
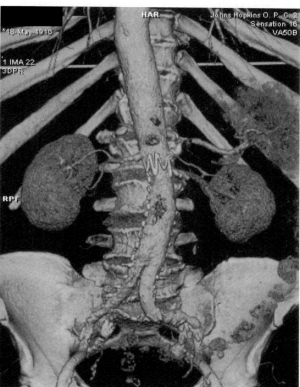

FIG. 2–21. Endovascular stent in color display. **A,B:** Imaging of endovascular stent in gray scale **(A)** and color **(B)** shows the advantage of color in defining the stent, whereas gray-scale image optimally shows the native aorta with aneurysm. (See Color Fig. 2–21B)

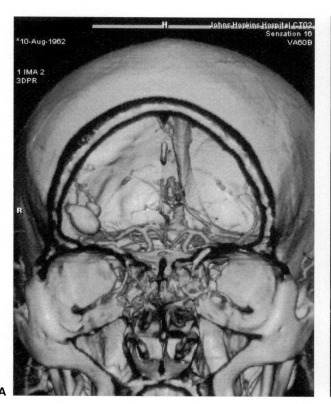
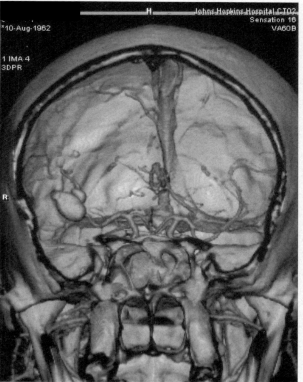

FIG. 2–22. Middle cerebral artery aneurysm in 3D volume display with color mapping. **A,B:** Detailed 3D mapping defines middle-cerebral-artery aneurysm. Color imaging in this case adds to the realism of the images and provides an increased 3D feel to the images. (See Color Fig. 2–22)

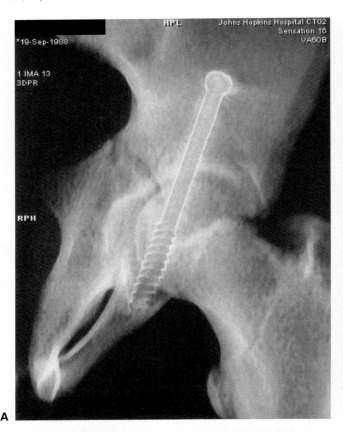

A

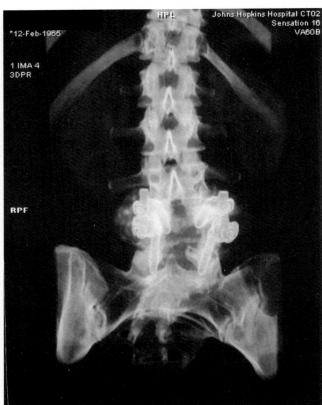

B

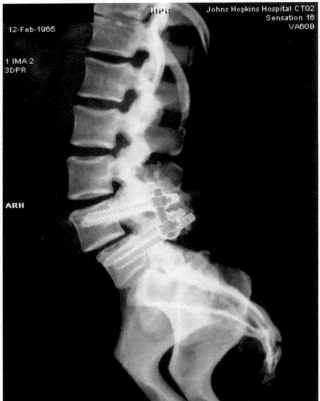

C

FIG. 2–23. Three-dimensional rendering of orthopedic hardware using color mapping to optimize image display. A: Screw in place for repair of acetabular fracture. Note detail of the ridges of the screw. B,C: Postoperative study following fusion of lower lumbar spine. Note detail of 3D volume-rendered images despite significant artifact on axial images (not shown). (See Color Fig. 2–23)

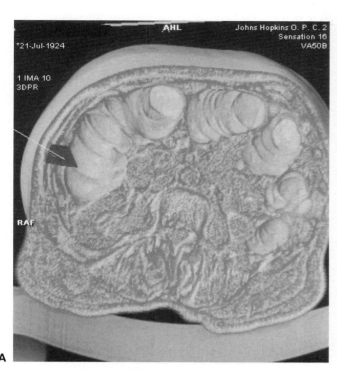
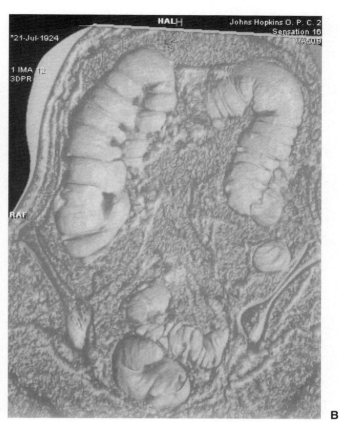

FIG. 2–24. Adjustment of lighting model to accentuate colonic folds. **A,B:** Lighting is adjusted to accentuate colonic folds. Interactive rendering allows real-time adjustment of parameters to optimize analysis and interpretation of CT dataset.

Finally, varying the lighting model can enhance images when applied in select applications, especially when imaging the skin in craniofacial imaging or when reviewing colonic folds (Figure 2-24).

CONCLUSION

The advent of 4-, 8-, and finally 16-slice helical CT has provided the impetus for many changes in CT applications and implementation of study protocols. In particular, the impact has been felt with the ability to acquire isotrophic datasets that can be visualized as true volume in a 3D environment. To take advantage of this revolution in CT, the radiologist must develop not only an understanding of the technical details of 3D imaging and the available rendering algorithms, but also a hands-on knowledge of how to apply it in clinical practice. Many of the chapters in this book will address these applications and focus on the changes this new technology is providing today. Equally exciting, however, is that these changes will continue to evolve and improve in the near future. In this brave new world, we believe that post processing of CT data will move from a secondary application to the primary technique for image display of analysis of CT datasets.

REFERENCES

1. Marsh JL, Vannier MW. Surface imaging from computerized tomographic scans. *Surgery* 1983;94:159–165.
2. Herman GT, Liu HK. Display of three-dimensional information in computed tomography. *J Comput Assist Tomogr* 1977;1:155–160.
3. Totty WG, Vannier MV. Complex musculoskeletal anatomy analysis using three-dimensional surface reconstruction. *Radiology* 1984;160:173–177.
4. Pate D, Resnick D, Andre M, et al. Perspective: three-dimensional imaging of the musculoskeletal system. *AJR Am J Roentgenol* 1986;147:545–551.
5. Burk DL Jr, Mears DC, Kennedy WH, et al. Three-dimensional computed tomography of acetabular fractures. *Radiology* 1985;155:183–186.
6. Fishman EK, Drebin RA, Magid D, et al. Volumetric rendering techniques: applications for three-dimensional imaging of the hip. *Radiology* 1987;163:737–738.
7. Fishman EK, Magid D, Drebin RA, et al. Three-dimensional imaging and display of musculoskeletal anatomy. *J Comput Assist Tomogr* 1988;12:465–467.
8. Drebin RA, Carpenter L, Hanrahan P. Volume rendering. *Comput Graph* 1988;22:65–74.
9. Fishman EK, Magid D, Ney DR, et al. Three dimensional imaging. *Radiology* 1991;181:321–337.
10. Levoy M. Display of surfaces from volume data. *IEEE Comput Graph Appl* 1988;8:29–37.
11. Scott WW Jr, Fishman EK, Magid D. Optimal imaging of acetabular fractures. *Radiology* 1987;11:1017–1020.
12. Magid D, Fishman EK. Imaging of musculoskeletal trauma in three dimensions. *Radiol Clin North Am* 1989;27:945–956.

13. Calhoun PS, Kuszyk BS, Heath DG, et al. Three-dimensional volume rendering of spiral CT data: theory and method. *Radiographics* 1999; 19:745–764.

14. Johnson PT, Heath DG, Kiuszyk BS, et al. CT angiography with volume rendering: advantages and applications in splanchnic vascular imaging. *Radiology* 1996;200:564–568.

15. Fishman EK. CT angiography: clinical applications in the abdomen. *Radiographics* 2001;21:S3–S16.

16. Kuszyk BS, Heath DG, Ney DR, et al. CT angiography with volume rendering: imaging findings. *AJR Am J Roentgenol* 1995; 165:445–448.

17. Magnusson M, Lenz R, Danielsson PE. Evaluation of methods for shaded surface display of CT volumes. *Comput Med Imaging Graph* 1991;15:247–256.

18. Kuszyk BS, Heath DG, Bliss DF, et al. Skeletal 3-D CT: advantages of volume rendering over surface rendering. *Skeletal Radiol* 1996; 25:207–214.

19. Napel S, Marks MP, Rubin GD, et al. CT angiography with spiral CT and maximum intensity projection. *Radiology* 1992;185:607–610.

20. Johnson PT, Halpern EJ, Kuszyk B, et al. Renal artery stenosis: CT angiography—comparison of real time volume rendering and maximum intensity projection algorithms. *Radiology* 1999;211:337–343.

21. Johnson PT, Heath DG, Duckwall JR, et al. Enhanced display of vascular anatomy with stereoscopic viewing. *J Diagn Radiogr Imaging* 1999; 21(1):25–28.

22. Smith PA, Marshall FF, Urban BA, et al. Three-dimensional CT stereoscopic visualization of renal masses: imapct on diagnosis and patient management. *AJR Am J Roentgenol* 1997;169:1331–1334.

23. Smith PA, Heath DG, Fishman EK. Virtual angioscopy using spiral CT and real-time interactive volume-rendering techniques. *J Comput Assist Tomogr* 1998;22:212–214.

24. Royster AP, Fenlon HM, Clarke PD, et al. CT colonoscopy of colorectal neoplasms: two-dimensional and three-dimensional virtual-reality techniques with colonoscopic correlation. *AJR Am J Roentgenol* 1997; 169:1237–1242.

25. McFarland EG, Brink JA. Helical CT colonography (virtual colonoscopy): the challenge that exists between advancing technology and generalizability. *AJR Am J Roentgenol* 1999;173:549–559.

26. Kim JK, Ahn JH, Park T, et al. Virtual cystoscopy of the contrast material filled bladder in patients with gross hematuria. *AJR Am J Roentgenol* 2002;179:763–768.

CHAPTER 3

Perspective Rendering and Virtual Endoscopy

Christopher F. Beaulieu, Geoffrey D. Rubin

INTRODUCTION

Not long after the introduction of spiral computed tomography (CT) in 1990 (1–3), new clinical applications such as CT angiography (4,5) and multiphasic and thin-section imaging of solid organs such as the liver and pancreas began to emerge (6–8). The new applications, in turn, stimulated interest in advanced means of data visualization (4,9) to take advantage of the excellent depiction of three-dimensional (3D) anatomy due to high-resolution overlapping sections (10). With even higher resolution in the longitudinal direction, multidetector CT (MDCT) further motivates the use of image displays other than traditional axial viewing (11).

In parallel with improvements in CT technology, rapid advances in computer-graphics hardware and software have enabled sophisticated image creation on inexpensive workstations. An important innovation of the spiral CT–computer-graphics era began with the recognition that the spatial position of the observer for 3D visualization need not be confined to locations outside the imaging volume. In other words, unlike the situation in the live patient, there are no risks or barriers to penetrating inside the ''virtual'' body represented by imaging data. Graphics tools that permit viewing of the data from inside, or so-called *perspective* techniques, have been embraced rapidly and have stimulated new data-interpretation methods that are loosely called ''virtual reality'' or ''virtual imaging,'' initially represented by virtual colonoscopy and virtual bronchoscopy (12,13).

This chapter provides an overview of perspective-rendering methods applied to spiral and MDCT data. While the fundamental principles of 3D rendering are covered elsewhere, key concepts of perspective graphics are discussed here. Current applications are illustrated for various organ systems, and potential future developments are discussed.

PRINCIPLES OF PERSPECTIVE VISUALIZATION

Volumetric Data

The primary image data—in this context, the group of reconstructed cross sections—are the most basic representa-

tion of the patient's anatomy and have a crucial influence on the quality of 3D renderings. As imaging times have decreased, it is now straightforward to obtain high-quality spiral CT data, even on patients with limited breath-holding capability. Another attribute of the input data relates to anisotropy in spatial resolution between the in-plane (x,y plane) and longitudinal (x,z or y,z plane) dimensions. Ideally, input data for a graphics computer would be isotropic, that is, contain the same voxel dimensions and spatial resolution in x,y as in x,z. Newer 4-, 8-, and 16-detector–row scanners enable routine acquisition of sections on the order of 1-mm thickness, approaching isotropic resolution. In fact, 16-row and higher scanners can produce sections on the order of 0.5-mm thickness, finally achieving true isotropic resolution (14). As with other forms of visualization, such as multiplanar reformations, maximum-intensity projections, and external 3D rendering, acquisition of the thinnest sections possible for a given longitudinal coverage and reconstruction of overlapping sections is highly desirable in the creation of perspective renderings, as long as image signal-to-noise is sufficient and radiation doses are reasonable. Further discussion on these issues is given elsewhere in this book and in publications by Kalender (14) and Wang et al. (15)

Perspective

Because human beings have binocular vision, they perceive the world in three dimensions. The visual field or ''cone of vision'' is approximately 37 degrees horizontal and 28 degrees vertical (16) and is determined by the physiological optics of the eye for reception of light rays converging on the retina. Traditional methods of 3D visualization have relied on the creation of models of the data in which the computed rays forming the rendering are parallel, and viewing is as if one were using magnification from an infinite distance. While creating renderings that have 3D cues owing to occlusion of far objects by near ones and shading/lighting effects, the observer's effective cone of vision amounts to tunnel vision, a situation in which further magni-

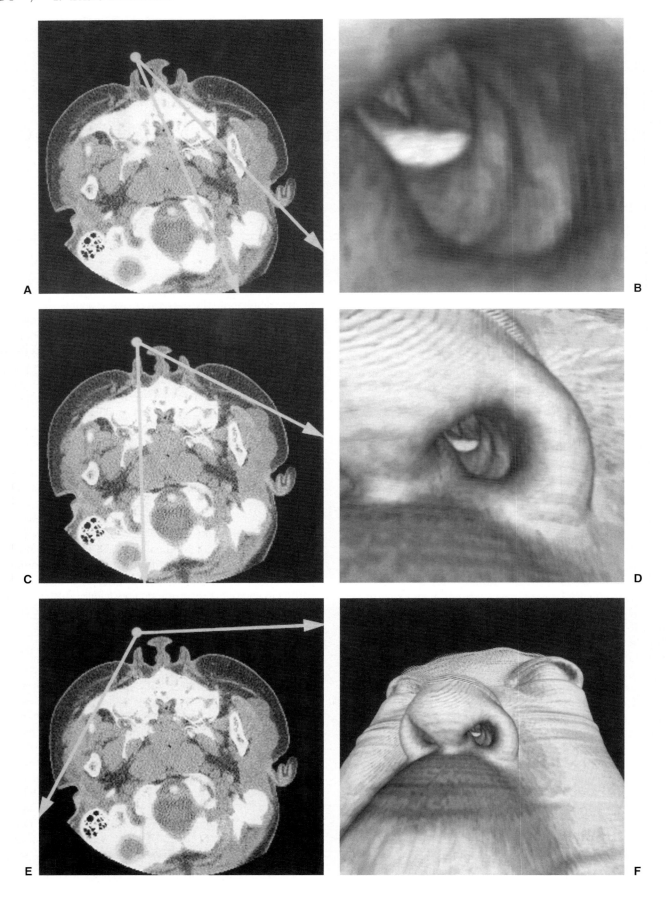

fication gives the impression of moving closer to the object, but spatial context is lost quickly as only a small fraction of the object becomes visible. Such close-up views are difficult to interpret and are largely part of the reason that internal exploration of datasets has not been useful in the past. In addition to the difficulties in exploring surfaces and objects from close range, visualization of parallel-ray renderings also is limited because unimportant anatomic structures may obscure visualization of the anatomy of interest. Removal of unwanted structures requires editing in the form of thresholding, segmentation, or manual editing. These processes are not only time consuming, but also inadvertently may result in the loss of important information about the patient or create artifacts that result in misinterpretation.

In art, *perspective* is defined as a means by which an impression of three dimensions is produced upon a two-dimensional (2D) plane (16). Similarly, in computer graphics, perspective rendering lends objects in the scene the impression of relative positions, shapes, and distance. Their appearance depends on the position of the eye or virtual camera (the viewpoint), as well as on the observer's *effective* cone or field of vision (FOV). Perspective effects are created by graphics software that uses divergent, rather than parallel, rays to generate the image. By adjusting the amount of divergence of the rendering rays, one can expand the FOV analogous to a wide-angle camera lens and capture more of the surrounding scene from a given viewpoint. Furthermore, a wider FOV results in the impression that objects appear further away than they actually are; this is the fundamental attribute of perspective rendering that enables exploration from within the volume and close to surfaces without loss of visual context. Figure 3-1 illustrates the effect of different degrees of rendering-ray divergence on 3D renderings of a facial CT study. From the same viewpoint, at a distance of approximately 1 cm from the tip of the nose, rays with wider divergence (a larger effective FOV) show more of the surrounding anatomy and make the nose and face appear further away.

When perspective effects are combined with other display features such as color and lighting models, varying a voxel's opacity in volume rendering, or simulated motion along a "flight path," one can create images that mimic naturally occurring anatomical scenes, with the possibility for visualization of nearly any surface or anatomic feature that has sufficient image contrast compared with neighboring structures. Another useful feature of perspective rendering lies in the ability to change the observer's viewpoint in order to "get around" structures that would otherwise obscure the line of sight; this can obviate the need for spatial editing and reduce the risk of information loss and artifact generation inherent to editing techniques in conventional 3D.

Rendering Techniques

Perspective-rendering techniques can be implemented with either shaded-surface display (SSD) or volume-rendering (VR) graphics systems. Many laboratories initially developed their own software for perspective rendering (17–20), and a multitude of systems for perspective surface rendering (PSR) and perspective volume rendering (PVR) now are available commercially. While a full discussion of rendering techniques is beyond the scope of this chapter, it is worth emphasizing that the same advantages/disadvantages of SSD and VR that apply to conventional external renderings also apply to perspective rendering with these algorithms (21,22). In addition, since the last writing of this chapter, there has been a major shift away from SSD towards VR, largely owing to improvements in hardware and software.

Shaded-surface displays rely on thresholding of the data to create a model in which a binary classification is made, where voxels are either kept or deleted from the data (9,23). Because the size of the dataset is reduced greatly when a surface model is created, SSDs can be computed rapidly. However, such displays cannot simultaneously represent voxels with a range of attenuation values, and artifacts such as surface discontinuities and "floating pixels" are common. Volume rendering has advantages in that simultaneous visualization of structures with a range of attenuation values is possible (12,21,24), and the effective display of interfaces between structures with different attenuation values can be achieved with few inherent artifacts. Computationally, however, VR techniques are much more intensive, as potentially all of the voxels in the dataset are being rendered to create

FIG. 3–1. Perspective rendering: effective visual field of view (FOV). Pairs of images representing the axial CT section and a corresponding 3D volume-rendered view are given for three different visual fields of view: 20 degrees, 60 degrees, and 120 degrees. Images are from a facial bone study with 1-mm collimation, pitch 1.5, reconstruction interval 1 mm, bone-reconstruction kernel, and reconstruction field of view (DFOV) 18 cm. **A:** Axial CT section with yellow arrows indicating 20-degree FOV. **B:** PVR view showing the nasal passage. Without prior knowledge, it might be difficult to identify the anatomy being displayed. **C:** Axial CT section with yellow arrows indicating 60-degree FOV. **D:** Corresponding 60-degree PVR image. Although the viewpoint is unchanged from that in **(A)**, more of the surrounding anatomy is visible, allowing recognition of anatomic features that represent the nose. **E:** Axial CT section with yellow arrows indicating 120-degree FOV. **F:** Corresponding 120-degree PVR image. At this wide camera angle, nearly the entire face becomes visible. Image distortion in the form of an elongated upper lip is evident. Similar concepts apply to perspective rendering inside the body, such that a wider FOV allows visualization of more surrounding anatomy and structures close to the observer appear further away than they actually are.

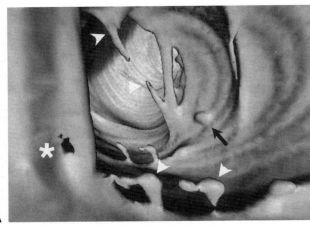
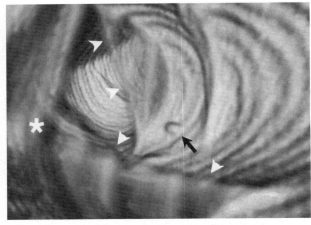

A   B

FIG. 3–2. Rendering techniques: PSR vs. PVR. **A:** Simulated endoscopic view of the ascending colon created with PSR, threshold −960 H.U. At this threshold, haustral folds that are thin and subject to partial volume averaging with adjacent air are rendered as incomplete structures that can take on a polypoid appearance (*arrowheads*). A 5-mm adenomatous polyp is depicted by the black arrow. Because of the thresholding inherent in PSR, haustra also may develop surface discontinuities (*asterisk*). **B:** Same view of the colon created with PVR, with an opacity table that renders the thin haustra as semitransparent (*arrowheads*). While depicting the 5-mm polyp, as well as PSR, carefully performed PVR is less susceptible to creating artifactual polypoid structures and holes (*asterisk*). In addition, PSR techniques typically compute the surface for a fixed threshold value and require complete recomputation to change the threshold. With PVR, the user can adjust interactively the opacity table to optimize the rendering and see the results almost immediately on current computers.

the image. Over the past several years, VR techniques have become interactive, with some laboratories having achieved "real-time" VR of large spiral CT datasets (25), and many commercial systems available. An example of the display differences between PSR and PVR is shown in Figure 3-2. Endoluminal perspective renderings of the colon effectively display a 5-mm polyp with both PSR and PVR, but the PSR image (at the selected threshold) exhibits surface artifacts that might be misleading for diagnostic interpretation.

Personal experience with perspective rendering has relied almost exclusively on PVR. While today the computational aspects are becoming trivial, in earlier works (12,26), it was believed that the superior display qualities of PVR outweighed the disadvantages of needing higher-priced workstations with relatively slow rendering times compared with PSR.

Animations and "Virtual Reality"

With perspective rendering, body cavities and hollow viscera can be viewed from a unique internal perspective that simulates fiberoptic endoscopy. Indeed, as long as sufficient image contrast is present for visualization, the "virtual" endoscope has no limitations on what spaces can be explored, unlike the mechanical device. When a series of images is strung together, the series representing a logical progression through the dataset, whether through spatial movement, changes in viewing direction, or through systematic variation of other rendering parameters, one obtains an animated sequence or movie that simulates flying through

the data. To consider that this represents "virtual reality" has a certain high-tech appeal and may be useful as a familiar term for communication. However, true virtual-reality displays assume that interaction with the data is a real-time computation/display experience, with scenes updating many times each second. [What constitutes "real-time" is a matter of debate. The concept is that the scene updates with a rate sufficient to allow user input to be displayed almost instantaneously, so that a truly interactive environment is simulated. Computer-graphics engineers often assume that the benchmark for real-time is the standard frame rate for video playback, or 30 frames per second (fps).] Perspective-rendering systems currently available are capable of real-time updating of the image display many times per second. With such fast rendering rates, the observer can use input devices such as the mouse, a joystick, or the keyboard to explore a dataset interactively.

Previously, slower rendering rates, varying from about 0.1 to 0.5 fps (image display every 2–10 seconds, or longer) necessitated precomputation of animations. To create such animations, the observer selected a series of "key frames" that formed a logical spatial progression through the dataset. Each key frame encoded a viewpoint, viewing direction and FOV, and sometimes other parameters such as opacity or lighting properties. Then a scripted animation was created by stringing together a series of key frames, and the graphics computer interpolated scenes between key frames to create an animation that is played back "interactively." The disadvantage of this method was that the observer is limited to precomputed views and can interact with the animation only in the form of selecting a playback rate and running the loop in a forward or reverse direction. In early work with perspective rendering, it often took many hours of interacting with the computer to generate key frames for animation. New tools were developed quickly that allowed a user to use a mouse to "point and click" on axial sections or reformatted sagittal or coronal sections to determine the viewpoint and view direction. This markedly simplified the flight planning, but left the often-tedious job of determining the flight path up to the observer. More recently, a number of semi-automated path-planning tools have been developed that use segmentation of the data and central-axis determination to generate automatically the key frames that are used for scripted animations (17,27,28). Such semi-automated paths also may be useful as "guidepaths" for real-time interactive navigation, in which the operator could fly along a prescribed flight path, but stop and "look around" by changing the camera angle or FOV at a selected point. Additionally, having a median-to-median throughout-axis path allows for computation of other useful quantitative features such as cross-sectional area, diameter, and local curvature (29,30).

Since initial implementations of perspective visualization in spiral CT often required precomputation of animations, they do not constitute virtual reality in the pure sense. For this reason, the terms "fly-through" and "fly-around" have been adopted as more broadly applicable, encompassing techniques that actually render in "real time," as well as precomputed animations. In this scheme, a "fly through" is usually visualization of a specific organ when confined within the organ's boundaries and "fly around" describes visualization of an organ from outside its boundaries, but from a viewpoint that remains within the boundaries of the volume (31).

"Virtual Endoscopy"

Some of the earliest and most promising techniques enabled by perspective visualization are those that create renderings that simulate the views traditionally obtained by inserting a fiberoptic endoscope into a body cavity. Alternatively, the virtual endoscope is not limited by the anatomic boundaries of the body, but relies on natural (or generated, with iodinated contrast enhancement) image contrast for visualization. The chief requirement to create an adequate endoscopic view is a sufficient attenuation difference (image contrast) between the voxels to be viewed and those comprising the viewpoint. The higher the image contrast, the less overlap exists between voxels of interest and voxels one wishes to make transparent. This is true whether the transparent voxels are assigned by thresholding, effectively eliminating them from the data, as in SSD, or by assignment of minimal or zero opacity to a range of attenuation in continuous VR. Several natural situations exist in which the image contrast is excellent for creation of endoscopic renderings from CT data. The roughly 1000 H.U. of attenuation difference between air (−1000 H.U.) and tissues (−100 to 100 H.U.)

provides high contrast and is used advantageously in applications such as virtual colonoscopy and virtual bronchoscopy. For orthopedic applications, the high attenuation of bone relative to neighboring structures serves as a high-contrast tissue relative to its surroundings. Finally, just as it increases conspicuity in axial CT imaging, the administration of intravenous (IV) iodine generates high contrast between enhancing structures and their neighbors.

The Overall Process

Computation of perspective renderings is only one step in the overall process of advanced visualization. For each type of study, there are four essential elements: patient preparation, data acquisition, rendering, and interpretation. Patient preparation may involve cleansing the colon of stool, fluid, and air insufflation for polyp detection, or ensuring adequate hydration when IV iodinated contrast is administered for evaluation of vascular structures or solid organs. Data acquisition is a critical phase in which the projection data are acquired and reconstructed into a series of cross sections. Rendering involves the transfer of data to a graphics workstation and the creation of images, whether snapshots, computed animations, or models, for real-time interactivity. Finally, interpretation of the newly generated information is necessary, whether the study is for scientific validation or clinical use. At present, there is no consensus on the optimal means of presentation of 3D data to provide the highest diagnostic accuracy. Issues such as the use of color, lighting, and motion cues are relatively foreign to diagnostic radiology, and the individual or collective value of these advance visual cues in depicting normality or pathology is unknown. As work progresses, developing insight into the visual psychophysical properties of these new displays and their diagnostic applications will become increasingly important.

APPLICATIONS OF PERSPECTIVE VISUALIZATION

Colon—"Virtual Colonoscopy"

The clinical rationale for examining the colon with spiral CT and computer graphics, known as "virtual colonoscopy" or "three-dimensional computed tomography colonography" (3DCTC), is that the technique may serve as a tool for detection of colonic polyps and masses that are malignant or premalignant (13). Lesions equal to 1.0 cm in diameter are the target size for detection because the risk of malignancy in lesions less than 1.0 cm is only 1%, but the risk of malignancy increases to 37% for a 2-cm polyp (32). A technique that could serve as a minimally invasive tool for detection of early cancers could be well accepted by patients and potentially eliminate fatal cases of colon carcinoma. Virtual colonoscopy has emerged as a very active research focus and early clinical tool; it is the subject of a dedicated chapter in this book. In this chapter, we use the colon as a model to illustrate the principles of perspective rendering.

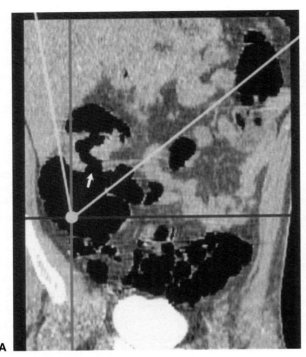
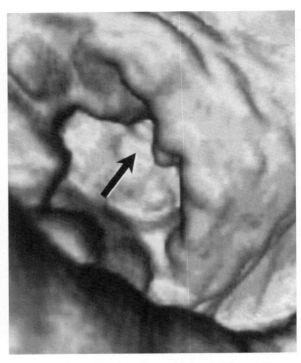

FIG. 3–3. Conceptual basis of virtual endoscopy (colonoscopy). Spiral CT data were obtained at 3-m collimation, pitch 2, and reconstructed at 1-mm intervals at a 36-cm DFOV. The patient had undergone colonic cleansing for fiberoptic colonoscopy and had air insufflated into the colon with a Foley catheter. **A:** Coronal reformation through the abdomen and pelvis indicating the viewpoint as a yellow circle and a 60-degree FOV for the virtual camera as delimited by the yellow lines. *Arrow,* lumen of constricting adenocarcinoma of the ascending colon. (Contrast in the urinary bladder is a result of a preceding hepatic CT acquisition.) **B:** PVR view of the carcinoma with 60-degree FOV. Note the nodularity of the inner colonic surface. *Arrow,* residual lumen through the lesion. Rendering a series of images obtained at viewpoints coursing through the lumen, one can create an animation simulating fiberoptic colonoscopy. In this patient, the virtual camera captured the proximal aspect of the lesion and permitted endoscopic views of the cecum; the fiberoptic scope could not be passed through the constricted lumen. (See Color Fig. 3–3B)

Figure 3-3A illustrates the process of selecting a viewpoint within the distended colon lumen and pointing the "camera" towards a structure of interest, such as a constricting adenocarcinoma in this patient. Figure 3-3B shows the resulting PVR image, which demonstrates a nodular mass with a constricted residual lumen. By systematically moving the viewpoint along the lumen of the colon and capturing successive PVR frames as a movie, a colon fly through is created.

It is important to recognize, however, that viewing of 3D images alone often is not sufficient for *characterization* of a colonic lesion. This is because 3D images usually are optimized to display the colon surface as a continuous opaque structure, whether created with PSR or PVR, such that the attenuation of the underlying tissue is not apparent on the 3D image. Examples of pitfalls that can be encountered with 3D display alone are given in Chapter 19—Multidetector CT of the Large Intestine: Virtual Colonoscopy.

Liver

Three-dimensional rendering of hepatic masses is performed in some centers to help guide surgical therapy and assess response of malignanices to medical therapy (21,25). To the best of our knowledge, perspective visualization of the liver has been applied only to anecdotal cases; systematic studies on any incremental value of the technique are lacking. An example of PVR of the liver in a patient with multiple masses due to focal nodular hyperplasia is shown in Figure 3-4. In this example, high CT contrast was achieved by acquisition of a spiral volume during the arterial phase of IV contrast injection. This permitted creation of high-quality PVR images because the voxels representing tumor and those representing normal liver had approximately 150 H.U. difference in attenuation, allowing assignment of high opacity to tumor voxels and low opacity to normal liver voxels. In general, as the lesion-to-background contrast decreases, it becomes increasingly difficult to classify voxels as either tumor or normal liver, in turn making it difficult (or impossible) to create meaningful renderings without the use of manual tracing of individual lesions. In Figure 3-4C, a different opacity table has been applied to the same data shown in Figures 4A and 4B, and a 50-mm-thick volume-rendered slab of the data is rendered as viewed in the conventional CT orientation. This type of visualization combines

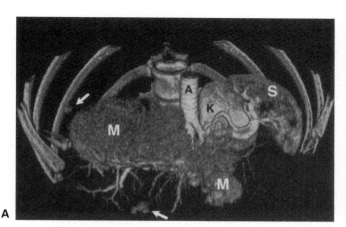

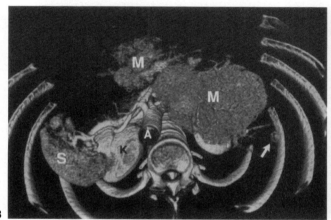

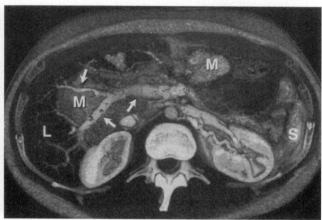

FIG. 3–4. Fly around of focal hepatic masses: focal nodular hyperplasia (FNH). **A,B:** Two different PVRs of hyperenhancing hepatic lesions imaged with 5-mm collimation, pitch 1.5, in the arterial phase of bolus IV contrast enhancement. Images were created with VoxelView 2.5 with a 60-degree FOV and the opacity table adjusted to emphasize contrast enhancement and osseous structures. Normal liver parenchyma is transparent. The relationship of the multiple masses (*M*) to the portal venous system can be visualized on static images or when a series of images is viewed as an animation. *Arrows,* small foci of FNH; *A,* abdominal aorta; *K,* left kidney; *S,* spleen. **C:** Volume-rendered view of a slab of data 50 mm thick from the same patient. In this view, normal liver parenchyma is semitransparent and the relationship of the FNH foci to the portal venous system (*arrows*) is illustrated. Note that the hepatic masses (*M*) are assigned the same color as the spleen, owing to similar attenuation values achieved with contrast enhancement. (See Color Fig. 3–4)

features of advanced visualization with conventional CT viewing and is somewhat analogous to sliding thin slab maximum intensity projection (STS-MIP) imaging (33). With sliding-slab VR, however, an individual image encodes depth information that is not available in MIP. Furthering applications to the hepatobiliary system, virtual CT cholangioscopy has been proposed as a means of viewing the biliary tree (34).

Airways—''Virtual Bronchoscopy''

For spiral CT of the tracheobronchial tree, no specific patient preparation is necessary, as the natural image contrast between the lumen and walls of airways is on the order of 1000 H.U. The clinical rationale for evaluating the airways lies in the potential to provide information beyond that provided by evaluation of routine cross sections and reformatted images, and ultimately, in the potential of the technique to replace fiberoptic bronchoscopy in some patients (35). We have experience with approximately 50 patients in performing virtual bronchoscopy for a number of indications. Examples of the types of images that can be created using PVR techniques are shown in Figure 3-5.

In a preliminary study by Vining and colleagues, spiral acquisitions with 3-mm collimation, pitch 2, and 1-mm reconstruction intervals were used to compare virtual bronchoscopy with fiberoptic bronchoscopy in 20 patients (20). Although virtual bronchoscopy accurately identified endobronchial tumor in five patients, airway distortion and/or ectasia in four patients, and an accessory bronchus in one case, suboptimal examinations limited evaluation in half the cases. Summers and colleagues used virtual bronchoscopy with 3-mm collimation, pitch 2, and 1-mm reconstruction intervals to evaluate 14 patients with a variety of airway abnormalities (36). These authors found that third-order bronchi were depicted in up to 90% of cases. However, only 82% of expected and 76% of segmental airways were identified. Axial CT and the virtual endoscopic images were of equal accuracy in estimating the maximal luminal diameter and cross-sectional area of the central airways (when the airways could be identified). Although many investigators initially relied on 3-mm collimation imaging, current technology favors the use of thinner sections on the order of 0.625 mm to 1.25 mm. Using such protocols, 6th- and 7th-order bronchial branches can be visualized, as shown in Figure 3-5H.

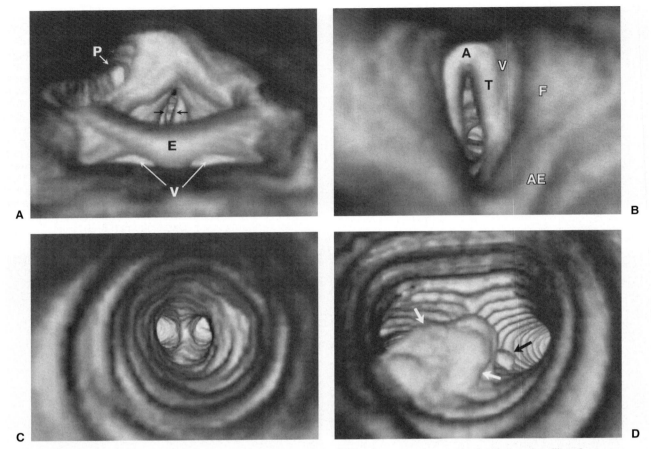

FIG. 3–5. Perspective rendering of the airways. Spiral CT volumes were acquired with 1-mm collimation, pitch 2, and reconstructed at 0.5-mm –1.0-mm intervals, unless indicated otherwise, and rendered with a 60-degree FOV. **A:** Orohypopharynx. Supero–inferior view from a viewpoint at the base of the tongue shows the epiglottis (*E*), lingual valleculae (*V*), and the right pyriform sinus (*P*). Further inferiorly, the true vocal cords are seen (*black arrows*). **B:** Larynx viewed from above. Aryepiglottic folds (*AE*), false (*F*) and true (*T*) vocal cords are seen along with the anterior commissure (*A*) and the laryngeal ventricle (*V*). **C:** Normal trachea. PVR of a scan with 3-mm collimation, pitch 2, shows carina and mainstem bronchi. Corrugations in the tracheal wall may represent normal cartilaginous rings; however, spatial variations in spiral CT noise also can cause a "ribbed" or corrugated appearance, especially with extended pitch scanning, requiring that the viewer appreciate spiral CT artifacts and the influence of scan parameters (35). **D:** Endobronchial coccidiomycosis. Inferior-viewing PVR image of a patient with a large tracheal lesion (*white arrows*) and several smaller endobronchial lesions, one of which is shown by the *black arrow*. *(Continued)*

There is potential for the virtual examination to replace fiberoptic bronchoscopy in some patients requiring frequent screening for bronchial anastomotic strictures, such as the pulmonary-transplant population (37), or in patients with other conditions affecting the airways (38, 39). In the immediate postoperative period, however, limitations in the ability of CT to detect bronchial dehiscence relative to fiberoptic bronchoscopy need to be considered (37). For initial diagnosis of airway abnormalities that are not detected on axial sections or routine reformatted tomograms, it remains to be established clearly that perspective imaging provides an incremental benefit (35); however, data are beginning to accrue that complementing other image displays with perspective views may improve overall diagnostic accuracy (40).

Preliminary studies have suggested that virtual bronchoscopy may aid in the planning of fiberoptic bronchoscopy by displaying simultaneously the airway walls and surrounding anatomy (41). By obtaining a 3D mental image of a particular patient's anatomy and disease, transbronchial biopsy of technically difficult or risky areas may be performed more safely (42). Ultimately, image fusion of virtual-endoscopy data with the actual invasive procedure may be possible and could be helpful for anatomically complex instrumentations. Finally, applications of virtual imaging in the pediatric patient population have begun to appear (40).

The nasal cavity and paranasal sinuses also are anatomical structures amenable to perspective visualization because of high image contrast inherent in the air-containing cavities.

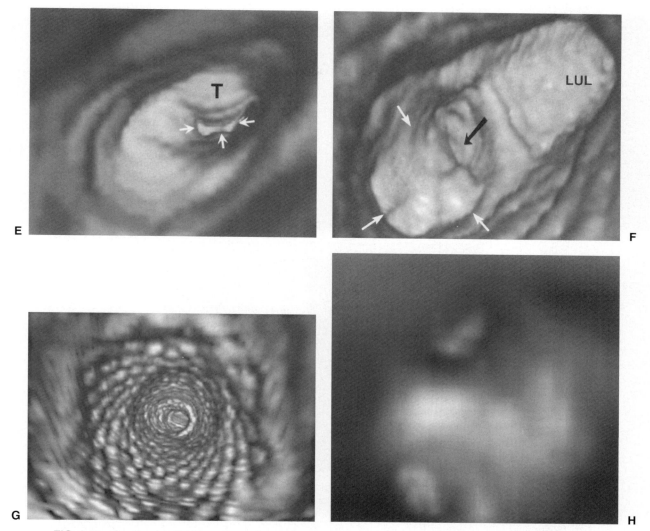

FIG. 3–5. *Continued.* **(E)** Bronchogenic carcinoma. Supero–inferior view of the left mainstem bronchus shows marked narrowing of the lumen (*arrows*) due to tumor (*T*). **F:** Bronchial carcinoid. Lobular endobronchial mass lesion (*white arrows*) is seen in the proximal bronchus intermedius. *Black arrow,* residual lumen; *LUL,* takeoff of normal upper-left lobe bronchus. **G:** Tracheal stent. Follow-up PVR view (80-degree FOV) of spiral CT in a patient with tracheal stenosis shows wide patency of the trachea after placement of expandable metallic stents. The stent could be assigned a different color than the tracheal wall because of the higher attenuation values in the metal, which aids in visualization. **H:** Small airways. Seventh-order bronchial branching is demonstrated within a subsegment of the anterior segment of the upper-right lobe. This level of detail is possible only with thin (1-mm) collimation. (**A,C, and E:** From Rubin et al. *Radiology* 1996;199:321–330, with permission, and **(D)** from Rubin et al. *Radiology* 1996; 200:312–317, with permission.) (See Color Fig. 3–5G)

Figure 3-6 illustrates some of the detailed anatomy that can be rendered with high-quality spiral CT data. Such renderings may be useful for planning or followup of endoscopic sinus surgery and for teaching the principles of sinus endoscopy to trainees (43). When affordable real-time display of perspective rendering becomes a reality, further innovations should be expected in the form of head-mounted displays, systems to detect collisions with walls or organ boundaries, and methods for realistic surgical simulation. In otolaryngology, virtual imaging has been applied further to vocal cord lesions (44) and the inner-ear ossicles (45).

As with the colon, initial results on perspective rendering of the airways are encouraging. To what extent the techniques will replace invasive procedures currently is not clear, nor is the extent to which the 3D endoluminal perspective influences the accuracy of interpretation of the CT study relative to more conventional means of CT interpretation.

Blood Vessels—"Virtual Angioscopy"

Whereas virtual colonoscopy and bronchoscopy have their fiberoptic correlates, there is no means of directly visu-

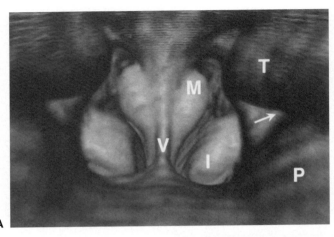

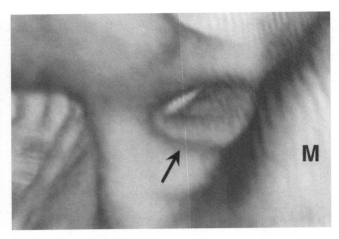

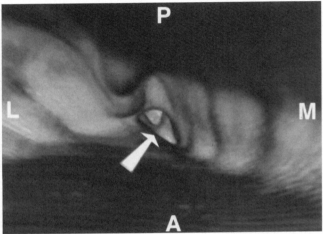

FIG. 3–6. Nasal cavity and paranasal sinuses. Spiral CT volume was acquired with 1-mm collimation, pitch 2, and reconstructed at 1-mm intervals. **A:** Nasal cavity viewed postero–anteriorly from the upper surface of the soft palate. The midline vomer (*V*), middle (*M*), and inferior (*I*) turbinates, torus tubarii (*T*), eustachian-tube hiatus (*arrow*), and the mucosal covering of the levator veli palatini muscles (*P*) are well depicted. **B:** Antero–posterior view of the ostium to the right maxillary sinus (*arrow*) as viewed from within the maxillary sinus. The ability to choose a perspective that looks into or outward from a sinus cavity may be valuable to plan endoscopic sinus surgery or reevaluate previously operated patients. **C:** Supero–inferior view from within the right frontal sinus demonstrates the ostium of the sinus (*arrow*). The anterior margin (*A*) that underlies the calvarial outer table, the posterior margin (*P*) that underlies the inner calvarial table, and the lateral (*L*) and medial (*M*) aspects of the sinus are labeled for orientation. Rendering was performed by Helmut Ringl, M.D. (From Rubin et al. *Radiology* 1996;199:321–330, with permission.)

alizing the inner walls of large blood vessels with an optical technique because of the opaqueness of blood. Fiberoptic angioscopes have been used in smaller vessels where a saline flush can replace sufficiently the blood within the lumen and enable visualization of more abnormalities. With administration of bolus IV iodinated contrast and spiral CT, sufficient image contrast is generated to enable simulated "angioscopy" (31, 46). This technique affords a unique perspective of intraluminal relationships of branch origins and various lesions, such as intimal flaps and atherosclerotic plaques, and, potentially, an improved means of interrogation of stents and stent grafts to determine their relationship to normal structures, adequacy of deployment, and complica-

tions (47, 48). A key feature of perspective rendering as applied to the cardiovascular system is that the time-intensive manual editing of source CT images to remove unwanted structures can be avoided; if ribs or other structures obscure the line of sight, one simply can move inside or around them to obtain the desired view. Figures 3–7 and 3–8 illustrate PVR techniques applied to the thoracic aorta and the abdominal aorta, respectively. Figure 3-9 illustrates the concept of "flying around" for viewing of spiral CT data from outside the structure of interest, but within the boundaries of the volume. Figure 3-10 shows PVR applied to the intracranial arteries. Such images may be helpful in determining the optimal surgical or endoluminal approach to aneurysms.

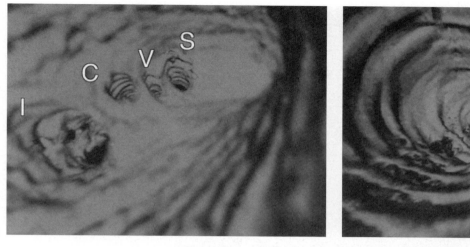

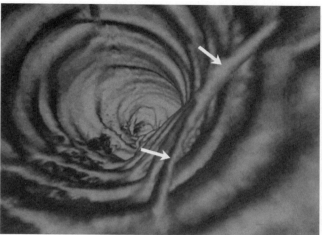

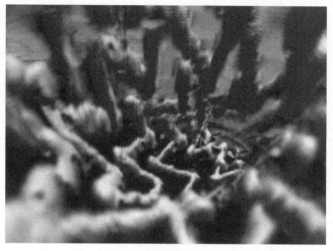

FIG. 3–7. Endoscopic imaging of the thoracic aorta. Images were acquired with 3-mm collimation, pitch 1.5–2.0, during bolus IV injection of iodinated contrast at 4–5 cc/sec and rendered with PVR. **A:** PVR view showing the innominate (*I*), left common carotid (*C*), left vertebral (*V*), and left subclavian (*S*) arteries arising from the aortic arch as viewed from the ascending aorta. **B:** Type-B aortic dissection. Infero–superior view from the descending thoracic aorta shows a dissection flap (*arrows*) demarcating the true and false lumina. Prominent corrugations in the aortic wall predominantly reflect pulsatility of the thoracic aorta during the CT acquisition. **C:** Aortic stent graft. Metallic struts of a covered thoracic aortic stent graft can be depicted along the aortic wall to visualize adequacy of stent deployment and the configuration of the aortic lumen. (See Color Fig. 3–7)

While perspective rendering of spiral CT-angiography data provides unique displays, systematic studies need to be performed to show that additional expense and effort provides either incremental diagnostic accuracy or uniquely valuable means of communication with treating physicians. In the majority of practices performing CT angiography, it is believed that the production of endoluminal vascular images is uncommon. As computer-hardware and -software technology continue to advance, we expect that semiautomated rendering and path-planning methods will become available, allowing the efficient creation of renderings from an endoluminal or extraluminal perspective. These renderings can then be compared directly with traditional CT review, other studies [such as magnetic resonance imaging (MRI) and en-dovascular ultrasound], and surgical findings to determine their relative values.

Kidneys and Urinary Collecting System

Pilot studies on perspective visualization applied to the genitourinary (GU) system have been reported. In the urinary bladder, distention with air, and potentially with iodinated contrast, can be used to generate surface-rendered displays (49) and VR displays (50) that depict the inner contour of the bladder. Figure 3-11 shows a VR display of a large bladder neoplasm obtained by imaging the bladder at 3-mm collimation, pitch 1.5 after distention of the bladder with air. Systematic clinical studies will be necessary to evaluate if

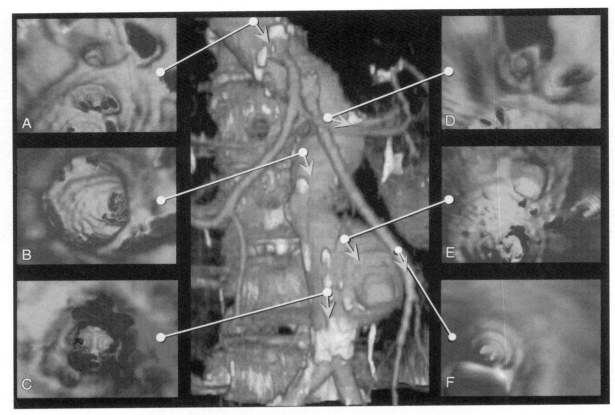

FIG. 3–8. Endoscopic imaging of the abdominal aorta. Multiple frames were captured from an endoscopic fly through of a patient with an infrarenal abdominal aortic aneurysm performed with PVR on spiral CT data obtained with 3-mm collimation, pitch 2, during injection of IV iodinated contrast at 5 cc/sec. Center image depicts the general morphology of the abdominal aorta. Calcific plaque has been assigned a white color and can be depicted as distinct from contrast column due to attenuation higher than the aortic lumen. Lines with arrows show viewpoint and viewing directions for multiple endoluminal views shown in **(A–F)**. **A:** Celiac and superior mesenteric artery (SMA) origins. Note foci of atherosclerotic plaque at the ostium of the SMA. **B:** Mid-aortic view showing plaque and proximal neck of aneurysm. **C:** Caudal aorta showing aortic bifurcation and heavy calcific plaque. **D:** Left renal artery origin with ostial plaque, but no significant stenosis. **E:** Endoluminal view of focal ulcer in the anterior/left aspect of the aneurysm. The aortic bifurcation is visible in the lower portion of image, but better shown in **(C)**. **F:** SMA fly through. Second- through fourth-order branch vessels can be viewed routinely from an endoscopic perspective provided there is adequate vascular enhancement. Focal calcific plaque in the distal SMA is seen in the lower portion of the image and branching is seen in the distance. Renderings performed by Yasayuki Kobayashi, MD. (See Color Fig. 3–8)

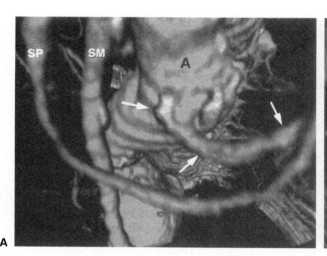
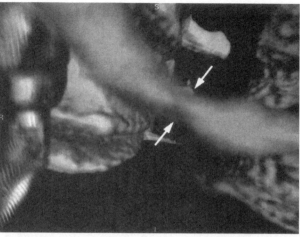

FIG. 3–9. Fly around of the abdominal aorta. By assuming a viewpoint inside the volume, a unique perspective can be obtained allowing the viewer to move around and between structures to optimize visualization of the anatomy of interest. **A:** Oblique supero–inferior view (60 degree) of the left renal artery (*arrows*) in a patient with an infrarenal abdominal aortic aneurysm. Calcific plaque at the ostium is evident. The splenic (*SP*) and superior mesenteric (*SM*) arteries also are visible. *A,* aorta. **B:** Antero–posterior view of the left renal artery (80-degree FOV) in a patient with moderate renal artery stenosis (*arrows*). In this case, early enhancement of the left renal vein obscured visualization of the renal artery, so the viewpoint was positioned *between* the renal artery and the vein, obviating the need to perform spatial editing of the data. (See Color Fig. 3–9)

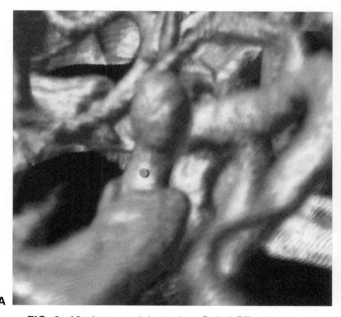
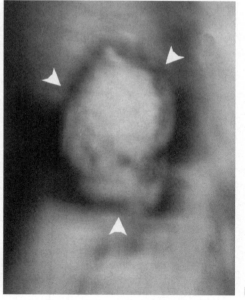

FIG. 3–10. Intracranial arteries. Spiral CT volume was acquired during IV contrast administration with 1-mm collimation, pitch 2, and image reconstruction at 0.5-mm intervals. **A:** Oblique PVR view of a supraclinoid carotid aneurysm. **B:** Endoluminal view of the broad aneurysm neck (*arrowheads*) viewed from the point in **(B)** indicated by the *circle.* Evaluation of the cerebrovascular system with spiral CT and perspective rendering may aid in detection of aneurysms and planning the surgical approach for optimal clipping of aneurysms.

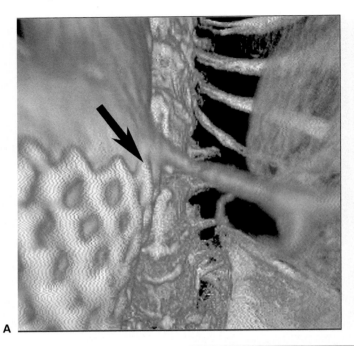

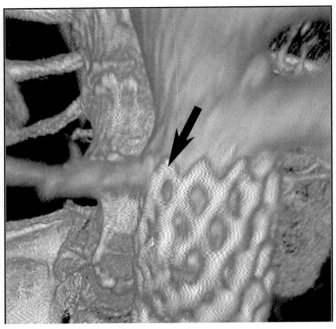

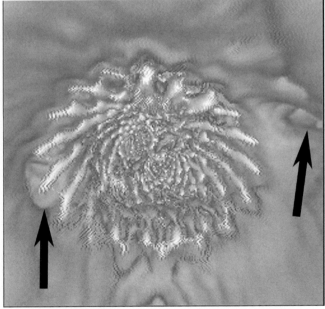

FIG. 3–11. Renal arteries. Multidetector CT reconstructed with 1.25-mm section thickness. **A,B:** Left and right renal arteries, respectively, with an aortic stent graft (*arrow*) that originated close to both renal ostea. The exact relationship between the stent graft and the renal artery ostea is difficult to ascertain. **C:** Perspective volume rendering within the suprarenal aorta, looking inferiorly. The *arrows* identify the renal artery ostea. From this perspective, the relationship of the renal artery ostea and the stent graft remains difficult to assess. *(Continued)*

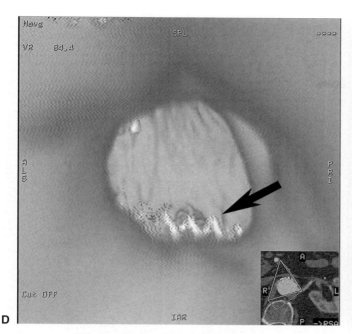
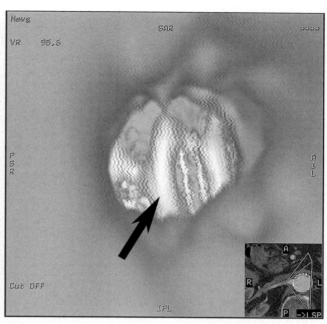

FIG. 3–11. *Continued.* **D,E:** Perspective volume rendering from within the left and right renal arteries, respectively, looking in to the aorta. The left renal artery origin is encroached upon minimally, but the right renal artery origin is obstructed nearly completely by the stent graft. (See Color Fig. 3–11)

the CT examination could replace or improve upon conventional cystoscopic evaluation in selected patients. Publications from several groups undertaking these issues are beginning to appear (51,52).

One important issue that has not been addressed carefully is the efficacy with which CT virtual examinations can depict relatively flat mucosal lesions, which can be malignant and need to be detected (49). The ability of perspective rendering, particularly with VR graphics, to depict relationships of masses to normal structures has been applied anecdotally to the kidneys (50). Figure 3-12 shows several images demonstrating the relationship of a renal cell carcinoma to the kidney and the renal collecting system in a patient with a horseshoe kidney. In Figure 3-12C–F, the use of perspective to create images that simulate the view of an endoscope in the renal pelvis is demonstrated, although mechanical endoscopy from this perspective would not be accomplished easily. In this example, the high image contrast afforded by dense iodine in the collecting system allows creation of effective renderings of the interface between the renal pelvis and surrounding structures, including the renal mass. In cases where complex surgical planning is necessary, exploration of the patient's anatomy and pathology with multiplanar reformations, 3D, and perspective techniques may improve the outcome. A significant problem, however, is that it is difficult to quantify how such displays change the surgeon's mental image or level of confidence when treating a given patient, so that it is not easy to design studies to help validate whether or not the additional effort and expense involved in creating advanced renderings is justified.

Joints—"Virtual Arthroscopy"

Initial applications of perspective rendering to articular disorders, particularly with MRI (53), have been encouraging. Since the majority of clinical imaging of joints is done with MRI, capitalizing on the ability to supplement routine MR examinations with acquisition of 3D Fourier volume datasets is appealing. In spiral CT, there is potential for virtual arthroscopic examination if iodinated contrast material or air is injected into the joint. Injection of the joint of interest is necessary to provide sufficient image contrast and to distend the joint capsule for visualization of its surface anatomy. Figure 3-13 shows a perspective image of the posterior glenohumeral joint obtained after injecting the joint with air. In Figure 3-13A, the opacity has been adjusted so that only bone-attenuation voxels are opaque; a posterior glenoid fracture is evident. By applying a new opacity table that makes the soft tissues of the glenoid labrum relatively more opaque, one can visualize how the posterior labrum is applied to the glenoid and ascertain that there is no significant labral injury (Fig. 3-13B). Virtual arthroscopy with spiral CT may be helpful in communicating results of studies to orthopedic surgeons and in surgical planning, though competition from volumetric MR arthrography can be expected. The improvements in longitudinal resolution with MDCT have led to the realization that ligaments and tendons are better seen on CT than previously recognized. In one study, the anterior cruciate ligament was diagnosed accurately as intact or torn in 21 patients with knee trauma who underwent arthroscopy (54). In another publication, the ability of VR to depict si-

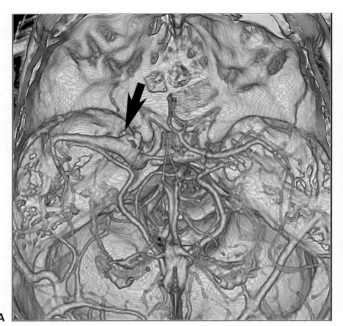

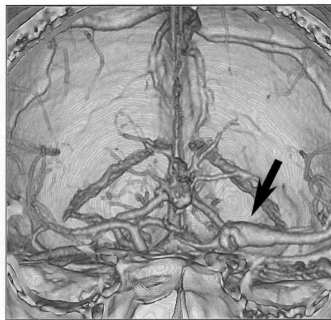

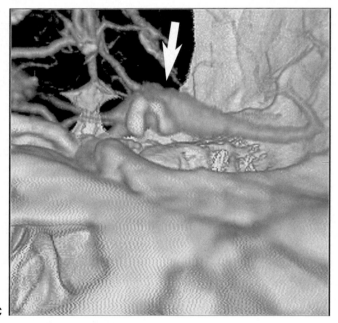

FIG. 3–12. Intracranial arteries. Multidetector CT reconstructed with 0.625-mm section thickness. **A:** Volume rendering viewed from above after the superior aspect of the skull has been removed. There is a fusiform aneurysm of the left-middle cerebral artery (*arrow*). **B:** Frontal view of the aneurysm shows the aneurysm (*arrow*) with the A1 segment originating medially. **C:** Perspective volume-rendered view seen from the floor of the anterior cranial fossa demonstrates the aneurysm (*arrow*) rendered from within the cranium. (See Color Fig. 3–12)

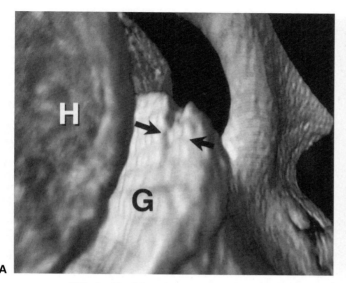
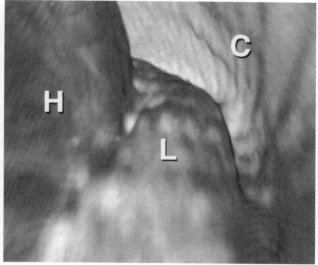

FIG. 3–13. Virtual arthroscopy. In a patient with subacute posterior dislocation of the glenohumeral joint, a spiral CT volume was acquired with 3-mm collimation, pitch 1, after injection of air into the shoulder joint under fluoroscopy. Images were reconstructed at 0.5-mm intervals with the standard reconstruction kernel. **A:** Perspective volume-rendered image of osseous structures. Opacity table adjusted to render only bone opaque, so that glenoid fossa (*G*) and humeral head (*H*) are depicted. Arrows denote posterior glenoid fracture. **B:** Perspective volume-rendered image of soft tissues. Opacity table adjusted to render the glenoid labrum (*L*) and air-distended capsule (*C*) from the same viewpoint as in **(A)**. By creating an animation that slowly alternates between osseous and soft tissue visualization, one obtains a unique understanding of how soft tissue anatomy relates to the underlying bones. Because the normal joint capsule is applied closely to the bones, adequate visualization requires distention of the joint with air or positive contrast.

multaneously tendons, muscle, and bone about joints was well demonstrated (55).

CONCLUSIONS

Improvements in scanner technology, coupled with affordable and powerful computer-graphics systems, have resulted in superb image generation and visualization tools for the radiologist and clinician. Perspective rendering of spiral CT data may be the best current example, but the concepts may be equally applicable to any imaging system providing a volumetric dataset, such as MRI and ultrasound. While the advanced visualization techniques do not actually create new anatomical *data* above and beyond the source cross sections, using these tools to display the data in new ways that more closely simulate natural 3D scenes may create additional new visual *information* about the patient. This new information now can be created efficiently and affordably, and the current challenge is to prove that the additional effort and expense is justified by improving patient care through more accurate diagnoses, improved patient outcomes, or measurably improved communication with referring physicians. When considering the more-distant future of computer graphics and spiral CT, we will be limited only by our imagination in terms of how imaging data will be manipulated and visualized. At the same time, we need to remain ever conscious of the fact that advanced visualization tools can never increase the quality of the source image data.

ACKNOWLEDGMENTS

We offer thanks to our scientific and physician collaborators, including Sandy Napel, R. Brooke Jeffrey, Jr., David Paik, Marta Davila, Scott Mitchell, Christopher Zarins, Craig Miller, James Mark, Norman Rizk, John Feller, and Gary Fanton. Support from the Lucas Foundation, the Society for Gastrointestinal Radiology, the Society of Computed Body Tomography and Magnetic Resonance, and National Institutes of Health Grant RO1 CA72023 also is appreciated. Finally, thanks to our wives, Patti and Rhesa, and to our children, Marielle, Elena, and Rainier, and Magellan, Giulianna, Elka, and Griffin, who help us keep things in perspective.

REFERENCES

1. Kalender WA, Vock P, Polacin A, et al. Spiral CT: a new technique for volumetric scans. I. Basic principles and methodology. *Rontgenpraxis* 1990;43:323–330.
2. Kalender WA, Seissler W, Klotz E, et al. Spiral volumetric CT with single-breath-hold technique, continuous transport, and continuous scanner rotation. *Radiology* 1990;176:181–183.
3. Crawford CR, King KF. Computed tomography scanning with simultaneous patient translation. *Med Phys* 1990;17:967–982.

4. Napel S, Marks MP, Rubin GD. CT angiography with spiral CT and maximum intensity projection. *Radiology* 1992;185:607–610.

5. Rubin GD, Dake MD, Napel SA, et al. Abdominal spiral CT angiography: initial clinical experience. *Radiology* 1993;186:147–152.

6. Honda H, Matsuura Y, Onitsuka H, et al. Differential diagnosis of hepatic tumors (hepatoma, hemangioma, and metastasis) with CT: value of two-phase incremental imaging. *AJR Am J Roentgenol* 1992; 159:735–740.

7. Bluemke DA, Soyer P, Fishman EK. Helical (spiral) CT of the liver. *Radiol Clin North Am* 1995;33:863–886.

8. Bluemke DA, Cameran JL, Hruban RH, et al. Potentially resectable pancreatic adenocarcinoma: spiral CT assessment with surgical and pathologic correlation. *Radiology* 1995;197:381–385.

9. Magnusson M, Lenz R, Danielsson PE. Evaluation of methods for shaded surface display of CT volumes. *Comput Med Imaging Graph* 1991;15:247–256.

10. Kalender WA, Polacin A, Suss C. A comparison of conventional and spiral CT: an experimental study on the detection of spherical lesions. *J Comp Assist Tomogr* 1994;18(2):167–176.

11. Rubin GD, Napel S, Leung AN. Volumetric analysis of volumetric data: achieving a paradigm shift. *Radiology* 1996;200:312–317.

12. Rubin GD, Beaulieu CF, Argiro V, et al. Perspective volume rendering of CT and MR images: applications for endoscopic imaging. *Radiology* 1996;199:321–330.

13. Vining DJ. Virtual endoscopy: Is it reality? *Radiology* 1996; 200:30–31.

14. Kalender WA. Thin-section three-dimensional spiral CT: is isotropic imaging possible? *Radiology* 1995;197:578–580.

15. Wang G, Vannier MW. Longitudinal resolution in volumetric x-ray computerized tomography—Analytical comparison between conventional and helical computerized tomography. *Med Phys* 1994;21(3): 429–433.

16. West K. *Basic perspective for artists.* New York: Watson–Guptill, 1995:10.

17. Summers RM. Navigational aids for virtual endoscopy. *Radiology* 1996;201(P):248(abst).

18. Lorensen WE, Jolesz FA, Kikinis R, Satara R, Morgan K, eds. The exploration of cross-sectional data with a virtual endoscope. In: *Interactive technology and the new paradigm for health care: medicine meets virtual reality III proceedings.* Amsterdam, Holland: IOS Press, 1995; 221–230.

19. Geiger B, Kikinis R. Simulation of endoscopy. In: *AAAI spring symposium series: applications of computer vision in medical image processing.* Stanford University, 1994;138–140.

20. Vining DJ, Liu K, Choplin RH, et al. Virtual bronchoscopy: relationships of virtual reality endobronchial simulations to actual bronchoscopic findings. *Chest* 1996;109:549–553.

21. Fishman EK, Magid D, Ney DR, et al. Three-dimensional imaging. *Radiology* 1991;181:321–337.

22. Heath DG, Soyer PA, Kuszyk BS, et al. Three-dimensional spiral CT during arterial portography: comparison of three rendering techniques. *Radiographics* 1995;15:1001–1011.

23. Rubin GD, Dake MD, Napel S, et al. Spiral CT of renal artery stenosis: comparison of three-dimensional rendering techniques. *Radiology* 1994;190:181–189.

24. Drebin RA, Carpenter L, Hanrahan P. Volume rendering. *Comp Graph* 1988;22:65–74.

25. Johnson PT, Heath HG, Bliss DF, et al. Three-dimensional CT: real-time interactive volume rendering. *Radiology* 1996;200:581–583.

26. Beaulieu CF, Baker ME, Chotas HG, et al. Volume rendering for 3D helical CT of the abdominal aorta. *Radiology* 1993;189(P):173(abst).

27. Paik DS, Beaulieu CF, Jeffrey RB, et al. Automated flight path planning for virtual endoscopy. *Med Phys* 1998;25(5):629–637.

28. Samara Y, Fiebich M, Dachman AH, et al. Automated calculation of the centerline of the human colon on CT images. *Acad Radiol* 1999; 6(6):352–359.

29. Hung PW, Paik DS, Napel S, et al. Quantification of distention in CT colonography: development and validation of three computer algorithms. *Radiology* 2002;222(2):543–554.

30. Rubin GD, Paik DS, Johnston PC, et al. Measurement of the aorta and its branches with helical CT. *Radiology* 1998;206(3):823–829.

31. Kobayashi Y, Rubin GD, Napel S, et al. Intraluminal and extraluminal images of the vasculature: perspective volume rendering of CT angiograms without editing or thresholding. *Radiology* 1996;201(P): 316(abst).

32. Hermanek P. Dysplasia–carcinoma sequence, types of adenomas and early colo-rectal carcinoma. *Eur J Surg Oncol* 1987;13:141–143.

33. Napel S, Rubin GD, RBJ Jr. STS-MIP: a new reconstruction technique for CT of the chest. *J Comput Tomogr* 1993;17:832–838.

34. Koito K, Namieno T, Hirokawa N, et al. Virtual CT cholangioscopy: comparison with fiberoptic cholangioscopy. *Endoscopy* 2001;33(8): 676–681.

35. Naidich DP, Gruden JF, McGuinness G, et al. Volumetric (helical/spiral) CT (VCT) of the airways. *J Thorac Imaging* 1997;12:11–28.

36. Summers RM, Feng DH, Holland SM, et al. Virtual bronchoscopy: segmentation method for real-time display. *Radiology* September 1996; 200:857–862.

37. McAdams HP, Palmer SM, Erasmus JJ, et al. Bronchial anastomotic complications in lung transplant recipients: virtual bronchoscopy for noninvasive assessment. *Radiology* 1998;209(3):689–695.

38. Summers RM, Aggarwal NR, Sneller MC, et al. CT virtual bronchoscopy of the central airways in patients with Wegener's granulomatosis. *Chest* 2002;121(1):242–250.

39. Hoppe H, Walder B, Sonnenschein M, et al. Multidetector CT virtual bronchoscopy to grade tracheobronchial stenosis. *AJR Am J Roentgenol* 2002;178(5):1195–1200.

40. Sorantin E, Geiger B, Lindbichler F, et al. CT-based virtual tracheo-bronchoscopy in children—comparison with axial CT and multiplanar reconstruction: preliminary results. *Pediatr Radiol* 2002;32(1):8–15.

41. McAdams HP, Erasmus JJ, Shahidi R, et al. Virtual bronchoscopy: principles, pitfalls and clinical applications. *Radiology* 1996;201(P): 480(abst).

42. Hopper KD, Lucas TA, Gleeson K, et al. Transbronchial biopsy with virtual CT bronchoscopy and nodal highlighting. *Radiology* 2001; 221(2):531–536.

43. Gilani S, Norbash AM, Ringl H, et al. Virtual endoscopy of the paranasal sinuses using perspective volume rendered helical sinus computed tomography. *Laryngoscope* 1997;107(1):25–29.

44. Walshe P, Hamilton S, McShane D, et al. The potential of virtual laryngoscopy in the assessment of vocal cord lesions. *Clin Otolaryngol* 2002;27(2):98–100.

45. Nakasato T, Sasaki M, Ehara S, et al. Virtual CT endoscopy of ossicles in the middle ear. *Clin Imaging* 2001;25(3):171–177.

46. Rubin GD, Napel S, Beaulieu CF, et al. Virtual angioscopy using volume rendered CT angiograms. Three-dimensional rendering without editing or thresholding. *Radiology* 1995;197(P):144(abst).

47. Neri E, Caramella D, Cioni R, et al. Pseudoaneurysm of the abdominal aorta: evaluation with virtual angioscopy of spiral CT data sets. *Eur Radiol* 1999;9(6):1227–1230.

48. Davis CP, Ladd ME, Romanowski BJ, et al. Human aorta: preliminary results with virtual endoscopy based on three-dimensional MR imaging data sets. *Radiology* 1996;199:37–40.

49. Vining DJ, Zagoria RJ, Liu K, et al. CT cystoscopy: an innovation in bladder imaging. *AJR Am J Roentgenol* 1996;166:409–410.

50. Sommer FG, Olcott EW, Ch'en IY, et al. Volume rendering of CT data: applications to the genitourinary tract. *AJR Am J Roentgenol* 1997; 168:1223–1226.

51. Bernhardt TM, Rapp-Bernhardt U. Virtual cystoscopy of the bladder based on CT and MRI data. *Abdom Imaging* 2001;26(3):325–332.

52. Fielding JR, Hoyte LX, Okon SA, et al. Tumor detection by virtual cystoscopy with color mapping of bladder wall thickness. *J Urol* 2002; 167(2 Pt 1):559–562.

53. Feller JF, Rubin GD, Tirman PF, et al. MR virtual arthroscopy. *Radiology* 1995;197(P):227(abst).

54. Irie K, Yamada T. Three-dimensional virtual computed tomography imaging for injured anterior cruciate ligament. *Arch Orthop Trauma Surg* 2002;122(2):93–95.

55. Pelc JS, Beaulieu CF. Volume rendering of tendon–bone relationships using unenhanced CT. *AJR Am J Roentgenol* 2001;176(4):973–977.

CHAPTER 4

Clinical Impact of Multidetector CT

R. Brooke Jeffrey, Jr.

INTRODUCTION AND HISTORICAL PERSPECTIVE

There can be little doubt that, compared to single-slice spiral computed tomography (CT), the recent development of multidetector CT (MDCT) represents a major hardware breakthrough for CT technology (1). Multidetector CT affords two major advantages that have impacted its clinical application: dramatically increased speed of scan acquisition and substantially improved spatial resolution through the routine use of thinner collimation. Currently available commercial MDCT scanners are capable of capturing 16 slices of spiral CT data with a single gantry rotation. Further enhancement of temporal resolution has been achieved via a reduction in the gantry rotation time from 1 second to 0.5 seconds. With the use of half-gantry rotation, the effective temporal resolution (250 milliseconds) is beginning to approximate that of electron-beam CT for such clinical applications as coronary calcium screening (2). To assess adequately this impressive second generation of spiral CT technology and its clinical impact, it is useful to view it first within the historical context of the development of CT, and then focus on the unique clinical application of MDCT.

Quite remarkably, the initial development of single-slice spiral (helical CT) was met with only tepid enthusiasm when first introduced into clinical practice in the early 1990s in the United States. At the time, few clinical authorities in CT clearly recognized this hardware innovation as a dramatic advance. While it was clear that the combination of continuous gantry rotation with continuous table translation would lead to reduced scanning time, few appreciated how revolutionary this technology would become. To be fair, the initial spiral acquisitions often were limited by their scanning parameters. The first spiral acquisitions were of relatively short duration (24 seconds) and could support relatively low milliamperage (mA) of the X-ray beam. However, the *rate-limiting step*, and perhaps the greatest challenge of the first generation of spiral scanners, was the lack of available software to support radically new clinical applications. It was only when dedicated workstations with image-processing software were introduced, in parallel with the improved performance of the spiral scanning acquisition, that completely new procedures such as CT angiography, three-dimensional (3D) endoscopic imaging, and computer-assisted diagnosis became possible (3,4). Viewed from the perspective of these new clinical applications, there is no doubt that the initial spiral CT technology represented a quantum leap in scanning acquisition from the days of dynamic (step-and-shoot) CT. Dynamic CT required up to 2 minutes to perform an abdominal acquisition, and therefore could not be performed with a single breath hold. Breath-held acquisitions with spiral CT eliminated the major limitation of the previous generation of CT, namely the inevitable motion and misregistration artifacts that result from multiple breath holds. The single-breath-held acquisition was a key first step in the development of volumetric datasets for CT free of these artifacts. The combination of continuous table translation with continuous tube rotation was in itself a remarkable achievement; however, it was only when the CT data could be processed and displayed with innovative software solutions into angiographic or 3D studies that the full advantage of spiral CT technology could be realized.

After nearly a decade of clinical use, a second major hardware upgrade was introduced with the development of MDCT. Now it has become possible to acquire multiple channels of CT data with a single gantry rotation, thus dramatically improving the speed of scan acquisition. With the use of thinner-slice collimation, imaging near isotropic voxels can be obtained. All of this can be achieved without paying a significant penalty in terms of scanning artifacts. In the past year, with the clinical introduction of 8- and 16-slice MDCT scanners, it is clear that this technology represents an important evolutionary step toward volumetric CT.

Even when compared with single-slice helical CT, multidetector technology has had a major clinical impact in a number of very important areas. It should be emphasized,

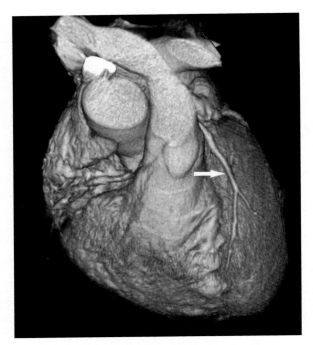

FIG. 4–1. Cardiac MDCT. Note normal left coronary artery on volume-rendered image (*arrow*). (See Color Fig. 4–1)

however, that there are relatively few entirely new scanning applications in MDCT (coronary CT angiography, peripheral vascular CT angiography, etc.) (Figs. 4–1 and 4–2). Rather, MDCT might best viewed as a technology that greatly improves many existing applications of single-slice spiral CT. With dynamic CT, misregistration artifacts and the slow speed of scan acquisition precluded any attempt at CT angiography or 3D imaging. Thus, despite all its limitations, single-slice spiral CT technology was truly revolutionary. It has resulted in many completely new clinical applications that have had a major effect on patient referrals and practice patterns. Computed tomography angiography, for example, is now a routine part of clinical practice that has achieved widespread clinical acceptance, and in many specific clinical areas, it has reduced dramatically the need for invasive catheter angiography. Similarly, the development of software to perform real-time volume rendering and computer-assisted diagnosis has rapidly transformed 3D imaging. Applications such as virtual colonoscopy (Figure 4-3) and virtual bronchoscopy have been introduced into clinical practice. Multidetector CT substantially improves the image quality of all these applications.

To summarize, the single most salient characteristic of MDCT is its increased speed of scan acquisition. Faster scanning technology results in several major diagnostic benefits

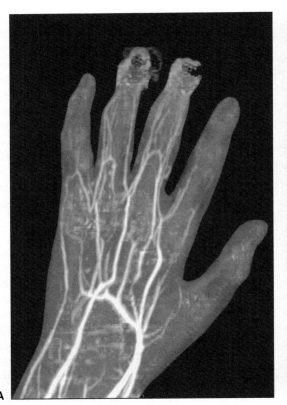

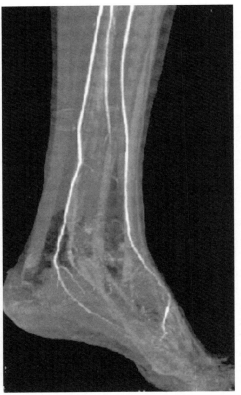

FIG. 4–2. A,B: Peripheral vascular CT angiography. Note fine detail of small vessels of the hand on MIP images. Patient had sustained soft tissue degloving injury to the digits. **B:** MIP image from a peripheral vascular study.

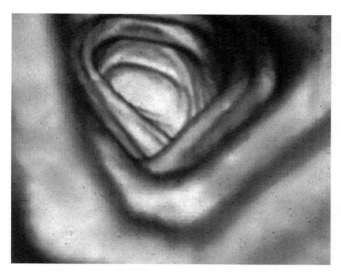

FIG. 4–3. Virtual endoscopic image of normal colon with MDCT colonography. (See Color Fig. 4–3)

for CT: (i) substantially improved anatomic coverage and ability to scan large regions of the abdomen and extremities with a single scan acquisition; (ii) the ability to scan at thinner collimation, to improve spatial resolution; and (iii) optimization of intravenous contrast enhancement achieved by scanning at the peak of vascular opacification. Restated in a more direct way, MDCT technology allows us to scan larger regions of the body with thinner collimation in a faster time.

LIMITATIONS OF MDCT: THE INFORMATION EXPLOSION

This new technology has some important drawbacks that must be kept in mind when assessing its overall clinical impact. There is a modest increase in radiation dosage with the use of very thinly collimated scans in MDCT technology. With the rapid proliferation of CT into clinical practice, limiting radiation exposure should be the goal of all radiologists using this new technology. Radiation dose is a key concern as MDCT evolves into the controversial area of screening low-risk populations (5). Some of the effects of the radiation dosage can be mitigated by judicious use of scanning parameters (such as lowering the milliamperage) (6); however, significant progress will be required on the part of manufacturers to ensure that the X-ray-detector systems are maximally efficient to avoid scatter and radiation dosage that has no diagnostic benefit. Some progress has been made already with the use of focal spot tracking to reduce scatter.

A second problematic aspect of MDCT, and perhaps one of its "unintended consequences," is that the use of thinner collimation over large areas of the body results in a "data explosion" with a dramatic increase in the number of CT images (7). For many clinical applications, it becomes impractical to view and interpret this technology with traditional filming or viewing the images with a traditional light box. A typical example in clinical practice has been the impact of MDCT on pancreatic imaging. For the local staging of pancreatic carcinoma, a dedicated protocol employing 1.25-mm collimated scans affords superior diagnostic images of the pancreas. At the same time, however, this examination creates datasets with hundreds of images. Peripheral vascular studies may have datasets with a thousand images. It becomes impractical for the radiologist or the referring physician to view all of these images in a time-efficient manner. As a consequence of this data explosion, there is a renewed emphasis

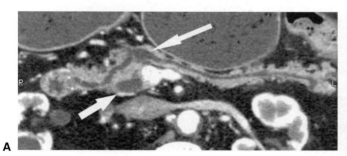

A

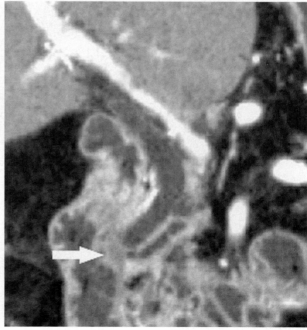

B

FIG. 4–4. A: Curved planar reformation of pancreatic duct. Note entire display of ductal system with focal dilatation of the main duct (*long arrow*) and uncinate process branch (*short arrow*) in a patient with an intraductal papillary and mucinous tumor. **B:** Curved planar reformation of mildly dilated common bile duct and pancreatic duct. Note enlarged ampulla from small tumor (*arrow*).

on soft copy reading from picture-archive-and-communication-system (PACS) workstations and the ability to survey rapidly key diagnostic views often obtained with multiplanar imaging or volume rendering.

A secondary benefit of very thin collimation is the high quality of anatomic resolution afforded by isotropic voxel datasets. When combined with overlapping reconstructions, these datasets greatly facilitate multiplanar reconstructions and volume rendering. Through unique imaging-processing display methods (curved planar reforma-

tions, minimum-intensity images, and volume-rendered images) (Figs. 4–4 and 4–5), a small selected number of key images can be reviewed quickly. These images displaying the entire pancreas and surrounding peripancreatic vasculature highlight the tumor and its local infiltration, greatly facilitating the efficient review of the images. Nevertheless, the fact remains that huge datasets are generated by MDCT, creating the necessity for a soft copy and/or PACS solution in conjunction with image-display methods for time-efficient viewing.

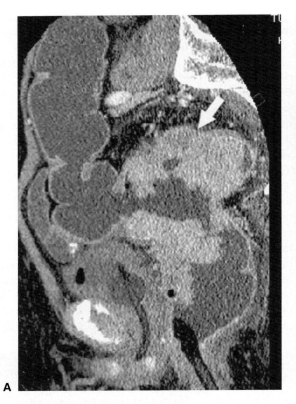

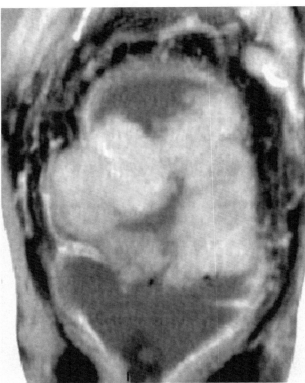

A

B

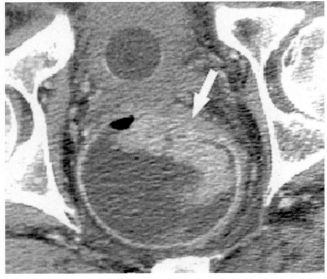

C

FIG. 4–5 A,B, and C: Multidetector CT image processing of rectal cancer. **A:** A curved planar reformation demonstrating a bulky intraluminal mass that proved to be a villous adenoma with invasive adenocarcinoma. **B:** A median intensity coronal image of the intraluminal mass. **C:** Deep mural invasion is evident on axial 1.25-mm scan (*arrow*).

AREAS OF GREATEST CLINICAL BENEFIT WITH MDCT

The Trauma Patient

The evaluation of patients with blunt trauma has been one of the major success stories in the clinical development of CT. With the advent of MDCT, this single examination has lead to "one-stop shopping" for a global assessment of cerebral, thoraco-abdominal, skeletal visceral, and vascular injuries (Figure 4-6). The rapid survey of the head, neck, chest, abdomen, pelvis, and vascular system afforded by MDCT is a truly remarkable achievement for this technology that is unmatched by any other modality. This fact is underscored by the growing recognition that MDCT scanners should be required instrumentation in all Level I trauma centers in this country. Multidetector CT has eliminated many difficult to obtain and technically limited plain radiographs in the emergency room, such as cervical spine views. It has dramatically reduced the need for thoracic angiography in patients with suspected aortic arch injuries. In patients with visceral injuries, MDCT greatly facilitates diagnosis of active arterial extravasation (Figure 4-7). This finding is of key importance in guiding patient management. Many renal, hepatic, and retroperitoneal areas of active arterial extravasation may be managed successfully with angiographic embolization rather than open surgery, thus reducing the overall morbidity.

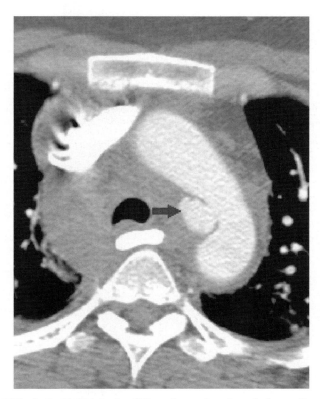

FIG. 4–6. Multidetector CT angiography of aortic laceration. Note large pseudoaneurysms of thoracic aorta (*arrow*).

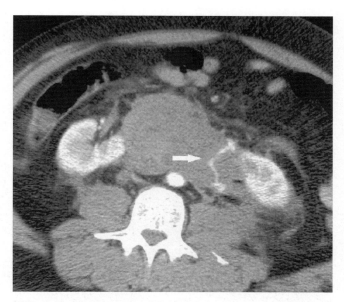

FIG. 4–7. Multidetector CT of active arterial extravasation. Note high-attenuation contrast (*arrow*) surrounded by lower-density hematoma at the isthmus of horseshoe kidney.

It should be emphasized, however, that CT evaluation still requires a hemodynamically stable patient. It often is difficult in the emergent trauma setting to monitor carefully patients in the CT suite. The scanning acquisition of MDCT is so fast that the most time-consuming aspect of examination is transporting the patient to the CT suite and placing the injured individual on and off the CT table. The use of portable ultrasound at the bedside remains an invaluable examination in the unstable patient who is not suitable for CT.

MDCT in the Oncology Patient

To date, there have been few prospective studies comparing single-slice spiral technology to MDCT in evaluation of the diagnosis and staging of malignancy. Nevertheless, the improved diagnostic benefits through improved spatial and temporal resolution afforded by MDCT make it likely that many areas of cancer imaging will improve. The use of thinner collimation as a routine reduces volume-averaging artifacts, which may aid in the specific diagnosis of focal hepatic lesions (8–11). Thinner collimation also improves evaluation of subtle vascular encasement by pancreatic tumors, which is a critical feature in determining surgical resectability. Similarly, the ability to rapidly acquire biphasic studies doing late arterial and venous phase of the liver is likely to improve detection of the small hepatocellular carcinomas at a size when they can be managed successfully with either minimally invasive ablative techniques or chemoembolization.

Evaluation of Vascular Pathology with MDCT

One new clinical application of MDCT is the evaluation of the peripheral vascular system with CT angiography

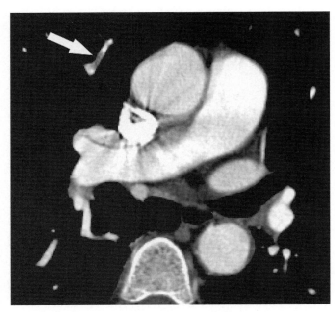

FIG. 4–8. Multidetctor CT of small pulmonary embolus. Note exquisite in-plane resolution of small right upper lobe pulmonary embolus (*arrow*).

(CTA) (12–14). Computed tomography angiography and magnetic resonance angiography (MRA) are likely to replace completely diagnostic catheter angiography merely for demonstration of arterial stenoses or occlusions. Because of the large volume of scan acquisition that is required to evaluate the aortoiliac and peripheral vascular runoff, this type of examination is simply not possible to perform with single-slice helical CT.

Other types of CT vascular procedures (pulmonary embolus studies, evaluation of aortic aneurysms, and aortic branch stenoses) all are facilitated with the use of thinner collimation (Figure 4-8). These types of studies, however, lend themselves to interpretation with soft copy image display on workstations, and 3D and multiplanar reconstructions for primary diagnosis.

MDCT for Screening

There is considerable debate about the clinical efficacy of CT in screening for various malignancies. Perhaps the most controversial is the use of CT for detection of lung cancer in patients with a history of smoking. Until larger prospective studies are performed with MDCT, one must reserve judgment before asserting that CT actually will lead to a survival benefit. It is far more likely that screening the colon with virtual colonoscopy will be a CT technique that will evolve into clinical practice in the near term. The detection and removal of adenomatous polyps has been shown clearly to improve survival. With data derived from single-slice helical CT demonstrating that clinically relevant polyps (1 cm or greater) can be detected with 90% sensitivity, it is likely that virtual colonoscopy performed with CT will be used in conjunction with fiberoptic colonoscopy in low-risk patients.

REFERENCES

1. Berland LL, Smith JK. Multidetector-array CT: once again, technology creates new opportunities. *Radiology* 1998;209(2):327–329.
2. Horiguchi J, Nakanishi T, Ito K. Quantification of coronary artery calcium using multidetector CT and a retrospective ECG-gating reconstruction algorithm. *Am J Radiol* 2001;177(6):1429–1435.
3. Fletcher JG, Luboldt W. CT colonography and MR colonography: current status, research directions and comparison. *Eur Radiol* 2000;10(5):786–801.
4. Behar JV, Nelson RC, Zidar JP, et al. Thin-section multidetector CT angiography of renal artery stents. *Am J Radiol* 2002;178(5):1155–1159.
5. Jakobs TF, Becker CR, Ohnesorge B, et al. Multislice helical CT of the heart with retrospective ECG gating: reduction of radiation exposure by ECG-controlled tube current modulation. *Eur Radiol* 2002;12(5):1081–1086.
6. Hamm M, Knopfle E, Wartenberg S, et al. Low dose unenhanced helical computerized tomography for the evaluation of acute flank pain. *J Urol* 2002;167(4):1687–1691.
7. Rubin GD. Data explosion: the challenge of multidetector-row CT. *Eur J Radiol* 2000;36(2):74–80.
8. Sze DY, Razavi MK, So SK, et al. Impact of multidetector CT hepatic arteriography on the planning of chemoembolization treatment of hepatocellular carcinoma. *Am J Radiol* 2001;177(6):1339–1345.
9. Kopp AF, Heuschmid M, Claussen CD. Multidetector helical CT of the liver for tumor detection and characterization. *Eur Radiol* 2002;12(4):745–752.
10. Murakami T, Kim T, Takahashi S, et al. Hepatocellular carcinoma: multidetector row helical CT. *Abdominal Imaging* 2002;27(2):139–146.
11. Ji H, McTavish JD, Mortele KJ, et al. Hepatic imaging with multidetector CT. *Radiographics* 2001; 21(special issue):S71–S80.
12. Rubin GD. Techniques for performing multidetector-row computed tomographic angiography. *Techniques Vasc Intervent Radiol* 2001; 4(1):2–14.
13. Raman R, Napel S, Beaulieu CF, et al. Automated generation of curved planar reformations from volume data: method and evaluation. *Radiology* 2002;223(1):275–280.
14. Rubin GD, Schmidt AJ, Logan LJ, et al. Multidetector-row CT angiography of lower extremity arterial inflow and runoff: initial experience. *Radiology* 2001;221(1):146–158.

SECTION II

Chest Applications

CHAPTER 5

Lung Cancer Screening

Ella A. Kazerooni

INTRODUCTION

Rapid advances in computed tomography (CT) technology, with faster acquisition speed of thin collimation images in a single breathhold throughout the lungs, reduces motion artifact and respiratory misregistration, thereby permitting reproducible high-resolution imaging of the lungs. This translates into greater sensitivity than obtained with previous generations of CT scanners for the detection of small lung nodules (1–3), which is further increased when soft copy workstations are used for interpretation (4). This has led to tremendous optimism regarding the ability of CT to detect lung cancer early. The basic premise of CT screening for lung cancer is that detecting small lung cancers may reduce lung cancer-specific mortality. In other words, size does matter. However, recent studies of clinically diagnosed lung cancer in which tumors less than 3 cm were studied have shown no significant relationship in either stage distribution of cancer or cancer survival among patients with smaller tumors, suggesting that size may not matter (5,6).

The application of CT technology to lung cancer screening in several prospective observational studies published from 1996 to the present has demonstrated the ability of CT to detect lung cancer when small, early in stage, and largely resectable (7–15). These data certainly raise hope. However, these same studies also raise concern because of the high false-positive rates encountered. The vast majority of nodules (approximately 99%) detected through CT screening are not cancerous and consequently result in patient anxiety. Furthermore, because it is not possible to differentiate between cancerous and noncancerous nodules, all nodules must be managed clinically, often with invasive procedures, resulting in increased morbidity and mortality, as well as considerable health-care expense (10,16). Postsurgical pain and functional health-status changes can persist for up to six months; in addition, studies have reported significant mortality within 6 months of lung cancer surgery (17). Factoring all these variables into a cost-effectiveness analysis has yielded mixed results (18,19). To date, no study has demonstrated that CT screening reduces lung cancer specific mortality (20). This chapter reviews these issues and summarizes the current level of knowledge about lung cancer screening with CT.

BACKGROUND AND RATIONALE FOR SCREENING

In the United States, lung cancer is the leading cause of cancer death in both men and women. More people die from lung cancer than from breast, colorectal, and prostate cancer combined (21). Screening tests exist for breast (mammography and physical breast examination), colorectal (fecal occult-blood tests, sigmoidoscopy, colonoscopy, and barium enema), and prostate cancer (prostate-specific antigen blood test and digital rectal examination) and have contributed to a reduction in mortality over the last few decades (21). Despite advances in medical care, including medical imaging, radiation therapy, and chemotherapy, lung cancer continues to have a high mortality rate, with 85% of patients dying from the disease (22). Although lung cancer represents only 13% of all new cancer cases, it is responsible for 28% of all cancer deaths. Over the last decade, its incidence has decreased among men, but increased considerably among women, largely due to increased cigarette smoking in women and a 30-year lag time between exposure and diagnosis.

Lung cancer screening is aimed at detection of non-small cell lung cancers, which represent nearly 75% of all lung cancers. The lower the stage at diagnosis, the better the prognosis. The five-year survival rate is 49% for patients presenting with localized cancer, compared to 22% if there is regional spread and 3% if there are distant metastases. Lung cancer is staged using a tumor, node, metastasis (TNM) classification scheme and an international staging system (23). The five-year survival rate for all lung cancers is 15% (21), and only 15% at one year with supportive therapy for patients presenting with Stage IV metastatic lung cancer, a rate only slightly improved with chemotherapy (24). In contrast, patients with Stage IA or Stage IB cancers have 5-year survival rates of 67% and 57%, respectively. Unfortunately, only 16% of patients present with local disease, the vast majority of these cancers being detected with regional or distant disease (21). Small cell cancer represents approximately 20% of all lung cancers and have a very poor prognosis with limited treatment options. Although they may be found incidentally in screening trials, they are not targeted by radiographic or CT screening.

LUNG CANCER RISK

Approximately 85% of lung cancers are caused by cigarette smoking, making it a largely preventable disease (25). Smoking is also a major risk factor for cardiovascular disease, emphysema, and many other cancers (larynx, oral cavity, esophagus, bladder, kidney, pancreas, and possibly cervix), with nearly one third of all cancer deaths directly attributable to cigarette smoking (26). In addition, more people die prematurely from smoking-related diseases than from automobile accidents, drug abuse, AIDS, and alcohol abuse combined (27). C. Everett Koop, the former Surgeon General, called cigarette smoking " . . . the chief, avoidable cause of death in our society and the most important public health issue of our time." The risk of smoking-related cancers is dose related and increases with greater exposure, including early onset, duration (packs per year), and intensity (cigarettes per day) of smoking (28,29). In addition to current and former smokers, individuals exposed to secondhand or passive smoke (known as environmental tobacco smoke or ETS) also are at risk (30). Nonsmokers who either live or work with smokers have a 30% to 50% greater risk of lung cancer, accounting for nearly 6000 deaths annually; this risk is estimated to be nearly 100 times higher than the risk of asbestos-related lung cancer. Even among smokers, there is a wide variation in lung cancer risk. A recent lung cancer prediction model demonstrated ten-year lung cancer risks as low as 0.8% for a 51-year-old woman with a one-pack-per-day history of smoking for 28 years who quit 8 years earlier, to as high as 15% for a 68-year old man with a two-pack-per-day smoking history for 50 years who continues to smoke (31).

Other risk factors for lung cancer include prior lung cancer (32), prior head and neck cancer (33), gender (greater for males than for females) (34), ethnicity (higher incidence in African Americans than Caucasians), lower socioeconomic status, occupational exposure, family history, and obstructive lung disease (four- to fivefold increase in risk) (35,36). To date, most lung cancer CT screening trials have included current or former smokers over age 50. The other risk factors described above have not been used as entry criteria. Interestingly, one CT screening study included nonsmokers and reported a similar lung cancer detection rate in both smokers (0.4%) and nonsmokers (0.44%). However, nonsmokers had a higher incidence of bronchoalveolar cell

carcinoma and well-differentiated adenocarcinoma than smokers (90% vs. 48%) (12).

SCREENING WITH CHEST RADIOGRAPHY

Currently, there are no accepted screening tests for lung cancer. While chest radiographs sometimes are performed to screen for lung cancer (Figure 5-1), a reduction in lung cancer specific mortality has not been demonstrated, and there are no general recommendations to perform them for this purpose.

The first large-scale chest radiography screening trial was performed in London in the 1960s. In this trial, 55,034 men underwent either chest radiography every 6 months for 3 years or radiography at baseline and again 3 years later (37). By obtaining more frequent radiographs, more lung cancers were identified (132 vs. 96) and more lung cancers were resectable (44% vs. 29%). However, no reduction in lung cancer-specific mortality was demonstrated.

With improvements in technology and development of sputum cytology, the National Cancer Institute funded a Cooperative Early Lung Cancer Group, which comprised studies at Johns Hopkins University, Memorial Sloan–Kettering Medical Center, and the Mayo Clinic, to evaluate lung cancer screening with both chest radiography and sputum cytology. Over 30,000 people were enrolled; no reduction in lung cancer mortality was demonstrated (38–41). The Mayo Lung Project included the most extensive chest radiographic protocol of the three studies. Men older than 45 years of age with at least a one-pack-per-day history were placed randomly into either a screened group that underwent chest radiography and sputum cytology every 4 months for 6 years or a control group that received usual care, consisting of an annual chest radiograph and sputum cytology. More cancers were detected in the screened group (206 vs. 160); these cancers were frequently Stage I or Stage II (48% vs. 32%) and more often resectable (46% vs. 32%) than those detected in the control group. The 5-year survival rate was higher in the screened group (33% vs. 15%). However, no significant difference in lung cancer-specific mortality was found, even with extended followup (median 20.5 years) (38,41).

Lung cancer screening trials that include radiography have been under considerable scrutiny since their inception. Reviews of the Memorial Sloan–Kettering Lung Project, the Johns Hopkins Lung Project, the Mayo Lung Project (MLP), as well as a Czechoslovakia Study performed during the same period, have suggested that screening with chest radiographs may improve lung cancer cure rates, and that the studies were statistically underpowered to detect clinically significant reductions in lung cancer mortality in the 10% to 20% range (42–45). Some questions exist regarding the study design, particularly the lack of a true control for radiography. For example, in the Hopkins and Memorial Sloan–Kettering studies, both the screened and control groups underwent annual chest radiography. The Mayo Lung

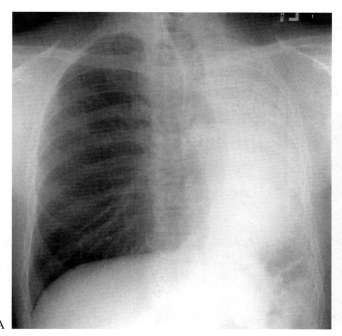

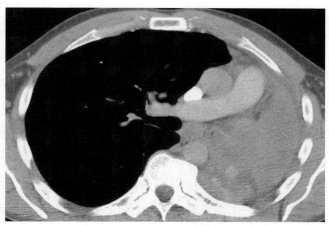

A   B

FIG. 5–1. Symptom-detected non-small cell lung cancer in 42-year-old man with a history of asthma and a 30-pack-year history of cigarette smoking. He was treated medically for bronchitis and pneumonia for 2 months, which failed to resolve despite several courses of antibiotics. He also has a nonproductive cough and night sweats, and recently developed dyspnea on exertion. A pneumonectomy was performed, documenting a T3, N1, M0 (Stage IIIA) poorly differentiated squamous cell carcinoma with vascular invasion. Maximum tumor diameter was 5.2 cm. **A:** Chest radiograph demonstrates complete collapse of the left lung. **B:** Computed tomography demonstrates complete collapse of the left lung with tumor occluding the left main bronchus and a heterogenously enhancing mass in the superior segment of the left lower lobe.

Project did not compare patients receiving radiography to those who did not. They compared patients receiving radiographs every 4 months to patients receiving usual care. Half of the control population underwent chest radiography. To date, it is still not clear that chest radiographs reduce lung cancer mortality. The answer may come in the next few years from the ongoing Prostate, Lung, Colorectal, and Ovarian Cancer Screening Trial (PLCO trial) sponsored by the National Cancer Institute (NCI). This trial is following 148,000 men and women for a minimum of 13 years, with annual chest radiographs in the screened group for 3 years and no radiographs in the control group (46). The large size of the PLCO trial, nearly five times the combined enrollment of the Cooperative Early Lung Cancer Group trials, is designed to detect at 10% or more reduction in lung cancer-specific mortality in the screened group versus the control group (47).

HELICAL CT TECHNIQUE FOR LUNG CANCER SCREENING

Computed tomography examinations in lung cancer screening trials began with single-detector CT scanners in Japanese screening trials, one of which was in a mobile van (9). The most recently reported screening trial from the Mayo Clinic included multidetector CT (MDCT) (10). Table 5–1 summarizes the scan acquisition, reconstruction, and viewing techniques used in the single-arm observation prospective cohort studies to date (7–13). The ongoing National Lung Screening Trial (NLST) of 50,000 subjects, randomized to either chest radiography or CT, uses MDCT scanners of 4 detector rows or greater. Detector collimation varies between 1.25 mm to 2.50 mm, with 1.25-mm to 2.00-mm reconstruction intervals. Scan acquisition times range from 13 seconds to 22 seconds, generating 200 to 320 axial reconstructed images per examination. Other parameters included 120 kVp, 50 milliamperes (mAs) to 160 mA, and mAs 20 to 80. The estimated CT dose index ranges from 2.6 mGy to 3.9 mGy. All examinations are interpreted soft copy on workstations.

Although CT protocols vary, particularly with the evolution of MDCT scanners with faster gantry rotation and additional detector rows, these screening trials share several elements. The examinations are performed in a single breath-hold to minimize respiratory motion and misregistration, and both lungs in their entirety are included in the scan range. Collimation has decreased with time, from 10 mm in initial trials to 5 mm in two of the most recent trials, and 2.5 mm or less in the NLST.

With the advances in CT technology, there has been

TABLE 5–1. *Low-dose helical CT techniques in screening trials*

Trial	Kaneko et al.	Sone et al.	Henschke et al.	Diederich et al.	Nawa et al.	Swensen et al.
Year published	1996	1998, 2001	1999	2002	2002	2003
Number of subjects	663	5483	1000	817	7986	1520
Scanner type	TCT-900S Superhelix; Toshiba	Mobile CT-W950SR; Hitachi Medical	HiSpeed Advantage; GE Medical	Tomoscan SR; Philips	Radix TURBO; Hitachi Medical	LightSpeed Qx/i; GE Medical
kvP	120	120	140	120	120	120
mA	50	50 (1996); 25 (1997–8)	40	NS	50	40
Gantry rotation speed	1 sec	2 sec	NS	NS	NS	0.8 sec
mAs	50	100 (1996); 50 (1997–8)	NS	50	NS	32
Collimation	10 mm	10 mm	10 mm	5 mm	10 mm	5 mm
Pitch	2	1	2	2	2	1.5
Table speed	20 mm/sec	10 mm/sec	NS	10 mm per rotation	NS	37.5 mm/sec
Scan range	30 cm; 2 cm above lung apex to diaphragm	Diaphragm to lung apex	Entire lungs	NS	Entire lungs	Sternal notch to iliac crests
Acquisition time	15 sec; single breath	30 sec; single breath	15–20 sec	15 sec; single breath	15 sec; single breath	Single breath
Reconstruction interval	10 mm	NS	5 mm	5 mm	1-mm interpolation	3.75 mm
Reconstruction algorithm	Lung	NS	Bone	NS	NS	NS
Average effective radiation dose	2.6 mGy	NS	NS	0.6 mSv men 1.1 mSv women	NS	0.65 mSv
Display method	Monitor and film	Monitor	Film; later monitor	Monitor and film	Monitor	Monitor
Display window width/level (H.U.)	2000/−700	1000/−700 1500/−550 & 300/20	1500/−650	1500/−600 & 400/40	1400/−700 & 400/60	Lung, soft tissue & bone

NS, not specified.

greater concern regarding radiation exposure, particularly with MDCT. All CT lung cancer screening trials use low-dose protocols, reducing the tube current compared to most diagnostic scanning. This keeps the radiation dose as low as possible without degrading image quality by introducing noise. The effective radiation dose in the earlier trials approximated 10 chest radiographs. In one of the more recent trials from Munster, Germany, radiation exposure was reported as 0.6 mSv in men and 1.1 mSv in women, equivalent to 3 and 5 two-view chest radiographs, respectively, and considerably lower than diagnostic thoracic CT (11). In the most recently reported Mayo Clinic Trial, the effective radiation dose was 0.65 mSv (10).

An important question to be answered is how low the minimum tube current can be to maintain good image quality. Several studies have reported that scanning with reduced tube current produces images of good diagnostic quality (48–51). In one study of 30 consecutive patients undergoing conventional CT using 400 mAs, four additional images were obtained at 20 mA, 80 mA, 140 mA, and 200 mA, at the level of the carina and the left atrium, and reviewed by

readers blinded to the mAs setting (50). Subjective image quality was maintained with mAs as low as 140 without reduction in underlying mediastinal or lung abnormalities, but degraded at 80 mAs and lower. Subject size in this study ranged from 75 pounds to 205 pounds (34 kg–93 kg), indicating that dose reductions can be accomplished using 140 mAs in average-weight adults for both lung and mediastinal window evaluation. The impact of lowering mAs on larger individuals is not known and may result in nondiagnostic examinations.

A recent study of 30 CT examinations of the lungs on seven healthy volunteers used tube currents ranging from 6 to 50 mAs, with computer-generated 6-mm nodules of ground-glass opacity (GGO) superimposed into the datasets (51). Readers, blinded to the mAs, subjectively judged the image quality obtained at 20 mAs and compared to images obtained at 50 mAs. Nodules were detectable, without any reduction in sensitivity, at mAs as low as 20 for the upper lobes, an area through which the shoulder girdles can produce image degradation. For the middle and lower lungs, sensitivity for nodule detection was maintained with mAs as low as 12 and 18, respectively. This study conducted in Nagoya, Japan, did not specify patient size. Large patient size may be a source of reduced image quality with low-dose techniques. Since the initial study, the same group of investigators has reported the feasibility of real-time tube-current modulation from 20 to 60 mAs during CT acquisition. This results in an equalization of image noise from lung apices to bases (52). Others have reported dose reductions of 20% to 40% with attenuation based on line modulation of tube current for body CT (53, 54). Since many subjects undergoing CT screening also will require serial CT examinations to follow any small indeterminate nodules, the cumulative radiation dose could be considerable. Keeping the dose as low as possible, following the ALARA principle, must be considered when determining scanning parameters (55).

The number of axial images reconstructed from lung CT screening depends on collimation and reconstruction intervals, with more recent protocols generating 200 to 300 images. With this large number of images, it is not feasible to interpret 15 to 20 images printed per 14 × 17'' sheets of film. Image size influences nodule detection. When images for lung-nodule detection are printed using six images to one sheet of 14 × 17'' film, readers are more sensitive than when progressively more images are printed per sheet of film (56). Most screening trials use computer workstations for image interpretation, and the results of the screening trials are therefore only applicable using that viewing method. Furthermore, workstation-based viewing increases reader sensitivity for nodule detection. In one study, in which simulated 3-mm to 5-mm nodules were introduced into 10-mm collimation lung CT datasets, there was significantly greater sensitivity for nodule detection with cine-based workstation viewing than with film interpretation (4,56).

HELICAL CT SCREENING TRIAL INCLUSION CRITERIA AND PATIENT POPULATIONS

Table 5–2 details the subject inclusion criteria in six published screening trials. Because individuals at greatest risk for cancer are older current and former smokers, most trials have targeted only this patient population. However, two trials had no smoking entry criteria. One of these studies demonstrated a similar cancer detection rate between smokers and nonsmokers; the other did not separate cancers by smoking history other than to identify all females between the age 55 and 64 with screening-detected lung cancer as

TABLE 5–2. *Helical CT screening study inclusion criteria and patient populations*

Trial	Kaneko et al.	Sone et al.	Henschke et al.	Diederich et al.	Nawa et al.	Swensen et al.
Year published	1996	1998, 2001	1999	2002	2002	2003
Number of subjects	1369	5483	1000	817	7986	1520
Inclusion criteria						
Age criterion (years)	38–83	≥40	≥60	≥40	50–69	≥50
Smoking criterion (pack per years)	>20	None	≥10	≥20	None	≥20
Other tests	Annual CXR & sputum cytology	Annual CXR & sputum cytology	Annual CXR	NS	NS	CT abdomen; blood for DNA analysis; spirometry
Study population						
Men : women	1232 (90%) : 137	2529 (46%) : 2954	540 (54%) : 460	588 (72%) : 229	6319 (79%) : 1637	785 : 735
Median age	60.4 (mean)	63 men; 64 women	67	53	NS; 76% age 50–59	59 (mean)
Median smoking history (pack—years)	NS; *median smoking index 960	NS	45	45	NS; 62% current or former smokers	45
Ethnicity	Location Japan; not otherwise specified	Location Nagano Prefecture, Japan; not otherwise specified	Location New York; 91% Caucasian; 5% African American; 2% Hispanic	Location Germany; not otherwise specified	Location Japan; not otherwise specified	Location Rochester, MN; not otherwise specified
Other	Anti-Lung Cancer Association (ACLA)	Telecommunications Advancement Organization of Japan	Early Lung Cancer Action Program (ELCAP) 14% asbestos exposure	2.4% asbestos esposure	Hitachi Employees Health Insurance Group (annual health examinations)	Mayo Clinic

* median smoking index = no. of cigarettes per day times number of years smoked.
NS, not specified.

nonsmokers (9,13). The risk of lung cancer from smoking increases with age. The German trial reported by Diederich et al. demonstrated a higher prevalence of screen-detected lung cancers with increasing age. In the entire screened population, the prevalence of lung cancer was 1.3% (11 out of 817) versus 2.1% (11 out of 519) for individuals older than 50 years of age, and 3.9% (8 out of 206) for individuals older than 60 years of age. Entry-criteria age ranges from 40 years to 60 years, with mean and median age of study populations ranging from 53 years to 67 years.

The Early Lung Cancer Action Program (ELCAP) has reported the highest cancer-detection rate to date among lung cancer screening trials using CT of 2.7%. Asbestos exposure was reported in 14% of these subjects, a known risk factor for lung cancer, particularly when combined with cigarette smoking (57). Ethnic differences in lung cancer risk also should be taken into account when reviewing the results of lung cancer screening trials. The largest reported number of CT-screened individuals has been from Japan, followed by the United States and Europe. Studies to date have not used other risk factors, such as family history or prior lung, head, or neck cancer, as inclusion criteria. While these individuals are at very high risk for developing lung cancer, studying this patient population concurrently would add confusion as to whether outcomes are related to new or preexisting cancers.

NODULES AND CANCERS FOUND IN HELICAL CT SCREENING TRIALS

Table 5–3 summarizes the prevalence data of published observational studies, while Table 5–4 summarizes the pub-

lished incidence-data results (9–13,15,58). The prevalence screens are the first annual screens performed, while incidence screens are those performed annually in subsequent years. The Anti-Lung Cancer Association (ALCA) member study reported by Kaneko et al. is not included here, as the data from 1975 to 1993 were based on a combination of chest radiography and sputum production, not CT (8).

Positive prevalence screens have been reported in up to 51% of screening trial participants (Figure 5-2). Among the United States screening trials, 23% of prevalence screens were positive in the New York ELCAP trial using single-detector CT at 10-mm collimation with 5-mm reconstruction intervals. A positive screen in the ELCAP trial was defined as the presence of 1 to 6 noncalcified pulmonary nodules. In the more recently published Mayo trial using MDCT at 5-mm collimation and 3.75-mm reconstruction intervals, 51% of prevalence screens were positive. In this trial, a positive screen included noncalcified nodules, and those above 6 per patient were not tracked. These differences in positive prevalence screens may be related to the CT technique, specifically the use of MDCT with thinner collimation and smaller reconstruction intervals. Additional explanations for the difference may include selection bias and patient-recruitment strategies, as well as differences in the definition of a positive test. Not only does the positive screen rate vary in lung cancer screening trials using CT, but the lung cancer detection rate also varies from as low as 0.4% in Japan and 0.44% in Germany to 1.7% in the Mayo trial, and a high of 2.7% in the ELCAP trial, a variation of nearly seven times. This also may be due to technical parameters influencing nodule detectability, as well as selection criteria for screening.

The majority of cancers detected with CT on prevalence

TABLE 5–3. *Helical CT screening trials: Baseline prevalence screen findings*

Trial	Sone et al.	Henschke et al.	Diederich et al.	Nawa et al.	Swensen et al.
Year published	1998, 2001	1999	2002	2002	2003
No. of subjects	5483	1000	817	7986	1520
No. of positive screens	279 (5%)	233 (23%)	350 (43%)	2099 (26%)	782 (51%)
No. patients with non-small-cell lung cancers	22	27	11	36	26**
No. non-small-cell lung cancers	23	31	12	37	27
No. non-small-cell lung cancers visible on radiography	9 (39%)	7 (23%)	NA	NA	NA
Cancer-detection rate	0.40%	2.7%	1.3%	0.44%	1.7%
Mean tumor size	15 mm	15 mm	25 mm	17 mm	17 mm
Cancer size					
1–5 mm	—	1 (4%)	0 (0%)	0 (0%)	1 (4%)
6–10 mm	6 (27%)*	14 (52%)	0 (0%)	6 (16%)	8 (30%)
11–20 mm	15 (68%)	8 (30%)	3 (27%)	24 (65%)	14 (52%)
>20	2 (9%)	4 (15%)	8 (73%)	7 (18%)	4 (15%)
Cancer stage					
IA	21 (91%)	22 (81%)	6 (54%)	28 (78%)	17 (63%)
IB	2 (9%)	1 (4%)	1 (9%)	3 (8%)	2 (7%)
II	0 (0%)	1 (4%)	2 (18%)	4 (11%)	4 (15%)
III	0 (0%)	3 (11%)	3 (27%)	1 (3%)	2 (7%)
IV	0 (0%)	0 (0%)	0 (0%)	0 (0%)	0 (0%)

* <10 mm, ** two additional small-cell carcinomas were detected.
NA, not applicable.

TABLE 5–4. *Helical CT screening trials: Incidence screen findings (subsequent annual screenings)*

Trial	Sone et al.		Henschke et al.	Nawa et al.	Swensen et al.	
Year Published	2001		2001	2002	2003	
Number of subjects	4425	3878	1000**	5568	1478	1438
	Year 1	Year 2			Year 1	Year 2
No. positive screens	173 (3.9%)	136 (3.5%)	30 (2.5%)	148 (2.7%)	207 (14%)	129 (9%)
No. patients with non-small-cell lung cancers	25	9	6	4	10	
No. non-small-cell lung cancers	27	10	6***	4	10***	
No. non-small-cell lung cancers visible on radiography	8 (30%) 5.4%	3 (30%) 2%	NA 0.5%	NA 0.07%	NA 0.3%	
Mean tumor size	12 mm	12 mm	10 mm	18 mm	16 mm	
Cancer size						
1–5 mm	—	—	3 (50%)	0 (0%)	2 (20%)	
6–10 mm	10 (36%)*	5 (55%)*	1 (17%)	0 (0%)	4 (40%)	
11–20 mm	17 (68%)	3 (33%)	2 (33%)	3 (75%)	3 (30)	
>20 mm	0 (0%)	1 (11%)	0 (0%)	1 (25%)	1 (10%)	
Cancer stage						
IA	24 (89%)	8 (80%)	5 (84%)	3 (75%)	5 (50%)	
IB	0 (0%)	1 (10%)	0 (0%)	1 (25%)	1 (10%)	
II	1 (4%)	0 (0%)	0 (0%)	0 (0%)	1 (10%)	
III	2 (7%)	0 (0%)	1 (17%)	0 (0%)	3 (30%)	
IV	0 (0%)	1 (10%)	0 (0%)	0 (0%)	1 (10%)	

* <10 mm, ** 1184 annual repeat screens performed in the 1000 subjects, *** an additional subject developed a new limited-stage small-cell carcinoma.
NA, not applicable.

screens are less than 2 cm in diameter, with tumors as small as 2 mm and as large as 5.5 cm detected. The majority is also Stage IA, ranging from 54% in the German trial to 63% in ELCAP and 81% in the Mayo trial. However, the overall staging ranged from Stage IA to Stage IV. Prevalence CT screens are more sensitive than chest radiography for the detection of these cancers, with radiography detecting only 23% to 39% of CT-detected cancers, reinforcing the greater sensitivity of CT. Although sensitivity increases with CT, specificity is reduced considerably owing to the large number of nonmalig-

nant nodules or false-positive lung cancers detected. For example, in the Mayo trial, 782 subjects had a positive test, of which only 25 subjects, or 1.7%, had lung cancer. In this trial, participants underwent baseline prevalence screening and two subsequent annual incidence screens. Over these three CT examinations, 69% of all subjects in the trial had at least one noncalcified nodule, totaling 2832 nodules.

Incidence screening results demonstrate a lower frequency of positive tests than prevalence screens, defined as new or growing nodules. Positive incidence tests range from

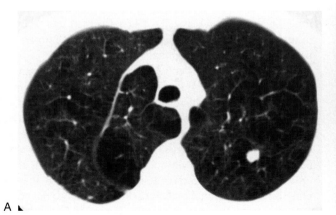
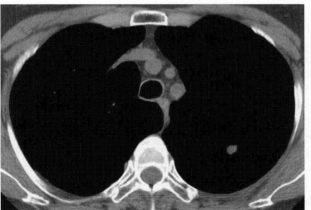

FIG. 5–2. Screen-detected bronchogenic carcinoma in a 66-year-old woman with long-standing chronic obstructive pulmonary disease and a 48-pack-year history of cigarette smoking. Pulmonary-function testing revealed a forced expiratory volume in 1 sec of 0.78 liters (43% of predicted). A 9-mm noncalcified nodule was identified on screening CT, as shown on **(A)** lung and **(B)** soft-tissue window settings, confirmed to be a T1, N0, M0 (Stage 1A) non-small cell lung cancer. Note the moderately severe underlying emphysema.

2.5% in ELCAP to 14% in the Mayo trial at the first incidence screen. The cancer-detection rate is also lower on incidence screens than prevalence screens, and less than 0.5% in several trials. Interval cancers represent those that develop between annual screenings and are detected symptomatically. Two incidence cancers were detected in ELCAP, including one Stage IIB squamous cell cancer that presented 5 months after screening, and one limited-stage small cell carcinoma that presented 6 months after screening. Two interval cancers also were reported in the Mayo trial, including one Stage IV non-small cell carcinoma, and a 20-mm limited-stage small cell carcinoma. These usually are aggressive, rapidly growing lung cancers with short volume-doubling times that present between annual screenings and may more likely lead to patient mortality in a shorter time frame.

The majority of lung cancers detected by CT screening (60%–80%) are adenocarcinomas, most of which are well differentiated, in contrast to clinically detected carcinomas, approximately 40% of which are adenocarcinomas (27). For example, in the ELCAP study, in which 27 cancers were detected, 18 (67%) were adenocarcinomas. In the study by Sone et al., in which 23 prevalence cancers were detected, 16 were described as adenocarcinoma (either bronchoalveolar cell carcinoma or well-differentiated adenocarcinoma) and 3 as moderately differentiated adenocarcinoma, representing 83% of screen-detected cancers. Of the 27 prevalence cancers in the Mayo trial, 17 (63%) were adenocarcinoma. This difference in cell type may be associated with a better clinical outcome and may artificially elevate survival statistics in observational trials without a control group for comparison.

NODULE TERMINOLOGY

Lung cancer screening with CT has created a new lexicon of terms for describing pulmonary nodules. Nodules should be described as solid, part solid, or nonsolid (Figure 5-3). Nonsolid nodules are ground glass in attenuation and previously were referred to as GGOs (ground glass opacities) or focal GGOs, while part-solid nodules are both solid and ground glass in attenuation. Early Lung Cancer Action Program investigators developed this terminology. Recognition of these elements within focal lung abnormalities is an important indicator of malignancy. For example, of 233 nodules in the ELCAP prevalence screen, 44 (19%) were either part solid ($n = 16$) or nonsolid ($n = 28$). The malignancy rate of these 44 nodules was 34% (15 out of 44), significantly higher than the 7% malignancy rate for solid nodules (59). The 63% (10 out of 16) malignancy rate for the part-solid nodules was higher than the 18% (5 out of 28) rate for the nonsolid nodules. These differences in morphology also are related to the underlying histology. Part-solid nodules were predominantly bronchoalveolar cell carcinoma or adenocarcinoma with bronchoalveolar cell carcinoma features, whereas solid nodules were predominantly other adenocarcinomas. In the ELCAP incidence screen, 7 of the first 30 positive screens were part-solid or nonsolid nodules.

MANAGING A POSITIVE CT SCREEN FOR LUNG CANCER

Computed tomography screening for lung cancer detects many lung nodules, the vast majority of which are benign (Figure 5-4). For nodules greater than 1 cm in diameter, biopsy and positron-emission-tomography (PET) scanning are useful for evaluation (60,61). Unfortunately, the majority of screen-detected nodules are less than 1 cm in diameter, presenting a diagnostic challenge. With improvements in PET technology over the last two decades, the sensitivity of 18-FDG (fluorodeoxyglucose) PET for malignancy in small nodules has improved. In a recent study of 192 malignancies, 0.5 cm to 3.0 cm in size (all T1), sensitivity of PET for malignancy was 95% (61). The 9 out of 192 (5%) false positives were 0.5 cm to 2.5 cm in size (mean 1.3 cm). They included four bronchoalveolar cell carcinomas, one adenocarcinoma, and one mixed large and nonsmall cell carcinoma, all Stage IA.

Many small nodules detected with CT screening are now being followed with serial CT scans to document stability in size over 2 years as evidence of nonmalignancy or nonprogressing malignancy (62). The recommendations used in the Mayo trial for the followup of screen-detected nodules advise that nodules less than 4 mm should undergo CT at 6-month intervals; nodules greater than 4 mm and less than 8 mm should undergo CT at 3-month intervals; and nodules 8 mm to 20 mm should undergo usual diagnostic testing for possible malignancy, which may include biopsy, PET-, or CT-nodule-enhancement studies. The initial phase of the ELCAP trial recommended CT at 3 months, 6 months, 12 months, and 24 months for nodules less than 5 mm; no growth at 2 years was classified as benign. For 6 mm to 10 mm nodules, evaluation may include biopsy (CT guided or thoracoscopy) or serial CT. Nodules 11 mm or larger were recommended for biopsy. Based on accumulated knowledge of the natural history of screening-detected nodules evaluated with serial CT, investigators have begun to increase the time interval at which repeat CT is performed. For example, in the NLST, subjects with nodules less than 4 mm are recommended to return to annual screening.

Recommendations for performing serial CT examinations with dedicated thin sections through the nodules is based on the natural history of lung cancer and tumor volume-doubling times. Lung cancers vary in biologic behavior, with doubling time ranging from 52 days to 1732 days in one study, mean 432 days (63). In another study, mean tumor doubling time was 181 days; 22% of cancers had doubling times greater than 465 days (64). For example, if the doubling time of a 4-mm diameter nodule is 60 days, the nodule will measure 5.7 mm at 3 months, 8 mm at 6 months, and 16.4 mm at 12 months. If the doubling time is 180 days, the nodule will measure 4.5 mm at 3 months, 5 mm at 6 months, and 6.4 mm at 12 months. If the doubling time is 240 days, the nodule measures only 4.4 mm at 3 months, 4.7 mm at 6 months, and 5.7 mm at 12 months (65). These small differ-

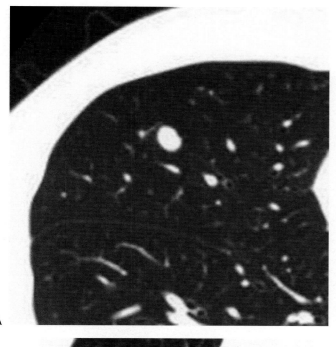

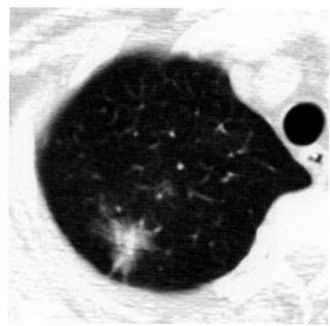

A

B

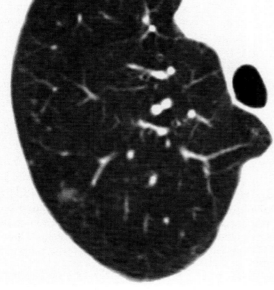

C

FIG. 5–3. Nodule characteristics. **A:** Solid nodule, **(B)** Part-solid with a central irregular solid component surrounded by GGO, **(C)** Nonsolid nodule (also known as a ground-glass nodule or focal ground-glass opacity).

ences in the diameter of small nodules with average doubling times reported for lung cancer are within the range of measurement error and interobserver reader error. The difficulty is compounded further by the small screen-detected cancers likely having longer doubling times than larger symptom-detected cancers. Nodules detected in nonsmokers participating in these trials have even longer doubling times, mean 813 days in one study (63). A 3-mm nodule with an 813 day doubling time would take 16 years to reach 15 mm. This not only creates difficulty in evaluating these small nodules on serial CT examinations, but also raises doubt as to the significance of such cancers to patient mortality.

High-resolution CT volumetric measurement of small pulmonary nodules has been developed to more accurately evaluate nodule growth in three dimensions and calculate nodule volume, allowing calculation of nodule doubling time between follow-up CT examinations as an indicator of the likelihood of malignancy (Figure 5-5) (66). Three-dimensional (3D) asymmetric changes in size and shape are measured more accurately with volumetric techniques than with traditional two-dimensional (2D) measurements.

MISSED LUNG CANCER ON CT SCREENING

Several investigators have reported their experience with missed lung cancers on screening CT examinations that

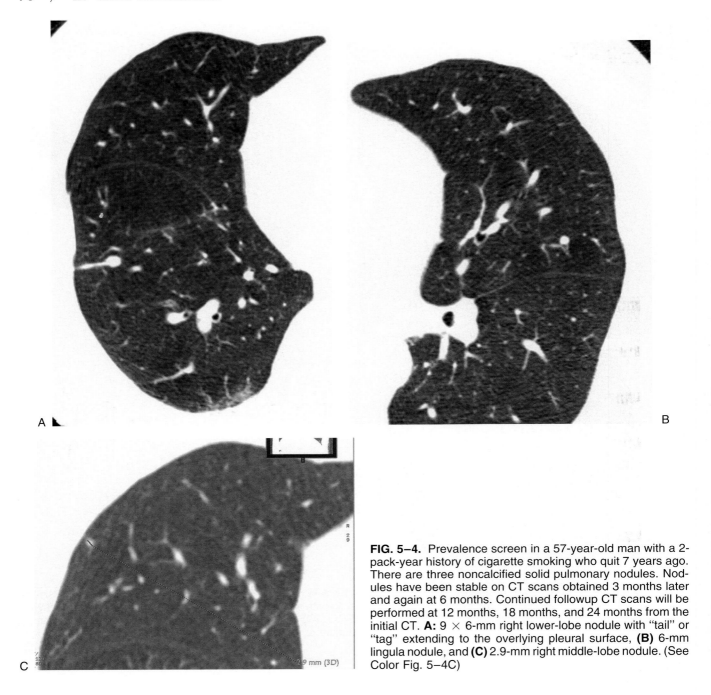

FIG. 5–4. Prevalence screen in a 57-year-old man with a 2-pack-year history of cigarette smoking who quit 7 years ago. There are three noncalcified solid pulmonary nodules. Nodules have been stable on CT scans obtained 3 months later and again at 6 months. Continued followup CT scans will be performed at 12 months, 18 months, and 24 months from the initial CT. **A:** 9 × 6-mm right lower-lobe nodule with "tail" or "tag" extending to the overlying pleural surface, **(B)** 6-mm lingula nodule, and **(C)** 2.9-mm right middle-lobe nodule. (See Color Fig. 5–4C)

are detected retrospectively (67,68). Knowledge of why these cancers were missed is important when reading screening CT examinations so that such pitfalls can be avoided when possible. Sone et al. evaluated missed cancers for an extended cohort undergoing cancer screening in which 83 total primary cancers were detected at combined prevalence and incidence screens; 32 of the cancers were visible in retrospect on a total of 39 CT screening examinations (67). They were all intrapulmonary cancers; none were endobronchial. The majority, 28 out of 32 (88%), was Stage IA. Errors were classified as detection errors in 62% (20) of cases, all of

which were adenocarcinomas, mean diameter 9.8 mm. Seventeen of these were well differentiated, and 11 (55%) occurred in nonsmoking women. Cancer-detection errors usually were due to overlap, obscuration, or similarity in appearance to normal structures. The remaining 12 errors were classified as interpretation errors. These cancers had a mean diameter of 15.9 mm, making them significantly larger than detection errors. Interpretation errors usually were due to findings that mimicked benign disease or occurred in subjects with underlying lung disease such as fibrosis, tuberculosis, or emphysema. In a report from the ALCA member

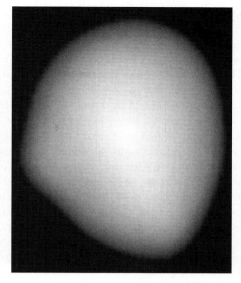

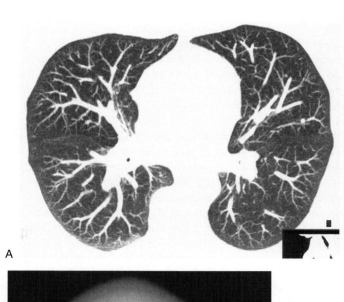

A

B

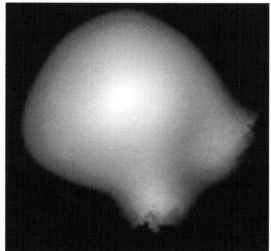

C

FIG. 5–5. Alternate imaging viewing methods. **A:** Sliding-slab maximum-intensity projection (MIP) image of the same nodule illustrated in Fig. 4**(B)**, in which the 1.25-mm images are stacked together to yield an image that shows the relationship of vessels to the nodule. These usually are viewed in cine-mode or scrolling-mode on a computer workstation, and may enhance the conspicuity of small nodules. **B,C:** Volumetric CT of the same nodule volume in the **(B)** anterior and **(C)** inferior projections. The Advance Lung Analysis software package displays nodule dimensions as $7.1 \times 5.6 \times 6.6$ mm, and calculates nodule volume as 67 mm^3. Serial measurements of nodule volume can be used to calculate tumor doubling time. By viewing the nodule in three dimensions, variations in shape may be appreciated that are not shown on two-dimensional images alone. (See Color Fig. 5–5)

cohort, seven lung cancers were visible in retrospect on prior CT (68). This included four detection errors; two subjects with minute faint nodules, and two subjects with nodules adjacent to vessels. Interpretation errors occurred in three subjects; two subjects with tuberculosis and one subject with a faint nodule that had high attenuation centrally.

Computer-aided diagnosis (CAD) applied to lung CT may be able to assist radiologists interpreting CT-screening examinations by serving as a second reader to identify candidate nodules for approval or rejection by the reader, similar to the way CAD is used for mammography in breast cancer screening. The potential value of this method is to reduce false negatives. Armato et al. applied automated lung nodule detection to a database of 38 low-dose lung cancer screening CT scans containing 50 nodules, 38 of which were biopsy-proven lung cancers not detected on initial screening CT. Results were very promising, with 84% of missed cancers detected with computer-assisted nodule detection (69). Automated lung-nodule detection has improved rapidly in the last 5 years, with a recent study demonstrating 100% sensitivity for the detection of nodules greater than 3 mm in diameter and 70% sensitivity for nodules less than 3 mm (70). The radiologist's sensitivity for the same nodules was 91% and 51%, respectively, improving to 95% and 74% with assistance from the automated system.

Computer-aided diagnosis may be used to provide automatic characterization of nodules, including nodule volume, shape, and attenuation characteristics. To facilitate followup with serial CT examinations, computer techniques have been developed to use a patient's baseline CT data to assist with image segmentation and registration, allowing changes in size and shape to be measured automatically (71).

FUTURE DIRECTIONS IN LUNG CANCER SCREENING

As stated earlier, lung cancer screening with CT rests on the premise that the detection of small nodules is sufficient to detect tumors before regional spread and distant metastases. However, size may prove to be unimportant. It is known that malignant cells may be found in normal-sized lymph nodes or in distant organs of patients with small lung cancers (72,73). Furthermore, lung cancer cells may be found in the peripheral blood and bone marrow of lung cancer patients of all stages, including individuals otherwise considered surgically resectable (74–76). Biomolecular and genetic markers for lung cancer, applied to blood, urine, or sputum samples ultimately may prove more accurate markers of lung cancer than anatomic imaging with CT, or may be used in conjunction with CT to identify ways to increase the specificity of CT screening alone (77,78). Several oncogenes for lung cancer have been identified that may be abnormal before other existing screening tests (78–82). Participants in the NLST give blood, urine, and sputum samples that are stored at a tissue bank to permit analysis for biomarkers in the future.

EXISTING SCREENING GUIDELINES FOR LUNG CANCER

To date, no public policy-setting body recommends lung cancer screening CT for subjects outside of clinical trials. A consensus statement by the Society of Thoracic Radiology states that ''mass screening for lung cancer with CT is not currently advocated'' and that ''suitable subjects who wish to participate should be encouraged to do so in controlled trials, so that the value of CT screening can be ascertained as soon as possible'' (83). Similarly, a publication by Bach et al. from the Health Outcomes Research Group graded the available guidelines related to screening and early detection of lung cancer, stating that, while early data are promising, ''we recommend that individuals should only be screened with LDCT (low dose CT) in the context of well-designed clinical trials'' (84). Furthermore, an update of American Cancer Society guidelines states that ''given the high rate of positive results that occur with CT screening for lung cancer and the complexity of algorithms for working up small nodules, there is reason to be concerned about broad dissemination of lung screening outside of experienced, multispecialty settings and prior to validation of these new technology,'' and that ''individuals interested in early detection should be encouraged to participate in trials'' (85).

TEN CRITERIA FOR LUNG CANCER SCREENING WITH CT

A recent perspective by Obuchowski et al. concisely describes ten criteria for effective lung cancer screening, summarized and adapted here for lung cancer screening with CT (86).

1. *Lung cancer has serious consequences:* Yes. Lung cancer is the leading cause of cancer death in the United States, with an overall 5-year survival rate of less than 15%.

2. *The population available for lung cancer screening has high prevalence of detectable preclinical phase:* Yes. The preclinical phase is the time from lung cancer onset to the first time that signs and symptoms of lung cancer manifest, such as a change in cough or hemoptysis, and ends when a patient seeks medical attention. Evidence from the observational CT screening trials confirms a high preclinical prevalence in an at-risk population that consists of older individuals, both current and former smokers, with a greater than 10-to-20-pack-year history of smoking. The age at which screening should begin is unclear, with some studies including individuals greater than or equal to 40, 50, 55, or 60 years of age.

3. *Screening CT for lung cancer detects little pseudodisease:* Controversial. Pseudodisease is defined as lung cancer that would never have manifested during an individual's lifespan, including nonprogressive and very slowly progressing cancers. If too much pseudodisease is detected with screening CT, cost effectiveness will be impacted negatively, even if a reduction in lung cancer-specific mortality is found. Pseudodisease in lung cancer may be uncommon, as untreated Stage I cancer results in death within 5 years to 10 years in 80% to 100% of patients (87,88). Alternatively, there is evidence that many lung cancers may be indolent and, in fact, pseudodisease based on autopsy studies and CT screening in nonsmokers (89,90). In one series, one sixth of autopsy-identified lung cancers were unrecognized before death and unrelated to death (89). Current CT techniques also may be more sensitive to detecting small cancers than sectioning of lungs at autopsy (90). Nonsmokers in one trial had a lung cancer detection rate equal to smokers, yet the majority of clinically diagnosed lung cancer that progresses and causes death occurs in smokers, suggesting that cancers detected in nonsmokers may be pseudodisease (12).

4. *Computed tomography lung screening has a high accuracy for detecting detectable preclinical disease:* Yes and no. Accuracy is a combination of sensitivity and specificity. While an ideal screening test would have sensitivity and specificity greater than 95%, in practice, most cancer screening tests have a high sensitivity and low specificity, resulting in a high rate of false-positive test results due to the low pretest prevalence of disease. The prevalence of lung cancer in populations targeted for lung cancer screening with CT is low, less than 5%. The high rate of false-positive CT results (up to 51%) markedly reduces specificity, as well as cost effectiveness. Computed tomography screening trials have demonstrated few interval or potentially missed cancers, confirming that sensitivity is high and potentially contributing to pseudodisease.

5. *Computed tomography lung screening detects disease before the critical point:* The critical point is that time

in the natural history of lung cancer before which therapy is more effective and after which it is less effective. A lung cancer that has metastases is already beyond the critical point. If the critical point occurs before the detectable preclinical phase, then the cancer is already beyond the critical point when it is first detectable by the screening test. The fact that most CT screen-detected cancers are Stage IA is favorable. However, if small size within all T1 tumors is not indicative of better survival or tumor stage, as suggested by two recent studies, then detection of even small nodules may be after the critical point (5,6).

6. *Computed tomography lung screening causes little morbidity:* Yes and no. Other than radiation exposure, which can be reduced to that of three to five chest radiographs, there is little risk from the screening CT examination itself. No intravenous contrast is used. If complications of tests performed in the evaluation of indeterminate pulmonary nodules are included in this determination, such as percutaneous, bronchoscopic, or surgical biopsy, then there may be considerable morbidity associated with screening. Serial diagnostic CT examinations using standard mAs to evaluate nodules found on screening CT add the burden of radiation exposure, which itself may be carcinogenic.

7. *Computed tomography lung screening is affordable and available:* Uncertain. The cost of CT lung screening depends on many variables, such as patient throughput on the CT scanner, the cost of additional tests required as a result of the screening CT examination, the frequency with which the screening test is performed (once a year, every 2 years; starting at a younger age versus an older age), and indirect variables such as lost work days because of anxiety or in order to have additional testing. In one observational lung cancer screening trial using CT, the total time spent by the patient in the CT room was only 3 minutes (13). While the single-detector CT scanners used in earlier screening trials are widely available in the United States today, faster MDCT scanners have been available only since 1998, and the recent 16-detector row scanners have been available for approximately 1 year; both, particularly the latter, have a lower installed base and are more expensive. By comparison, stool guaiac testing for colon cancer is much less expensive that lung cancer screening CT, whereas colonoscopy is more expensive. The NLST is tracking closely medical-resource use and impact of screening on quality of life in order to obtain more information on these factors.

8. *Treatment exists for lung cancer:* Yes. In the case of lung cancer, surgical resection of lower-stage cancers is the therapy of choice. Screening is aimed at detecting disease for which there is available treatment; otherwise there is nothing that can be done after the disease is found.

9. *Treatment for lung cancer is more effective when ap-*

plied before symptoms begin: Probably. Early stage cancers have better prognosis than symptom-detected cancers, and, in general, there are fewer symptoms with early stage cancers than with advanced-stage cancers. Treatment for screen-detected lung cancers needs to be initiated during the preclinical detectable phase.

10. *Treatment for lung cancer is not too risky or toxic:* Uncertain. The risk or toxicity of treatment should be less than that of the lung cancer itself. The same treatment for a patient with a true cancer may be unacceptable for the treatment of pseudodisease. If there is a high rate of pseudodisease, the risks may outweigh the benefits. In the case of lung cancer, complications of lung biopsy, such as pneumothorax and hemoptysis, complications of radiation and chemotherapy, and excess cancers due to radiation exposure from serial CT examinations also should be considered as risks or toxicity related to lung cancer screening with CT.

SUMMARY

Rapid advances in CT technology, combined with its widespread availability, have led to tremendous optimism regarding the ability of CT to detect lung cancer early in hopes of decreasing lung cancer mortality. Recently, prospective cohort studies of patients screened with CT for lung cancer have documented the ability of CT to detect early stage lung cancer. To date, no group of investigators has demonstrated reduced lung cancer mortality in a large screening population compared to a nonscreened group of control subjects. The use of CT for lung cancer screening remains controversial, and it will require careful study and time to understand whether it is beneficial. The NLST, an expensive and lengthy randomized controlled trial of 50,000 subjects funded by the NCI, is currently underway to determine whether CT screening reduces lung cancer specific mortality versus chest radiography. This endpoint should provide substantial evidence to either support or refute the use of CT for lung cancer screening.

What we do know is that CT screening detects many small nodules, thereby converting asymptomatic individuals into "patients" requiring further diagnostic evaluations, such as followup CT, PET scanning, biopsy, and even resection. There may be a negative psychologic impact on otherwise healthy people who now have an "abnormality" on their lungs that is too small to biopsy, too small for PET, and is very likely benign. Only a very few nodules (1% to 2%) detected with CT screening are malignant, and these are most commonly Stage I adenocarcinomas. Computed tomography screening involves radiation exposure and, if a small nodule is found and requires serial CT follow up, results in repeated radiation exposure.

What is not known is who to screen (At what age to begin? Is there a history of smoking? Is there a family history?) or how often to screen (Annually? Every 2 years?).

The optimal CT protocol for maximizing the sensitivity for cancer detection with as low a radiation dose as possible is not yet known. It is not known if lung cancer screening with CT reduces lung cancer specific mortality.

Ultimately, lung cancer screening with CT may prove to reduce lung cancer-specific mortality and become adopted widely, similar to mammography for breast cancer. There is insufficient information to make that determination at this time. Individuals interested in obtaining lung cancer screening do so within the context of well-designed clinical trials. Anyone choosing to seek lung cancer screening with CT outside of such trials should be counseled about the potential risks and benefits of obtaining a CT examination for this yet unproven indication.

REFERENCES

1. Naidich DP, Rusinek H, McGuinness G, et al. Variables affecting pulmonary nodule detection with computed tomography: evaluation with three-dimensional computer simulation. *J Thorac Imaging* 1993; 8:291–299.
2. Remy-Jardin M, Remy J, Giraud F, et al. Pulmonary nodules: detection with thick-section spiral CT versus conventional CT. *Radiology* 1993; 187:513–520.
3. Costello P, Anderson W, Blume D. Pulmonary nodule: evaluation with spiral volumetric CT. *Radiology* 1991;179:875–876.
4. Seltzer SE, Judy PF, Adams DF, et al. Spiral CT of the chest: comparison of cine and film-based viewing. *Radiology* 1995;197:73–78.
5. Patz EF Jr, Rossi S, Harpole DH Jr, et al. Correlation of tumor size and survival in patients with stage IA non-small cell lung cancer.[comment]. *Chest* 2000;117:1568–1571.
6. Heyneman LE, Herndon JE, Goodman PC, et al. Stage distribution in patients with a small (< or = 3 cm) primary nonsmall cell lung carcinoma. Implication for lung carcinoma screening. *Cancer* 2001; 92:3051–3055.
7. Henschke CI, McCauley DI, Yankelevitz DF, et al. Early lung cancer action project: overall design and findings from baseline screening [see comments]. *Lancet* 1999;354:99–105.
8. Kaneko M, Eguchi K, Ohmatsu H, et al. Peripheral lung cancer: screening and detection with low-dose spiral CT versus radiography. *Radiology* 1996;201:798–802.
9. Sone S, Takashima S, Li F, et al. Mass screening for lung cancer with mobile spiral computed tomography scanner [see comments]. *Lancet* 1998;351:1242–1245.
10. Swensen SJ, Jett JR, Hartman TE, et al. Lung cancer screening with CT: Mayo Clinic experience. *Radiology* 2003;226:756–761.
11. Diederich S, Wormanns D, Semik M, et al. Screening for early lung cancer with low-dose spiral CT: prevalence in 817 asymptomatic smokers. *Radiology* 2002;222:773–781.
12. Sone S, Li F, Yang CF, et al. Results of three-year mass screening programme for lung cancer using mobile low-dose spiral computed tomography scanner. *Br J Cancer* 2001;84:25–32.
13. Nawa T, Nakagawa T, Kusano S, et al. Lung cancer screening using low-dose spiral CT*: results of baseline and 1-year follow-up studies. *Chest* 2002;122:15–20.
14. Bach PB, Kelley MJ, Tate RC, et al. Screening for lung cancer: a review of the current literature. *Chest* 2003;123:72S–82S.
15. Henschke CI, McCauley DI, Yankelevitz DF, et al. Early lung cancer action project: a summary of the findings on baseline screening. *Oncologist* 2001;6:147–152.
16. Casarella WJ. A patient's viewpoint on a current controversy. *Radiology* 2002;224:927.
17. Handy JR Jr, Asaph JW, Skokan L, et al. What happens to patients undergoing lung cancer surgery? Outcomes and quality of life before and after surgery [comment]. *Chest* 2002;122:21–30.
18. Mahadevia PJ, Fleisher LA, Frick KD, et al. Lung cancer screening with helical computed tomography in older adult smokers: a decision and cost-effectiveness analysis. *JAMA* 2003;289:313–322.
19. Chirikos TN, Hazelton T, Tockman M, et al. Screening for lung cancer sith CT*: a preliminary cost-effectiveness analysis. *Chest* 2002; 121:1507–1514.
20. Black W, Welch H. Screening for disease. *AJR Am J Roentgenol* 1997; 168:3–11.
21. American Cancer Society. *Cancer facts and figure*. Atlanta: American Cancer Society. 2000.
22. Fry WA, Menck HR, Winchester DP. The national cancer data base report on lung cancer. *Cancer* 1947;77:1947–1955.
23. Mountain CF. Revisions in the international system for staging lung cancer [see comments]. *Chest* 1997;111:1710–1717.
24. Anonymous. Chemotherapy in non-small cell lung cancer: a meta-analysis using updated data on individual patients from 52 randomised clinical trials. Non-small cell lung cancer collaborative group [see comments]. *BMJ* 1995;311:899–909.
25. Doll R. *Tobacco: an overview of health effects*. Lyon, France: IARC Scientific Publications, 1986;11–22.
26. Shopland DR, Eyre HJ, Pechacek TF. Smoking-attributable cancer mortality in 1991: is lung cancer now the leading cause of death among smokers in the United States? [see comments]. *J Natl Cancer Inst* 1991; 83:1142–1148.
27. Swensen SJ. CT screening for lung cancer.[comment]. *AJR Am J Roentgen* 2002;179:833–836.
28. Rogot E, Murray JL. Smoking and causes of death among U.S. veterans: 16 years of observation. *Public Health Rep* 1980;95:213–222.
29. Mattson ME, Pollack ES, Cullen JW. What are the odds that smoking will kill you?[erratum appears in *Am J Public Health* 1987;77(7):818]. *Am J Public Health* 1987;77:425–431.
30. Peto J, Doll R. Passive smoking. *Br J Cancer* 1986;54:381–383.
31. Bach PB, Kattan MW, Thornquist MD, et al. Variations in lung cancer risk among smokers. *J Natl Cancer Inst* 2003;95:470–478.
32. Martini N, Bains MS, Burt ME, et al. Incidence of local recurrence and second primary tumors in resected stage I lung cancer. *J Thorac Cardiovasc Surg* 1995;109:120–129.
33. Jones AS, Morar P, Phillips DE, et al.. Second primary tumors in patients with head and neck squamous cell carcinoma [comment]. *Cancer* 1995;75:1343–1353.
34. Zang EA, Wynder EL. Differences in lung cancer risk between men and women: examination of the evidence [comment]. *J Natl Cancer Inst* 1996;88:183–192.
35. Kishi K, Gurney JW, Schroeder DR, et al. The correlation of emphysema or airway obstruction with the risk of lung cancer: a matched case-controlled study. *Eur Respir J* 1093;19:1093–1098.
36. Nomura A, Stemmermann GN, Chyou PH, et al. Prospective study of pulmonary function and lung cancer. *Am Rev Respir Dis* 1991; 144:307–311.
37. Brett GZ. The value of lung cancer detection by six-monthly chest radiographs. *Thorax* 1968;23:414–420.
38. Fontana RS, Sanderson DR, Taylor WF, et al. Early lung cancer detection: results of the initial (prevalence) radiologic and cytologic screening in the Mayo Clinic study. *Am Rev Respir Dis* 1984;130:561–565.
39. Flehinger BJ, Melamed MR, Zaman MB, et al. Early lung cancer detection: results of the initial (prevalence) radiologic and cytologic screening in the Memorial Sloan–Kettering study. *Am Rev Respir Dis* 1984; 130:555–560.
40. Frost JK, Ball WC Jr, Levin ML, et al. Early lung cancer detection: results of the initial (prevalence) radiologic and cytologic screening in the Johns Hopkins study. *Am Rev Respir Dis* 1984;130:549–554.
41. Marcus PM, Bergstralh EJ, Fagerstrom RM, et al. Lung cancer mortality in the Mayo lung project: impact of extended follow-up. *J Natl Cancer Inst Cancer Spectrum* 2000;92:1308–1316.
42. Strauss GM. Screening for lung cancer: an evidence-based synthesis. *Surg Oncol Clin N Am* 1999;8:747–774, viii.
43. Flehinger BJ, Kimmel M, Polyak T, et al. Screening for lung cancer. The Mayo lung project revisited. *Cancer* 1993;72:1573–1580.
44. Fontana RS, Sanderson DR, Woolner LB, et al. Screening for lung cancer. A critique of the Mayo lung project. *Cancer* 1991; 67:1155–1164.
45. Kubik A, Polak J. Lung cancer detection. Results of a randomized prospective study in Czechoslovakia. *Cancer* 1986;57:2427–2437.
46. Prorok PC, Andriole GL, Bresalier RS, et al. Design of the prostate, lung, colorectal and ovarian (PLCO) cancer screening trial. *Control Clin Trials* 2000;21:2735–3095.
47. Kramer BS, Gohagan J, Prorok PC, et al. A National Cancer Institute

sponsored screening trial for prostatic, lung, colorectal, and ovarian cancers. *Cancer* 1993;71:589–593.

48. Naidich D, Marshall C, Gribbin C, et al. Low-dose CT of the lungs: preliminary observations. *Radiology* 1990;175:729–601.

49. Zwirewich CV, Mayo JR, Muller NL. Low-dose high-resolution CT of lung parenchyma. *Radiology* 1991;180:413–417.

50. Mayo JR, Hartman TE, Lee KS, et al. CT of the chest: minimal tube current required for good image quality with the least radiation dose. *AJR Am J Roentgenol* 1995;164:603–607.

51. Itoh S, Ikeda M, Arahata S, et al. Lung cancer screening: minimum tube current required for helical CT. *Radiology* 2000;215:175–183.

52. Itoh S, Ikeda M, Mori Y, et al. Lung: feasibility of a method for changing tube current during low-dose helical CT. *Radiology* 2002; 224:905–601.

53. Kalender WA, Wolf H, Suess C, et al. Dose reduction in CT by on-line tube current control: principles and validation on phantoms and cadavers. *Eur Radiol* 1999;9:323–328.

54. Greess H, Nomayr A, Wolf H, et al. Dose reduction in CT examination of children by an attenuation-based on-line modulation of tube current (CARE Dose). *Eur Radiol* 2002;12:1571–1576.

55. Cascade PN, Webster EW, Kazerooni EA. Ineffective use of radiology: the hidden cost. *AJR Am J Roentgenol* 1998;170:561–564.

56. Seltzer SE, Judy PF, Feldman U, et al. Influence of CT image size and format on accuracy of lung nodule detection. *Radiology* 1998; 206:617–622.

57. Omenn GS, Merchant J, Boatman E, et al. Contribution of environmental fibers to respiratory cancer. *Environ Health Perspect* 1986; 70:51–56.

58. Henschke CI, Naidich DP, Yankelevitz DF, et al. Early lung cancer action project: initial findings on repeat screenings. *Cancer* 2001; 92:153–159.

59. Henschke CI, Yankelevitz DF, Mirtcheva R, et al. CT Screening for lung cancer: frequency and significance of part-solid and nonsolid nodules. *AJR Am J Roentgenol* 2002;178:1053–1057.

60. Shaffer K. Role of radiology for imaging and biopsy of solitary pulmonary nodules. *Chest* 1999;116:519S–522S.

61. Marom EM, Sarvis S, Herndon JE 2nd, et al. T1 lung cancers: sensitivity of diagnosis with fluorodeoxyglucose PET. *Radiology* 2002; 223:453–459.

62. Yankelevitz DF, Henschke CI. Does 2-year stability imply that pulmonary nodules are benign? *AJR Am J Roentgenol* 1997;168:325–328.

63. Hasegawa M, Sone S, Takashima S, et al. Growth rate of small lung cancers detected on mass CT screening. *Br J Radiol* 2000; 73:1252–1259.

64. Winer-Muram HT, Jennings SG, Tarver RD, et al. Volumetric growth rate of stage I lung cancer prior to treatment: serial CT scanning. *Radiology* 2002;223:798–805.

65. Aberle DR. Personal communication. 2003.

66. Yankelevitz DF, Reeves AP, Kostis WJ, et al. Small pulmonary nodules: volumetrically determined growth rates based on CT evaluation. *Radiology* 2000;217:251–256.

67. Li F, Sone S, Abe H, et al. Lung cancers missed at low-dose helical CT screening in a general population: comparison of clinical, histopathologic, and imaging findings. *Radiology* 2002;225:673–683.

68. Kakinuma R, Ohmatsu H, Kaneko M, et al. Detection failures in spiral CT screening for lung cancer: analysis of CT findings. *Radiology* 1999; 212:61–66.

69. Armato SG III, Li F, Giger ML, et al. Lung cancer: performance of automated lung nodule detection applied to cancers missed in a CT screening program. *Radiology* 2002;225:685–683.

70. Brown MS, Goldin JG, Suh RD, et al. Lung micronodules: automated method for detection at thin-section CT—initial experience. *Radiology* 2003;226:256–262.

71. Brown MS, McNitt-Gray MF, Goldin JG, et al. Patient-specific models for lung nodule detection and surveillance in CT images. *IEEE Trans Med Imaging* 2001;20:1242–1250.

72. Chen ZL, Perez S, Holmes EC, et al. Frequency and distribution of occult micrometastases in lymph nodes of patients with non-small cell lung carcinoma. *J Natl Cancer Inst* 1993;85:493–498.

73. Izbicki JR, Passlick B, Hosch SB, et al. Mode of spread in the early phase of lymphatic metastasis in non-small cell lung cancer: significance of nodal micrometastasis. *J Thorac Cardiovasc Surg* 1996; 112:623–630.

74. Cote RJ, Beattie EJ, Chaiwun B, et al. Detection of occult bone marrow micrometastases in patients with operable lung carcinoma. *Ann Surg* 1995;222:415–423; 423–415 (discussion).

75. Peck K, Sher YP, Shih JY, et al. Detection and quantitation of circulating cancer cells in the peripheral blood of lung cancer patients. *Cancer Res* 1998;58:2761–2765.

76. Pantel K, Izbicki J, Passlick B, et al. Frequency and prognostic significance of isolated tumour cells in bone marrow of patients with non-small cell lung cancer without overt metastases. *Lancet* 1996; 347:649–653.

77. Toyooka S, Fukuyama Y, Wistuba II, et al. Differential expression of FEZ1/LZTS1 gene in lung cancers and their cell cultures. *Clin Cancer Res* 2002;8:2292–2297.

78. Tockman MS, Mulshine JL, Piantadosi S, et al. Prospective detection of preclinical lung cancer: results from two studies of heterogeneous nuclear ribonucleoprotein A2/B1 overexpression [comment]. *Clin Cancer Res* 1997;3:2237–2246.

79. Mao L, Hruban RH, Boyle JO, et al. Detection of oncogene mutations in sputum precedes diagnosis of lung cancer. *Cancer Res* 1994; 54:1634–1637.

80. Chen G, Gharib TG, Huang CC, et al. Proteomic analysis of lung adenocarcinoma: identification of a highly expressed set of proteins in tumors. *Clin Cancer Res* 2002;8:2298–2305.

81. Beer DG, Kardia SL, Huang CC, et al. Gene-expression profiles predict survival of patients with lung adenocarcinoma. *Nat Med* 2002; 8:816–824.

82. Giordano TJ, Shedden KA, Schwartz DR, et al. Organ-specific molecular classification of primary lung, colon, and ovarian adenocarcinomas using gene expression profiles. *Am J Pathol* 2001;159:1231–1238.

83. Aberle DR, Gamsu G, Henschke CI, et al. A consensus statement of the Society of Thoracic Radiology: screening for lung cancer with helical computed tomography. *J Thorac Imaging* 2001;16:65–68.

84. Bach PB, Niewoehner DE, Black WC, American College of Chest Phys. Screening for lung cancer: the guidelines. *Chest* 2003; 123:835–885.

85. Smith RA, von Eschenbach AC, Wender R, et al. American Cancer Society guidelines for the early detection of cancer: update of early detection guidelines for prostate, colorectal, and endometrial cancers. Also: update 2001—testing for early lung cancer detection.[erratum appears in *CA Cancer J Clin* 2001;51(3)(May–June):150]. *CA Cancer J Clin* 2001;51:38–75, quiz 77–80.

86. Obuchowski NA, Graham RJ, Baker ME, et al. Ten criteria for effective screening: their application to multislice CT screening for pulmonary and colorectal cancers [comment]. *AJR Am J Roentgenol* 2001; 176:1357–1362.

87. Sobue T, Suzuki T, Matsuda M, et al. Survival for clinical stage I lung cancer not surgically treated. Comparison between screen-detected and symptom-detected cases. The Japanese lung cancer screening research group. *Cancer* 1992;69:685–692.

88. Flehinger BJ, Kimmel M, Melamed MR. The effect of surgical treatment on survival from early lung cancer. Implications for screening. *Chest* 1992;101:1013–1018.

89. Chan CK, Wells CK, McFarlane MJ, et al. More lung cancer but better survival. Implications of secular trends in ''necropsy surprise'' rates. *Chest* 1989;96:291–296.

90. Dammas S, Patz EF Jr, Goodman PC. Identification of small lung nodules at autopsy: implications for lung cancer screening and overdiagnosis bias [comment]. *Lung Cancer* 2001;33:11–16.

CHAPTER 6

Spiral CT of Venous Thromboembolism

Ann N. Leung

INTRODUCTION

Venous thromboembolism is a complex vascular disease that affects approximately one in 1000 persons yearly in North America and Europe (1). Of its two most common clinical manifestations, deep venous thrombosis (DVT) is the more common, whereas pulmonary embolism (PE) is the more serious. Pulmonary embolism occurs in 30% to 60% of patients with DVT, with more than 90% of emboli believed to originate from a lower extremity source (1,2).

The clinical presentations of PE can be categorized broadly into three groups. The first and most common presentation is dyspnea, with or without associated chest pain and hemoptysis; the second presentation consists of hemodynamic instability and syncope, usually related to massive embolism; and the last and least-common presentation mimics indolent pneumonia or heart failure (1). However, because the majority of patients present with nonspecific signs and symptoms, clinical diagnosis is notoriously unreliable. As with DVT, when PE is suspected clinically, only one in four patients will prove to have the condition (3). Appropriate patient management requires the performance of additional tests that can confirm or exclude the diagnosis.

CT PULMONARY ANGIOGRAPHY

In 1992, Remy-Jardin and colleagues (4) proposed that spiral computed tomography (CT) pulmonary angiography (CTPA) could be used as a fast and relatively noninvasive technique to detect pulmonary emboli. In their seminal study, CTPA was found to have a sensitivity of 100% and a specificity of 96% for emboli lodged in main, lobar, and segmental pulmonary arteries (4). However, the inability to assess adequately subsegmental pulmonary arteries was recognized as a potential limitation to the accuracy of the technique (5,6) (Figure 6-1).

Over the ensuing decade, advances in spiral CT technology, including X-ray tubes with higher heat capacity,

faster gantry rotation periods, and multidetector row scanners, have allowed for significant refinements in CTPA protocols. With the overall increase in speed of image acquisition, volumetric thin-section (1.0 mm–2.0 mm) imaging of the pulmonary arterial system now can be performed within a tolerable breath-hold period; the resultant decrease in volume-averaging effects has been reported to improve both visualization of subsegmental pulmonary arteries (7,8) (Figure 6-2) and detection of peripheral emboli (9) (Figure 6-3).

SCANNING TECHNIQUE

The specific CTPA protocol that is performed should be tailored to the type of spiral scanner used. The minimum requirements of a diagnostic study consist of visualization of well-opacified main, lobar, and segmental pulmonary arteries of the upper, middle, and lower lobes, a volume of interest that extends from the level of the aortic arch to 2 centimeters below the inferior pulmonary veins. On a single-detector row spiral CT with a gantry rotation period of 1 second and scanning at a pitch of 2, the minimum collimation that can be prescribed to cover this 12-cm to 15-cm length within a tolerable breath-hold period (20 seconds–25 seconds) is 3 mm. On a 4-detector row spiral CT scanner, z-axis resolution can be improved by setting collimation to 1.0 mm to 1.25 mm; with a 0.5 second gantry rotation period and scanning at a pitch of 6, a 20-cm volume of interest extending from 2 centimeters above the aortic arch to the level of the diaphragm can be covered in 14 seconds to 17 seconds. Images should be reconstructed using a low-noise (standard) reconstruction kernel and the smallest field of view that contains the structures of interest. Generation of overlapping transverse images at an interval of one-half to two-thirds collimator width further improves longitudinal resolution and optimizes the dataset for multiplanar display, if desired.

An optimized-contrast administration protocol for CTPA requires that scanning of the pulmonary arterial sys-

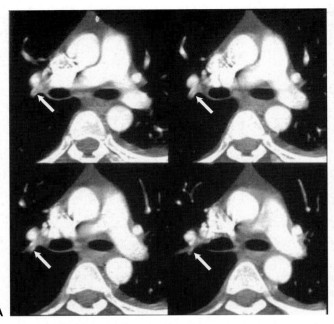

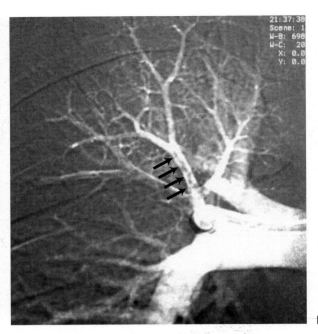

FIG. 6–1. Thirty-four-year-old woman, one week postpartum, suspected of having PE. **A:** Spiral CT scan (3-mm collimation/2-mm reconstruction interval) shows possible filling defect (*white arrow*) in the posterior segmental artery of the right upper lobe. **B:** Pulmonary angiogram definitively shows embolus (*black arrows*) in the same location.

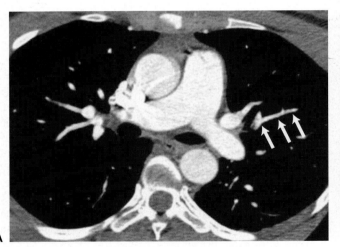

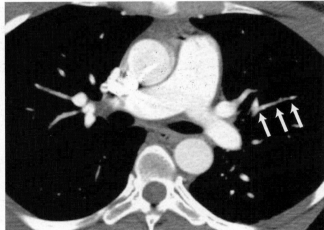

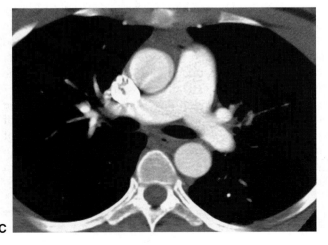

FIG. 6–2. Computed tomography pulmonary angiography study acquired on an 8-detector-row spiral CT scanner shows improved visualization of subsegmental pulmonary arteries (*arrows*) on 1.25-mm collimation spiral CT image **(A)** as compared to 2.5-mm **(B)** and 5.0-mm **(C)** collimation images due to decreased volume-averaging effects.

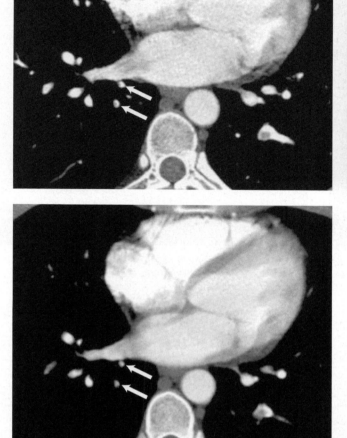
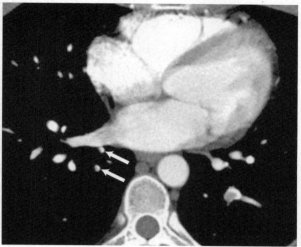

FIG. 6–3. Computed tomography pulmonary angiography study acquired on an 8-detector-row CT scanner shows improved detection of subsegmental pulmonary emboli (*arrows*) on 1.25-mm collimation spiral CT image **(A)** as compared to 2.5-mm **(B)** and 5-mm **(C)** collimation images.

tem be timed to the period of peak vascular opacification, which is maintained during the entire spiral acquisition using a power injector. A consistently high level of arterial opacification (greater than 200 HU in central pulmonary arteries) can be achieved using a high concentration (300 mg I/mL)/ high flow (4 mL/s–5 mL/s) protocol usually administered via an 18- or 20-gauge antecubital intravenous (IV) catheter. The total volume of required contrast medium is minimized by selecting a bolus duration equivalent to scan duration. The optimal delay time between start of contrast administration and initiation of scanning can be determined by performing a test bolus; 15 milliliters of contrast is injected at the same rate as for the CTPA. Five-millimeter collimated sections [120 kV, 80 milliampere (mA)] beginning 4 seconds after initiation of the bolus are acquired every 2 seconds at the level of the main pulmonary artery for a total of 10 images (Figure 6-4A). A time–density curve (Figure 6-4B) then is generated from a region of interest drawn within the

main pulmonary artery; the appropriate scan delay time is 2 seconds to 4 seconds added to the time corresponding to the peak of the curve. In patients with normal right-sided cardiac function, delay times typically range from 12 seconds to 16 seconds.

In order to facilitate high-quality pulmonary arterial enhancement and minimize motion artifacts, patients ideally should be scanned at either full inspiration or near the end of expiration during a period of strict apnea (10). Patients who are unable to maintain a breath hold should be instructed to take slow shallow breaths. Scanning in the caudocranial direction also may help to minimize motion artifacts, as the degree of respiratory excursion is less in the upper than lower lobes. In sedated intubated patients, suspension of ventilation for the duration of the CTPA study can improve significantly study quality and usually is well tolerated.

As part of a comprehensive work up for venous thromboembolic disease, a spiral CT venogram extending from

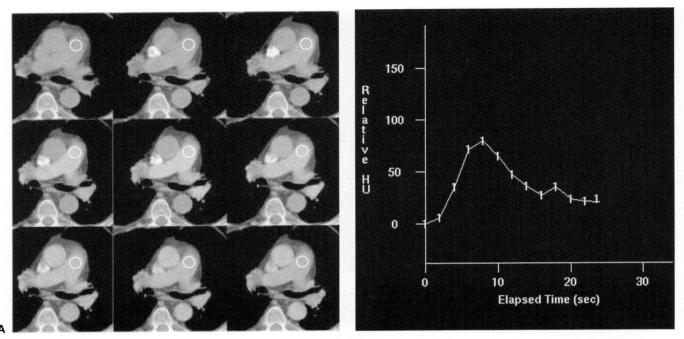

A

B

FIG. 6–4. Determination of optimal delay time using a test bolus. **A:** Five-millimeter collimation spiral CT images at level of main pulmonary artery are acquired every 2 seconds beginning 4 seconds after administration of a 15-mL test bolus. **B:** Time–density curve peaks at 12 seconds; optimal delay time is 14 seconds to 16 seconds.

the popliteal veins to the inferior vena cava is performed in each patient referred for the indication of PE at our institution. In order to ensure adequate opacification (greater than 85 H.U. in common femoral veins) of the deep venous system, a total of 150 mL of 300 mg I/mL nonionic contrast medium is administered for the CTPA study. Although the time to peak venous enhancement in the lower extremities is variable and dependent on patient circulation, consistently diagnostic results have been obtained with delay times (from time of initiation of contrast infusion) of 180 seconds to 210 seconds (2,11,12). Volumetric imaging using a collimator width of 5 mm to 10 mm is preferable to noncontiguous protocols, which can miss short thrombosed segments (13).

INTERPRETATION AND FINDINGS

Interpretation of CTPA and CT venogram studies should begin with an overall assessment of the diagnostic quality of the acquired examination. Suboptimal or inconclusive studies have been reported to occur in up to 11% to 13% of cases in some series (14,15). The three most common causes of suboptimal studies are: i) inadequate enhancement of the vascular structures of interest due to problems in delivery of contrast medium or inappropriate delay times, ii) excessive breathing or motion artifacts, and iii) excessive image noise in patients of large-body habitus.

Standard mediastinal (width = 400 H.U., level = 40 H.U.) or angiographic (width = 500 H.U., level = 100 H.U.) display-window settings usually are adequate for rou-

tine interpretation. However, because partial filling defects may be obscured by dense contrast material using these standard windows, Brink et al. (16) have proposed using window settings optimized to the degree of pulmonary arterial enhancement in individual patients. Using a porcine model, these investigators found that emboli were most conspicuous when displayed with a modified window referenced to the right or left pulmonary artery attenuation (width = measured mean attenuation plus two standard deviations, level = half of width attenuation value) (16) (Figure 6-5).

Familiarity with bronchovascular anatomy is a requirement for accurate interpretation of CTPA studies. A systematic approach incorporates visualization and assessment of all opacified subsegmental, segmental, lobar, and main pulmonary arteries. Differentiation between pulmonary arteries and veins can be made by tracking vessels to their proximal origin on serial images or by searching for the accompanying bronchus to a pulmonary artery on lung window settings (Figure 6-6). Both of these methods are facilitated greatly by review of images on a cathode ray tube monitor, which is the preferred method of viewing and has been shown to improve the detection rate of pulmonary emboli as compared with hard-copy review (17). Although multiplanar reformations have been advocated as a useful adjunct for evaluation of obliquely oriented arteries (18), transverse images usually are sufficient, particularly if acquired using a thin-collimation (1.0 mm–1.25 mm) protocol.

On CTPA studies, the diagnosis of pulmonary embolism is made on the basis of direct visualization of intravas-

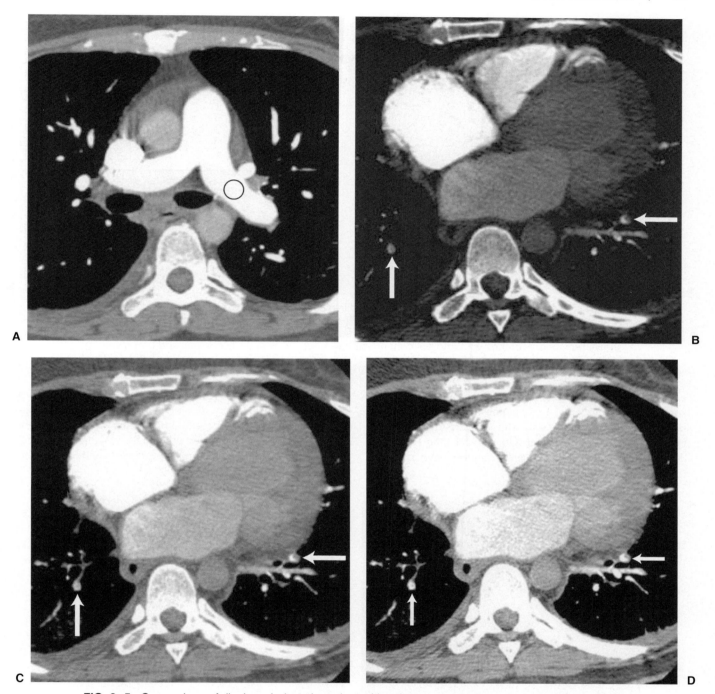

FIG. 6–5. Comparison of display windows in patient with subsegmental pulmonary emboli (*arrows*). **A:** Mean attenuation in left pulmonary-artery measures 620 ± 20 Hounsfield units. **B:** Optimized window setting, width = 660 HU, level = 330. **C:** Angiographic window setting, width = 500, level = 100. **D:** Standard window setting, width = 400, level = 40.

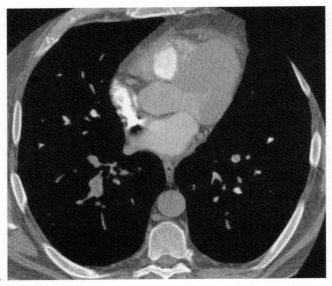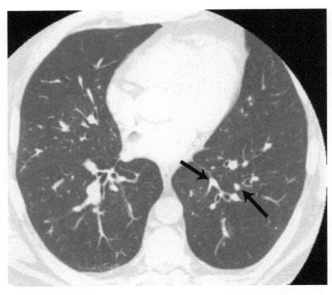

FIG. 6–6. Differentiation between arteries and veins in a patient with multiple bilateral lower lobe emboli. **A:** One-and-a-quarter-millimeter collimation spiral CT image displayed on angiographic windows shows low-attenuation regions in bilateral lower-lobe vessels. **B:** Same image displayed on lung windows shows pulmonary arteries with and pulmonary veins without (*arrows*) an accompanying bronchus.

cular clot; the filling defect may be partial or complete, sometimes filling or even expanding the occluded pulmonary artery (19) (Figure 6-7). Although the distribution of emboli typically is multifocal with a lower lung zonal predominance, isolated subsegmental emboli have been re-

ported to occur with a frequency of 6% to 36% of cases (5,14,20) and uniquely may involve an upper lobe subsegmental branch (Figure 6-8). In patients with a large clot burden resulting in elevated pulmonary vascular resistance, associated findings of pulmonary-artery hypertension such

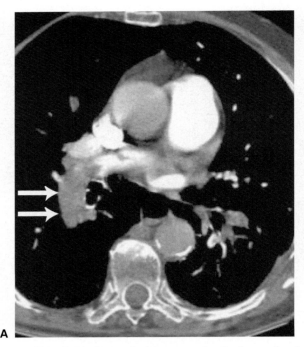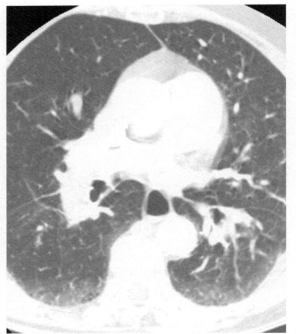

FIG. 6–7. Computed tomography findings of pulmonary embolism. **A:** One-and-a-quarter-millimeter collimation spiral CT image shows expansion of right interlobar artery (*arrows*) by embolus. **B:** Same image displayed on lung windows shows relative hypovascularity of right lung (Westermark sign).

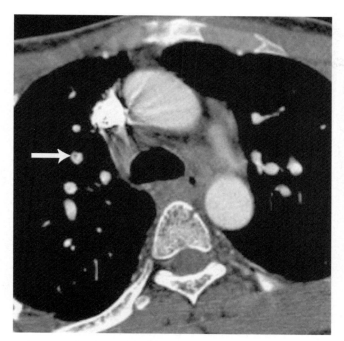

FIG. 6–8. One-and-a-quarter-millimeter collimation spiral CT image shows embolus (*arrow*) in right upper lobe subsegmental pulmonary artery. No other emboli were identified on the remainder of this CTPA study.

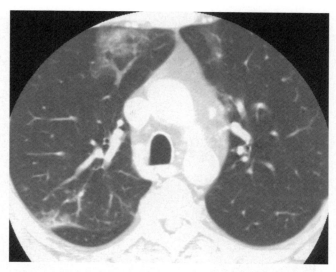

FIG. 6–10. One-and-a-quarter-millimeter collimation spiral CT image of a 31-year-old man with pulmonary embolism shows peripheral areas of ground-glass attenuation (Hampton hump) in bilateral upper lobes.

as a dilated main pulmonary artery (diameter greater than 29 mm) and interventricular septal deviation to the left may be seen (Figure 6-9).

Peripheral wedge-shaped opacities (Hampton hump) (Figure 6-10) are the only parenchymal findings on CT that

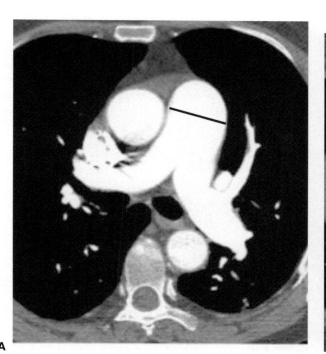

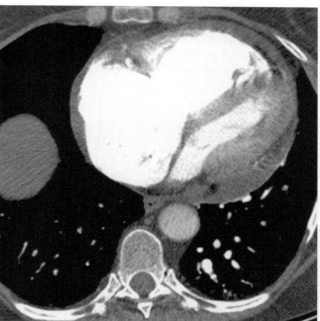

A

B

FIG. 6–9. Computed tomography findings of pulmonary hypertension. **A:** One-and-a-quarter-millimeter collimation spiral CT image shows dilatation of main pulmonary artery, which measures 35 mm. **B:** Enlargement of the right atrium and right ventricle is present, associated with straightening of the interventricular septum and a small pericardial effusion.

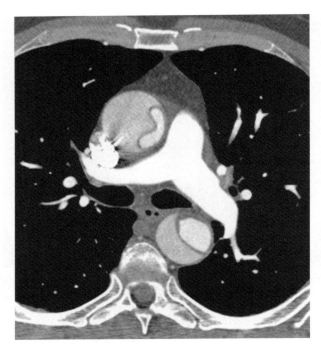

FIG. 6–11. One-and-a-quarter-millimeter collimation spiral CT image of a 62-year-old man suspected of having PE shows an intimal flap in the ascending and descending thoracic aorta consistent with a Type A dissection.

have been found consistently to be significantly more common in patients with PE than without (19,21). Other findings such as atelectasis, areas of decreased attenuation (Westermark sign), and pleural effusion have no discriminative value and are found with equal frequency in affected and unaffected patients presenting with dyspnea (21). In patients without PE, the performance of CTPA may provide additional information that suggests or confirms an alternate clinical diagnosis in 39% to 67% of patients (21,22) (Figure 6-11).

On CT venography, the diagnosis of DVT can be made confidently based on direct visualization of an intraluminal-filling defect, sometimes found in association with venous expansion, a high-contrast ringlike rim of enhancement, and perivenous stranding (23,24) (Figure 6-12). Poorly defined ''smudgy'' areas of low attenuation, particularly if seen on only one image, should not be mistaken for thrombus; these findings may arise from either volume averaging of valves (25) or flow artifacts due to nonhomogeneous mixing of contrast-enhanced and unenhanced blood (23, 24).

DIAGNOSTIC PITFALLS

Interpretation of CTPA studies requires recognition of a number of diagnostic pitfalls, which can result in falsely positive or negative studies. As previously stated, the minimum requirement for a diagnostic study consists of visualization of well-opacified main, lobar, and segmental pulmonary arteries of all lobes. Inadequate arterial enhancement can result in pseudofilling defects and usually occurs because of delay times that are too short (lack of contrast on earlier images) or too long (lack of contrast on later images). Regional differences in pulmonary vascular resistance, which usually is due to extensive parenchymal or pleural disease, also can lead to false-positive diagnoses (4,5). These pleuroparenchymal abnormalities result in slow arterial flow through the involved lung regions and the impression of emboli (26) (Figure 6-13). Flow-related causes of pseudofilling defects can be confirmed by performing a second spiral CT acquisition through the area of interest with a longer scan delay to demonstrate vessel patency (Figure 6-14).

Volume averaging of opacified subsegmental pulmonary arteries oriented horizontally or obliquely to the plane of section with adjacent lung often results in regions of arterial hypoattenuation that may mimic intraluminal filling defects. These partial volume effects are most pronounced

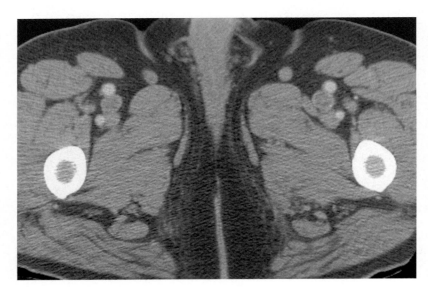

FIG. 6–12. Five-millimeter collimation spiral CT image shows intraluminal filling defects in bilateral superficial and deep femoral veins consistent with bilateral deep venous thrombosis.

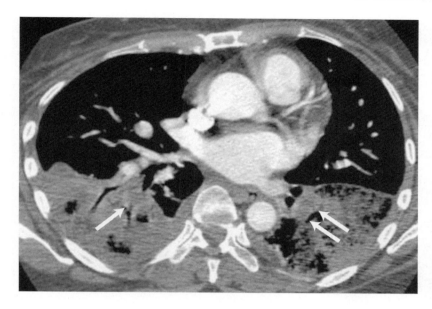

FIG. 6–13. One-and-a-quarter-millimeter collimation spiral CT image of a 40-year-old woman with lupus pneumonitis shows slow flow in bilateral lower lobe pulmonary arteries (*arrows*) simulating filling defects.

when using protocols of thicker collimation and reconstruction interval (Figure 6-2B). In severely tachypneic or agitated patients, breathing or motion can create additional partial volume-averaging effects as moving vessels occupy variable portions of the section width on successive images (26). In patients of large body habitus, an increase in image noise can cause an inhomogeneous appearance to opacified vessels; this effect, particularly when seen in conjunction with either a suboptimal bolus or significant motion artifacts, can cause pseudo-filling defects.

Lymphatic and connective tissue located between central bronchi and pulmonary arteries are a common pitfall in the interpretation of CTPA studies (Figure 6-15). Familiarity with the size and location of normal hilar lymph nodes is

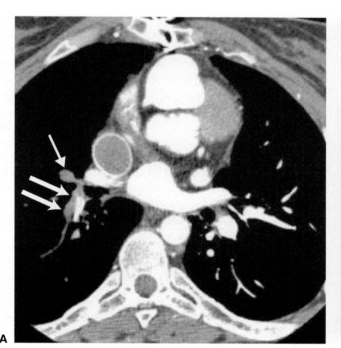
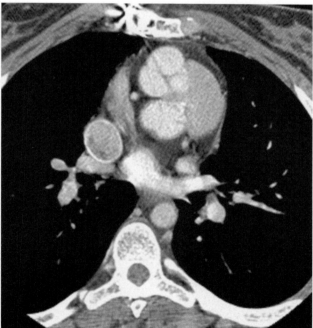

A
B

FIG. 6–14. Pseudofilling defects arising from mixing artifacts in a 40-year-old woman status post-Fontan procedure with transposition of great vessels, tricuspid atresia, and ventricular septal defect. **A:** One-and-a-quarter-millimeter collimation spiral CT image shows low-attenuation regions (*arrows*) involving the pulmonary arteries of the right middle and lower lobes. **B:** Delayed image shows homogeneous opacification of arteries previously suspected of containing emboli.

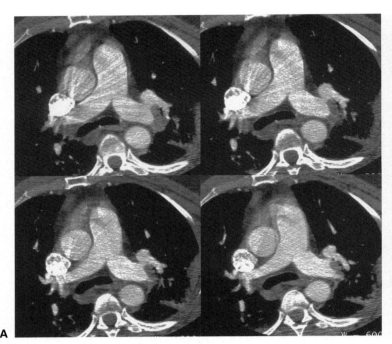 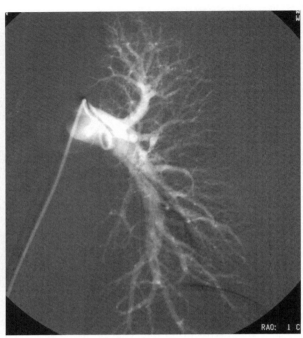

A   **B**

FIG. 6–15. Hilar lymph nodes simulating pulmonary embolus in a 50-year-old woman presenting with dyspnea. **A:** One-and-a-quarter-millimeter collimation spiral CT images reconstructed at 0.8-mm intervals show soft tissue attenuation near distal end of left main pulmonary artery. **B:** Corresponding angiogram of left pulmonary artery is normal.

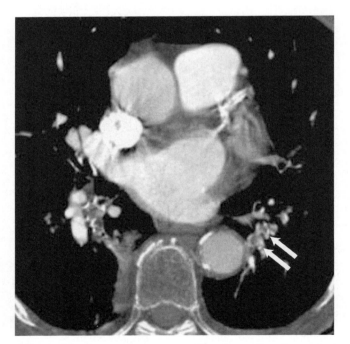

FIG. 6–16. One-and-a-quarter-millimeter collimation spiral CT image shows mucus impaction in calcified lower lobe segmental bronchi (*arrows*), which may simulate pulmonary emboli.

helpful in distinguishing between normal findings and emboli (27); in most situations, following the areas of low attenuation on sequential images will allow clear differentiation between an intraarterial or extraarterial location. Mucus plugging of calcified segmental bronchi also can simulate the appearance of an endoluminal clot (Figure 6-16). Again, sequentially following the area of abnormality on successive images allows recognition of the correct diagnosis of an impacted bronchus.

Pulmonary-artery sarcoma, a rare tumor, may present with CT findings identical to that of acute or chronic embolism. This tumor is diagnosed most commonly at surgery or autopsy and is associated with a poor prognosis (28). The diagnosis of pulmonary-artery sarcoma should be considered when intraarterial filling defects cause distension of the vascular lumen, are associated with transmural extension of soft tissue, or increase in size on follow-up studies.

ACCURACY OF CTPA FOR EMBOLIC DISEASE

Over the past decade, a number of studies have been performed to evaluate the accuracy of CTPA in the diagnosis of pulmonary embolism (Table 6–1). Due to differences in patient entry criteria and CT scanning protocols, results vary considerably (4,5,14,22,29–35). However, for those studies in which CTPA was performed with a maximum collimation of 3 millimeters, sensitivity and specificity values generally are on the order of 85% and 90%, respectively (Table 6–1).

TABLE 6–1. *Accuracy of CT pulmonary angiography in diagnosis of acute pulmonary embolism*

Reference	Year	No. of patients in study	Collimation (mm)	Sensitivity (%)	Specificity (%)	K value
Remy-Jardin et al. (4)	1992	42	5	100	96	—
Goodman et al. (5)	1995	20	5	63	89	—
van Rossum et al. (35)	1996	149	5	82–94	93–96	0.77
Remy-Jardin et al. (34)	1996	75	3–5	91	78	—
Mayo et al. (32)	1997	142	3	87	95	0.85
Drucker et al. (30)	1998	47	5	53–60	81–97	—
Herold et al. (31)	1998	401	3	88	94	0.72
Kim et al. (22)	1999	110	3	92	96	—
Qanadli et al. (14)	2000	157	2.5	90	94	0.86
Blachere et al. (29)	2000	179	2–3	94	94	0.72
Perrier et al. (33)	2001	299	3	70%	91%	0.82–0.90

Qanadli et al. (14) have reported the first results related to multidetector CT (MDCT) technology; using a dual-detector system to evaluate prospectively 157 patients with suspected pulmonary embolism, CTPA was found to have a sensitivity of 90% and a specificity of 94%.

While continuing innovations in CT technology likely will improve further depiction of small peripheral pulmonary arteries, the current major limitation of CTPA is inadequate sensitivity in detection of subsegmental emboli. Despite this drawback, CTPA is used commonly as a first-line screening study because its performance compares favorably with other diagnostic tests used to evaluate for PE. Mayo and colleagues (32) compared spiral CT with ventilation-perfusion scintigraphy in a prospective study of 142 patients suspected of PE; sensitivities, specificities, and K values with spiral CT and scintigraphy were 87%, 95%, and 0.85, and 65%, 94%, and 0.61, respectively. A similar comparison performed in 123 consecutive patients by van Rossum et al (36) found a significantly higher sensitivity (75% vs. 49%) and specificity (90% vs. 74%) of spiral CT as compared to scintigraphy (P = 0.01). This latter study also showed that CTPA provided a conclusive diagnosis in a significantly larger proportion of patients (P < 0.001), as well as more alternate diagnoses (P < 0.001) than scintigraphy (36).

Pulmonary angiography, generally regarded as the gold standard in the diagnosis of PE, is more invasive and more expensive than CTPA, may be impractical or unavailable in some clinical settings, and is associated with cardiac or pulmonary complications in 3% to 4% of patients (37). Similar to CTPA, interobserver agreement in interpretation of pulmonary angiograms is influenced strongly by the magnitude and site of the embolus, ranging from 98% for lobar pulmonary emboli to 66% for subsegmental pulmonary emboli (38). Baile and colleagues (39) compared spiral CT to pulmonary angiography for detection of subsegmental pulmonary emboli in an animal model of PE in which colored methacrylate beads were injected into the pulmonary circulation of 16 juvenile pigs. Using a methacrylate cast of the porcine pulmonary vessels as an independent gold standard, no significant difference (P > .05) in either sensitivity (82% vs. 87%) or positive predictive value (94% vs. 88%) was found between 3-mm collimation spiral CTPA and pulmonary angiography (39).

The utility of a negative CTPA study in patients suspected of having acute PE has been assessed in three prospective clinical-outcome studies (40–42). Ferretti et al. (40) examined 164 consecutive patients suspected of having acute PE who had an intermediate probability ventilation-perfusion scan and negative duplex ultrasound studies of the lower extremities. After three months of follow up, recurrent pulmonary embolism was detected in 6 of 112 patients (5%) who had negative spiral CT studies and had not received anticoagulation therapy (40). Goodman and colleagues (41) compared the outcome of 198 patients with negative CTPA to 350 patients with either normal (n = 188) or low-probability (n = 162) ventilation-perfusion studies. Subsequent PE was found in 2 (1%) patients with negative CTPA, 0 patients with normal ventilation-perfusion study, and 5 (3.1%) patients with low probability ventilation-perfusion study (not statistically significant) (41). Ost et al. (42) examined 103 consecutive patients with high clinical suspicion of PE and intermediate or low probability ventilation-perfusion scans. After 6 months of follow up, recurrent embolism was detected in 3 of 71 patients (4%) who had negative CTPA and 2 of 10 patients (20%) who had indeterminate CT scans (42).

ACCURACY OF CT VENOGRAPHY FOR DEEP VENOUS THROMBOSIS

Computed tomography venography has been shown to be a highly accurate method in the evaluation of deep venous thrombosis with both sensitivity and specificity on the order of 90% to 95% (Table 6–2) (13,23,25,43,44). Interobserver agreement in the interpretation of these studies has been reported to range from moderately good (K value, 0.56) (45) to excellent (K value, 0.88) (43). The performance of CT venography in conjunction with CTPA can increase the diag-

TABLE 6–2. *Accuracy of CT venography in diagnosis of deep venous thrombosis*

Reference	Year	No. of patients in study	Collimation (mm)	Reconstruction Interval (mm)	Sensitivity (%)	Specificity (%)	K value
Loud et al. (44)	2000	71	5–10	50	100	100	—
Garg et al. (23)	2000	70	10	20	100	97	—
Duwe et al. (25)	2000	74	10	10	89	94	—
Coche et al. (43)	2001	65	6.5	5	93	97	0.88
Loud et al. (13)	2001	308	5–10	50	97	100	—

nostic yield in the CT assessment of patients with suspected PE by identification of the approximately one-quarter of patients who manifest on CT with deep venous thrombosis alone (13).

INCIDENTAL VENOUS THROMBOEMBOLISM

Unsuspected pulmonary emboli can be detected in approximately 1% of patients who undergo a routine contrast-enhanced spiral CT scan of the thorax, with the prevalence of disease higher in the inpatient than outpatient population (17,46) (Figure 6-17). Similarly, Shah et al. (24) have reported a 1% prevalence of unsuspected deep venous thrombosis in patients undergoing routine pelvic spiral CT scans. In the reported series, affected patients typically had a known predisposing risk factor such as cancer and were treated for thromboembolic disease as a consequence of the CT findings (17,24,46).

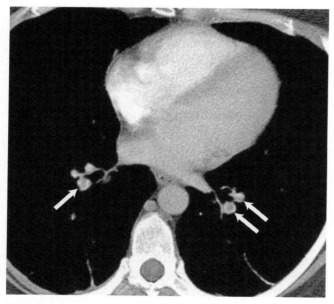

FIG. 6–17. Seven-millimeter collimation contrast-enhanced spiral CT study shows unsuspected emboli (*arrows*) in bilateral lower lobe pulmonary arteries of a 45-year-old woman with known history of breast cancer.

REFERENCES

1. Hyers TM. Venous thromboembolism. *Am J Respir Crit Care Med* 1999;159:1–14.
2. Bruce D, Loud PA, Klippenstein DL, et al. Combined CT venography and pulmonary angiography: how much venous enhancement is routinely obtained? *AJR Am J Roentgenol* 2001;176:1281–1285.
3. The PIOPED Investigators. Value of the ventilation/perfusion scan in acute pulmonary embolism. Results of the prospective investigation of pulmonary embolism diagnosis (PIOPED). *JAMA* 1990; 263:2753–2759.
4. Remy-Jardin M, Remy J, Wattinne L, et al. Central pulmonary thromboembolism: diagnosis with spiral volumetric CT with the single-breath-hold technique—comparison with pulmonary angiography. *Radiology* 1992;185:381–387.
5. Goodman LR, Curtin JJ, Mewissen MW, et al. Detection of pulmonary embolism in patients with unresolved clinical and scintigraphic diagnosis: helical CT versus angiography. *AJR Am J Roentgenol* 1995; 164:1369–1374.
6. Woodard PK. Pulmonary arteries must be seen before they can be assessed. *Radiology* 1997;204:11–12.
7. Remy-Jardin M, Remy J, Artaud D, et al. Peripheral pulmonary arteries: optimization of the spiral CT acquisition protocol. *Radiology* 1997; 204:157–163.
8. Remy-Jardin M, Baghaie F, Bonnel F, et al. Thoracic helical CT: influence of subsecond scan time and thin collimation on evaluation of peripheral pulmonary arteries. *Eur Radiol* 2000;10:1297–1303.
9. Schoepf UJ, Holzknecht N, Helmberger TK, et al. Subsegmental pulmonary emboli: Improved detection with thin-collimation multi-detector row spiral CT. *Radiology* 2002;222:483–490.
10. Remy-Jardin M, Remy J. Spiral CT angiography of the pulmonary circulation. *Radiology* 1999;212:615–636.
11. Loud PA, Grossman ZD, Klippenstein DL, et al. Combined CT venography and pulmonary angiography: a new diagnostic technique for suspected thromboembolic disease. *AJR Am J Roentgenol* 1998; 170:951–954.
12. Yankelevitz DF, Gamsu G, Shah A, et al. Optimization of combined CT pulmonary angiography with lower extremity CT venography. *AJR Am J Roentgenol* 2000;174:67–69.
13. Loud PA, Katz DS, Bruce DA, et al. Deep venous thrombosis with suspected pulmonary embolism: detection with combined CT venography and pulmonary angiography. *Radiology* 2001;219:498–502.
14. Qanadli SD, Hajjam ME, Mesurolle B, et al. Pulmonary embolism detection: prospective evaluation of dual-section helical CT versus selective pulmonary arteriography in 157 patients. *Radiology* 2000; 217:447–455.
15. Remy-Jardin M, Remy J, Baghaie F, et al. Clinical value of thin collimation in the diagnostic workup of pulmonary embolism. *AJR Am J Roentgenol* 2000;175:407–411.
16. Brink JA, Woodard PK, Horesh L, et al. Depiction of pulmonary emboli with spiral CT: optimization of display window settings in a porcine model. *Radiology* 1997;204:703–708.
17. Gosselin MV, Rubin GD, Leung AN, et al. Unsuspected pulmonary embolism: prospective detection on routine helical CT scans. *Radiology* 1998;208:209–215.
18. Remy-Jardin M. Diagnosis of central pulmonary embolism with helical CT: role of two-dimensional multiplanar reformations. *AJR Am J Roentgenol* 1995;165:1131–1138.

19. Coche EE, Muller NL, Kim KI, et al.. Acute pulmonary embolism: ancillary findings at spiral CT. *Radiology* 1998;207:753–758.
20. de Monye W, van Strijen MJ, Huisman MV, et al. Suspected pulmonary embolism: prevalence and anatomic distribution in 487 consecutive patients. Advances in New Technologies Evaluating the Localisation of Pulmonary Embolism (ANTELOPE) Group. *Radiology* 2000; 215:184–188.
21. Shah AA, Davis SD, Gamsu G, et al. Parenchymal and pleural findings in patients with and patients without acute pulmonary embolism detected at spiral CT. *Radiology* 1999;211:147–153.
22. Kim KI, Muller NL, Mayo JR. Clinically suspected pulmonary embolism: utility of spiral CT. *Radiology* 1999;210:693–697.
23. Garg K, Kemp JL, Wojcik D, et al. Thromboembolic disease: comparison of combined CT pulmonary angiography and venography with bilateral leg sonography in 70 patients. *AJR Am J Roentgenol* 2000; 175:997–1001.
24. Shah AA, Buckshee N, Yankelevitz DF, et al. Assessment of deep venous thrombosis using routine pelvic CT. *AJR Am J Roentgenol* 1999;173:659–663.
25. Duwe KM, Shiau M, Budorick NE, et al. Evaluation of the lower extremity veins in patients with suspected pulmonary embolism: a retrospective comparison of helical CT venography and sonography. *AJR Am J Roentgenol* 2000;175:1525–1531.
26. Remy-Jardin M, Remy J, Artaud D, et al.. Spiral CT of pulmonary embolism: diagnostic approach, interpretive pitfalls and current indications. *Eur Radiol* 1998;8:1376–1390.
27. Remy-Jardin M. Hilar lymph nodes: identification with spiral CT and histologic correlation. *Radiology* 1995;196:387–394.
28. Dennie CJ, Veinot JP, McCormack DG, et al. Intimal sarcoma of the pulmonary arteries seen as a mosaic pattern of lung attenuation on high-resolution CT. *AJR* 2002;178:1208–1210.
29. Blachere H, Latrabe V, Montaudon M, et al. Pulmonary embolism revealed on helical CT angiography: comparison with ventilation-perfusion radionuclide lung scanning. *AJR Am J Roentgenol* 2000; 174:1041–1047.
30. Drucker EA, Rivitz SM, Shepard JA, et al. Acute pulmonary embolism: assessment of helical CT for diagnosis. *Radiology* 1998;209:235–241.
31. Herold CJ, Remy-Jardin M, Grenier PA, et al. Prospective evaluation of pulmonary embolism: initial results of the European Multicenter Trial (ESTIPEP). *Radiology* 1998;209(P):299.
32. Mayo JR, Remy-Jardin M, Muller NL, et al. Pulmonary embolism: prospective comparison of spiral CT with ventilation-perfusion scintigraphy. *Radiology* 1997;205:447–452.
33. Perrier A, Howarth N, Didier D, et al. Performance of helical computed tomography in unselected outpatients with suspected pulmonary embolism. *Ann Intern Med* 2001;135:88–97.
34. Remy-Jardin M, Remy J, Deschildre F, et al. Diagnosis of pulmonary embolism with spiral CT: comparison with pulmonary angiography and scintigraphy. *Radiology* 1996;200:699–706.
35. van Rossum AB, Pattynama PM, Ton ER, et al. Pulmonary embolism: validation of spiral CT angiography in 149 patients. *Radiology* 1996; 201:467–470.
36. van Rossum AB, Pattynama PM, Mallens WM, et al. Can helical CT replace scintigraphy in the diagnostic process in suspected pulmonary embolism? A retrolective-prolective cohort study focusing on total diagnostic yield. *Eur Radiol* 1998;8:90–96.
37. Rathbun SW, Raskob GE, Whitsett TL. Sensitivity and specificity of helical computed tomography in the diagnosis of pulmonary embolism: a systematic review. *Ann Intern Med* 2000;132:227–232.
38. Stein PD, Athanasoulis C, Alavi A, et al. Complications and validity of pulmonary angiography in acute pulmonary embolism. *Circulation* 1992;85:462–468.
39. Baile EM, King GG, Muller NL, et al. Spiral computed tomography is comparable to angiography for the diagnosis of pulmonary embolism. *Am J Respir Crit Care Med* 2000;161:1010–1015.
40. Ferretti GR, Bosson JL, Buffaz PD, et al. Acute pulmonary embolism: role of helical CT in 164 patients with intermediate probability at ventilation-perfusion scintigraphy and normal results at duplex US of the legs. *Radiology* 1997;205:453–458.
41. Goodman LR, Lipchik RJ, Kuzo RS, et al. Subsequent pulmonary embolism: risk after a negative helical CT pulmonary angiogram—prospective comparison with scintigraphy. *Radiology* 2000;215:535–542.
42. Ost D, Rozenshtein A, Saffran L, et al. The negative predictive value of spiral computed tomography for the diagnosis of pulmonary embolism in patients with nondiagnostic ventilation-perfusion scans. *Am J Med* 2001;110:16–21.
43. Coche EE, Hamoir XL, Hammer FD, et al. Using dual-detector helical CT angiography to detect deep venous thrombosis in patients with suspicion of pulmonary embolism: diagnostic value and additional findings. *AJR Am J Roentgenol* 2001;176:1035–1039.
44. Loud PA, Katz DS, Klippenstein DL, et al. Combined CT venography and pulmonary angiography in suspected thromboembolic disease: diagnostic accuracy for deep venous evaluation. *AJR Am J Roentgenol* 2000;174:61–65.
45. Garg K, Kemp JL, Russ PD, et al. Thromboembolic disease: variability of interobserver agreement in the interpretation of CT venography with CT pulmonary angiography. *AJR Am J Roentgenol* 2001; 176:1043–1047.
46. Winston CB, Wechsler RJ, Salazar AM, et al. Incidental pulmonary emboli detected at helical CT: effect on patient care. *Radiology* 1996; 201:23–27.

CHAPTER 7

Other Thoracic Applications Including 3D Airway Imaging and Aortic Dissection

Leo P. Lawler, Elliot K. Fishman

INTRODUCTION

The potential for superior image quality and alternate methods of data display and analysis continues to evolve and provide us with novel approaches to noninvasive thoracic evaluation, which may improve on the already high diagnostic accuracy and yield of helical computed tomography (CT). Multidetector CT (MDCT) technology has improved many of the parameters of helical scanning and image acquisition, with rapid progress towards isotropic (cubic) voxels of data (1–6). Newer methodologies in post-processing techniques seek to realize the full potential of this MDCT data and to create new avenues for the understanding and interpretation of disease pathophysiology, as well as influencing the design of new management algorithms and therapeutic strategies (7). The first section of this chapter will look at these developments as they relate to the airways, lung parenchyma, chest wall, and diaphragm. The second part will address the spectrum of abnormalities in aortic dissection as imaged through newer CT techniques. In both sections there will be an initial discussion of MDCT acquisition and three-dimensional (3D) post-processing specific to each area, followed by a review of clinical conditions.

PART I. 3D CHEST AIRWAY, LUNG, CHEST WALL, AND DIAPHRAGM

MDCT—Airway- and Lung-Imaging Technique

Patients are scanned supine in a cranial to caudal direction, and the clinical history will dictate the coverage required. If the problem concerns the intrathoracic airways, coverage will be from the thoracic inlet to below the diaphragm; if the area of concern is above the thoracic inlet, coverage is usually from the glottis (C5 vertebral body) or supraglottic airway (8,9). For the majority of 3D airway and diffuse lung-parenchyma studies, noncontrast examinations will suffice. Contrast-enhanced studies are employed when

there are questions regarding airway bronchovascular relationships (e.g., rings and slings), mediastinal involvment, or focal lung disease (10). Dynamic imaging of the airway with MDCT (11) is possible but, in an effort to reduce radiation exposure, inspiration and expiration imaging is reserved for those patients in whom there is a high index of suspicion for tracheobronchomalacia or air trapping and a clear management benefit (12,13). One hundred milliamperes (mAs) and 140 kV are standard scanner settings, but they are adjusted for body size. Though low-dose techniques using 50 mA to 80 mA may be employed without significant loss of anatomic detail due to the high inherent contrast of the lungs, this must be balanced against the need for narrower slice widths with greater quantum mottle (8,9).

Volumetric CT (14–17) as applied to the airway represents significant progress over sequential scanning (8,9,18–20), and MDCT breath-hold imaging allows for scanning parameters (1,3,4) better suited to both optimal 3D-airway and lung-parenchyma reconstruction (21). From the thoracic MDCT raw data, various parenchymal-reconstruction-slice positions, thicknesses, intervals, and kernels (e.g., edge enhancing or soft tissue) may be generated from a single study acquisition. With the beam collimated to four 1-mm detectors with a pitch of 6, 1.25-mm slice thicknesses can depict the airways to their sixth-order branches (21) and image the secondary pulmonary lobules without significant broadening of the slice-sensitivity profile or effective slice width. Rapid MDCT acquisition (22), such as with 2.5-mm detectors providing 3-mm slice widths, will give faster coverage with less noisy images adequate for airway interpretation with coverage of the entire chest in 10 seconds or less. This is especially advantageous in patients with respiratory disease in whom breath holding presents a major challenge, and in whom dynamic alterations of airways otherwise might introduce interpretative difficulties through misregistration (23). By using a dedicated airway protocol with 20% to 30%

overlapping reconstruction intervals to generate optimal 3D reconstructions, subsequently larger slice widths or alternate kernels can be obtained for routine parenchymal and mediastinal images, or whole-lung high-resolution images. Multi-detector CT improves temporal resolution (24), reduces or eliminates breathing misregistration, and cardiac pulsation in the medial lung, while overlapping thin sections reduce volume averaging (19,25).

Post-processing—3D Airway and Lung CT

Although CT is an established standard for airway imaging, the value of an individual chest CT and its relevance to the specific needs of bronchoscopists and the individual patient may be increased through the use of an increasing number of post-processing applications (7,19,26,27). The potentially isotropic voxels (volume elements equal in size in all dimensions) of data produced by MDCT scanners afford a choice of image-display perspectives independent of the original acquisition plane and the variable anatomic-airway orientation, such that the volume acquired also may be interpreted as a volume. Earlier attempts at 3D CT of the airway were not accepted widely because the images were not of sufficient quality. The quality of 3D images now obtained with MDCT can provide a credible correlation with flexible bronchoscopy, and one that can be generated in routine radiologic practice (28).

Airway and lung CT reconstructions have been per-

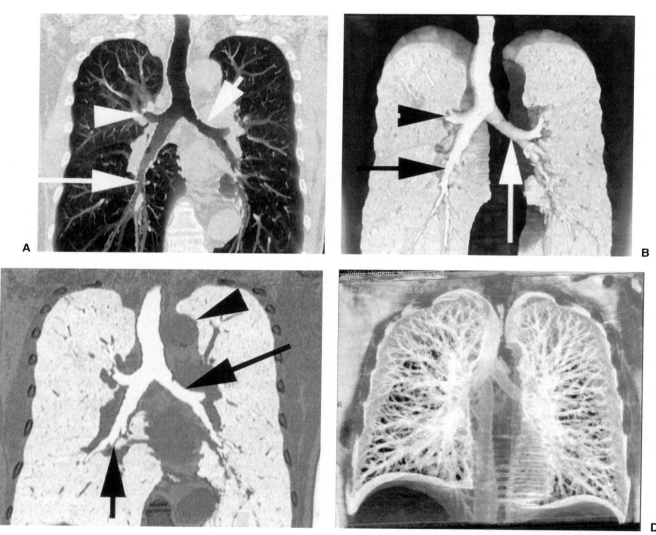

FIG. 7–1. A: Volume-rendered luminal-trapezoid anteroposterior (AP) view showing the right upper-lobe bronchus (*arrowhead*), right lower lobe bronchus (*long arrow*), and left lower lobe bronchus (*short arrow*). **B:** Volume-rendered solid-trapezoid AP view showing the right upper lobe bronchus (*arrowhead*), right lower-lobe bronchus (*black arrow*), and left lower-lobe bronchus (*white arrow*). **C:** Volume-rendered solid-airway and soft-tissue trapezoid AP view showing the aortic arch (*arrowhead*), left lower lobe bronchus (*long arrow*), and right lower lobe bronchus (*short arrow*). **D:** Volume-rendered bronchography trapezoid AP view of both lungs. *(continued)*

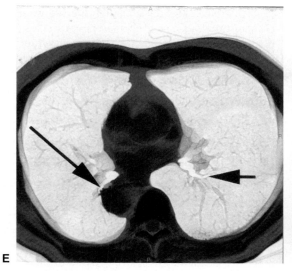
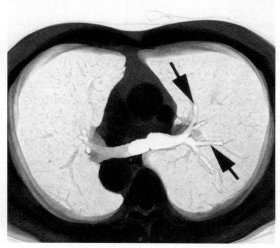

FIG. 7–1. *Continued.* **E:** Volume-rendered solid-trapezoid superior view with clip planes depicting left (*long arrow*) and right (*short arrow*) superior segment bronchi of the lower lung. **F:** Volume-rendered solid-trapezoid superior view with clip planes depicting the medial and lateral segment bronchi of the middle lobe (*arrows*).

formed largely by straight and curved multiplanar reconstruction (MPR and CMPR), maximum- and minimum-intensity projections (MIP and MinIP), shaded-surface display (SSD), and volume-rendering techniques (VRT) (8,9,29–33). Straight and curved multiplanar reconstructions are not computer intensive and produce 1-voxel thick tomographic sections, which can provide cross-sectional or longitudinal images (34–36) useful for demonstrating airway stenoses (18, 37). Maximum- and minimum-intensity projections with sliding thin slabs provide specific information through a projection of attenuation values at the highest and lowest range at the expense of much of the data in between. Although they have a role in interstitial lung disease, these techniques are not applicable for airway stenoses (34). Shaded-surface display depicts the airway by simulating the boundary between air and soft tissue and segmenting it as a series of polygons with lighting models. Shaded-surface display is an effective method for diagnosing central stenoses, but it is less useful for evaluating the lung periphery, and it may obscure high-density structures such as stents or broncholiths. Therefore, it has little advantage over multiplanar approaches (9,25,36,38).

Volume rendering is the latest approach to 3D tracheobronchial imaging (31,32,39–41), and is a technique that maintains high fidelity to the originally acquired data (40,42–45). All the density values within the chest may be manipulated through the application of various VRT tools to a histogram representation (i.e., a trapezoid) of all the Hounsfield values contained within the MDCT image (40,44,45). Unlike previous methods of image display, the final volume-rendered image with this approach shows tissues according to their original representation in the data. The spatial relationship of tracheobronchial structures is pre-

served with depth cues and opacity settings and infinite permutations of airway image editing. Perspective and trapezoid applications can be performed and tailored to individual cases. Clip-plane editing can remove slabs of data rapidly, such as the overlying chest wall or lung, and with appropriate perspective settings, individual bronchi may be isolated. Both internal and external perspectives may be depicted with a range of opacity settings from solid to nearly transparent and can be segmented in isolation or illustrated in relation to the soft tissues within the thorax. For example, the solid airway, air bronchography, and soft-tissue or luminal views, among others, may be selected depending on the case in question. Virtual bronchoscopy (VB) depicts the airways from an endoluminal perspective using SSD or volume rendering (VR) (46) with increased opacity settings (Figure 7-1) (8,9,14,31,32,35,42,43,47–53). Fly-through tools that automatically determine the centerline facilitate endobronchial navigation. Color-coded SSD combined with VR has been suggested to depict complex anatomy in virtual endoscopic renderings (54), and attempts have been made to register real and CT-derived bronchoscopic data to optimize the yield of both (55). Contemporary workstations also allow real-time image processing and display, which is essential for radiologic interpretation and clinician consultation.

3D Airway CT—Role in Clinical Practice

The natural contrast of the air–airway interface is well suited to the properties of CT, which include high-contrast resolution. Axial planar CT and bronchoscopy have largely replaced conventional bronchography for whole lung, central, and peripheral airway imaging. In many cases, conventional two-dimensional (2D) axial CT will suffice, providing information about the status of the lumen, the airway wall, and the extraluminal structures (8,9,54). Airways that course perpendicular to the imaging plane, although well seen for the most part, may have subtle changes in caliber that are not appreciated without 3D reconstruction (42,43,56). Other complex airway-branching patterns oblique to the imaging plane also have limitations with 2D planar axial CT (8,42,43,56). Three-dimensional airway imaging reformats the data in novel ways more suited to individual tracheobronchial anatomy and a range of pathologies (33,34). Moreover, many bronchoscopists find the 3D perspective to be more intuitive for endoscopic findings than the conventional cross-sectional axial images. When derived from an MDCT-acquisition protocol, it is a simple matter to supplement 2D studies with additional 3D reconstructions when indicated in routine practice.

There have been many studies positively reflecting the diagnostic accuracy of bronchoscopy or laryngoscopy compared with 3D CT (13,25,27,30,48,57), but perhaps this comparative approach alone underestimates some of the intrinsic properties and advantages of both modalities. Although it can produce compelling endoscopic simulations (31,32,47, 50–52), 3D-CT bronchoscopy will not replace the direct visualization, diagnostic sampling, and interventional capabilities of bronchoscopy, which directly visualizes and faithfully represents the mucosa both in hue and in duration. Virtual bronchoscopic imaging is uniquely valuable when used to display both the internal airway findings and those beyond the airway together. This can be achieved either by applying increased transparency or through the simultaneous display of endoluminal and multiplanar views (9,47). Software developments have matched VB images to flexible bronchoscopy images (55). The added value of 3D airway CT lies in its unique potential to noninvasively produce whole-lung tracheobronchial images together with precise measurements, functional assessment, and extraluminal information about the lung and mediastinum (51,58,59).

The current clinical role of 3D CT is for those patients who require additional noninvasive airway and lung evaluation that cannot be provided by axial planar 2D CT alone (26). Although it may increase diagnostic sensitivity in select cases, its role in the majority of patients is to provide more sophisticated interpretation, measurement accuracy, and improved appreciation of the subtleties of airway or lung disease for radiologists and nonradiologists alike. Three-dimensional airway CT aids patient triage for bronchoscopy, helps in planning the bronchoscopy procedure, and can be of value when endoscopy is inconclusive (25,48,50,51). Although the full impact of VB on endoscopy management has not been evaluated yet, it may obviate the need for bronchoscopy in certain cases. Three-dimensional airway CT is of particular value in measuring the length of airway abnormalities and in delineating their location in relation to endoluminal and extraluminal landmarks and pathology. A preprocedure review of 3D-volume-rendered images may provide a road map for bronchoscopy with or without fluoroscopic guidance, offering preparation that potentially increases the effi-

ciency or reduces the duration of the procedure. Virtual bronchoscopy tools also have been proposed as a technique to aid novice trainees in gaining the skills required for performing bronchoscopy (60).

3D Airway CT—Pediatric Airway

Many of the principles of airway imaging apply equally to the adult and pediatric population, with appropriate protocol dose modification for body size. Helical scanning improved airway imaging in younger infants who were less able to cooperate with breath holding (61). The brevity of scanning time with MDCT (22) also has decreased the need for pediatric sedation (62,63). In at-risk patients, such as children with small or malacic airways where the bronchoscope may occlude the airway, 3D CT can provide a safer noninvasive alternative (64–67) with objective evidence of the extent of expiratory collapse (11,12). Multidetector CT recently has been shown to be of some value in this area (11). The ability to generate 3D-CT angiograms and image relations beyond the airway wall is beneficial for identifying pulmonary vascular anomalies that lead to airway compromise (68) and has facilitated surgical planning.

Although there is some overlap in airway pathology, there are distinct conditions in the pediatric population that deserve special mention. Congenital airway anomalies are a more common reason for referral in children (69,70), for whom 2D and 3D CT have been used effectively for delineating pathology (61,64,71–74) (Table 7-1A). Older forms of 3D spiral CT have been applied successfully to cases of anomalous branching patterns, stenosis (73,75,76), bronchiectasis (72), pulmonary rings and slings (Figures 7–2 and 7–3) (67,68,74,76,77), and extrinsic tracheal compression from mediastinal masses (71). Anomalous branching patterns that may be unclear with a limited endoscopic-luminal

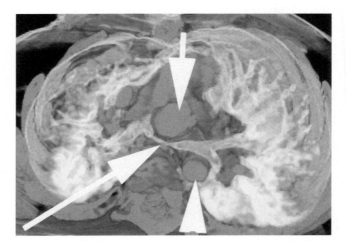

FIG. 7–2. Volume-rendered inferior view of a corrected TGA showing how the narrowed distance between ascending aorta (*short arrow*) and descending aorta (*arrowhead*) contributed to left lower-lobe bronchomalacia (*long arrow*).

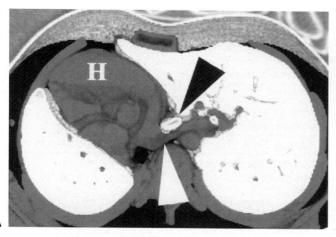

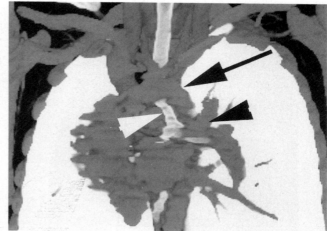

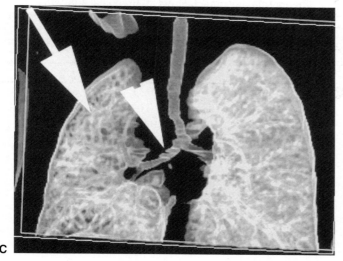

FIG. 7–3. A: Volume-rendered inferior view of a pulmonary sling (*white arrowhead*) behind the trachea (*black arrowhead*) with dextroposition (*H*). **B:** Volume-rendered AP view of a deviated trachea (*white arrowhead*) encased by aortic arch anteriorly (*black arrow*) and left pulmonary sling posteriorly (*arrowhead*). **C:** Volume-rendered AP view of the inferior origin of a bridging bronchus (*arrowhead*) in the setting of pulmonary sling. Note the absence of a right upper-lobe bronchus and subsequent loss of right lung volume (*arrow*).

view or that may be volume averaged on axial reconstructions may be obvious on whole-lung 3D renderings, which clearly depict the orientation and relation of bronchi. Subtle abnormal bronchial origins or angulations such as a bridging bronchus (Figure 7-3C) are quite difficult to appreciate with bronchoscopy or 2D CT, but the relationships and angles are measured easily with volume rendering. Bronchial atresia and its segmental effect are seen with tailored images that show the paucity of lung markings (Figure 7-4). The exact location of congenital tracheoesophageal fistulas can be rendered for surgical planning (Figure 7-5), and diffuse lung diseases specific to the pediatric age group may be depicted in a whole lung distribution (Figure 7-6).

3D-Airway CT—Airway Focal Abnormalities

Airway-filling defects may be classified as true or pseudolesions, benign or malignant (primary and secondary), and can be single or multiple (Table 7-1B). Three-dimensional airway CT has been used to assess endobronchial lesions and, although secondary invasion is the most common indi-

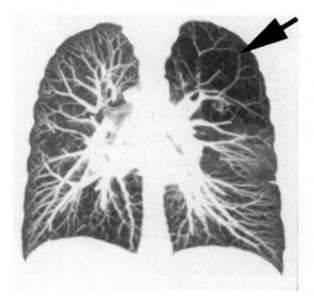

FIG. 7–4. Volume-rendered AP view of bronchial atresia with a paucity of lung markings noted in the left upper lung (*arrow*).

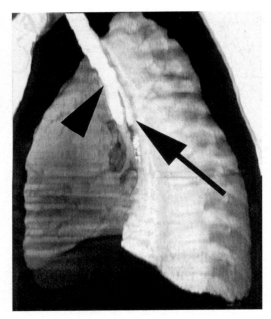

FIG. 7–5. Lateral volume-rendered perspective. A pouch remnant (*arrow*) of congenital tracheoesophageal-fistula (TEF) repair is noted arising from the posterior trachea (*arrowhead*).

cation, it has been performed for a wide range of conditions, such as primary neoplasms, metastatic disease, and broncholith erosion (35,48,49).

Three-dimensional-airway CT findings are quite nonspecific for isolated filling defects and cannot reliably differ-

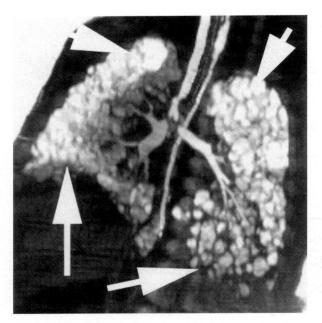

FIG. 7–6. Whole lung volume-rendered perspective demonstrates the cystic changes of bronchopulmonary dysplasia (*arrows*).

TABLE 7–1A. *Congenital airway anomalies*

Laryngotracheobronchomalacia
Complete cartilage rings
Vascular rings/slings
Accessory or anomalous bronchi, situs anomalies
Tracheal/bronchial atresia
Tracheobronchomegally (Mounier Khun/ cystic fibrosis)
Tracheo-esophageal fistula
Bronchogenic duplication cysts
Masses, e.g., hemangioma, laryngeal papillomata

TABLE 7–1B. Tracheobronchial filling defects—differential

Pseudotumor (mucus)
Foreign body
Web
Primary malignant neoplasm, e.g., squamous cell, adenoid cystic carcinoma, adenocarcinoma, carcinoid
Primary benign neoplasm, e.g., hemangioma, papilloma, chondroma, fibrovascular polyp, bronchial adenoma
Direct invasion, e.g., esophageal, thyroid, bronchogenic carcinoma
Multiple defects, e.g., metastases (melanoma), larygotracheal papillomatosis

TABLE 7–1C. Tracheobronchial stenosis-differential

Extrinsic
Mediastinal mass
Goiter, thymic carcinoma
Bronchogenic carcinoma
Radiation fibrosis, fibrosing mediastinitis
Rings and slings
Intrinsic
Post-intubation granulation tissue
Trauma/toxic insult, infection
Tracheomalacia, intubation, radiation
Complete cartilage ring
Tracheal thickening (see above)
Inflammation-epidermolysis bullosa
Primary carcinoma
Transplant or reconstruction anastamosis

TABLE 7–1D. Tracheal wall-thickening—differential

Relapsing polychondritis
Amyloid
Tracheopathia osteochrondroplastica
Sarcoid
Wegener's
Toxic inhalation
Infection, e.g., TB

entiate mucous (pseudomass) from benign or malignant masses (8,53). Sensitivity to tumor generally is limited to detecting lesions that distort the caliber or lumen of airways, rather than submucosal or superficial spreading neoplasms (53,78). Reformations parallel to an airway may be more sensitive to detect irregularities from early peribronchial-tumor invasion, and perspectives perpendicular to the airway better demonstrate thin weblike filling defects (e.g., tracheal web) (Figure 7-7). Volume rendering usually is employed for accurate localization and enumeration of filling defects and to define any transmural extent. The 3D interpretation

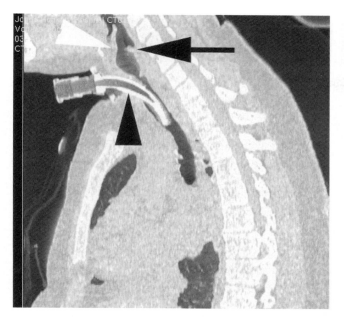

FIG. 7–7. Volume-rendered lateral view of a supraglottic web (*arrow*) occurring superior to a tracheostomy (*arrowhead*).

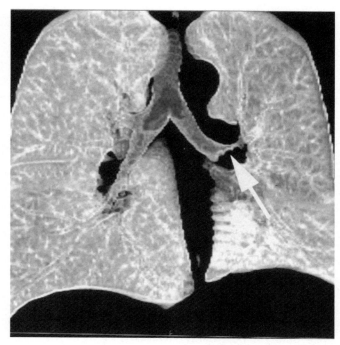

FIG. 7–9. Volume-rendered AP view of filling defects (*arrow*) in the left upper-lobe bronchus due to melanoma metastases.

provides measurements from landmarks that can be cross referenced to plain films, fluoroscopy, or endoscopy, and may increase the pulmonologist's confidence in CT interpretation (50,53) and aid the radiation oncologist in planning the therapeutic field (Figures 7–8 and 7–9)(79). Broncholiths may be identified and removed at endoscopy, but it is important to document any extraluminal attachment to pulmonary vessels on 2D and 3D CT to surgically avoid catastrophic hemorrhage (Figure 7-10). Three-dimensional renderings can evaluate the trachea site for possible resection and reconstruction after tracheoesophageal fistula repair (Figure 7-11).

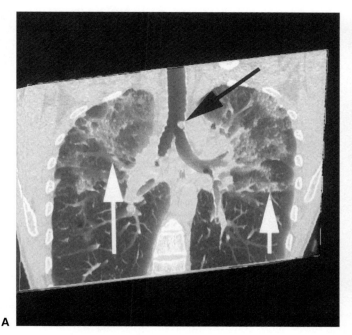

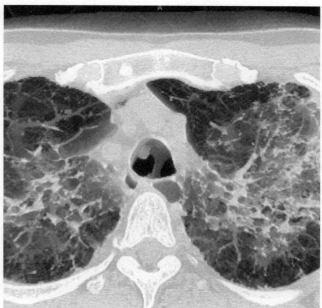

FIG. 7–8. A: Volume-rendered AP view of a polyp (*black arrow*) in the trachea. Upper lobe fibrosis noted (*white arrows*). **B:** Volume-rendered internal view of the tracheal polyp.

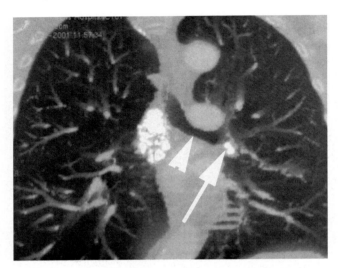

FIG. 7–10. An eroding broncholith causing hemoptysis was depicted on this volume-rendered AP view (*arrow*) at the left lower-lobe bronchus (*arrowhead*).

3D-Airway CT—Airway Stenosis

Airway stenoses may be discrete or diffuse and may be mural or extramural (Figure 7-12) in origin (Table 7-1). Three-dimensional-airway-CT imaging has been applied to the full spectrum of congenital and acquired stenosis both benign (Figures 7–13, 7–14, and 7–15)(80–86) and malignant (25,27,75,87) (Table 7-1C). Thin-section MDCT over longer areas of coverage facilitates depiction of more peripheral stenoses (88).

Etiologies resulting in airway wall thickening usually are well appreciated on 2D imaging (Table 7-1D). However, discrete or subtle airway tapering may not be appreciated on axial planar imaging alone, particularly in airways oblique to the imaging plane (Figure 7-16). In particular, measuring the length and cross-sectional area of the stenosis, as well as its distance from anatomical landmarks, is difficult with both 2D planar CT and endoluminal-endoscopic views. These measurements are best made with customized clip planes along the individual airway and true orthogonal projections (Figure 7-17) (26,34,37,42,43). Three-dimensional-CT interpretation involves comprehensive description of the number of lesions, their whole-lung distribution, wall thickness, and extraluminal relationships, together with the length of lesions and their degree of lumen compromise (27,43,78). Multiplanar reconstruction and MinIP reformatting do provide additional information to the 2D study (26,34,37), but VR is preferred for more complex pathologies (34,42). For high-grade stenosis, this 3D information is assimilated with 2D data to assess the lung parenchyma beyond and, in particular, air trapping and the likelihood of reexpansion of a postobstructive collapse once the stenosis has been relieved. Signs of drowned lung with fluid-filled bronchi or areas of necrosis imply that reexpansion is less likely and indicates that aggressive interventions are unwarranted. Customized multidimensional images are used to assess better the response or progression of inflammatory airway conditions, such as Wegener's granulomatosis (84) or post-lung-transplant stenoses (80), through consistent serial-tailored reconstructions. Similarly, volume-rendered images can provide

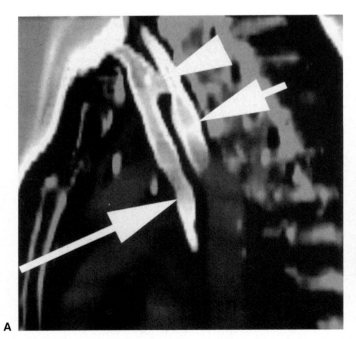

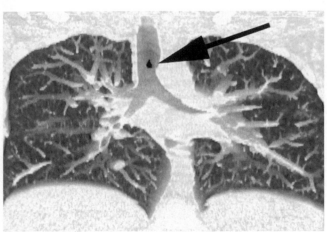

A **B**

FIG. 7–11. A: Volume-rendered lateral view of a TEF (*arrowhead*) between trachea (*long arrow*) and esophagus (*short arrow*) secondary to squamous-cell carcinoma. **B:** Volume-rendered AP view of the ostium of the TEF (*black arrow*).

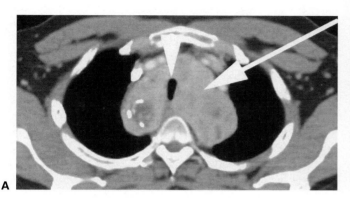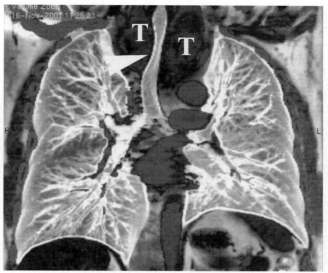

A   B

FIG. 7–12. A: Axial 2D view of a large substernal goiter (*long arrow*) causing tracheal narrowing (*arrowhead*). **B:** Volume-rendered AP view showing the relation of the goiter (*T*) to the narrowed trachea (*arrowhead*).

objective and reproducible evidence of response to bronchoscopic interventions such as tumor shaving or laser photocoagulation, electrocautery, or cryotherapy.

3D-Airway CT—Airway Stents

There is an increasing role for self-expandable metal endoprostheses to restore and maintain airway patency (84,89–91) in patients with major airway obstruction. Air-

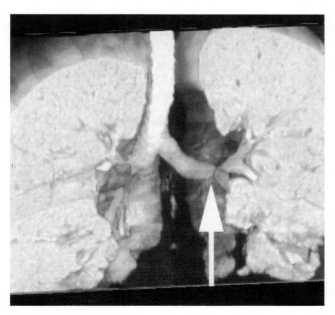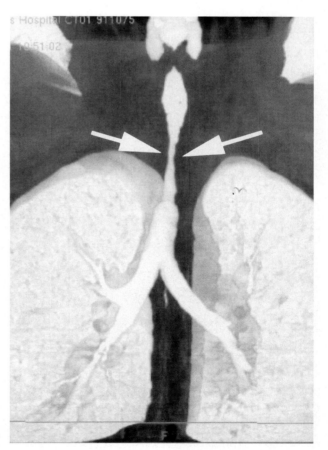

FIG. 7–13. Focal stricture of the left bronchial anastomosis (*arrow*) seen on volume-rendered images of this transplant patient.

FIG. 7–14. A long segment tracheal stenosis occurred secondary to chemical inhalation in this patient and is seen on a volume-rendered AP view (*arrows*).

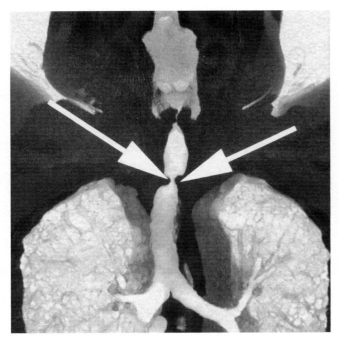

FIG. 7–15. A volume-rendered AP view with solid trapezoid shows a focal annular-subglottic stenosis (*arrows*).

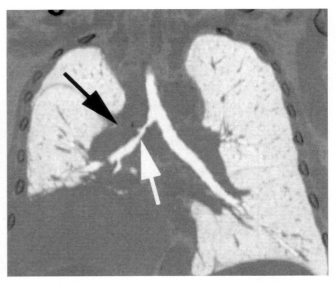

FIG. 7–17. Malignant irregularity and narrowing of the right lower-lobe bronchus (*white arrow*) is seen on a volume-rendered image of this patient with a right hilar mass (*black arrow*). Note the right-lung volume loss.

way CT has been used widely for assessing cancer patients for such stents (87) and for those patients with nonneoplastic airway disease (e.g., following chemical aspiration and anastamotic strictures in lung-transplantation recipients) (30). Three-dimensional-airway CT helps identify suitable patients and has replaced conventional bronchography in this role (23). Once planar CT has established that there is sal-

vageable lung parenchyma, the main questions to be answered by a 3D-airway study are: i) the distance from the cricoid or carina to beyond the stenosis and ii) the likelihood of the bronchoscopist being able to traverse the stenosis. Once the patient is selected, the scan aids in the choice of optimal stent design and size (92). After a stent has been placed, an immediate 3D CT documents the baseline positioning and reexpansion, often better than an endoluminal approach. It then is possible to reproduce the same imaging

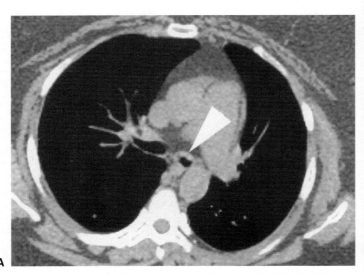

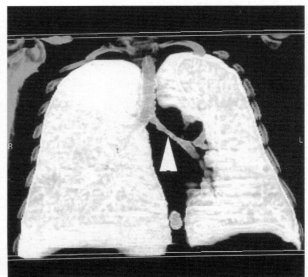

A B

FIG. 7–16. A: Axial 2D planar image of thickened left lower lobe bronchus due to Wegener's granulomatosis. B: The long segment nature of the stenosis is appreciated on this volume-rendered AP view (*arrowhead*).

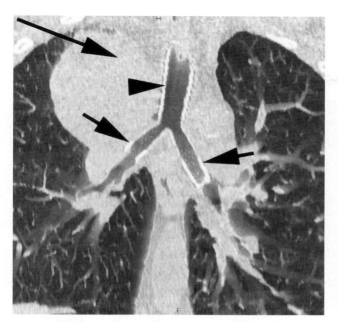

FIG. 7–18. Tracheal (*arrowhead*) and bilateral bronchial (*short arrows*) stents were placed in this patient to palliate an encroaching right-lung mass (*long arrow*).

perspective in a series of studies so that any subtle migration or collapse of the stent can be detected and quantified. Similarly, any stent-lumen compromise due to benign granulation tissue or tumor encroachment may be seen, so that bronchoscopy then may be reserved for those cases where CT suggests intervention for salvage is indicated (Figures 7–18 and 7–19).

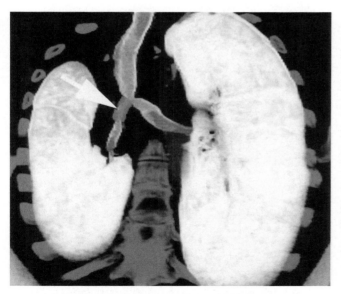

FIG. 7–19. Right lung-volume loss and airway irregularity is noted in this patient on a volume-rendered AP view. A short stent has been placed at the origin of the right lower-lobe bronchus (*arrow*).

3D-Airway CT—Airway Bronchiectasis

Bronchiectasis is a permanent abnormal dilatation of the airway and CT examination and is part of the diagnostic work up (72). Transient dilatation can be seen in the setting of an acute inflammatory process. It may be congenital (Mounier–Khun, cystic fibrosis) or acquired. Acquired conditions include infection [e.g., *Mycobacterium avium-intracellulare* (MAI), allergic bronchopulmonary aspergillosis (ABPA)], and traction from adjacent fibrosis (e.g., radiation) or usual interstitial pneumonitis. Volumetric helical CT is quite advantageous for diagnosing bronchiectasis (93,94) and when characterization of bronchiectatic change is limited with axial planar interpretation alone. Transparent bronchography-like images are used to depict the bronchiectatic change alone, and classic lung-parenchyma trapezoids show the bronchiectasis in relation to other lung disorders, such as interstitial diseases. Unlike airway stenosis, bronchiectasis is more commonly a multisegmental process, and for this reason the 3D volume rendered whole-lung images are well suited to mapping the extent of the disease process. In patients with cystic fibrosis, for example, the distribution of disease and its relative severity in different lung locations can be depicted better with selected oblique coronal and sagittal views. Whole-lung display with clip planes oriented along airways of interest is optimal for appreciation of bronchiectatic change in an individual airway or segment of lung. This approach also may be valuable in the future to assess better response to therapies (42,43) and to map localized disease for possible resection (Figure 7-20).

3D CT and Diffuse Lung Disease

Many diffuse lung diseases can affect the lung in variable but characteristic patterns of distribution between the upper and lower lobes and can be quite asymmetric between lungs. Some conditions such as bronchiolitis obliterans and organizing pneumonia (BOOP) may demonstrate spontaneous temporal change in distribution, and involved areas may change their imaging features in response to therapy or due to disease progression. An appreciation of whole or partial lung distribution of such diseases readily is apparent with coronal and sagittal reformatted images that display the abnormal and normal lung in a single image (Figures 7–21, 7–22, and 7–23). Subtle disease that may not be apparent on axial images may become more conspicuous when, for example, upper-lung-predominant disease is seen on the same imaging slice as normal lower lung. For interstitial lung disease, volume-rendered classic lung-parenachyma-like settings are useful for appreciating the distribution of disease, and MinIP images display the low densities of centrilobular emphysema, cysts, air trapping, or ground glass opacities (GGOs) (Figures 7–24, 7–25, 7–26, and 7–27) (93,95,96). Minimum-intensity projections can be applied to MPRs or to user-defined sliding slabs of data, which reduce data from a greater proportion of lung to a single slice that

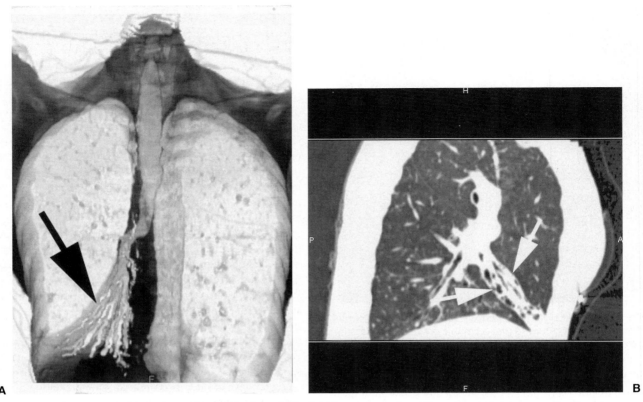

FIG. 7–20. A: Volume-rendered AP view of the right lung shows focal bronchiectatic change affecting the right middle lobe (*arrow*). **B:** Volume-rendered right lateral view of the focal bronchiectasis in the right middle lobe (classic lung trapezoid).

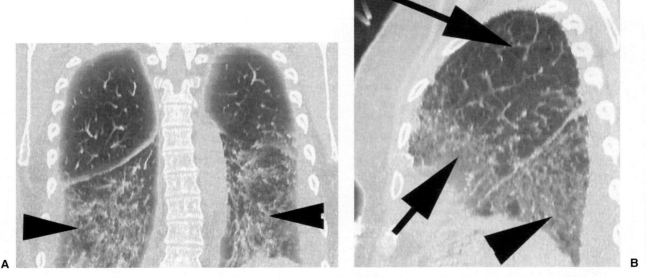

FIG. 7–21. A: Volume-rendered AP view of interstitial fibrosis predominantly affecting both lower lobes (*arrowheads*). **B:** Volume-rendered left lateral view of interstitial fibrosis in the lingula (*short arrow*) and left lower lobe (*arrowhead*) with relative sparing of the upper lung (*long arrow*).

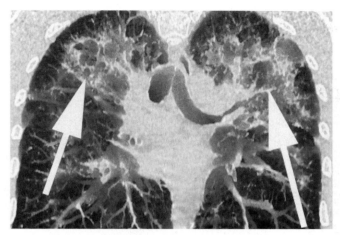

FIG. 7–22. Volume-rendered AP view with interstitial fibrosis mainly in an upper lung distribution (*arrows*).

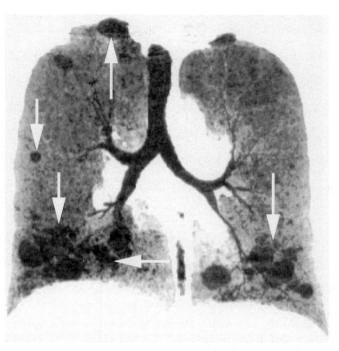

FIG. 7–24. Cystic change due to tuberous sclerosis is depicted on this AP MinIP (*arrows*).

may be more sensitive (95–98). Remy-Jardin et al. have suggested that MIPs may increase sensitivity to centrilobular-micronodular change and may delineate better their location in the secondary pulmonary lobule compared with high-resolution CT (95). Prone, supine, and dynamic inspiratory and expiratory images are performed, which then can be reformatted into 3D for direct comparison. Together with multidimensional nuclear ventilation and perfusion imaging with dynamic volume measurements, CT ultimately may provide a comprehensive morphological, functional, and quantitative (99–101) evaluation (25,99,101,102) of the entire lung with information on distribution of disease, gas transfer, and perfusion derangements (103). When lung-vol-

ume-reduction surgery is considered, 3D reformatted images can be consulted when contemplating removal of an anatomic area of air trapping (104).

3D CT—Focal Lung Disease

There is currently great interest in assessing the role of MDCT in screening for lung nodules in the hope of reducing

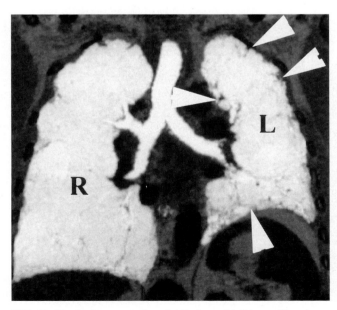

FIG. 7–23. Volume-rendered AP view of left lung (*L*) volume loss in this right lung (*R*) transplant recipient. Note the septal lines (*arrowheads*).

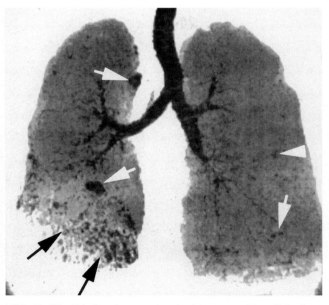

FIG. 7–25. Cystic change due to honeycombing (*black arrows*) is noted in the right lower lung on this AP view MinIP.

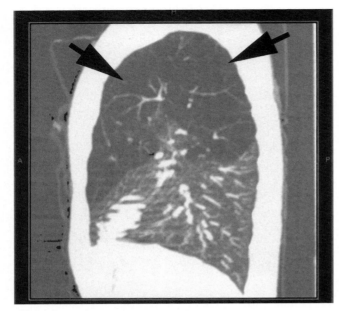

FIG. 7–26. Upper-lobe predominant emphysema is seen on this right lateral volume-rendered view (*arrows*) with paucity of lung markings.

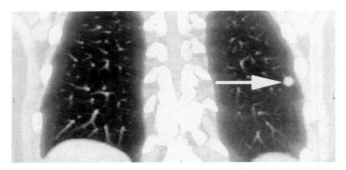

FIG. 7–28. Coronal volume-rendered view of a discrete left lung nodule (*arrow*).

lung-cancer mortality (105,106). Differentiating benign nodules from malignant nodules involves assessment of the morphology, density, activity (fluorodeoxyglucose uptake), temporal change, and contrast dynamics. However, in smaller lung nodules, much of the 2D morphological features of malignancy are not present, and other features must be looked to. Three-dimensional CT images may be a useful

adjunct to whole body positron-emission tomography (PET) and CT PET images to localize abnormal activity for diagnostic accuracy, and to help plan resection when indicated (Figures 7–28, 7–29, and 7–30). Often, nodules are not perfect spheres, and measurement differences between 2D and 3D may have significant clinical impact. Three-dimensional segmentation has been shown to have the spatial resolution to measure accurately nodule volumes within 3% and to detect volumetric change for doubling times 30 day to 180 days and nodules larger than 5 mm (107). Furthermore, it has been suggested these volume measurements may be more consistent with final pathology than 2D techniques (107) and may be better suited to longitudinal follow up to assess for potential malignancy and response to therapy.

For tissue diagnosis, 3D CT further exploits the "CT bronchus sign," facilitating the path into lesions far in the periphery (108,109) and choosing safe avenues for tissue

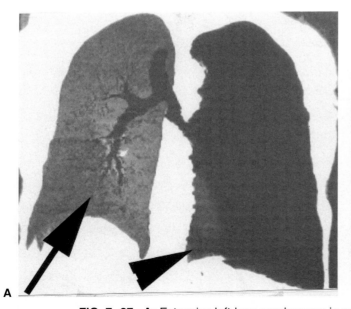

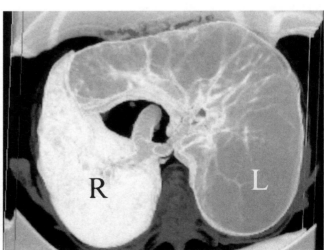

FIG. 7–27. **A:** Extensive left-lung emphysema is noted on this MinIP view (*arrowhead*) compared with the normal right lung (*arrow*). **B:** The extensive left lung emphysema (*L*) has caused marked hyperinflation compared with the right (*R*) side.

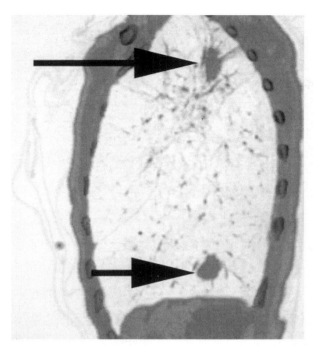

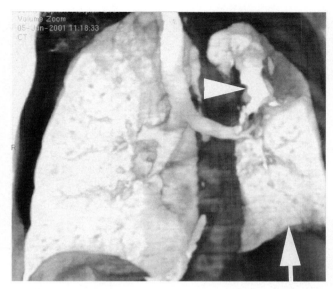

FIG. 7–31. The relation of this cavitary mass (*arrowhead*) in the left lung (*arrow*) to the left airway is seen on this volume-rendered view.

FIG. 7–29. Two synchronous lung masses are depicted on this left lateral volume-rendered view in the upper (*long arrow*) and lower lungs (*short arrow*).

sampling for transbronchial-biopsy sampling (85,86), with identification of the shortest needle path into mediastinal nodes and those nodes amenable to endoscopic ultrasound-guided biopsy. Computed tomography may help identify those with small lung nodules who more likely would benefit from either bronchoscopic tissue sampling or percutaneous approach (108,109). It also has been suggested that VB guid-

ance of ultrathin bronchoscopes may improve the accuracy and duration of conventional bronchosopy for peripheral lung lesions (110). Three-dimensional renderings designed to depict medial lung neoplasms are more intuitive for assessing suitability for sleeve resection, showing the tumor in relation to the bronchus or pulmonary vessels in their entirety, together with the medial extent of tumor (Figure 7-31). If a patient has poor respiratory reserve, the 3D CT can be interpreted with the ventilation perfusion for anatomic segmentation to quantify what proportion of normal lung will be removed by tumor resection and what lung-parenchyma-preserving approaches are feasible (111,112). Although once the preserve of magnetic-resonance imaging (MRI), current coronal and sagittal 3D images can define equally superior sulcus tumors, differentiate basal lung tumor from hepatic dome masses, and demonstrate the distribution of mesothelioma (Figures 7–32 and 7–33). Radiation

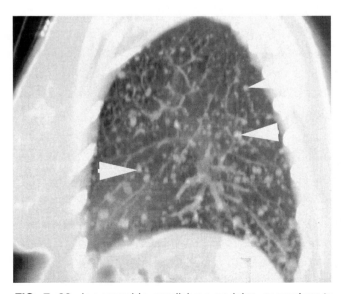

FIG. 7–30. Innumerable small lung nodules secondary to cervical cancer metastases are seen in a whole-lung distribution on this left lateral volume-rendered view (*arrowheads*).

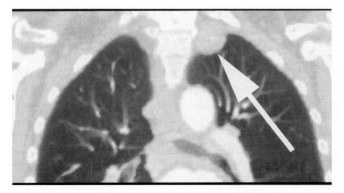

FIG. 7–32. An apical lesion (nerve-sheath tumor) (*arrow*) is best depicted on this AP volume-rendered view.

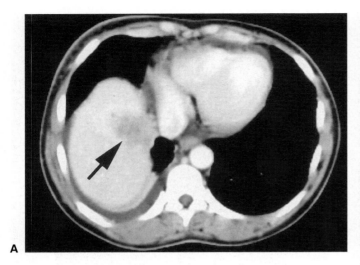

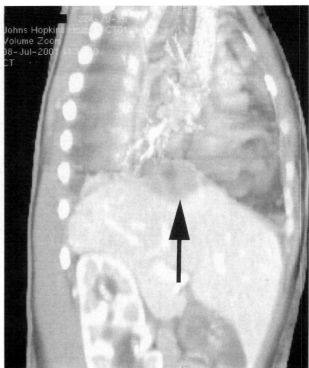

FIG. 7–33. A: A base of lung mass appears as an intrahepatic lesion (*arrow*) on this axial 2D view. **B:** A right lateral volume-rendered view shows the mass to be in the base of lung impinging upon the liver (*arrow*).

therapy requires an anatomically accurate field for focal lung disease (113), and images have been found useful (79) in planning the portal for delivery of external-beam irradiation by providing measurements and thoracic landmarks that then can be applied to a conventional radiograph to maximize tumor dose and minimize injury to normal tissue.

3D CT—Chest Wall and Diaphragm

The orientation of the bone and muscle of the chest wall is not seen well with 2D imaging, and the specific ribs and their orientation are difficult to localize, so that any deformity of curvature is hard to appreciate or measure. Three-dimensional chest-wall CT is requested to evaluate congenital abnormalities, such as *pectus excavatum* or "acquired Jeune's syndrome" (114), or resection and reconstruction of chest-wall tumors, such as direct invasion of lung carcinoma, primary-rib osteosarcoma, or infection (Figures 7–34 and 7–35) (114–117). Optimal trauma renderings, such as for sternal or clavicle fractures, are seen better on sagittal or coronal reconstructions, respectively, and multidimensional views have been favored for diaphragm imaging, including cases of rupture (Figure 7–36) (118–120). Color trapezoids can depict better sternotomy repairs (Figure 7-37). Volume rendering is preferred over MIP or SSD, as it preserves the densities of costochondral cartilage, bone, and muscle, and does not require laborious editing (116, 121–123).

PART II. AORTIC DISSECTION

Aortic Dissection—Introduction

The aorta has limited ways of manifesting disease states, and although penetrating atherosclerotic ulcer, intra-

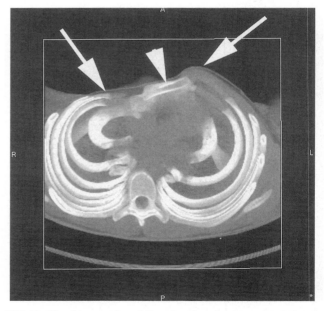

FIG. 7–34. Asymmetry of the chest wall (*arrows*) relative to the sternum (*arrowhead*) is seen on this volume-rendered inferior view.

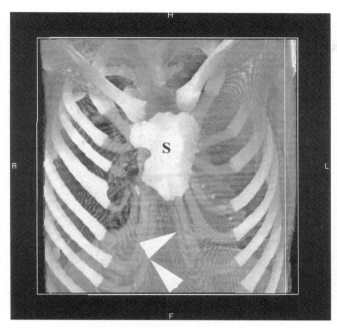

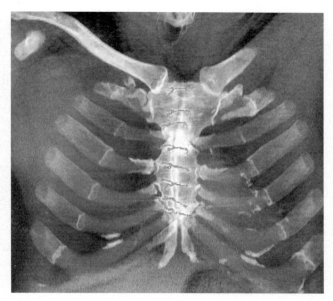

FIG. 7–37. Sternotomy wires are depicted on a volume-rendered AP view with color trapezoid.

FIG. 7–35. Sternal anomaly (*S*) noted on this AP volume-rendered view. Costochondral cartilages (*arrowheads*).

mural hematoma, and classic aortic dissection each can represent distinct pathological entities, their clinical assessment is imprecise and their pathophysiology and morphological expression clearly lie upon an imaging spectrum (124–128). Transesophageal echo (TEE), MRI, and CT all have proven efficacious in aortic-dissection imaging, but CT is the initial test in two thirds of cases and is the second test in the majority of those who have multimodality evaluation (129–133). The accessibility of CT, together with its rapid and accurate evaluation, has changed the understanding of aortic-dissection disease and may have reduced its mortality (134–137). Multidetector-CT acquisition and VRT permit high-quality CT angiography (CTA) of aortic dissection through volume-data acquisition and interpretation (5,6,39,138–142).

Aortic Dissection—MDCT-Imaging Technique and Protocols

Careful attention to patient preparation is important for optimal image quality to confirm or exclude dissection. Possible sources of beam-hardening artifact should be removed from the field of view with alternate placement of metallic leads and placement of the arms above the head. Eighteen- to twenty-two-gauge venous access through a *right* antecubital vein is preferred for power injection of contrast that causes minimal opacification of the left brachiocephalic vein as it crosses the aortic arch. Femoral-vein injection (143) also has been advocated for this reason, but is less favored by patients.

Routine coverage for thoracic aortic-dissection CT is from the celiac axis to the proximal great vessels with a caudal-to-cranial scan direction, which allows for some clearance of high-density contrast from the upper thoracic veins (144). The superior field may be extended if there is concern for carotid involvement. Likewise, when there is concern for further dissection propagation below the diaphragm and organ involvement, or if there are plans for an endovascular approach, the scanning range is extended inferiorly. Unlike single-detector systems, the high pitch of

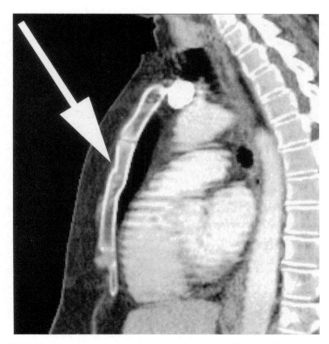

FIG. 7–36. An occult sternal fracture on 2D axial images is seen on sagittal MPR (*arrow*).

MDCT and the heat-loading capacity of its ceramic detectors permits imaging from the aortic arch to the femoral vessels in a single acquisition while still within peak contrast enhancement (145). If abdominopelvic imaging is performed, negative oral contrast is preferred to aid post processing.

Noncontrast studies are not performed as a matter of routine, but they have value in discriminating displaced intimal calcification, displaying high-density acute intramural hematoma, or depicting acute mediastinal or pleural blood. Most of these diagnoses will not be missed, however, with careful evaluation of a contrast-enhanced study. On occasion, noncontrast studies are requested to assess the extent of atherosclerosis prior to placing an intraaortic balloon pump, or when cross clamping the aorta is anticipated. Noncontrast studies are recommended for endovascular stent follow up to assess for endoleak. When used, dose exposure for noncontrast studies may be reduced with 10-mm slice widths, 2-mm to 3-mm interslice gaps and high pitch values ($\sim$1.7–2.0), and low mAs ($\sim$50 mA–80 mA) (140,143, 146,147).

Computed-tomography angiography for aortic dissection is performed with 200 mA to 300 mA and 120 kV to 140 kV, depending on patient size. A maximum 1 cc/kg of 350-mg/L iodinated nonionic contrast is administered at a rate of 3 cc to 5 cc/second (140,143,148–151) with a power injector for optimal lumen opacification. Timing is a critical factor in accurate dissection interpretation. Larger contrast volumes or a saline chaser (151) do prolong the contrast plateau, but with fast MDCT acquisition, bolus timing is not necessary, even for iliofemoral-vessel visualization, unless there is large-body habitus. Two hundred HU measurements have been found with doses as low as 80 cc (152), and further refinement of MDCT techniques promises decreased contrast doses (140,146,153). The initial HU within the aorta rises linearly with early injection. The contrast plateau is, in fact, an asymmetric hump formed during continued injection combined with the onset of contrast recirculation. After the total volume has been administered, there is a precipitous fall in density of the true lumen as slower opacification in the false lumen or systemic veins develops (131,148–150, 154,155). The high injection rates do give high arterial contrast (148–150), and although they do shorten the acquisition-time window, this is not usually a problem with the fast data acquisition of MDCT. A minimum true-lumen-contrast plateau of 2 to 300 HU (143,156) should be placed consistently within the MDCT-scan duration of 13 seconds to 20 seconds (144) using an empiric scan delay of 25 seconds to 30 seconds from the start of injection. Approximately 4-second scan delays are added for perceived diminished-cardiac output (148–150), manual injections (e.g., central lines), or injections in the far periphery, such as the foot. Injection rates should be slowed for tenuous access or access in tight limb compartments (e.g., dorsum of hand). A timed bolus can be designed from a time–density curve obtained from a 10-cc to 20-cc test bolus administered at 4 cc/s to 5 cc/s, with sequential single-level imaging every 2 seconds

after an 8-second delay (157). Although a tailored test bolus (157) or automated bolus tracking and triggering (140, 143,151,156) and tailored multiphasic-injections techniques (154,158–160) are advocated by some, and do give some numerical improvement in consistency, uniformity, and duration of opacification, they require additional contrast and radiation dose (17). Empiric delays will suffice in most cases for consistent opacification (161,162) and delineation of a dissection flap. The peak opacification level may be increased by increasing the rate of contrast administration or increased iodine concentration, but there is little to be gained diagnostically with attenuation values greater than 300 HU. Indeed, in many cases, the MDCT capture of the bolus is so good that the windows need to be adjusted from the conventional settings so as not to miss the flap. Seventy-second delayed post-contrast imaging is performed to assess for delayed flow in the false lumen or graft leak.

Multidetector CT continues to build on the advances in breath-hold imaging made with slip-ring technology (5,6,14–17,163–166). Rubin et al. have shown that multidetector systems benefit CTA of the arterial system in terms of scan duration, contrast use, thinner sections, and cost savings (153) in comparison with single-detector systems. Multidetector CT provides improved z-axis spatial resolution for similar coverage and extended coverage for smaller resolution (1,3,5,6,22). Smaller slice widths and high pitch values provide higher-quality images than larger slice widths with smaller pitch. Fusion of small slices into a broader slice minimizes the artifact of wider slice widths and diminishes interslice misregistration. For optimal 2D imaging and for a good 3D substrate, a beam collimated to four 1-mm detectors of an adaptive-array design ($\sim$ four 1.25-mm matrix-array detectors) is employed to provide 1.25-mm slice thickness with overlapping 1-mm reconstruction interval and a 25 cm to 30 cm field of view (165). The higher MDCT pitch values (pitch defined as table increment per gantry rotation divided by single-slice collimation) required for aortic imaging come without the single-detector penalty in widened slice-sensitivity profile and effective slice width through (167) the use of multiple detectors and weighted interpolation (3,4). Temporal resolution of 130 ms to 250 ms is attainable with simultaneous 4-detector acquisition systems, somewhat reducing pulsation artifacts. The dissection flap is clearly defined by a 512 in-plane matrix and narrow z-axis resolution. Tube current and patient-dose exposure is modulated according to body habitus, with diminished dose for anteroposterior imaging compared to transverse imaging. The penumbra of focal spot wobble of the MDCT cone beam of wasted irradiation is reduced proportionally with the use of larger detector arrays, such as 16-detector compared with 4-detector systems. Near isotropic data with overlapping reconstruction suffices for most dissection evaluations with 4-detector systems, although 16-detector designs likely will permit routine true-isotropic data with 0.5-mm detectors. For patients who are poor breath-holders, or for those in whom greater coverage is required, 2.5-mm detectors can be used, and the image quality still is better than with single-detector systems. For hard-copy interpretation, larger slice widths are assimilated from smaller ones to limit the amount of film required for the 500 to 600 slices acquired. Data are sent to both a PACS workstation for scrolling and a 3D workstation for post processing.

Aortic-dissection CT-image Processing and Data Evaluation

Three-dimensional CTA has become a useful adjunct to a well-performed 2D CT for dissection evaluation (31,32,144,166,168,169). Whatever post-processing techniques are employed to generate 3D CTA, they must be real time (frame rate over 20F/s) without laborious editing for clinical practicality, and current options include: MPR and CMPR reconstructions, MIP, SSD, and VRT (10,44,45,140, 166,170,171). Multiplanar and CMPR techniques are on many CT consoles and require minimal computer power (140). These are not true 3D techniques, but rather a reordering of voxels into a tomographic section, which can be of value, but often are limited by a tortuous nonplanar aorta and dissection flap (169). Maximum-intensity projection (172) displays only density values above a chosen threshold and reduces the length of data encountered by the ray to a single plane. Maximum-intensity projection is similar to digital-subtraction angiography (DSA) projectional technique and lacks depth cues without movement. Maximum-intensity projection also may be problematic in evaluating complex-enhancing mediastinal vascular structures. The chest wall must be edited from the projection or it will be included in the reconstruction of the vessels. Shaded-surface display will reconstruct the data of an assigned interface through polygon building blocks and uses lighting models for perspective. Both MIP and SSD use only 10% to 20% of the acquired data, but they will obscure the intimal flap and internal lumen information on thrombus burden (169).

Volume-rendered techniques now are preferred for 3D CTA of dissection (39,44,45,138,140–142). This method is of high fidelity to the original dataset, and all density values are preserved in the final segmentation (10,40,44, 45). Since VR uses a percentage-based classification of the values encountered by the ray, including the intimal flap, slow flow, or thrombus, is represented, as well as areas of volume averaging. Areas of interest such as intimal calcification, thrombus, and flaps are highlighted through trapezoid-histogram manipulation of the level, width, opacity, and brightness (171). Multidetector-CT acquisition, together with infinite VRT clip-planes editing, projections, and trapezoids, permits visualization of the differential aortic enhancement, the dissection flap, and branch vessels with perspectives that are independent of the acquisition plane and tailored to the individual patient. When there are associated aneurysms, true orthogonal measurement can be obtained and consistent reproducible views can be generated for follow-up studies. Although endoscopic modes for 3D display can be per-

formed, they may not add to the 2D interpretation (141,173). Conventional perspectives such as anterior and left-anterior oblique views, which the surgeons are used to, are produced routinely. These are supplemented with the unique tailored views for the individual patient and include information on branch vessels and end-organ supply where indicated. With 3D post processing, surgical consultation with simulation of the possible approaches to therapy becomes part of routine practice, and tables of required-operative measurements become standard.

Dissection Epidemiology and Pathophysiology

As the body ages, the elastic fibers of the aorta fragment and the smooth muscle cells diminish in number with increasing collagen fibers and mucoid ground substance, resulting in multidimensional dilatation (ectasia). Atherosclerosis results in lipid deposition, fibrosis, and calcification of the *tunica intima*, with underlying *tunica media* atrophy (128).

A classic aortic dissection is defined as a disruption of the aortic wall, forming an intimal flap and therefore separating into a true and false lumen (135,174). It is the most common life-threatening disease of the aorta, with rupture occurring twice as often as with aneurysms (175). Most risk factors for dissection are those entities that cause weakening of the aortic wall (Table 7-2A). Ninety percent of patients are hypertensive, which increases transmural pressure and may lead to aortic sclerosis and stiffer vessels more vulnerable to wall stress (134,135,146). Other risk factors include congenital abnormalities (connective-tissue disorders, valve abnormalities, cystic-medial necrosis), atherosclerosis [Penetrating atherosclerotic ulcer (PAU) or intramural hematoma (IMH)], inflammation (176), toxic agents (e.g., cocaine)(177), trauma [acute traumatic aortic injury (ATAI) or iatrogenic] (178,179), third trimester of pregnancy (180), and more rare conditions, such as neurofibromatosis (181). Fewer than 10% of Marfans patients suffer dissection, but it accounts for a large proportion of their deaths. Traumatic-deceleration dissections tend to occur at points of fixation, such as the aortic root or isthmus, and account for up to 20% of high-speed-deceleration fatalities (182). Iatrogenic etiologies are due largely to catheter manipulation, cardiac bypass, balloon pump, or cross clamping. Aortic dissection is not thought to be related to atherosclerosis unless it is the sequela of PAU or IMH. This explains its preponderance in the relatively atherosclerosis-free ascending aorta (174,183). Dissection is considered acute if diagnosed within 14 days of symptom onset; dissections diagnosed beyond 14 days are considered chronic (184). It has a population prevalence of 0.5 to 2.95/100,000/year with an incidence of 2.95/100,000 (185–187). The mortality is 3.25 to 3.6 deaths 100,000, three times higher in men than women, with a high acute mortality of 1.4% per hour. The overall mortality rate is 21% within the first 24 hours, 60% within 2 weeks, and 90% within 3 months (188–191). Eighty percent of deaths are due to aortic rupture, with tamponade, massive aortic regurgitation, and coronary or carotid compromise accounting for the rest. Thinning of the aortic wall, aneurysmal dilatation, hypertensive transmural pressure, and cystic medial necrosis associated with dissection are all factors that can predispose to rupture according to the Law of Laplace. Aortic rupture is found in 0.9% of cases of sudden death, and 62% of these patients are found to have dissection (192).

Dissection usually begins in the thoracic aortic as a transverse intimal tear involving 25% to 50% of the circumference (128). Primary abdominal dissections are rare except for iatrogenic etiologies. There may be an entry site and a more distal reentry site; there also may be multiple sites, allowing multidirectional flow (193) with a pressure gradient of 10 mmHg to 25 mmHg (135). Blood flow and dissection propagation tend to be antegrade, and reentry tears are common in the abdominal aorta or iliac vessels. Retrograde dissection occurs in fewer than 20% of patients (194). The fibrous pericardium blends with the ascending aortic wall, and both the ascending arch and pulmonary trunk are contained within a common sleeve of serous pericardium. The distal extent of a dissection flap is thought to be limited by atherosclerosis, media scarring or atrophy, and branch points or coarctation (128,183). In Marfan patients with limited scarring of the aorta, it is common to find the entire aorta involved.

The false lumen is located in the outer half of the media, giving a thinner outer wall than inner wall (128), and it has high pressure and wall stress (135). Since the outer wall of the false lumen lacks smooth muscle, it tends to be larger and to compress the true lumen. False-lumen flow is quite variable and may be less than or equal to the true lumen, or thrombosed. Rarely does it have greater flow than the true lumen. Although the false lumen may provide blood flow to organs, thrombosed false lumens generally are thought to be more stable. By definition, the wall of the false lumen is thinner than the normal aorta and thus, according to the Law of Laplace, more prone to continued expansion and pseudoaneurysm formation under the influence of systemic transmural pressure. Aneurysms with communicating dissections will enlarge at a rate of 2 mm to 3 mm per year with systemic transmural pressure, and those with noncommunicating dissection will enlarge at a rate of 1 mm per year (135).

Dissection Classification

Dissections initially were categorized based on site, which largely dictates management. The Stanford classification (195) is the most widely used, where all dissections involving the ascending aorta are Type A, regardless of the site of tear or distal extent (same as DeBakey Type I/II) (196), and all dissections limited to origin beyond the left subclavian artery are Type B, regardless of distal extent [same as DeBakey Type III (196)]. The DeBakey classification further subdivided the Type-B dissections into those that involve the thoracic aorta only (IIIa) or both the thoracic and abdominal aorta (IIIb)(Table 7.2B, Figure 7-38A,B).

TABLE 7–2A. Risk factors for aortic dissection

Inherited	Connective tissue disorders (Ehlers Danlos and Marfan's syndromes)
	Polycystic kidney disease
	Annuloaortic ectasia and familial aortic dissection
	Coarctation, biscuspid or stenotic aortic valves
Inflammatory	Third trimester of pregnancy
	SLE, giant cell arteritis
	Cushing's syndrome
Toxic	Cocaine use
	Weight lifters
	Secondary to trauma iatrogenic or noniatrogenic
	Secondary to penetrating atherosclerotic ulcer or intramural hematoma

TABLE 7–2B. *Dissection Classification*

De Bakey (site)	
Type I	Ascending and descending aorta
Type II	Isolated ascending aorta
Type III	Isolated descending aorta
Type IIIa	Isolated descending thoracic aorta
Type IIIb	Isolated descending thoracic and abdominal aorta

Stanford (site)	
Type A	Ascending aorta regardless of distal extent
Type B	Isolated to descending aorta regardless of distal extent

Svensson (etiology)	
Class I	Classic aortic dissection with intimal flap between true and false lumen (communicating and non-communicating)
Class 2	Medial disruption with formation of intramural hematoma or hemorrhage (IMH)
Class 3	Discrete/subtle dissection without hematoma, eccentric bulge at tear site
Class 4	Plaque rupture leading to aortic ulceration, penetrating aortic atherosclerotic ulcer with surrounding hematoma usually adventitial
Class 5	Iatrogenic and traumatic dissection

Sixty-five percent of dissections are of the ascending aorta, with an entrance tear 2 centimeters above the sinotubular junction (128), 10% involve the arch, 20% affect the descending thoracic aorta, and 5% are abdominal. The one-year survival rate for Type-A dissections is around 30%, with 60% mortality at 24 hours (188), reflecting their greater propensity to propagate retrogradely into the pericardium, interrupting coronary- or carotid-artery flow, or massive aor-

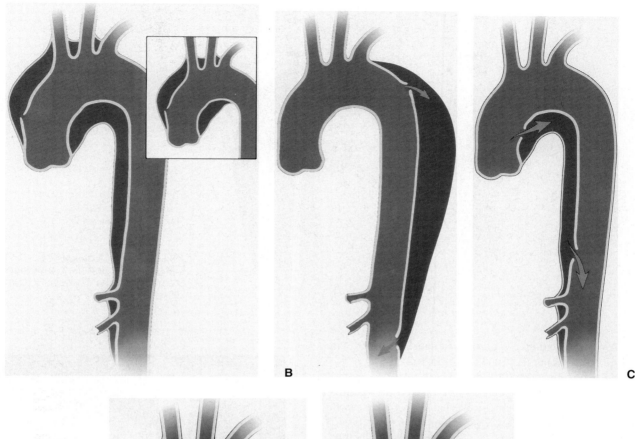

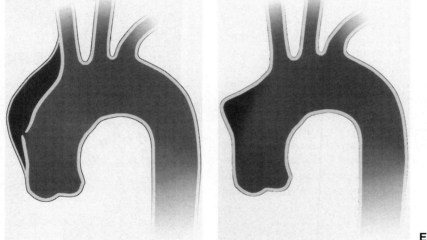

FIG. 7–38. A: Type-A dissection. An entry tear proximal to the left subclavian regardless of its distal extent. DeBakey Type I (*large figure*) and Type II (*inset figure*). **B:** Type-B dissection (DeBakey Type III). An entry tear distal to the left subclavian artery. **C:** Svenson Class I. Classic dissection with entry and reentry tears and a clear intimal flap. **D:** Svenson Class II. An intramural hematoma. No tears identified and no flowing blood in the media. **E:** Svenson Class III. A focal bulge possibly represents an abortive dissection. *(continued)*

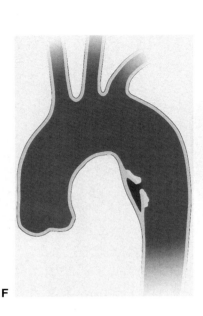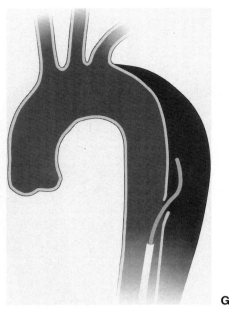

F G

FIG. 7–38. *Continued.* **F:** Svenson Class IV. Penetrating atherosclerotic ulcer. **G:** Svenson Class V. Traumatic dissection.

tic-valve regurgitation. Type-B dissections fare better, with an 85% one-year survival rate (134,135,197–199).

Svenson more recently attempted to classify dissections based on etiology in an attempt to reconcile the multiple conditions that are thought to overlap with classic aortic dissection (200) (Figure 7-38C–G). This is a useful classification for clinical interpretation, as it goes beyond the morphological system alone. Under this classification, a Class-I dissection is the classic aortic dissection with an identifiable flap and true and false lumen with or without communication of the two lumina. A Class-II dissection represents an IMH. Class-III dissections are subtle wall bulges and are thought by some to represent an abortive dissection with a subtle tear and healing thrombus overlying it. Under this classification, PAU is named a Class-IV dissection. Finally, tears in the intima due to iatrogenic or noniatrogenic trauma are assigned to Class-V dissections, although they can lead to Class-I or Class-II dissections.

Class-I, Class-III, and Class-IV Dissection—CT-Imaging Interpretation

There are two fundamental rules for aortic-dissection CT interpretation: (i) survival is related directly to the timeliness of diagnosis, and (ii) imaging always should be interpreted finally in the clinical context for correct triage and management although all suspected dissections must be treated initially as potentially fatal acute processes. A comprehensive CTA for aortic dissection permits a high degree of accuracy of diagnosis and classification, localization of tears, and documentation of the nature of false lumen flow. The status of branch vessels and the viscera or bowel must be established. The need for therapy and the type of surgical or endovascular approach are determined in large part by

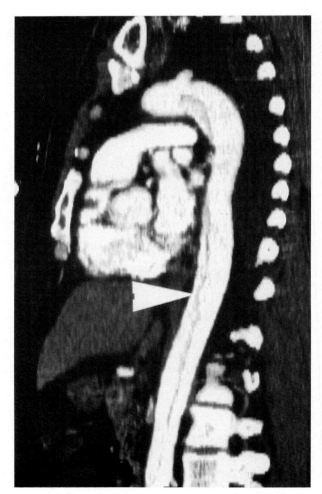

FIG. 7–39. Sagittal MPR demonstrates the intimal flap (*arrowhead*) of this Type-B dissection.

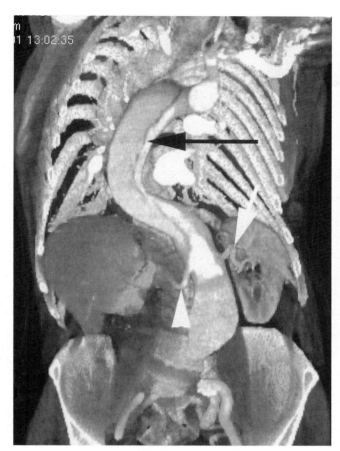

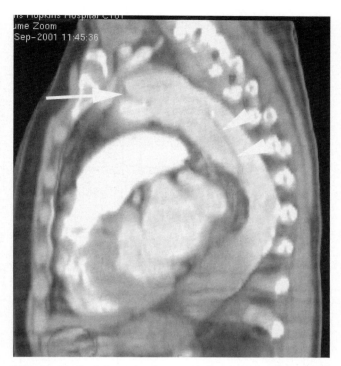

FIG. 7–41. Left lateral volume-rendered view of a Type-B dissection flap (*arrowheads*) with an origin at the left subclavian artery (*arrow*).

FIG. 7–40. Coronal volume-rendered view of a Type-B dissection shows the relationship of the false lumen (*black arrow*) to the right renal artery (*white arrowhead*) and left renal artery (*short white arrow*).

this CT interpretation. Multidetector CT and 3D volume rendering may not add greatly to the established sensitivity and specificity of single detector CT (SDCT), but they will add to the sophistication and precision of interpretation and measurements (Figures 7–39, 7–40, 7–41, 7–42, and 7–43).

The intimal flap usually appears as a single homogeneously low-density linear or curvilinear structure with or without intimal calcification. The flap can appear more complex or as more than two lumens with more extensive tears, intimal redundancy, or greater infolding (184,201). It also may appear as falsely multiple flaps due to pulsation artifact, but these usually are apparent from their parallel nature. The flap tends to spiral posterolaterally for a variable distance and can extend into and divide among the ostia of branch vessels (169,202) (Figures 7–44, 7–45, 7–46, and 7–47).

Accurate discrimination of the true and false lumen has become increasingly important with the use of interventional therapies. The true lumen is usually along the inner curvature of the aorta in continuity with the diseased aorta. It often is under lower pressure than the false lumen and thus may be compressed partially. The false lumen tends to be larger and under higher pressure, although it may be compressed in

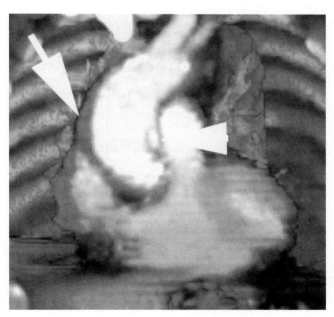

FIG. 7–42. Coronal volume-rendered view of a Type-A dissection in the proximal ascending aorta (*arrowhead*). Mural thrombus is noted (*arrow*).

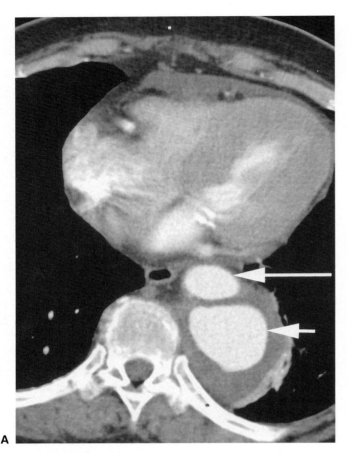

A

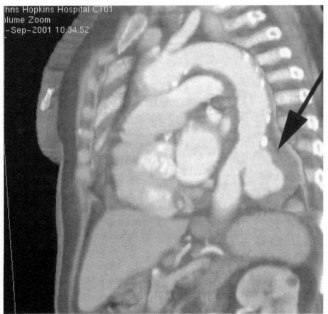

B

FIG. 7–43. A: An axial 2D image suggests a focal dissection with two lumen (*long and short arrows*). **B:** A left sagittal volume-rendered view shows this appearance to be due to a pseudoaneurysm (*arrow*).

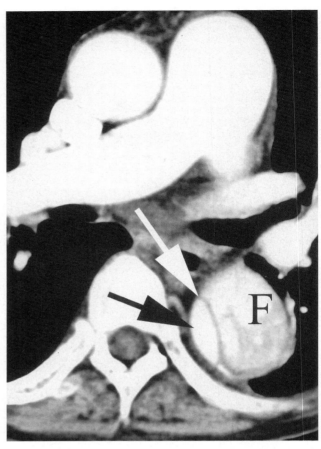

FIG. 7–44. Classic Type-B dissection with large false lumen (*F*), intimal flap (*white arrow*), and compressed true lumen (*black arrow*).

systole. It tends to be posterolateral in the chest, posterior at the level of the common iliac arteries, and is noted deep to any intimal calcification (Figures 7–48, 7–49, and 7–50). Calcification may be a useful sign for acute dissection, but it becomes less reliable with chronic dissections where reendothelialization occurs, and can calcify within the false lumen (203). It has a more variable flow rate dependent on the size of the entry and reentry tears, and this can manifest as a swirling pattern of contrast or thrombus formation in the form of the *beak* sign, *cobweb* sign, or complete thrombosis (203). It is important to document whether the dissection is *communicating* (flow present in the false lumen) or *noncommunicating*. The former may serve to supply some branch vessels, but it has a greater tendency to progress and rupture.

Computed-tomography angiography sensitivity and specificity is over 95% for assessment of branch-vessel involvement by the dissection process (82,204). The true lumen usually supplies the celiac axis, superior mesenteric artery, and right renal artery, with the false lumen supplying the left renal artery (Figure 7-51)(146). True- or false-lumen caliber may be compromised in diastole or systole, respectively. On occasion, the false lumen remains as the sole sup-

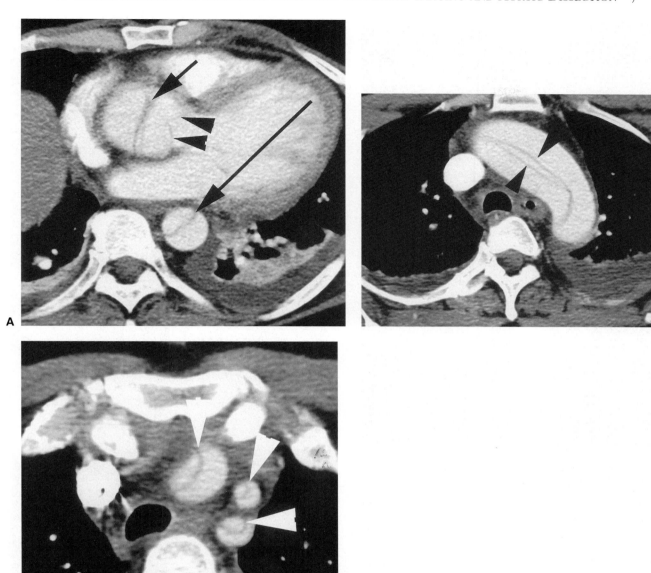

FIG. 7–45. A: Type-A dissection with flap in the ascending aorta (*short arrow*) and descending aorta (*long arrow*). Note the proximity of the aortic-valve leaflets (*arrowheads*). **B:** Type-A dissection. The double flap (*arrowheads*) is due to motion artifact. **C:** Type-A dissection with involvement of the great vessels of the neck (*arrowheads*).

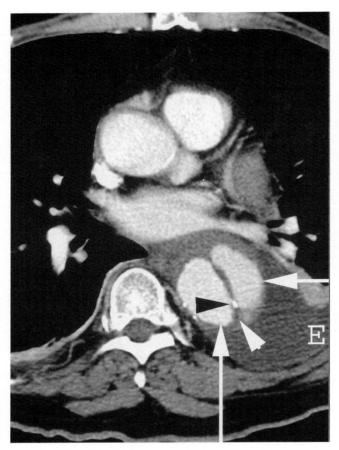

FIG. 7–46. A low-attenuation dissection flap (*white arrow-head*) is seen in the descending aorta with a small amount of calcification (*black arrowhead*) separating the false lumen (*short arrow*) and true lumen (*long arrow*). A pleural effusion is present (*E*).

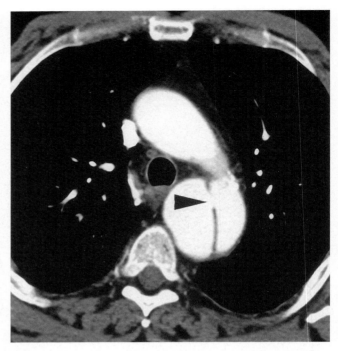

FIG. 7–47. An entry tear is noted in the proximal descending aorta (*arrowhead*).

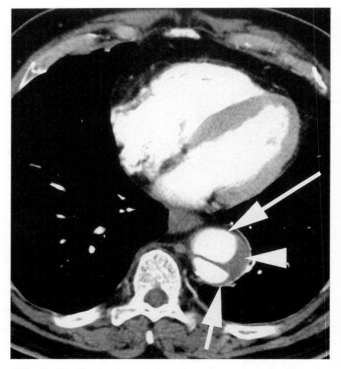

FIG. 7–48. Beak sign of thrombus (*arrowhead*) within the false lumen (*long arrow*). True lumen (*short arrow*).

ply of blood to the organ, and it may be inadequate due to slow flow or obstruction. There are two types of branch-vessel compromise: *static* and *dynamic* (184). Static obstruction is due to the actual dissection flap or thrombosis extending into the vessel ostium, and dynamic obstruction is due to a ball-valve effect of the intimal flap covering the ostium. Such branch-vessel compromise is associated with a poor outcome due to dissection (205). Renal-artery involvement is most commonly reported, whereas clinical mesenteric ischemia is found in 2.5% of cases, and superior mesenteric artery (SMA) or celiac involvement is found in 10% of autopsies (Figures 7–52 and 7–53) (205). Mortality in aortic dissection is due to renal insufficiency in 50% to 70% (205)(206) of patients, and mesenteric ischemia in 87% of patients (205). Asymmetric renal perfusion is suggestive but not confirmatory of renal ischemia, and bowel ischemia is suggested by mural thickening, abnormal enhancement, and mesenteric stranding, with infarct suggested by pneumatosis or air in the portal system. Any involvement of iliofemoral vessels must be documented carefully to aid planning of endovascular approaches, and the relatively small iliofem-

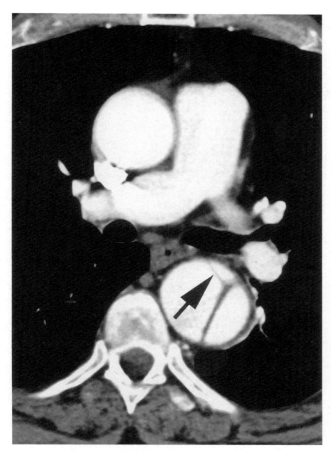

FIG. 7–49. Web sign of thrombus (*arrow*) in the false lumen.

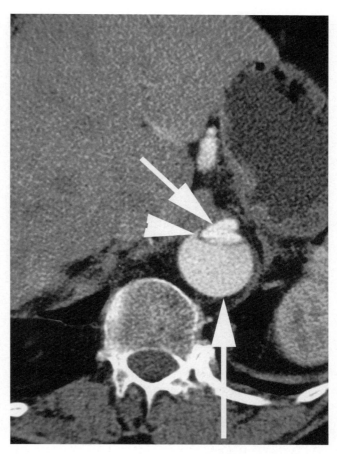

FIG. 7–51. The celiac origin (*short arrow*) supplied by a small true lumen. Note the flap (*arrowhead*) and large false lumen (*long arrow*).

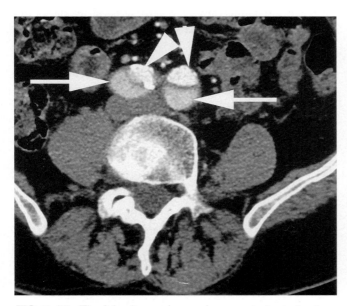

FIG. 7–50. The false lumen (*arrows*) are posterior to the true lumen (*arrowheads*) below the birfurcation.

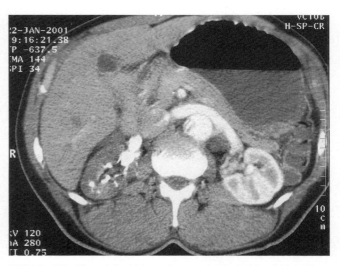

FIG. 7–52. The right kidney is not perfused in this patient with a Type-B dissection extending into the abdomen.

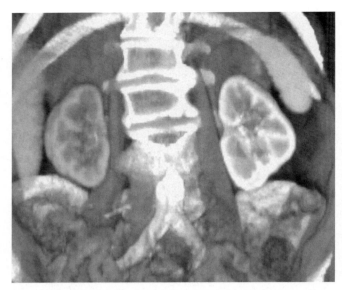

FIG. 7–53. The right kidney is not perfused in this patient with a Type-B dissection extending into the abdomen.

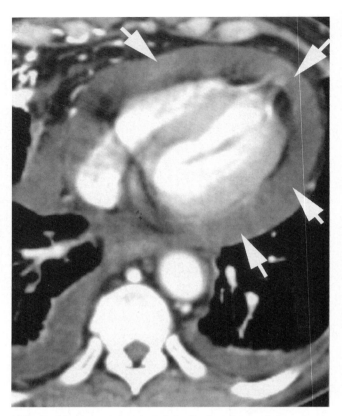

FIG. 7–54. A large pericardial effusion (*arrows*) is seen in this patient with a Type-A dissection.

oral vessels can be occluded with diastolic collapse of the true lumen, which may require a bypass procedure. Those with peripheral vascular compromise have high mortality (175,207,208). Coronary-artery involvement is rare, but cardiac ischemia is seen in 3% to 4% of patients, which can be multifactorial (135).

Features of aortic rupture include an irregular aortic wall, high-attenuation blood around the aorta or in the serosal spaces, or active extravasation of contrast. Pericardiac, mediastinal, or pleural fluid do not necessarily imply impending rupture, but are ominous signs, as they are seen frequently in cases of sudden death (209,210) and have been associated with higher mortality (135). Fluid greater than 1 centimeter around the aorta separating it from the left atrium and esophagus, or pericardial effusion (Figure 7-54) separating epicardium and pericardium, are associated with 50% mortality (210).

Acute traumatic aortic injury from blunt chest trauma may manifest as a Class-I, Class-II, or Class-V dissection. When there is a focal transection, it is a transverse laceration and may appreciated on axial images as a focal-wall irregularity and caliber change, and on 3D imaging may demonstrate a distinctive kink in the aorta and focal outpouching (56,182,211–214) (Figure 7-55).

A discordant CT result with no evidence of Class–I classic dissection in the presence of classic history, symptoms, and signs should lead to a search for more subtle IMH or PAU variants of dissection, as well as other causes of acute chest pain.

Class-II Dissection—Aortic Intramural Hematoma

The *tunica intima* and inner one third of the *tunica media* are supplied by diffusion of nutrients from the circu-

lating blood, with the *vasa vasorum* supplying the remaining wall. Aortic intramural hematoma (AIH) is a hemorrhagic dissection of the media (Class II) without an intimal tear (193) or intramural flow (215,216) and will remain occult on conventional angiography. Aortic intramural hematoma has been found in 13% to 27% of suspected dissection cases (193,204,217–219). In 1920, Krukenberg first ascribed this to spontaneous rupture of the *vasa vasorum* in the outer layers of the media. Traumatic etiologies previously have been described (38). There are two nontraumatic etiological types: *cystic medial necrosis Erdheim–Gsell* or *atherosclerosis* (193). Traumatic etiologies tend to have a better prognosis than nontraumatic etiologies, and all do worse in aneurysmal aortas (218). Unlike Class-I dissection, AIH occurs in older hypertensive patients with an equal male:female ratio (220) and is found in anatomic areas of atherosclerosis; therefore, it is more likely to occur in the descending thoracic aorta. It is classified and managed like Type-A and Type-B classic dissections and carries a high mortality (~80%), with a wide range reported (221,222) and higher mortality for Type-A (50%–100%) than Type-B (20%–40%) AIH (193,223), usually due to rupture through the *adventitia*. The natural history is that 15% to 41% will convert to Class-I dissection, 5% to 26% will rupture, and 11% to 75% will heal spontaneously (38,135,193,218,221,223,224), with progression more likely in an aorta greater than 5 centimeters

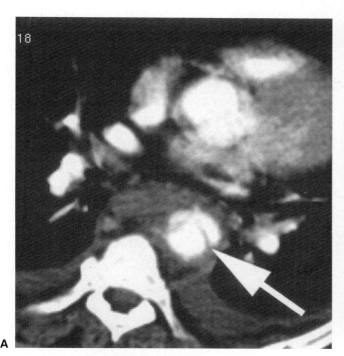
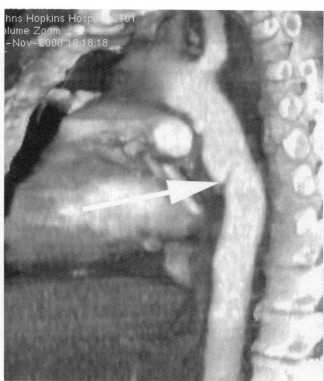

FIG. 7–55. A: A focal irregularity of the descending thoracic aorta (*arrow*) is noted in this patient after trauma. There is also some fluid around the aorta. **B:** The nature of the aortic injury is appreciated on this left lateral volume-rendered view that shows the focal kink (*arrow*).

(210,225). The hematoma may progress longitudinally and in a circumferential manner and, by weakening the aortic wall, can subsequently lead to aneurysmal dilatation (210,218,224,226). Findings such as Type-A AIH, thick hematoma, compression of the true lumen, or the presence of pleural or pericardial effusions are thought to predict progression to overt dissection (225). Aortic intramural hematoma can be missed with DSA and may not be appreciated with SSD or MIP techniques.

On axial 2D and 3D volume-rendered interpretation, AIH appears as a circular or eccentric discrete crescentic segmental thickening of the aortic wall (>0.5 cm) (83,193), which may be high in attenuation on noncontrast study, may displace the intimal calcification, and does not enhance. It maintains a constant anatomical relation to the aorta and may extend over multiple slices, but it does not cause significant lumen compromise. Associated pleural (75%) and pericardial (88%) effusions are common (193,224) and, although not necessarily indicative of a leak, all should be viewed with caution for impending rupture. Aortic intramural hematoma may be distinguished from mural thrombus by its location beneath the *intima* and its smooth inner surface, but it can be difficult to distinguish from a Class-I dissection with thrombosed false lumen (noncommunicating dissection) (83,217). The thickness of the aortic wall will vary over time, reflecting resorption or progression (218), and resolution can

occur within 7 days to 10 days (193,210). The full longitudinal extent is best appreciated on sagittal 3D reconstructions (Figure 7-56).

Class-IV Dissection—Penetrating Atherosclerotic Ulcer

PAU, like AIH, is an entity appreciated on CT, although often not diagnosed with aortography (227–231). It is a Class-IV dissection, by Svenson's criteria, due to a focal violation of the internal elastic lamina by plaque rupture and washout of the lipid core. It is principally a disease of elderly men (232), first attributed to atherosclerotic ulceration of the internal elastic lamina by Stanson in 1986 with incidence in 2.3% of patients who had aortography for suspected dissection (228).

On CT, PAU typically is manifested as a single focal *collar-button* ulcer with perhaps a small rind of thrombus extending beyond the expected circumference of the aortic wall (218,230,233)(Figure 7-57). There is no dissection flap or false lumen, and it usually is seen in the setting of extensive atherosclerotic disease of the aorta. It tends not to extend far longitudinally, unlike AIH, possibly due to the limitations imposed by the atherosclerosis present. PAU is uncommon in the ascending aorta and is found most commonly in the middescending thoracic aorta (233). Axial 2D and cine

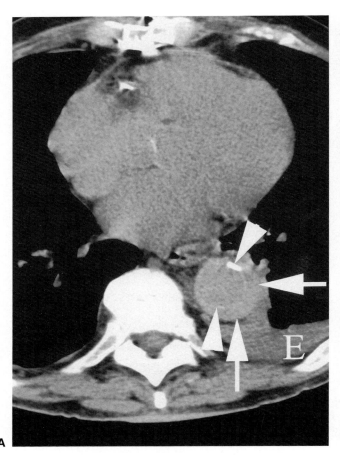
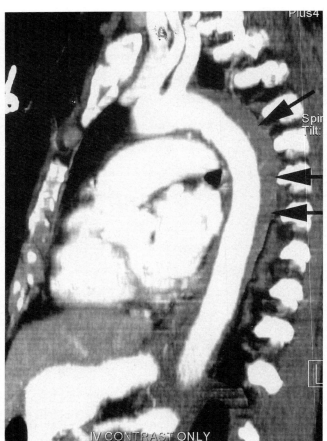

FIG. 7–56. A: Intramural hematoma. A noncontrast study demonstrates a high-attenuation crescent (*short arrows*) external to the intima (*arrowheads*). **B:** Intramural hematoma. After intravenous contrast the AIH is seen (*arrows*) on this sagittal MPR.

scrolling are ideal for their detection, but their anatomic location is depicted best with 3D imaging. PAU has a high incidence of complications (234), and it is thought to be more likely to rupture than Class-I classic aortic dissection (218,228,229,231,232). Although the risk of PAU rupture is greater in larger aortas (232) or in the ascending aorta (233,235), it may occur in normal-sized aorta as well (218). It may resolve spontaneously, progress to AIH (87%) or pseudoaneurysm (26%), or rupture (8%) (235); 10% to 20% become Class-I aortic dissections (216,218,227,233, 234,236). Any sign of progression or embolic phenomena may require resection of the ulcer and graft interposition (229). Endovascular repair has been reported with some success (99,237).

DISSECTION CTA—THE DATA

Computed-tomography angiography is accurate for diagnosis of dissection (~96%–100%), with sensitivity over 90% and specificity over 85%, even with older CT technologies (82,184,204,238). It seldom is compared to DSA. The negative predictive value of a normal study is close to 100%,

although minimal aortic injury (MAI) (239), which represents a slight intimal disruption without blood in the media, can be overlooked. Computed-tomography angiography is changing our understanding of diseases and can detect injuries limited to the intimal and inner media (239). This latter condition, however, tends to be self-limited. Computed tomography has proven efficacious in the emergency-room setting with rapid triage of those with traumatic and nontraumatic dissections (137,213,214), and 3D CTA is useful in preoperative assessment (168). Even with the accuracy of today's CTA, false positives and needless sternotomies exist, although they are rare. Four-detector acquisition systems are not adequate for coronary-flow assessment, but 16-detector systems show great promise in this area. Transesophageal echo still is favored to quantify and establish the flow direction across the proximal intimal tears, and both TEE and MRI can assess better aortic regurgitation. Computed tomography is reliable in excluding aortic injury in the trauma setting (240) and diagnosing it (241), with 90% to 100% sensitivity, 82% to 99% specificity, and 47% to 90% positive predictive value (213,214,241), although aortography still may be required in the setting of extensive mediastinal hema-

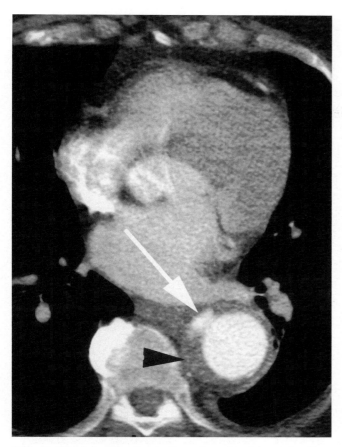

FIG. 7–57. A focal collar button of contrast (*arrow*) with a small AIH (*arrowhead*) represents a penetrating atherosclerotic ulcer.

toma with no evidence of ATAI of obvious cause for bleeding (242). Small or subtle injuries can be problematic for all modalities (182), but may not have great clinical significance.

False positives may be minimized by attention to suboptimal technical factors, recognition of common pitfalls, including artifact and periaortic normal structures, and variant anatomy (243). Streak artifacts are a common cause of a false-positive diagnosis due to either metallic leads, arms, or venous streak artifact due to transmitted pulsation and beam hardening at high-contrast interfaces. Proper patient preparation, appropriate scan direction, and larger volumes of lower-concentration contrast will minimize some of the more common causes. Streak artifacts can be discriminated by their arbitrary trajectory on sequential slices in parallel lines, or radiation from a single point, and on occasion artifacts can be followed clearly beyond the vessel wall. They tend to be less serpiginous than intimal flaps. In patients with problematic artifacts, MPR or alternate 3D reconstructions may help.

Ghosting artifact (aortic motion artifact) (244–248) due to vessel-wall misregistration is the next most common false positive, seen on almost 60% of patients, usually between 12 o'clock and 1 o'clock or between 6 o'clock and 7 o'clock (246). It occurs when nongated scanning occurs arbitrarily in the systolic and diastolic phases of the cardiac cycle R–R interval and there is up to 1-cm-motion artifact of the ascending aorta, even with gantry rotation times of 0.5 seconds. It usually is not contiguous on serial images, and is curvilinear and ill defined, often sited beyond the aortic wall. Sagittal 3D reconstructions may reveal the repetitive nature of this artifact on serial images. Ghosting artifact can be minimized with the improved temporal resolution of MDCT or 180-degree linear interpolation (244,245). Prospective or retrospective electrocardiogram (ECG) gating also will reduce this artifact. As yet, CT cannot evaluate precisely and quantify aortic-valve or coronary-artery involvement, and although the intima tears may be localized, their size, quantity of flow, and flow direction cannot be estimated accurately. An imaging result, regardless of modality, should never be treated in isolation. The symptom of dissection pain in particular is an important measure of the significance of many signs on CT.

Dissection Therapy and Follow Up

Follow-up studies are recommended at 1-month, 3-month, 6-month, and 12-month intervals after the acute event (Figure 7-58). Surgery is thought to reduce the mortality of Type-A dissections (249–252). For blunt chest trauma, surgery is indicated to repair transection. Surgery has a 20%

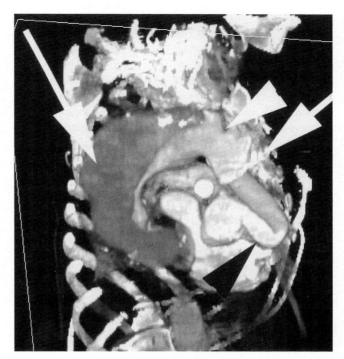

FIG. 7–58. Post-surgical repair of a Type-A dissection. The graft suture line (*short arrow*) is seen. There remains a dissection with true lumen (*arrowhead*) and false lumen (*long arrow*).

to 35% perioperative mortality rate (250,253), which has been reduced 50% by newer imaging techniques (135). Many Type-B dissections may heal spontaneously, leaving only wall thickening in 31% of patients (254). Dissections proximal to the left subclavian usually are treated surgically by graft or composite valved conduit graft (130,207,250,253, 255). Conduit grafts replace the entire aortic root, occlude the entry tear, induce false-lumen thrombosis, and prevent the 2% retrograde extension (256). If the root is not compromised, repair may be limited to the area of abnormality (257–259). This conventional wisdom has been challenged with the use of medical therapies for Type-A dissections. The false lumen is patent after surgery in 90% of cases (135) and should be monitored for progression (260). Dissections limited to the descending aorta usually can be treated by medical therapy aimed at reducing the underlying hypertension, with surgery considered in the setting of persistent pain, aortic expansion, or any suggestion of rupture or organ compromise (128,205,206,250,251,261,262). Surgery for Type-B dissections has a high rate of mortality and paraplegia (253). When surgery is required, PAU usually is treated with interposition graft (216,235). Aortic intramural hematoma is treated much like Class-I dissection, but older patients are thought to do better on medical therapy, as the atherosclerotic process may limit expansion (193).

The use of endovascular approaches is in the early stages (204,263–265), but it already has been applied for thoracic aneurysms and trauma (265,266). Stents have been applied for Class-I, Class-IV, and Class-V acute and subacute Type-B dissections (134,135,204,237,252,263,265, 267,268) to occlude the entry tear. They have been used to fenestrate a flap to cause communication between true and false lumen that is causing dynamic limitation of organ blood flow (206,269,270) with operative mortality 21% to 67% (270–272), or to create a reentry tear where false-lumen thrombosis would lead to organ compromise. Stents are not used to push back the *intima*, but to occlude entry tears, buttress a flap and prevent propagation into a branch vessel, or to maintain vessel patency in the face of an encroaching false-lumen static obstruction (270). Endovascular stenting has been suggested for PAU patients considered too frail for surgery (232). The blooming artifact of wire components can limit MRI studies for follow up, but they are less of a problem for CT. It is important in these cases to assess for failure of the stent to prevent progression or complication of dissection, and to evaluate the stent for failure such as endoleak, migration, or thrombosis. Ninety percent of the false lumen will be patent at follow up, and 20% will have pseudoaneurysm formation (273) and, less commonly, aneurysms of the true lumen. Survival rates for surgically repaired Type-A dissections are better when the false lumen is thrombosed (260). Fifteen percent to thirty percent of those surgically treated for aortic dissection will have aortic disease, leading to life-threatening conditions that require surgery after 10 years. Large reentry tears promote flow, preventing thrombosis and emobolism formation (262), but also

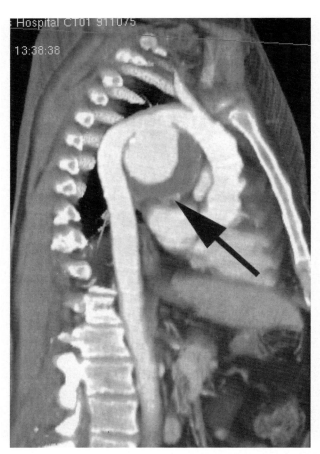

FIG. 7–59. A right sagittal view of a pseudoaneurysm (*arrow*) occurring after a remote history of traumatic injury to the aorta.

increase the likelihood of pseudoaneurysm formation and rupture. Noncommunicating dissections are thought to be more stable over time (132). Aneurysms of the aorta in association with dissection enlarge at a rate proportionate to their size and require 3D true orthogonal measurements to detect accurately 1-mm to 3-mm changes. Through 3D post-processing, consistent views may be produced that are better for assessing stent migration, kinking, or device failure. For the most part, AIH is treated like Type-A and Type-B Class-I dissections, depending on its site (193), although there have been some recent reports suggesting that medical therapy can be successful for selected cases affecting the ascending aorta (217). Particular attention must be given to measurements and angulation for thoracic-stent-clarity placement (264). Traumatic dissections may develop pseudoaneurysm remote from the inciting event (Figure 7-59).

CONCLUSION

Any current assessment of 3D-airway and aortic CT must address the latest developments in MDCT and volume rendering post-processing, which are the imaging standards for the foreseeable future. Together they represent improved image quality and a means to manage the large datasets produced (Rubin, 2000 #113). Successful studies require appropriate protocol design and radiologist experience in the use of rendering software and the virtual-imaging concept of anatomy and disease (21). Novel imaging perspectives will continue to evolve with and contribute to new minimally invasive procedures for diagnosis and therapy. It is hoped that advances in MDCT imaging soon will allow comprehensive lung and cardiovascular evaluations in single studies (105,274–280), and that detailed *in vivo* studies will change our understanding of disease and its outcome. The future will see continued refinements, including larger detector arrays, greater temporal resolution, new dose-reduction strategies, and preventive care through screening.

REFERENCES

1. Berland LL, Smith JK. Multidetector-array CT: once again, technology creates new opportunities. *Radiology* 1998;209:327–329.
2. Rubin GD. Data explosion: the challenge of multidetector-row CT. *Eur J Radiol* 2000;36:74–80.
3. Klingenbeck-Regn K, Schaller S, Flohr T, et al. Subsecond multislice computed tomography: basics and applications. *Eur J Radiol* 1999;31:110–124.
4. Fuchs T, Kachelriess M, Kalender WA. Technical advances in multislice spiral CT. *Eur J Radiol* 2000;36:69–73.
5. Rydberg J, Kopecky KK, Fleiter TR. Multislice CT improves diagnosis, management of aortic disease. *Diagn Imaging (San Franc)* 2000; 22:159–163, 165.
6. Rydberg J, Buckwalter KA, Caldemeyer KS, et al. Multisection CT: scanning techniques and clinical applications. *Radiographics* 2000; 20:1787–1806.
7. Kirchgeorg MA, Prokop M. Increasing spiral CT benefits with postprocessing applications. *Eur J Radiol* 1998;28:39–54.
8. Naidich DP, Harkin TJ. Airways and lung: CT versus bronchography through the fiberoptic bronchoscope. *Radiology* 1996;200:613–614.
9. Naidich DP, Gruden JF, McGuinness G, et al. Volumetric (helical/spiral) CT (VCT) of the airways. *J Thorac Imaging* 1997;12:11–28.
10. Remy-Jardin M, Remy J. Spiral CT angiography of the pulmonary circulation. *Radiology* 1999;212:615–636.
11. Gilkeson RC, Ciancibello LM, Hejal RB, et al. Tracheobronchomalacia: dynamic airway evaluation with multidetector CT. *AJR Am J Roentgenol* 2001;176:205–210.
12. Goldin JG, Aberle DR. Functional imaging of the airways. *J Thorac Imaging* 1997;12:29–37.
13. Gluecker T, Lang F, Bessler S, et al. 2D and 3D CT imaging correlated to rigid endoscopy in complex laryngo-tracheal stenoses. *Eur Radiol* 2001;11:50–54.
14. Kalender WA, Vock P, Polacin A, et al. Spiral-CT: a new technique for volumetric scans. I. Basic principles and methodology. *Rontgenpraxis* 1990;43:323–330.
15. Kalender WA, Seissler W, Klotz E, et al. Spiral volumetric CT with single-breath-hold technique, continuous transport, and continuous scanner rotation. *Radiology* 1990;176:181–183.
16. Kalender WA, Polacin A. Physical performance characteristics of spiral CT scanning. *Med Phys* 1991;18:910–915.
17. Kalender WA, Wedding K, Polacin A, et al. Basic principles of vascular imaging with spiral CT. *Aktuelle Radiol* 1994;4:287–297.
18. Newmark GM, Conces DJ Jr, Kopecky KK. Spiral CT evaluation of the trachea and bronchi. *J Comput Assist Tomogr* 1994;18:552–554.
19. Zeiberg AS, Silverman PM, Sessions RB, et al. Helical (spiral) CT of the upper airway with three-dimensional imaging: technique and clinical assessment. *AJR Am J Roentgenol* 1996;166:293–299.
20. Vock P, Soucek M, Daepp M, et al. Lung: spiral volumetric CT with single-breath-hold technique. *Radiology* 1990;176:864–867.
21. Neumann K, Winterer J, Kimmig M, et al. Real-time interactive virtual endoscopy of the tracheo-bronchial system: influence of CT imaging protocols and observer ability. *Eur J Radiol* 2000;33:50–54.
22. Hu H, He HD, Foley WD, et al. Four multidetector-row helical CT: image quality and volume coverage speed. *Radiology* 2000; 215:55–62.
23. Doi M, Miyazawa T, Mineshita M, et al. Three-dimensional bronchial imaging by spiral computed tomography as applied to tracheobronchial stent placement. *J Bronchol* 1999;6:155–158.
24. Taguchi K, Anno H. High temporal resolution for multislice helical computed tomography. *Med Phys* 2000; 27:861–672.
25. Kauczor HU, Wolcke B, Fischer B, et al. Three-dimensional helical CT of the tracheobronchial tree: evaluation of imaging protocols and assessment of suspected stenoses with bronchoscopic correlation. *AJR Am J Roentgenol* 1996;167:419–424.
26. Remy J, Remy-Jardin M, Artaud D, Fribourg M. Multiplanar and three-dimensional reconstruction techniques in CT: impact on chest diseases. *Eur Radiol* 1998;8:335–351.
27. Fleiter T, Merkle EM, Aschoff AJ, et al. Comparison of real-time virtual and fiberoptic bronchoscopy in patients with bronchial carcinoma: opportunities and limitations. *AJR Am J Roentgenol* 1997; 169:1591–1595.
28. Lawler LP, Fishman EK. Multi-detector row CT of thoracic disease with emphasis on 3D volume rendering and CT angiography. *Radiographics* 2001;21:1257–1273.
29. LoCicero J 3rd, Costello P, Campos CT, et al. Spiral CT with multiplanar and three-dimensional reconstructions accurately predicts tracheobronchial pathology. *Ann Thorac Surg* 1996;62:818–822; discussion 822–823.
30. Lee KS, Yoon JH, Kim TK, et al. Evaluation of tracheobronchial disease with helical CT with multiplanar and three-dimensional reconstruction: correlation with bronchoscopy. *Radiographics* 1997; 17:555–567; discussion 568–570.
31. Rubin GD, Napel S, Leung AN. Volumetric analysis of volumetric data: achieving a paradigm shift. *Radiology* 1996;200:312–317.
32. Rubin GD, Beaulieu CF, Argiro V, et al. Perspective volume rendering of CT and MR images: applications for endoscopic imaging. *Radiology* 1996;199:321–330.
33. Silverman PM, Zeiberg AS, Sessions RB, et al. Helical CT of the upper airway: normal and abnormal findings on three-dimensional reconstructed images. *AJR Am J Roentgenol* 1995;165:541–546.
34. Remy-Jardin M, Remy J, Deschildre F, et al. Obstructive lesions of the central airways: evaluation by using spiral CT with multiplanar and three-dimensional reformations. *Eur Radiol* 1996;6:807–816.
35. Summers RM, Shaw DJ, Shelhamer JH. CT virtual bronchoscopy of simulated endobronchial lesions: effect of scanning, reconstruction, and display settings and potential pitfalls. *AJR Am J Roentgenol* 1998; 170:947–950.
36. Lacrosse M, Trigaux JP, Van Beers BE, et al. 3D spiral CT of the tracheobronchial tree. *J Comput Assist Tomogr* 1995;19:341–347.
37. Quint LE, Whyte RI, Kazerooni EA, et al. Stenosis of the central airways: evaluation by using helical CT with multiplanar reconstructions. *Radiology* 1995;194:871–877.
38. Murray JG, Manisali M, Flamm SD, et al. Intramural hematoma of the thoracic aorta: MR image findings and their prognostic implications. *Radiology* 1997;204:349–355.
39. Fishman EK, Magid D, Ney DR, et al. Three-dimensional imaging. *Radiology* 1991;181:321–337.
40. Calhoun PS, Kuszyk BS, Heath DG, et al. Three-dimensional volume rendering of spiral CT data: theory and method. *Radiographics* 1999; 19:745–764.
41. Ney DR, Kuhlman JE, Hruban RH, et al. Three-dimensional CT-volumetric reconstruction and display of the bronchial tree. *Invest Radiol* 1990;25:736–742.
42. Remy-Jardin M, Remy J, Artaud D, et al. Volume rendering of the tracheobronchial tree: clinical evaluation of bronchographic images. *Radiology* 1998;208:761–770.
43. Remy-Jardin M, Remy J, Artaud D, et al. Tracheobronchial tree: assessment with volume rendering—technical aspects. *Radiology* 1998; 208:393–398.
44. Johnson PT, Heath DG, Bliss DF, et al. Three-dimensional CT: real-time interactive volume rendering. *AJR Am J Roentgenol* 1996; 167:581–583.
45. Johnson PT, Fishman EK, Duckwall JR, et al. Interactive three-dimensional volume rendering of spiral CT data: current applications in the thorax. *Radiographics* 1998;18:165–187.
46. Hopper KD, Iyriboz AT, Wise SW, et al. Mucosal detail at CT virtual

reality: surface versus volume rendering. *Radiology* 2000; 214:517–522.

47. Becker HD. Heading into a virtual world—bronchoscopy at the turn of the century. *J Bronchol* 1999;6:151–152.

48. Vining DJ, Liu K, Choplin RH, et al. Virtual bronchoscopy. Relationships of virtual reality endobronchial simulations to actual bronchoscopic findings. *Chest* 1996;109:549–553.

49. Summers RM, Aggarwal NR, Sneller MC, et al. CT virtual bronchoscopy of the central airways in patients with Wegener's granulomatosis. *Chest* 2002;121:242–250.

50. Ferretti GR, Bricault I, Coulomb M. Virtual tools for imaging of the thorax. *Eur Respir J* 2001;18:381–392.

51. Ferretti GR, Vining DJ, Knoplioch J, et al. Tracheobronchial tree: three-dimensional spiral CT with bronchoscopic perspective. *J Comput Assist Tomogr* 1996;20:777–781.

52. Ferretti GR, Knoplioch J, Bricault I, et al. Central airway stenoses: preliminary results of spiral-CT-generated virtual bronchoscopy simulations in 29 patients. *Eur Radiol* 1997;7:854–859.

53. Ferretti GR, Thony F, Bosson JL, et al. Benign abnormalities and carcinoid tumors of the central airways: diagnostic impact of CT bronchography. *AJR Am J Roentgenol* 2000;174:1307–1313.

54. Seemann MD, Claussen CD. Hybrid 3D visualization of the chest and virtual endoscopy of the tracheobronchial system: possibilities and limitations of clinical application. *Lung Cancer* 2001;32:237–246.

55. Bricault I, Ferretti G, Cinquin P. Registration of real and CT-derived virtual bronchoscopic images to assist transbronchial biopsy. *IEEE Trans Med Imaging* 1998;17:703–714.

56. White CS, Mirvis SE. Pictorial review: imaging of traumatic aortic injury. *Clin Radiol* 1995;50:281–287.

57. Liewald F, Lang G, Fleiter T, et al. Comparison of virtual and fiberoptic bronchoscopy. *Thorac Cardiovasc Surg* 1998;46:361–364.

58. Aquino SL, Vining DJ. Virtual bronchoscopy. *Clin Chest Med* 1999; 20:725–730, vii–viii.

59. Haponik EF, Aquino SL, Vining DJ. Virtual bronchoscopy. *Clin Chest Med* 1999;20:201–217.

60. Colt HG, Crawford SW, Galbraith O 3rd. Virtual reality bronchoscopy simulation: a revolution in procedural training. *Chest* 2001; 120:1333–1339.

61. Gustafson LM, Liu JH, Link DT, et al. Spiral CT versus MRI in neonatal airway evaluation. *Int J Pediatr Otorhinolaryngol* 2000; 52:197–201.

62. Pappas JN, Donnelly LF, Frush DP. Reduced frequency of sedation of young children with multisection helical CT. *Radiology* 2000; 215:897–899.

63. Donnelly LF, Frush DP, Nelson RC. Multislice helical CT to facilitate combined CT of the neck, chest, abdomen, and pelvis in children. *AJR Am J Roentgenol* 2000;174:1620–1622.

64. Konen E, Katz M, Rozenman J, et al. Virtual bronchoscopy in children: early clinical experience. *AJR Am J Roentgenol* 1998; 171:1699–1702.

65. Contencin P, Gumpert LC, de Gaudemar I, et al. Non-endoscopic techniques for the evaluation of the pediatric airway. *Int J Pediatr Otorhinolaryngol* 1997;41:347–352.

66. Salvolini L, Bichi Secchi E, Costarelli L, et al. Clinical applications of 2D and 3D CT imaging of the airways—a review. *Eur J Radiol* 2000;34:9–25.

67. Dunham ME, Wolf RN. Visualizing the pediatric airway: three-dimensional modeling of endoscopic images. *Ann Otol Rhinol Laryngol* 1996;105:12–17.

68. Hopkins KL, Patrick LE, Simoneaux SF, et al. Pediatric great vessel anomalies: initial clinical experience with spiral CT angiography. *Radiology* 1996;200:811–815.

69. Carpenter LM, Merten DF. Radiographic manifestations of congenital anomalies affecting the airway. *Radiol Clin North Am* 1991; 29:219–240.

70. Mahboubi S, Kramer SS. The pediatric airway. *J Thorac Imaging* 1995;10:156–170.

71. Kirks DR, Fram EK, Vock P, et al. Tracheal compression by mediastinal masses in children: CT evaluation. *AJR Am J Roentgenol* 1983; 141:647–651.

72. Kornreich L, Horev G, Ziv N, et al. Bronchiectasis in children: assessment by CT. *Pediatr Radiol* 1993;23:120–123.

73. Sagy M, Poustchi-Amin M, Nimkoff L, et al. Spiral computed tomographic scanning of the chest with three dimensional imaging in the diagnosis and management of paediatric intrathoracic airway obstruction. *Thorax* 1996;51:1005–1009.

74. Nicotra JJ, Mahboubi S, Kramer SS. Three-dimensional imaging of the pediatric airway. *Int J Pediatr Otorhinolaryngol* 1997; 41:299–305.

75. Toki A, Todani T, Watanabe Y, et al. Spiral computed tomography with 3-dimensional reconstruction for the diagnosis of tracheobronchial stenosis. *Pediatr Surg Int* 1997;12:334–336.

76. Manson D, Babyn P, Filler R, et al. Three-dimensional imaging of the pediatric trachea in congenital tracheal stenosis. *Pediatr Radiol* 1994;24:175–179.

77. Katz M, Konen E, Rozenman J, et al. Spiral CT and 3D image reconstruction of vascular rings and associated tracheobronchial anomalies. *J Comput Assist Tomogr* 1995;19:564–568.

78. Rodenwaldt J, Kopka L, Roedel R, et al. 3D virtual endoscopy of the upper airway: optimization of the scan parameters in a cadaver phantom and clinical assessment. *J Comput Assist Tomogr* 1997; 21:405–411.

79. Armstrong JG. Target volume definition for three-dimensional conformal radiation therapy of lung cancer. *Br J Radiol* 1998; 71:587–594.

80. Schafers HJ, Haydock DA, Cooper JD. The prevalence and management of bronchial anastomotic complications in lung transplantation. *J Thorac Cardiovasc Surg* 1991;101:1044–1052.

81. Lee KW, Im JG, Han JK, et al. Tuberculous stenosis of the left main bronchus: results of treatment with balloons and metallic stents. *J Vasc Interv Radiol* 1999; 10:352–358.

82. Sommer T, Fehske W, Holzknecht N, et al. Aortic dissection: a comparative study of diagnosis with spiral CT, multiplanar transesophageal echocardiography, and MR imaging. *Radiology* 1996; 199:347–352.

83. Sommer T, Abu-Ramadan D, Busch M, et al. Intramural hematoma of the thoracic aorta: diagnostic imaging and differential diagnosis. *Rofo Fortschr Geb Rontgenstr Neuen Bildgeb Verfahr* 1996; 165:249–256.

84. Ward S, Muller NL. Pulmonary complications following lung transplantation. *Clin Radiol* 2000;55:332–339.

85. McAdams HP, Palmer SM, Erasmus JJ, et al. Bronchial anastomotic complications in lung transplant recipients: virtual bronchoscopy for noninvasive assessment. *Radiology* 1998;209:689–695.

86. McAdams HP, Goodman PC, Kussin P. Virtual bronchoscopy for directing transbronchial needle aspiration of hilar and mediastinal lymph nodes: a pilot study. *AJR Am J Roentgenol* 1998; 170:1361–1364.

87. Nicholson DA. Tracheal and oesophageal stenting for carcinoma of the upper oesophagus invading the tracheo-bronchial tree. *Clin Radiol* 1998;53:760–763.

88. Curtin JJ, Innes NJ, Harrison BD. Thin-section spiral volumetric CT for the assessment of lobar and segmental bronchial stenoses. *Clin Radiol* 1998;53:110–115.

89. Wilson GE, Walshaw MJ, Hind CR. Treatment of large airway obstruction in lung cancer using expandable metal stents inserted under direct vision via the fibreoptic bronchoscope. *Thorax* 1996; 51:248–252.

90. Lehman JD, Gordon RL, Kerlan RK Jr, et al. Expandable metallic stents in benign tracheobronchial obstruction. *J Thorac Imaging* 1998; 13:105–115.

91. Mehta AC, Dasgupta A. Airway stents. *Clin Chest Med* 1999; 20:139–151.

92. Zwischenberger JB, Wittich GR, vanSonnenberg E, et al. Airway simulation to guide stent placement for tracheobronchial obstruction in lung cancer. *Ann Thorac Surg* 1997;64:1619–1625.

93. Engeler CE, Tashjian JH, Engeler CM, et al. Volumetric high-resolution CT in the diagnosis of interstitial lung disease and bronchiectasis: diagnostic accuracy and radiation dose. *AJR Am J Roentgenol* 1994; 163:31–35.

94. Lucidarme O, Grenier P, Coche E, et al. Bronchiectasis: comparative assessment with thin-section CT and helical CT. *Radiology* 1996; 200:673–679.

95. Remy-Jardin M, Remy J, Artaud D, et al. Diffuse infiltrative lung disease: clinical value of sliding-thin-slab maximum intensity projection CT scans in the detection of mild micronodular patterns. *Radiology* 1996;200:333–339.

96. Remy-Jardin M, Remy J, Gosselin B, et al. Sliding thin slab, minimum

intensity projection technique in the diagnosis of emphysema: histo-pathologic-CT correlation. *Radiology* 1996;200:665–671.

97. Napel S, Rubin GD, Jeffrey RB Jr. STS-MIP: a new reconstruction technique for CT of the chest. *J Comput Assist Tomogr* 1993;17:832–838.

98. Bhalla M, Naidich DP, McGuinness G, et al. Diffuse lung disease: assessment with helical CT—preliminary observations of the role of maximum and minimum intensity projection images. *Radiology* 1996;200:341–347.

99. Mergo PJ, Williams WF, Gonzalez-Rothi R, et al. Three-dimensional volumetric assessment of abnormally low attenuation of the lung from routine helical CT: inspiratory and expiratory quantification. *AJR Am J Roentgenol* 1998;170:1355–1360.

100. Brown MS, McNitt-Gray MF, Goldin JG, et al. Automated measurement of single and total lung volume from CT. *J Comput Assist Tomogr* 1999;23:632–640.

101. Park KJ, Bergin CJ, Clausen JL. Quantitation of emphysema with three-dimensional CT densitometry: comparison with two-dimensional analysis, visual emphysema scores, and pulmonary function test results. *Radiology* 1999;211:541–547.

102. Kinsella M, Muller NL, Abboud RT, et al. Quantitation of emphysema by computed tomography using a "density mask" program and correlation with pulmonary function tests. *Chest* 1990;97:315–321.

103. Thurnheer R, Engel H, Weder W, et al. Role of lung perfusion scintigraphy in relation to chest computed tomography and pulmonary function in the evaluation of candidates for lung volume reduction surgery. *Am J Respir Crit Care Med* 1999;159:301–310.

104. Holbert JM, Brown ML, Sciurba FC, et al. Changes in lung volume and volume of emphysema after unilateral lung reduction surgery: analysis with CT lung densitometry. *Radiology* 1996;201:793–797.

105. Schoepf UJ, Becker CR, Obuchowski NA, et al. Multi-slice computed tomography as a screening tool for colon cancer, lung cancer and coronary artery disease. *Eur Radiol* 2001;11:1975–1985.

106. Obuchowski NA, Graham RJ, Baker ME, et al. Ten criteria for effective screening: their application to multislice CT screening for pulmonary and colorectal cancers. *AJR Am J Roentgenol* 2001;176:1357–1362.

107. Yankelevitz DF, Reeves AP, Kostis WJ, et al. Small pulmonary nodules: volumetrically determined growth rates based on CT evaluation. *Radiology* 2000;217:251–256.

108. Aoshima M, Chonabayashi N. Can HRCT contribute in decision-making on indication for flexible bronchoscopy for solitary pulmonary nodules and masses. *J Bronchol* 2001;8:161–165.

109. Midthun DE. Pulmonary nodules: reach for the imaging—not the scope. *J Bronchol* 2001;8:159–160.

110. Asano F, Matsuno Y, Matsushita T, et al. Transbronchial diagnosis of a pulmonary peripheral small lesion using an ultrathin bronchoscope with virtual bronchoscopic navigation. *J Bronchol* 2002;9:108–111.

111. Ravenel JG, McAdams HP, Remy-Jardin M, et al. Multidimensional imaging of the thorax: practical applications. *J Thorac Imaging* 2001;16:269–281.

112. Wu MT, Pan HB, Chiang AA, et al. Prediction of postoperative lung function in patients with lung cancer: comparison of quantitative CT with perfusion scintigraphy. *AJR Am J Roentgenol* 2002;178:667–672.

113. Leibel SA, Kutcher GJ, Mohan R, et al. Three-dimensional conformal radiation therapy at the Memorial Sloan–Kettering Cancer Center. *Semin Radiat Oncol* 1992;2:274–289.

114. Haller JA Jr, Colombani PM, Humphries CT, et al. Chest wall constriction after too extensive and too early operations for pectus excavatum. *Ann Thorac Surg* 1996;61:1618–1624; discussion 1625.

115. Pretorius ES, Haller JA, Fishman EK. Spiral CT with 3D reconstruction in children requiring reoperation for failure of chest wall growth after pectus excavatum surgery. Preliminary observations. *Clin Imaging* 1998;22:108–116.

116. Pretorius ES, Fishman EK. Volume-rendered three-dimensional spiral CT: musculoskeletal applications. *Radiographics* 1999;19:1143–1160.

117. Pretorius ES, Fishman EK. Spiral CT and three-dimensional CT of musculoskeletal pathology. Emergency room applications. *Radiol Clin North Am* 1999;37:953–974, vi.

118. Israel RS, McDaniel PA, Primack SL, et al. Diagnosis of diaphrag-

matic trauma with helical CT in a swine model. *AJR Am J Roentgenol* 1996;167:637–641.

119. Brink JA, Heiken JP, Semenkovich J, et al. Abnormalities of the diaphragm and adjacent structures: findings on multiplanar spiral CT scans. *AJR Am J Roentgenol* 1994;163:307–310.

120. Killeen KL, Mirvis SE, Shanmuganathan K. Helical CT of diaphragmatic rupture caused by blunt trauma. *AJR Am J Roentgenol* 1999;173:1611–1616.

121. Kuszyk BS, Heath DG, Bliss DF, et al. Skeletal 3-D CT: advantages of volume rendering over surface rendering. *Skeletal Radiol* 1996;25:207–214.

122. Leitman BS, Firooznia H, McCauley DI, et al. The use of computed tomography in evaluating chest wall pathology. *J Comput Tomogr* 1983;7:399–405.

123. Kuriyama K, Tateishi R, Kumatani T, et al. Pleural invasion by peripheral bronchogenic carcinoma: assessment with three-dimensional helical CT. *Radiology* 1994;191:365–369.

124. Waller BF, Clary JD, Rohr T. Nonneoplastic diseases of aorta and pulmonary trunk—Part V. *Clin Cardiol* 1997;20:1026–1028.

125. Waller BF, Clary JD, Rohr T. Nonneoplastic diseases of aorta and pulmonary trunk—Part IV. *Clin Cardiol* 1997;20:964–966.

126. Waller BF, Clary JD, Rohr T. Nonneoplastic diseases of aorta and pulmonary trunk—Part III. *Clin Cardiol* 1997;20:879–884.

127. Waller BF, Clary JD, Rohr T. Nonneoplastic diseases of aorta and pulmonary trunk—Part II. *Clin Cardiol* 1997;20:798–804.

128. Waller BF, Clary JD, Rohr T. Nonneoplastic diseases of aorta and pulmonary trunk—Part I. *Clin Cardiol* 1997;20:730–734.

129. Treasure T, Raphael MJ. Investigation of suspected dissection of the thoracic aorta. *Lancet* 1991;338:490–495.

130. Cigarroa JE, Isselbacher EM, DeSanctis RW, et al. Diagnostic imaging in the evaluation of suspected aortic dissection. Old standards and new directions. *N Engl J Med* 1993;328:35–43.

131. Petasnick JP. Radiologic evaluation of aortic dissection. *Radiology* 1991;180:297–305.

132. Flachskampf FA, Daniel WG. Aortic dissection. *Cardiol Clin* 2000;18:807–817, ix.

133. Hartnell GG. Imaging of aortic aneurysms and dissection: CT and MRI. *J Thorac Imaging* 2001;16:35–46.

134. Erbel R. Diseases of the thoracic aorta. *Heart* 2001;86:227–234.

135. Erbel R, Alfonso F, Boileau C, et al. Diagnosis and management of aortic dissection. *Eur Heart J* 2001;22:1642–1681.

136. Ledbetter S, Stuk JL, Kaufman JA. Helical (spiral) CT in the evaluation of emergent thoracic aortic syndromes. Traumatic aortic rupture, aortic aneurysm, aortic dissection, intramural hematoma, and penetrating atherosclerotic ulcer. *Radiol Clin North Am* 1999;37:575–589.

137. Novelline RA, Rhea JT, Rao PM, et al. Helical CT in emergency radiology. *Radiology* 1999;213:321–339.

138. Fishman EK. High-resolution three-dimensional imaging from subsecond helical CT data sets: applications in vascular imaging. *AJR Am J Roentgenol* 1997;169:441–443.

139. Fishman EK. From the RSNA refresher courses: CT angiography: clinical applications in the abdomen. *Radiographics* 2001;21 Spec No:S3–S16.

140. Prokop M. Multislice CT angiography. *Eur J Radiol* 2000;36:86–96.

141. Smith PA, Heath DG, Fishman EK. Virtual angioscopy using spiral CT and real-time interactive volume-rendering techniques. *J Comput Assist Tomogr* 1998;22:212–214.

142. Smith PA, Fishman EK. Clinical integration of three-dimensional helical CT angiography into academic radiology: results of a focused survey. *AJR Am J Roentgenol* 1999;173:445–447.

143. Prokop M, Schaefer C, Kalender WA, et al. Vascular imaging with spiral-CT. The path to CT-angiography. *Radiologe* 1993;33:694–704.

144. Rubin GD, Dake MD, Semba CP. Current status of three-dimensional spiral CT scanning for imaging the vasculature. *Radiol Clin North Am* 1995;33:51–70.

145. Katz DS, Hon M. CT angiography of the lower extremities and aortoiliac system with a multi-detector row helical CT scanner: promise of new opportunities fulfilled. *Radiology* 2001;221:7–10.

146. Coulam CH, Rubin GD. Acute aortic abnormalities. *Semin Roentgenol* 2001;36:148–164.

147. Jeffrey RB Jr. CT angiography of the abdominal and thoracic aorta. *Semin Ultrasound CT MR* 1998;19:405–412.

148. Bae KT, Heiken JP, Brink JA. Aortic and hepatic contrast medium

enhancement at CT. Part II. Effect of reduced cardiac output in a porcine model. *Radiology* 1998;207:657–662.

149. Bae KT, Heiken JP, Brink JA. Aortic and hepatic contrast medium enhancement at CT. Part I. Prediction with a computer model. *Radiology* 1998;207:647–655.

150. Bae KT, Heiken JP, Brink JA. Aortic and hepatic peak enhancement at CT: effect of contrast medium injection rate—pharmacokinetic analysis and experimental porcine model. *Radiology* 1998;206:455–464.

151. Prokop M, Schaefer-Prokop C, Galanski M. Spiral CT angiography of the abdomen. *Abdom Imaging* 1997;22:143–153.

152. Costello P, Dupuy DE, Ecker CP, et al. Spiral CT of the thorax with reduced volume of contrast material: a comparative study. *Radiology* 1992;183:663–666.

153. Rubin GD, Shiau MC, Leung AN, et al. Aorta and iliac arteries: single versus multiple detector-row helical CT angiography. *Radiology* 2000;215:670–676.

154. Bae KT, Tran HQ, Heiken JP. Multiphasic injection method for uniform prolonged vascular enhancement at CT angiography: pharmacokinetic analysis and experimental porcine model. *Radiology* 2000;216:872–880.

155. Burbank FH, Brody WR, Bradley BR. Effect of volume and rate of contrast medium injection on intravenous digital subtraction angiographic contrast medium curves. *J Am Coll Cardiol* 1984;4:308–315.

156. Prokop M, Schaefer-Prokop C, Galanski M. Spiral CT of the lung. Technique, findings, value. *Radiologe* 1996;36:457–469.

157. van Hoe L, Marchal G, Baert AL, et al. Determination of scan delay time in spiral CT-angiography: utility of a test bolus injection. J Comput Assist Tomogr 1995; 19:216–220.

158. Fleischmann D, Rubin GD, Bankier AA, Hittmair K. Improved uniformity of aortic enhancement with customized contrast medium injection protocols at CT angiography. *Radiology* 2000;214:363–371.

159. Fleischmann D, Hittmair K. Mathematical analysis of arterial enhancement and optimization of bolus geometry for CT angiography using the discrete fourier transform. *J Comput Assist Tomogr* 1999;23:474–484.

160. Tello R, Hartnell G. Tailored timing as a critical factor in CT angiography. *AJR Am J Roentgenol* 1994;162:997–999.

161. Sheiman RG, Raptopoulos V, Caruso P, et al. Comparison of tailored and empiric scan delays for CT angiography of the abdomen. *AJR Am J Roentgenol* 1996;167:725–729.

162. Macari M, Israel GM, Berman P, et al. Infrarenal abdominal aortic aneurysms at multi-detector row CT angiography: intravascular enhancement without a timing acquisition. *Radiology* 2001;220:519–523.

163. Mesurolle B, Qanadli SD, Merad M, et al. Dual-slice helical CT of the thoracic aorta. *J Comput Assist Tomogr* 2000;24:548–556.

164. Heiken JP, Brink JA, Vannier MW. Spiral (helical) CT. *Radiology* 1993;189:647–656.

165. Fleischmann D, Rubin GD, Paik DS, et al. Stair-step artifacts with single versus multiple detector-row helical CT. *Radiology* 2000;216:185–196.

166. Kalender WA, Prokop M. 3D CT angiography. *Crit Rev Diagn Imaging* 2001;42:1–28.

167. Brink JA, Heiken JP, Balfe DM, et al. Spiral CT: decreased spatial resolution in vivo due to broadening of section-sensitivity profile. Radiology 1992; 185:469–474.

168. Adachi H, Ino T, Mizuhara A, Yamaguchi A, Kobayashi Y, Nagai J. Assessment of aortic disease using three-dimensional CT angiography. *J Card Surg* 1994;9:673–678.

169. Zeman RK, Berman PM, Silverman PM, et al. Diagnosis of aortic dissection: value of helical CT with multiplanar reformation and three-dimensional rendering. *AJR Am J Roentgenol* 1995;164:1375–1380.

170. Addis KA, Hopper KD, Iyriboz TA, et al. CT angiography: in vitro comparison of five reconstruction methods. *AJR Am J Roentgenol* 2001;177:1171–1176.

171. Wu CM, Urban BA, Fishman EK. Spiral CT of the thoracic aorta with 3-D volume rendering: A pictorial review of current applications. *Cardiovasc Intervent Radiol* 1999;22:159–167.

172. Schreiner S, Paschal CB, Galloway RL. Comparison of projection algorithms used for the construction of maximum intensity projection images. *J Comput Assist Tomogr* 1996;20:56–67.

173. Kimura F, Shen Y, Date S, et al. Thoracic aortic aneurysm and aortic dissection: new endoscopic mode for three-dimensional CT display of aorta. *Radiology* 1996;198:573–578.

174. Nakashima Y, Kurozumi T, Sueishi K, et al. Dissecting aneurysm: a clinicopathologic and histopathologic study of 111 autopsied cases. *Hum Pathol* 1990;21:291–296.

175. Miller DC, Mitchell RS, Oyer PE, et al. Independent determinants of operative mortality for patients with aortic dissections. *Circulation* 1984;70:I153–I164.

176. DeSanctis RW, Doroghazi RM, Austen WG, et al. Aortic dissection. *N Engl J Med* 1987;317:1060–1067.

177. Chang RA, Rossi NF. Intermittent cocaine use associated with recurrent dissection of the thoracic and abdominal aorta. *Chest* 1995;108:1758–1762.

178. Crawford ES, Svensson LG, Coselli JS, et al. Aortic dissection and dissecting aortic aneurysms. *Ann Surg* 1988;208:254–273.

179. Fisher A, Holroyd BR. Cocaine-associated dissection of the thoracic aorta. *J Emerg Med* 1992;10:723–727.

180. Oskoui R, Lindsay J Jr. Aortic dissection in women < 40 years of age and the unimportance of pregnancy. *Am J Cardiol* 1994;73:821–823.

181. Chew DK, Muto PM, Gordon JK, et al. Spontaneous aortic dissection and rupture in a patient with neurofibromatosis. *J Vasc Surg* 2001;34:364–366.

182. Patel NH, Stephens KE Jr, Mirvis SE, et al. Imaging of acute thoracic aortic injury due to blunt trauma: a review. *Radiology* 1998;209:335–348.

183. Roberts WC. Aortic dissection: anatomy, consequences, and causes. *Am Heart J* 1981;101:195–214.

184. Sebastia C, Pallisa E, Quiroga S, et al. Aortic dissection: diagnosis and follow-up with helical CT. *Radiographics* 1999;19:45–60, quiz 149–150.

185. Asfoura JY, Vidt DG. Acute aortic dissection. *Chest* 1991;99:724–729.

186. Fuster V, Halperin JL. Aortic dissection: a medical perspective. *J Card Surg* 1994;9:713–728.

187. Fuster V, Andrews P. Medical treatment of the aorta. I. *Cardiol Clin* 1999;17:697–715, viii.

188. Dmowski AT, Carey MJ. Aortic dissection. *Am J Emerg Med* 1999;17:372–375.

189. Pretre R, Von Segesser LK. Aortic dissection. *Lancet* 1997;349:1461–1464.

190. Fowkes FG, Macintyre CC, Ruckley CV. Increasing incidence of aortic aneurysms in England and Wales. *BMJ* 1989;298:33–35.

191. Meszaros I, Morocz J, Szlavi J, et al. Epidemiology and clinicopathology of aortic dissection. *Chest* 2000;117:1271–1278.

192. Young J, Herd AM. Painless acute aortic dissection and rupture presenting as syncope. *J Emerg Med* 2002;22:171–174.

193. Mohr-Kahaly S. Aortic intramural hematoma: from observation to therapeutic strategies. *J Am Coll Cardiol* 2001;37:1611–1613.

194. Erbel R, Oelert H, Meyer J, et al. Effect of medical and surgical therapy on aortic dissection evaluated by transesophageal echocardiography. Implications for prognosis and therapy. The European Cooperative Study Group on Echocardiography. *Circulation* 1993;87:1604–1615.

195. Daily PO, Trueblood HW, Stinson EB, et al. Management of acute aortic dissections. *Ann Thorac Surg* 1970;10:237–247.

196. DeBakey ME, McCollum CH, Crawford ES, et al. Dissection and dissecting aneurysms of the aorta: twenty-year follow-up of five hundred twenty-seven patients treated surgically. *Surgery* 1982;92:1118–1134.

197. Glower DD, Speier RH, White WD, et al.. Management and long-term outcome of aortic dissection. *Ann Surg* 1991;214:31–41.

198. Masuda Y, Yamada Z, Morooka N, et al. Prognosis of patients with medically treated aortic dissections. *Circulation* 1991;84:III7–III13.

199. Eagle KA, DeSanctis RW. Aortic dissection. *Curr Probl Cardiol* 1989;14:225–278.

200. Svensson LG, Labib SB, Eisenhauer AC, et al. Intimal tear without hematoma: an important variant of aortic dissection that can elude current imaging techniques. *Circulation* 1999;99:1331–1336.

201. Karabulut N, Goodman LR, Olinger GN. CT diagnosis of an unusual aortic dissection with intimointimal intussusception: the wind sock sign. *J Comput Assist Tomogr* 1998;22:692–693.

202. Quint LE, Francis IR, Williams DM, et al. Evaluation of thoracic aortic disease with the use of helical CT and multiplanar reconstructions: comparison with surgical findings. *Radiology* 1996;201:37–41.

203. LePage MA, Quint LE, Sonnad SS, et al. Aortic dissection: CT features that distinguish true lumen from false lumen. *AJR Am J Roentgenol* 2001;177:207–211.

204. Nienaber CA, Fattori R, Lund G, et al. Nonsurgical reconstruction of thoracic aortic dissection by stent-graft placement. *N Engl J Med* 1999;340:1539–1545.

205. Cambria RP, Brewster DC, Gertler J, et al. Vascular complications associated with spontaneous aortic dissection. *J Vasc Surg* 1988;7:199–209.

206. Laas J, Heinemann M, Jurmann M, Borst HG. Surgical aspects of acute aortic dissection. *Herz* 1992;17:348–356.

207. Fann JI, Smith JA, Miller DC, et al. Surgical management of aortic dissection during a 30-year period. *Circulation* 1995;92:II113–II121.

208. Miller DC. Surgical management of acute aortic dissection: new data. *Semin Thorac Cardiovasc Surg* 1991;3:225–237.

209. McDonald GR, Schaff HV, Pyeritz RE, et al. Surgical management of patients with the Marfan syndrome and dilatation of the ascending aorta [author's transl]. *J Thorac Cardiovasc Surg* 1981;81:180–186.

210. Kaji S, Nishigami K, Akasaka T, et al. Prediction of progression or regression of type A aortic intramural hematoma by computed tomography. *Circulation* 1999;100:II281–II286.

211. Kuhlman JE, Pozniak MA, Collins J, et al. Radiographic and CT findings of blunt chest trauma: aortic injuries and looking beyond them. *Radiographics* 1998;18:1085–1106, discussion 1107–1108, quiz 1.

212. Marotta R, Franchetto AA. The CT appearance of aortic transection. *AJR Am J Roentgenol* 1996;166:647–651.

213. Gavant ML, Flick P, Menke P, et al. CT aortography of thoracic aortic rupture. *AJR Am J Roentgenol* 1996;166:955–961.

214. Gavant ML, Menke PG, Fabian T, et al. Blunt traumatic aortic rupture: detection with helical CT of the chest. *Radiology* 1995;197:125–133.

215. Banning AP, Ruttley MS, Musumeci F, et al. Acute dissection of the thoracic aorta. *BMJ* 1995;310:72–73.

216. Harris JA, Bis KG, Glover JL, et al. Penetrating atherosclerotic ulcers of the aorta. *J Vasc Surg* 1994;19:90–98, discussion 98–99.

217. Song JK, Kim HS, Kang DH, et al. Different clinical features of aortic intramural hematoma versus dissection involving the ascending aorta. *J Am Coll Cardiol* 2001;37:1604–1610.

218. Vilacosta I, San Roman JA, Ferreiros J, et al. Natural history and serial morphology of aortic intramural hematoma: a novel variant of aortic dissection. *Am Heart J* 1997;134:495–507.

219. Kang DH, Song JK, Song MG, et al. Clinical and echocardiographic outcomes of aortic intramural hemorrhage compared with acute aortic dissection. *Am J Cardiol* 1998;81:202–206.

220. Sawhney NS, DeMaria AN, Blanchard DG. Aortic intramural hematoma: an increasingly recognized and potentially fatal entity. *Chest* 2001;120:1340–1346.

221. Ide K, Uchida H, Otsuji H, et al. Acute aortic dissection with intramural hematoma: possibility of transition to classic dissection or aneurysm. *J Thorac Imaging* 1996;11:46–52.

222. Alfonso F, Goicolea J, Aragoncillo P, et al. Diagnosis of aortic intramural hematoma by intravascular ultrasound imaging. *Am J Cardiol* 1995;76:735–738.

223. Maraj R, Rerkpattanapipat P, Jacobs LE, et al. Meta-analysis of 143 reported cases of aortic intramural hematoma. *Am J Cardiol* 2000;86:664–668.

224. Sueyoshi E, Matsuoka Y, Sakamoto I, et al. Fate of intramural hematoma of the aorta: CT evaluation. *J Comput Assist Tomogr* 1997;21:931–938.

225. Choi SH, Choi SJ, Kim JH, et al. Useful CT findings for predicting the progression of aortic intramural hematoma to overt aortic dissection. *J Comput Assist Tomogr* 2001;25:295–299.

226. Ohmi M, Tabayashi K. Long-term surgical results of acute aortic dissection. *Kyobu Geka* 1998;51:665–669.

227. Quint LE, Williams DM, Francis IR, et al. Ulcerlike lesions of the aorta: imaging features and natural history. *Radiology* 2001;218:719–723.

228. Stanson AW, Kazmier FJ, Hollier LH, et al. Penetrating atherosclerotic ulcers of the thoracic aorta: natural history and clinicopathologic correlations. *Ann Vasc Surg* 1986;1:15–23.

229. Cooke JP, Kazmier FJ, Orszulak TA. The penetrating aortic ulcer: pathologic manifestations, diagnosis, and management. *Mayo Clin Proc* 1988;63:718–725.

230. Hayashi H, Matsuoka Y, Sakamoto I, et al. Penetrating atherosclerotic

231. Welch TJ, Stanson AW, Sheedy PF 2nd, et al. Radiologic evaluation of penetrating aortic atherosclerotic ulcer. *Radiographics* 1990;10:675–685.

232. Troxler M, Mavor AI, Homer-Vanniasinkam S. Penetrating atherosclerotic ulcers of the aorta. *Br J Surg* 2001;88:1169–1177.

233. Kazerooni EA, Bree RL, Williams DM. Penetrating atherosclerotic ulcers of the descending thoracic aorta: evaluation with CT and distinction from aortic dissection. *Radiology* 1992;183:759–765.

234. Coady MA, Rizzo JA, Elefteriades JA. Pathologic variants of thoracic aortic dissections. Penetrating atherosclerotic ulcers and intramural hematomas. *Cardiol Clin* 1999;17:637–657.

235. Movsowitz HD, Lampert C, Jacobs LE, et al. Penetrating atherosclerotic aortic ulcers. *Am Heart J* 1994;128:1210–1217.

236. Hussain S, Glover JL, Bree R, et al. Penetrating atherosclerotic ulcers of the thoracic aorta. *J Vasc Surg* 1989;9:710–717.

237. Dake MD, Kato N, Mitchell RS, et al. Endovascular stent-graft placement for the treatment of acute aortic dissection. *N Engl J Med* 1999;340:1546–1552.

238. Vasile N, Mathieu D, Keita K, et al. Computed tomography of thoracic aortic dissection: accuracy and pitfalls. *J Comput Assist Tomogr* 1986;10:211–215.

239. Malhotra AK, Fabian TC, Croce MA, et al. Minimal aortic injury: a lesion associated with advancing diagnostic techniques. *J Trauma* 2001;51:1042–1048.

240. Dyer DS, Moore EE, Mestek MF, et al. Can chest CT be used to exclude aortic injury? *Radiology* 1999;213:195–202.

241. Mirvis SE, Shanmuganathan K, Miller BH, et al. Traumatic aortic injury: diagnosis with contrast-enhanced thoracic CT—five-year experience at a major trauma center. *Radiology* 1996;200:413–422.

242. Scaglione M, Pinto A, Pinto F, et al. Role of contrast-enhanced helical CT in the evaluation of acute thoracic aortic injuries after blunt chest trauma. *Eur Radiol* 2001;11:2444–2448.

243. Batra P, Bigoni B, Manning J, et al. Pitfalls in the diagnosis of thoracic aortic dissection at CT angiography. *Radiographics* 2000;20:309–320.

244. Loubeyre P, Angelie E, Grozel F, et al. Spiral CT artifact that simulates aortic dissection: image reconstruction with use of 180 degrees and 360 degrees linear-interpolation algorithms. *Radiology* 1997;205:153–157.

245. Loubeyre P, Grozel F, Carrillon Y, et al. Prevalence of motion artifact simulating aortic dissection on spiral CT using a 180 degree linear interpolation algorithm for reconstruction of the images. *Eur Radiol* 1997;7:320–322.

246. Duvernoy O, Coulden R, Ytterberg C. Aortic motion: a potential pitfall in CT imaging of dissection in the ascending aorta. *J Comput Assist Tomogr* 1995;19:569–572.

247. Posniak HV, Olson MC, Demos TC. Aortic motion artifact simulating dissection on CT scans: elimination with reconstructive segmented images. *AJR Am J Roentgenol* 1993;161:557–558.

248. Posniak H, Olson M, Demos T. Motion artifact simulating aortic dissection. *AJR Am J Roentgenol* 1993;160:420.

249. Kouchoukos NT, Dougenis D. Surgery of the thoracic aorta. *N Engl J Med* 1997;336:1876–1888.

250. Chang Q, Sun L, Wu Q. Surgical treatment of DeBakey type I and II aortic dissection. *Zhonghua Yi Xue Za Zhi* 2001;81:1187–1189.

251. Walker WE. Surgery for acute aortic dissection in octogenarians. *J Thorac Cardiovasc Surg* 2001;122:1049–1050.

252. Kang SG, Lee DY, Maeda M, et al. Aortic dissection: percutaneous management with a separating stent-graft—preliminary results. *Radiology* 2001;220:533–539.

253. Hagan PG, Nienaber CA, Isselbacher EM, et al. The international registry of acute aortic dissection (IRAD): new insights into an old disease. *JAMA* 2000;283:897–903.

254. Hara K, Yamaguchi T, Wanibuchi Y, et al. The role of medical treatment of distal type aortic dissection. *Int J Cardiol* 1991;32:231–240.

255. Riley P, Rooney S, Bonser R, et al. Imaging the post-operative thoracic aorta: normal anatomy and pitfalls. *Br J Radiol* 2001;74:1150–1158.

256. Mohr-Kahaly S, Erbel R, Rennollet H, et al. Ambulatory follow-up of aortic dissection by transesophageal two-dimensional and color-coded Doppler echocardiography. *Circulation* 1989;80:24–33.

257. Borst HG. Aortic dissection. *Rev Port Cardiol* 2000;19:763–769.

258. Lemole GM. Operation for type A aortic dissection. *Ann Thorac Surg* 1995;60:1863–1864.

259. Najafi H, Dye WS, Javid H, et al. Proceedings: Aortic insufficiency secondary to aortic root aneurysm and/or dissection. *J Cardiovasc Surg (Torino)* 1976;17:91.

260. Ergin MA, Phillips RA, Galla JD, et al. Significance of distal false lumen after type A dissection repair. *Ann Thorac Surg* 1994; 57:820–824, discussion 825.

261. Elefteriades JA, Lovoulos CJ, Coady MA, et al. Management of descending aortic dissection. *Ann Thorac Surg* 1999;67:2002–2005, discussion 2014–2019.

262. Elefteriades JA, Hartleroad J, Gusberg RJ, et al. Long-term experience with descending aortic dissection: the complication-specific approach. *Ann Thorac Surg* 1992;53:11–20, discussion 20–21.

263. Bortone AS, Schena S, Mannatrizio G, et al. Endovascular stent-graft treatment for diseases of the descending thoracic aorta. *Eur J Cardiothorac Surg* 2001;20:514–519.

264. Milner R, Bavaria JE, Baum RA, et al. Thoracic aortic stent grafts. *Semin Roentgenol* 2001;36:340–350.

265. Taylor PR, Gaines PA, McGuinness CL, et al. Thoracic aortic stent grafts—early experience from two centres using commercially available devices. *Eur J Vasc Endovasc Surg* 2001;22:70–76.

266. Mita T, Arita T, Matsunaga N, et al. Complications of endovascular repair for thoracic and abdominal aortic aneurysm: an imaging spectrum. *Radiographics* 2000;20:1263–1278.

267. Sailer J, Peloschek P, Rand T, et al. Endovascular treatment of aortic type B dissection and penetrating ulcer using commercially available stent-grafts. *AJR Am J Roentgenol* 2001;177:1365–1369.

268. Ide K, Kichikawa K, Uchida H, et al. Stent-graft treatment of dissecting aneurysm in association with aortic intramural hematoma: when should the procedure be performed? *J Endovasc Ther* 2001; 8:144–149.

269. Elefteriades JA, Hammond GL, Gusberg RJ, et al. Fenestration revisited. A safe and effective procedure for descending aortic dissection. *Arch Surg* 1990;125:786–790.

270. Williams DM, Lee DY, Hamilton BH, et al. The dissected aorta: percutaneous treatment of ischemic complications—principles and results. *J Vasc Interv Radiol* 1997;8:605–625.

271. Walker PJ, Dake MD, Mitchell RS, et al. The use of endovascular techniques for the treatment of complications of aortic dissection. *J Vasc Surg* 1993;18:1042–1051.

272. Saito S, Arai H, Kim K, et al. Percutaneous fenestration of dissecting intima with a transseptal needle. A new therapeutic technique for visceral ischemia complicating acute aortic dissection. *Cathet Cardiovasc Diagn* 1992;26:130–135.

273. Kawamoto S, Johnson PT, Fishman EK. Three-dimensional CT angiography of the thorax: clinical applications. *Semin Ultrasound CT MR* 1998;19:425–438.

274. Schroeder S, Kopp AF, Ohnesorge B, et al. Virtual coronary angioscopy using multislice computed tomography. *Heart* 2002; 87:205–209.

275. Knez A, Becker CR, Leber A, et al. Usefulness of multislice spiral computed tomography angiography for determination of coronary artery stenoses. *Am J Cardiol* 2001;88:1191–1194.

276. Janowitz WR. Current status of mechanical computed tomography in cardiac imaging. *Am J Cardiol* 2001;88:35E–38E.

277. Cline H, Coulam C, Yavuz M, et al. Coronary artery angiography using multislice computed tomography images. *Circulation* 2000; 102:1589–1590.

278. Becker CR, Ohnesorge BM, Schoepf UJ, et al. Current development of cardiac imaging with multidetector-row CT. *Eur J Radiol* 2000; 36:97–103.

279. Fallenberg M, Juergens KU, Wichter T, et al. Coronary artery aneurysm and type-A aortic dissection demonstrated by retrospectively ECG-gated multislice spiral CT. *Eur Radiol* 2002;12:201–204.

280. Achenbach S, Ulzheimer S, Baum U, et al. Noninvasive coronary angiography by retrospectively ECG-gated multislice spiral CT. *Circulation* 2000;102:2823–2828.

CHAPTER 8

Cardiac MDCT

Frandics P. Chan

INTRODUCTION

Since the development of computed tomography (CT) in the early 1970s, CT has undergone numerous technological revolutions. With each significant innovation, there was a quantum leap in performance resulting in faster scan acquisition and increased spatial resolution. Most recently, CT scanners have benefited from parallel imaging with multidetector CT (MDCT). With MDCT, the shortened scan time makes more efficient use of intravenous (IV) contrast medium and, in most applications, reduces the total amount of contrast medium needed, limiting the effects of nephrotoxicity in susceptible patients. The rapid scan time also promotes patient compliance, allowing consistent breath-hold even in very ill patients. The increased spatial resolution permits visualization of ever finer anatomical details. With decreasing slice thickness, a voxel approaches the same size in all three dimensions, which enables high-quality three-dimensional (3D) image reconstruction. As a whole, these attributes enable new clinical applications not feasible before, and the latest beneficiary is cardiac MDCT imaging.

Cardiac-gated tomographic imaging of the heart had been tried with CT scanners in the early 1980s (1,2), but they did not progress beyond experimental stages. Clinical cardiac imaging became viable with the development of cardiac magnetic-resonance imaging (MRI) and electron-beam computed tomography (EBCT), both begun in the mid-1980s. The experience learned from EBCT directly influenced the development of cardiac MDCT (3,4). The EBCT design eliminates the mechanically driven gantry by electromagnetically steering a beam of electrons through a vacuum funnel onto a focal spot on a fixed 210-degree arc of tungsten target. Since there are no moving parts, the X-ray source can move about rapidly (5). After passing through a subject, the X-ray is detected by a fixed 240-degree arc of detectors. Current EBCT scanners permit multislice imaging at a rate of 100 ms per slice and a slice width of 3 mm. The rapid scan rate helps freeze the cardiac motion. Electrocardiographic (ECG) triggering is added to synchronize cardiac phases

from slice to slice. These features make EBCT suitable for cardiac imaging. In the current implementation, however, EBCT is beset by limited X-ray-power output, such that scanning at top speed and thinnest slice in adults produces images with poor signal-to-noise ratio. In addition, EBCT is a costly specialized machine with limited install base. Consequently, despite being available for over a decade, EBCT has not contributed significantly to the routine management of heart disease, with the notable exception of coronary calcium scoring.

Cardiac MDCT overcomes many shortcomings of EBCT. Technically, cardiac MDCT produces images with better signal-to-noise ratio at a thinner slice thickness, although at a lower scan rate and increased radiation dose. In addition, most MDCT implementations for general imaging can be adapted relatively simply to perform cardiac imaging. This makes cardiac imaging available to a large and growing community of MDCT scanners at a relatively low additional cost. It is expected that in the near future, MDCT will become the dominant CT modality for cardiac imaging.

The development of clinical applications for cardiac MDCT parallels those attempted with EBCT (6). The two most important applications deal with adult ischemic heart disease. They are coronary calcium scoring (7) and coronary angiography (8). In addition, cardiac MDCT shows promise in coronary-plaque characterization (9). The differentiation of stable versus unstable plaques has important prognostic implications. The high spatial resolution of cardiac MDCT can provide a detailed look at various valvular structures, during the cardiac phase when the valves are relatively stationary (10). Cardiac MDCT is useful in presurgical planning for valve replacement and detection of valvular vegetation responsible for endocarditis. With the development of cardiac endovascular procedures requiring access to the coronary venous system, such as placement of a biventricular pacemaker, cardiac MDCT can be helpful in mapping the cardiac veins and detecting unexpected venous anomalies (11). Using the retrospective gating technique, cardiac

MDCT records the motion of the heart, which can be used to evaluate ventricular volumes and functions (12). In congenital heart disease, cardiac MDCT can provide an accurate 3D evaluation of intracardiac and extracardiac structural anomalies (13,14). Evaluation of the extracardiac congenital anomalies is particularly important because they are not seen well by echocardiography. Lastly, cardiac MDCT is used to evaluate postinterventional or postsurgical complications. Although cardiac MDCT is still in its infancy, more clinical applications undoubtedly will evolve in the future.

PRINCIPLES OF CARDIAC MDCT

The scan time required to cover the volume of the heart, even with the fastest MDCT scanner currently available, is significantly longer than a heartbeat. By necessity, the imaging of a volume takes place over multiple heartbeats. To maintain a consistent cardiac phase throughout the volume, data acquisition is broken up into small segments, with each segment synchronized to a specific cardiac phase. This principle of cardiac synchronization, or gating, is employed extensively in cardiac MRI and EBCT. To minimize motion artifact, the data-acquisition period of each segment must be kept short to insure that cardiac movement is minimal. In cardiac EBCT and MDCT, this period defines the temporal resolution of the scanner. As will be seen, the choices of cardiac-synchronization method and temporal resolution have a profound influence on spatial resolution, artifact, total scan time, radiation dose, and overall image quality (15).

Methods of Cardiac Synchronization

There are two main cardiac-synchronization strategies: prospective gating and retrospective gating. In most scanners, ECG signal is used as a surrogate marker for the periodic motion of the heart. In prospective gating, the user prescribes a specific cardiac phase to image before the scan. This cardiac phase can be specified as an absolute time delay after an ECG trigger, usually at the R-wave, or as a percentage of the time interval between adjacent R-waves. The scanner advances the table to the prescribed starting position and waits for the arrival of the predetermined cardiac phase. Once the cardiac phase arrives, the scanner acquires parallel axial slices equal to the number of detector rows. The table then advances to a new position by an increment equal to the slice width times the number of detector rows. There, the scanner waits for the arrival of the next cardiac phase, and the cycle repeats until the whole volume is scanned. This procedure is called aptly the ''step-and-shoot'' method. Figure 8-1 graphically depicts the movement of the detector rows as a function of time.

The main advantage of prospective gating is its simplicity. The total scan time is inversely proportional to heart rate, slice width, and the number of detector rows. Since the X-ray source is activated only during image acquisition, the radiation dose to the patient is limited. On the other hand,

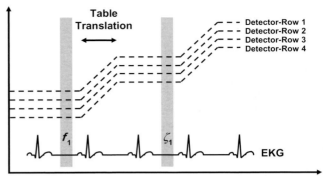

FIG. 8–1. Timing diagram of prospective gating. The scanner moves the table to a predetermined position and acquires images at cardiac phase ϕ_1. The scanner then moves the table to the next position and acquires images at the next cardiac phase ϕ_1. This process repeats until the entire volume is scanned.

prospective gating is susceptible to irregularities in the heart rhythm. Only one cardiac phase can be imaged per scan. To date, prospective gating finds its greatest use in coronary calcium imaging.

In retrospective gating, the scanner continuously acquires data in spiral mode while the table travels at a constant speed. For MDCT, pitch is defined as the table distance traveled in one gantry rotation divided by the total scan width, or the detector width multiplied by the number of detector rows. For retrospective gating, the pitch is kept low deliberately to ensure that a different detector row scans the same cardiac location at a different time during a different cardiac phase. This pitch can be as low as a third or quarter of the pitch used in nongated spiral scans. Electrocardiographic (ECG) tracing is recorded independently and used only during image reconstruction.

The process of reconstruction is illustrated best by the example in Figure 8-2, which depicts the position of four detector rows plotted against time. They are represented by four straight lines whose slopes are determined by the pitch. The lower the pitch is, the flatter the lines are. The ECG tracing is laid out along the time axis. To reconstruct an image at table position z_1 and cardiac phase ϕ_1, using Figure 8-2 the reconstruction algorithm looks for the intersections between z_1 and ϕ_1, which recur periodically over time. The algorithm determines that detector-row 2 passes closest to one of these intersections at cardiac-cycle 2. Data from detector-row 2 acquired at that moment are retrieved to reconstruct the slice at z_1. For the next slice at z_2 and the same cardiac-phase ϕ_1, the algorithm goes through the same steps and finds that detector-row 1 passes nearby at cardiac-cycle 2. This piece of data is retrieved to reconstruct the slice at z_2. For the next slice at z_3, the algorithm finds that detector-row 2 passes near an intersection at the next cardiac cycle, which is cycle 3. This piece of data is retrieved to reconstruct

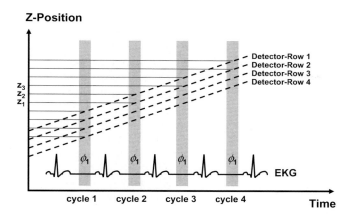

FIG. 8-2. Timing diagram of retrospective gating. The scanner table moves at a constant speed while data are being acquired continuously by all detector rows. To reconstruct a slice at position z_1 and cardiac phase ϕ_1, the algorithm looks for data recorded by the closest detector row, which is detector-row 2 in cardiac-cycle 2 in this example.

TABLE 8–1. *Comparison between prospective and retrospective gating*

	Prospective gating	Retrospective gating
Radiation	Low	High
Temporal resolution*	333 ms	250 ms
Multisector reconstruction	No	Yes
Multiphase reconstruction	No	Yes
Slice misregistration	Greater	Less

* Assuming 60-degree fan angle, 0.5-second gantry rotation, and single-sector reconstruction for retrospective gating.

the slice at z_3. This process repeats until the whole volume is reconstructed. In practice, detector data usually do not fall exactly on the desired position z and cardiac-phase ϕ. In these cases, images are reconstructed from interpolated data from adjacent detector rows (16).

The choice of pitch is important. If the pitch is too high and the heart rate too low, there could be gaps in the table position where no data are available to reconstruct a given cardiac phase. If the pitch is too low, the scan will be slow, exposing the patient to increased radiation. The optimal choice of pitch depends on heart rate and, as will be seen, it also depends on the reconstruction algorithm.

The main advantage of retrospective gating over prospective gating is its ability to reconstruct arbitrary cardiac phases after the scan. This capability can be used to identify a cardiac phase with minimal motion and to reduce artifacts. This adjustment is important for the detection of small lesions such as coronary stenoses (17,18). In addition, multiple cardiac phases may be reconstructed at regular intervals to produce a movie of the heart, during which wall motion can be visualized and ventricular functions can be quantified. Retrospective gating also has the entire history of cardiac rhythm available for optimal image reconstruction. Knowledge of the rhythm permits removal of inconsistent data acquired during arrhythmic beats. A major drawback of retrospective gating is the increased radiation dose, since the X-ray source must be turned on throughout the scan. For images of the same noise level and spatial resolution, the radiation dose imparted by retrospective gating can be four times higher than that by prospective gating (19). Table 8.1 compares the capabilities of prospective gating and retrospective gating.

Temporal Resolution and Heart Rate

Artifacts caused by cardiac motion are a unique problem of cardiac MDCT and may seriously degrade visualization of small anatomic structures. The severity of motion artifacts can be reduced by improving temporal resolution or by decreasing movement of the heart. For prospective gating, temporal resolution is determined by the time it takes the CT gantry to sweep the minimum angle of data needed to reconstruct one image slice. For nonspiral imaging, this minimum angle is 180 degrees plus the fan angle of the gantry, typically 60 degrees. Therefore, at a gantry-rotation period of 0.5 second, the temporal resolution is 333 ms. The minimum angle is 180 degrees for retrospective gating (20), yielding a temporal resolution of 250 ms. Even at a low heart rate of 60 beats per minute, the temporal resolutions occupy a third and a quarter of the cardiac cycle, respectively. Thus, motion artifacts can be expected to occur commonly in cardiac MDCT, especially during systole when heart motion is fast (21).

Temporal resolution can be improved either by increasing the gantry rotation rate or by reducing the amount of data acquired per heartbeat. Although conceptually simple, the first proposition is difficult to achieve technically. Physics dictates that the centrifugal forces experienced by components mounted on a CT gantry scale to the square of the rotation rate. Thus, force increases rapidly with rotation rate. The component most sensitive to this force is the X-ray tube. The structural reinforcement needed to tolerate this increased stress is costly. Furthermore, a higher scan rate necessitates a proportionally higher X-ray-power output to maintain a constant signal-to-noise ratio. Thus, the cost to achieve a significant increase in gantry rotation may be prohibitive. At present, the shortest gantry-rotation period of a commercially available MDCT scanner is 0.42 second (22). While small incremental gains can be expected, large-scale improvement is unlikely in the near future.

Alternatively, the 180-degree scan may be divided into smaller sectors. Each sector is scanned at a different heartbeat and reassembled before image reconstruction. This process is schematically shown in Figure 8-3. The multisector reconstruction technique assumes that heart motion is periodic and reproducible. It further requires that the heart at a table position z and a cardiac-phase ϕ is imaged multiple times by different detector rows. These concepts can be incorporated into the retrospective gating scheme, represented in Figure 8-4. The temporal resolution is defined by the time

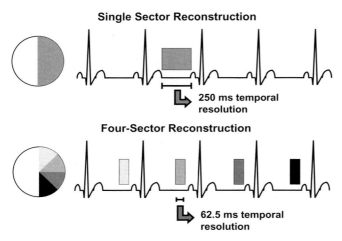

Single Sector Reconstruction

250 ms temporal resolution

Four-Sector Reconstruction

62.5 ms temporal resolution

FIG. 8–3. Schematic representation of a four-sector reconstruction. Assuming a 0.5-second gantry-rotation period, a single-sector reconstruction would have a temporal resolution of 250 ms. The 180 degrees of data needed to reconstruct an image are divided into four sectors. Each sector is recorded in a different heartbeat. Although it takes four times as long as single-sector reconstruction to image one slice, the temporal resolution is shortened fourfold. (Diagram courtesy of Dr. Curtis Coulam)

it takes to scan one sector. Using a two-sector or four-sector reconstruction algorithm, the temporal resolution for a scanner with a 0.5-second gantry rotation is reduced to 125 ms and 63 ms, respectively, comparable to the temporal resolution of an EBCT scanner. Figure 8-5 demonstrates the improved visualization of the right coronary artery using four-sector reconstruction. The gain in temporal resolution comes at a cost, however. As demonstrated in Figure 8-4, the need to image the same slice location multiple times forces a low

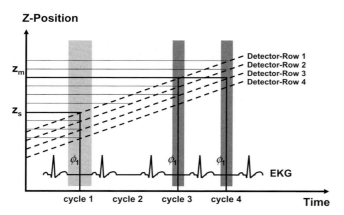

FIG. 8–4. Single-sector versus two-sector reconstruction in retrospective gating. For single-sector reconstruction, the image at position z_s is reconstructed with data acquired by detector-row 1 in cardiac-cycle 1. For two-sector reconstruction, the image at position z_m is reconstructed with data pieced together from detector-row 1 in cardiac-cycle 3 and detector-row 3 in cardiac-cycle 4. The temporal resolution of two-sector reconstruction is half that of single-sector reconstruction.

pitch value, prolonging scan time and exposing the patient to increased radiation. In general, multisector reconstruction is useful when the heart rhythm is regular and equal and the heart rate is high. In some scanner implementations, the reconstruction can switch adaptively between single- and multisector reconstruction, depending on the instantaneous heart rate (23).

Decreasing heart movement also can reduce motion artifacts. Multiple studies have demonstrated that superior image quality is associated with a lower heart rate, and detection of coronary-artery stenosis is more sensitive at a lower heart rate, ideally less than 65 beats per minute (24–26). Some investigators advocate the reduction of heart rate through administration of a β_1 receptor antagonist, such as metoprolol, before each scan. A typical oral regimen is 50 mg of metoprolol at 30-minute intervals for up to two doses. Alternatively, an IV regimen is 3 mg metoprolol at 10-minute intervals for up to three doses. The target heart rate is 60 beats per minutes or below. Contraindications to β_1 receptor antagonist are asthma, atrioventricular heart block, aortic valvular stenosis, hypotension, and severe heart failure.

Spatial Resolution

Like conventional spiral CT, the in-plane spatial resolution of cardiac MDCT is determined by the size of the X-ray focal spot, the detector width in the plane of the fan beam, and the back-projection reconstruction filter. Typical in-plane spatial resolution is on the order of 0.5 mm or less. Successive generations of MDCT scanners produce an increasing number of detector rows at a decreasing detector width, thus keeping the overall scan time unchanged or even reduced. For the currently available 16-slice scanners, the minimum slice thickness is about 0.7 mm. At a typical pitch of 0.3 and gantry rotation of 0.5 second, a heart that spans 18 cm can be scanned in 30 seconds. A finer slice thickness allows discrimination of smaller structures and improves the quantity of 3D reconstruction (27). This is important because optimal viewing of the heart often requires reformation of the imaging plane to the cardiac axes. The quality improvement of 3D-processed images through successive generations of cardiac MDCT scanners is illustrated in Figure 8-6.

Radiation Exposure

Computed tomography, like other X-ray-based imaging modalities, exposes the patient to harmful ionizing radiation. In the current understanding of radiation safety, there is no threshold below which exposure to X-ray is deemed harmless. Radiation dose is a special concern for pediatric patients, whose lifetime cumulative dose can be substantial. For these reasons, a patient who undergoes a cardiac CT examination must have defined indications where the diagnostic benefit outweighs the risks and the maximum amount of diagnostic information is extracted.

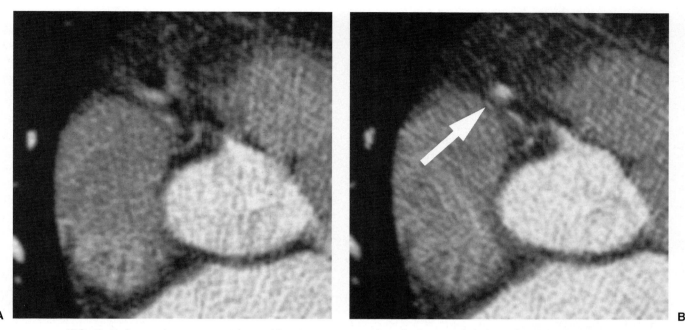

FIG. 8–5. Image improvement by multisector reconstruction. **A:** In an axial view, the right coronary artery (RCA) is blurred by motion in single-sector reconstruction. **B:** Visualization of the RCA (*arrow*) is improved by four-sector reconstruction.

Using an anthropomorphic phantom, Hunold et al. measured the radiation dose expected from typical protocols employed by cardiac MDCT, EBCT, and conventional coronary angiography (28). Using manufacturer-recommended protocol, calcium scoring with prospectively gated MDCT yields effective doses of 1.5 mSv for men and 1.8 mSv for women. In comparison, calcium scoring using EBCT yields an effec-

tive dose of 1.0 mSv for men and 1.3 mSv for women. Thus, radiation doses for calcium scoring are similar between MDCT and EBCT. For a 4-slice MDCT scanner operating at 1-mm detector width, contrast-enhanced coronary angiography with retrospective gating gives effective doses as high as 10.9 mSv for men and 13.0 mSv for women. The highest organ doses occur in the breast (44.0 mSv) and lung (37.6

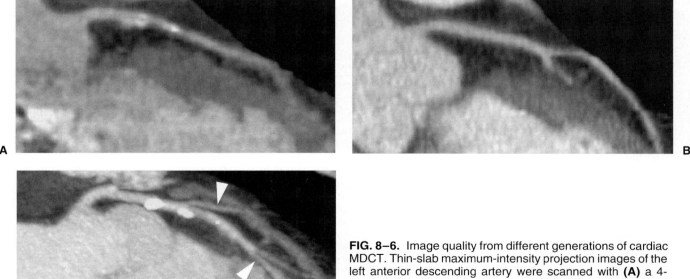

FIG. 8–6. Image quality from different generations of cardiac MDCT. Thin-slab maximum-intensity projection images of the left anterior descending artery were scanned with **(A)** a 4-slice MDCT at 1.25-mm detector width, **(B)** an 8-slice MDCT at 1.25-mm detector width, and **(C)** a 16-slice MDCT at 0.625-mm detector width, where definitions of small branch vessels (*arrowheads*) are improved.

mSv). These values vary substantially depending on tube voltage, tube current, and pitch value. In contrast, EBCT coronary angiography at 3-mm slice thickness imparts 1.5 mSv for man and 2.0 mSv for women. It should be noted that EBCT operates in prospective gating mode, where retrospective reconstruction at different cardiac phases is not possible. Other investigators reported similar results (29–31).

To put these numbers in perspective, fluoroscopic coronary angiogram produces 3 mSv to 10 mSv of radiation dose, depending on the size of the patient and whether a ventriculogram is performed. Thus, a CT coronary angiogram can exceed the radiation dose of fluoroscopic coronary angiogram (32,33). Computed-tomography coronary angiogram also exceeds the radiation dose of a routine chest CT, which ranges from 5 mSv to 7 mSv (34,35). A CT coronary angiogram is 50 to 100 times the radiation dose of a two-view chest radiograph and 3 times the average annual background radiation in the United States. Newer-generation MDCT scanners equipped with submillimeter slice thickness require even higher radiation doses to maintain the same signal-to-noise ratio.

Clearly, the radiation dose produced in MDCT coronary angiography is substantial. In pediatric examinations, it is crucial to lower the exposure technique appropriate to the patient's size. Techniques have been described to reduce radiation dose by spatial modulation or temporal modulation of the X-ray output. In spatial modulation, the tube current decreases when the X-ray travels through a thinner section of the body, typically in the anterior–posterior direction (36). This method of X-ray-dose reduction is applicable to noncardiac and cardiac CT scanning. A 50% reduction of radiation dose has been demonstrated on phantom studies. In temporal modulation, the tube current is reduced during the cardiac phase when images are not expected to be reconstructed (37). This technique

is useful in retrospectively gated CT coronary angiography, in which image reconstruction takes place mostly at diastole. A 45% to 50% reduction of radiation dose has been demonstrated with this technique. It potentially is possible to combine both modulation techniques to reduce further radiation dose.

Protocols

Cardiac MDCT applications can be grouped into coronary calcium scoring, cardiac morphology and function imaging, coronary angiography, and cardiac venography. Table 8.2 lists suggested imaging protocols for these applications. Iodinated contrast is used in all protocols except coronary calcium scoring. Cardiac morphology imaging and coronary angiography call for timed first-pass contrast enhancement similar to noncardiac CT angiography. Either a timing bolus or bolus triggering may be employed. In the former, a test bolus of approximately 20-cc contrast is injected and the region of interest is monitored at regular intervals, typically 1 second to 2 seconds. The contrast arrival time determines the scan delay of the actual CT angiography. In bolus triggering, the entire volume of contrast is injected. The region of interest is monitored again at regular intervals. Once the contrast material arrives, the patient is instructed to hold his or her breath and the CT angiography begins immediately.

Multidimensional Reconstruction

A routine cardiac MDCT scan produces 100 to 300 images per cardiac phase. Examining 10 cardiac phases, or 3000 primary images, is time consuming and exhausting. The amount of images would tax even the most capable picture-archive communication system (PACS) (38). Three-dimensional or four-dimensional (4D) image reconstruction may ameliorate this situation by focusing our attention on the

TABLE 8–2. *Typical cardiac MDCT protocols*

	Coronary calcium score	Cardiac morphology or function	Coronary angiography	Coronary vein mapping
Contrast volume	None	60 cc	120 cc	135 cc
Injection rate	None	4 cc/sec	4 cc/sec	3 cc/sec
Scan delay	None	Timing or Bolus trigger	Timing or Bolus trigger	50 sec Fixed delay
Scan mode	Prospective	Restrospective	Retrospective	Retrospective
Detector width	2.5 mm	1.25 mm	0.625 mm	1.25 mm
Gantry rotation	0.5 sec	0.5 sec	0.5 sec	0.5 sec
Pitch*	None	0.30–0.38	0.30–0.38	0.30–0.38
Scan direction	Top-down	Top-down	Top-down	Bottom-up
kVp	120	120	120	120
mA	300	300	400	300
Cardiac phase	70%	0%–90 %	40%–80%	50%–70%
% RR-interval	Prospective	at 10% interval	at 5% interval	at 10% interval

* Pitch is defined as distance traveled by table in one gantry rotation divided by the combined scan width, which is the detector width times the number of detect rows used.

relevant anatomy by highlighting functional abnormalities. When static anatomy is displayed, one or several cardiac phases with the best image quality are selected for traditional 3D-image-reconstruction techniques. For example, multiplanar reconstructions (MPR) can be used to generate the cardiac short-axis and long-axis views, which can be compared with echocardiography (Figure 8-7). Reformatted images parallel and perpendicular to a coronary vessel are valuable to assess coronary stenoses (39). Curved planar reformation (CPR), another 3D reformation technique, is helpful in laying out a long segment of coronary vessel on a single image (Figure 8-8). When technically adequate, CPR images succinctly convey information about stenoses and aneurysms (40). Virtual rendering provides a realistic depiction of the cardiac vessels, including the aorta, vena cavae, pulmonary artery and veins, and coronary artery and veins. Virtual rendering images particularly are useful for surgical planning (41). Even endoscopic views, popular in virtual

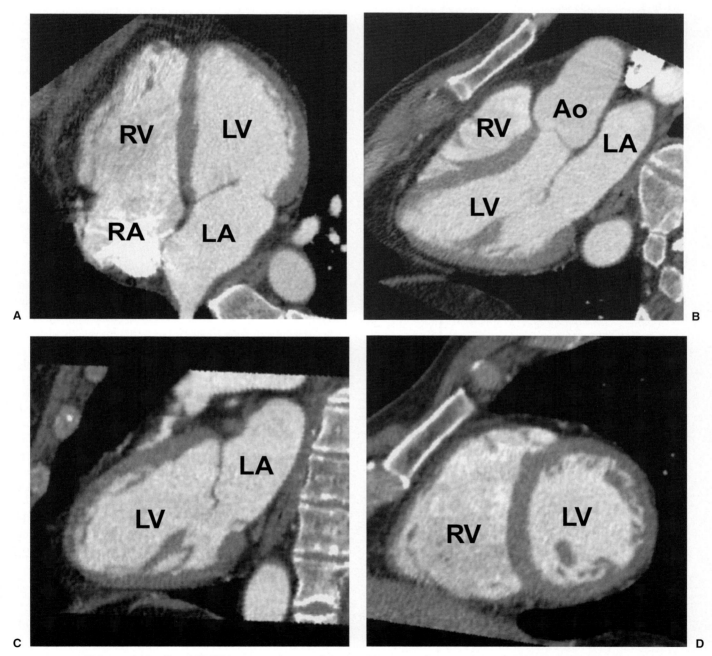

FIG. 8–7. Cardiac MDCT images planar reformatted into standard cardiac-axis views. **A:** Horizontal long-axis view, **(B)** three-chamber view, **(C)** vertical long-axis view, and **(D)** short-axis view. Labels are right ventricle (RV), left ventricle (LV), right atrium (RA), left atrium (LA), and aorta (Ao).

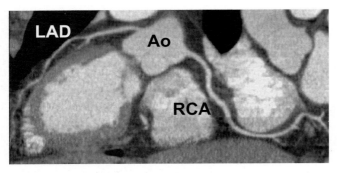

FIG. 8–8. Curved planar reformation of the coronary arteries. Curved planar reformation allows both coronary arteries to be seen on one image. Labels are right coronary artery (RCA), left anterior descending artery (LAD), and aorta (Ao).

colonoscopy and bronchoscopy, are helpful in the visualization of shunts and wall defects, such as atrial septal defect and aortopulmonary window.

Cardiac imaging is unique in that it contains temporal information that can be incorporated into image reconstruction. All the 3D reconstruction techniques discussed can be extended to the temporal domain and display dynamic movies of the beating heart in 3D (42). Dynamic MPR in the short-axis plane can be used to quantify ventricular volumes, ejection fractions, ventricular masses, and wall motion (43). Therefore, multidimensional reconstruction helps visualize both structural and functional abnormalities.

ISCHEMIC HEART DISEASE

Coronary artery disease (CAD) is the leading cause of death in developed countries. In the United States, CAD accounts for over 30% of deaths. The economic burden of CAD is in excess of 60 billion dollars a year (44). In the past thirty years, great strides have been made in understanding the molecular and genetic underpinnings of this disease. Technologies in diagnostic imaging and therapeutic intervention also have progressed tremendously. Together, these advances promise to help clinicians provide optimized care for their patients. There are numerous imaging studies for CAD. Some studies, such as coronary angiography, focus on the detection of structural lesions responsible for CAD. Others, such as stress myocardial-perfusion imaging, focus on the detection of myocardial ischemia. Multidetector CT and EBCT contribute to the CAD work up in three areas: coronary calcium scoring, coronary angiography, and coronary plaque characterization.

Coronary Calcium Scoring

Pathophysiology of Coronary Calcium

Coronary calcium is a product of systemic atherosclerosis, which is responsible for CAD. While there is no consensus, the prevailing theory for the genesis of atherosclerosis is the "response-to-injury" hypothesis (45). According to this hypothesis, an initial injury to the endothelium of the coronary arteries incites an inflammatory response. The nature of this injury is not defined well; it may be mechanical, biochemical, immunologic, or infectious in nature. The earliest detectable atherosclerotic lesions are fatty streaks in the arterial wall, composed of fat-laden monocytes residing beneath the intima. These lesions are asymptomatic and appear in individuals as early as the teens and twenties. The fatty streaks may progress to fibrofatty plaques composed of a large cholesterol core covered by a thin fibrous cap. The amount of calcium deposit in fibrofatty plaques is relatively small. Fibrofatty plaques, however, may evolve to a primarily fibrous plaque after reduction of their cholesterol core and resultant thickening of their fibrous cap. These lesions may calcify, and repeated hemorrhage and clotting may lead to complex plaques. This progression of atherosclerotic plaques generally is associated with luminal narrowing of the coronary arteries that may result in myocardial ischemia and infarction.

Recent investigations suggest a "vulnerable plaque" hypothesis, which proposes a distinction between unstable and stable plaques (46). In this hypothesis, unstable plaques are identified with early fibrofatty plaques. Their thin fibrous caps are thought to have a greater risk of rupture than the caps of later fibrous plaques. By exposing the clotting receptors underneath the endothelium, the rupture heralds a catastrophic thrombosis and occlusion of the coronary artery. This hypothesis may explain in part why a substantial number of patients who present with acute myocardial infarction have no previous history or symptoms of CAD. Note that calcium deposits are associated more closely with later more stable coronary plaques than earlier less stable plaques (47).

If the "response-to-injury" hypothesis and the "vulnerable plaque" hypothesis hold true, it may then be concluded that while coronary calcium does indicate the presence of atherosclerosis, it does not identify the location of a hemodynamically significant stenosis, the risk of catastrophic occlusion at the site, or the timing of the occlusion. In general, the amount of coronary calcium correlates with the overall severity of atherosclerosis, calcific and noncalcific plaques included. Therefore, coronary calcium is a marker for the unseen, potentially more dangerous, noncalcified or soft plaque. The quantification of coronary calcium then allows the assigning of an overall risk to a patient that assesses the probability of significant coronary atherosclerosis.

Coronary Calcium Imaging

Before the clinical introduction of CT, attempts had been made to detect coronary calcium with fluoroscopy, but this imaging method proved to have low sensitivity. Compared to EBCT, only 52% of the calcific lesions were detected by fluoroscopy and only lesions greater than 546

Hounsfield units (HU) could be seen (48). Fluoroscopic detection of coronary calcium was complicated further by considerable interobserver variability and a lack of standardized quantification method.

Objective characterization of coronary calcium became possible after the introduction of EBCT. Image quality improved with the rapid-scanning and cardiac-synchronization capabilities of EBCT. In a typical protocol, each image is obtained in a 100-ms acquisition at 3-mm slice thickness. Thirty to forty adjacent axial images are obtained by table incrementation similar to the prospective gating scheme of MDCT. Typically, image acquisition occurs at 80% RR interval, selected near the end of diastole when cardiac motion is at a minimum; the images are then postprocessed to calculate the overall calcium score. Over a decade, a large amount of clinical data has been accumulated for calcium scoring using EBCT; in fact, coronary calcium scoring has become a defining application for EBCT.

The recent development of cardiac MDCT offered an alternative to EBCT for coronary calcium imaging. Multidetector CT calcium images can be acquired with either prospective or retrospective gating (49). Prospective gating has the advantage of delivering a lower radiation dose, an important consideration in the screening of an asymptomatic population. A typical protocol acquires images at 2.5-mm slice thickness and 300-ms temporal resolution during diastole. Figure 8-9 shows examples of coronary calcium imaged with prospectively gated MDCT. With four-detector rows or more, the entire heart can be scanned in a single breath hold. Some investigators advocate the use of retrospective gating for better image quality and reproducibility of the calcium score (50,51). A retrospectively gated protocol acquires images at 2.5-mm detector width, a pitch of 0.38, and image reconstruction at 3.0-mm slice thickness. Improved reproducibility of calcium scoring is important in comparing serial studies of a patient. Presently, there is no standardized MDCT protocol for calcium imaging.

Scoring Methods

Standardization of the calcium scoring method provides a consistency that permits meaningful comparison among longitudinal studies or cross-sectional studies. The most common quantification indices are calcium volume, calcium mass, and the Agatston score. The simplest index is calcium volume. To measure calcium volume, an operator outlines and selects the expected regions of the coronary arteries on the CT images. A threshold is applied to discriminate the coronary calcium. The total volume is calculated by adding the number of pixels multiplied by the product of the pixel area and the slice thickness. The calculation of calcium mass is similar, except that each pixel first is weighted by the calcium density of that pixel. The absolute value of calcium density can be related to the CT number of a pixel by imaging with the patient a phantom containing calcium of known densities (52).

In 1990, Agatston et al. published a calcium scoring scheme that would become known as the Agatston score (53). The Agatston scoring scheme assumes a standardized EBCT protocol as described above. To be considered a calcium deposit, the lesion on an image must have density greater than 130 HU and must have an area greater than 1 mm^2. The latter requirement usually means three or more contiguous pixels. These criteria help filter out EBCT image noise that otherwise would be included as calcium. On each image, the area of calcific lesion is recorded, along with the maximum CT number measured in Hounsfield units within that lesion. A per-lesion score is determined from the maximum CT number according to Table 8.3. The area of the lesion is multiplied by the corresponding per-lesion score. This then is summed over all lesions in all image slices to produce the final Agatston score. The physical interpretation of the Agatston score is complex. When the overall calcification is severe, where most pixels have values greater than 400 HU, the Agatston score correlates with calcium volume. Conversely, when the calcification is mild, where most pixels have values less than 400 HU, the Agatston score correlates with calcium mass.

MDCT versus EBCT

For over a decade, a large amount of clinical and epidemiological data related to coronary calcium has been collected using the Agatston score on EBCT images. The choice of the Agatston scoring scheme created two problems. First, the computation algorithm of the Agatston score assumes certain performances of the EBCT scanner that are not true in MDCT scanners. For the same patient, the Agatston scores calculated from MDCT and EBCT images may not be the same. This problem is compounded further by a lack of standard imaging protocol for MDCT. Early studies suggested that the EBCT Agatston scores correlate with those obtained with prospectively gated MDCT (54) and retrospectively gated MDCT (55). However, the MDCT and EBCT scores do not always match, especially at low score values. This discrepancy may be due to differences in noise characteristics, differences in temporal resolution, or mismatch between image slices. Unfortunately, the absence of coronary calcium is a clinically important observation because it helps exclude CAD as the cause of symptoms. Inconsistency at low calcium score can jeopardize the interpretation. In addition, there are studies that suggest that the Agatston score may not be as reproducible as other calcium indices, such as volume and mass (56,57). For these reasons, some investigators advocate moving away from the traditional Agatston scoring scheme and replacing it with a scanner-independent scoring system, such as calcium mass calibrated by phantom. However, epidemiological data would have to be collected again using the new scoring system to guide clinical interpretation.

To date, there are no clinical studies relating MDCT calcium score directly to clinical outcomes. In the following discussion, data are derived from EBCT studies.

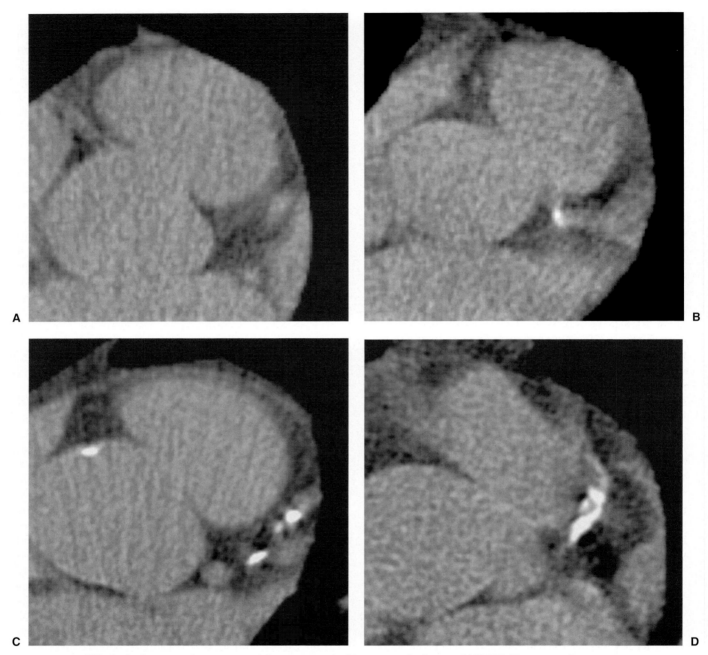

FIG. 8–9. Images of coronary calcium scanned with prospectively gated MDCT. Shown are four examples of the left anterior descending artery with increasing calcium burden. Their Agatston scores are **(A)** 0, **(B)** 41, **(C)** 380, and **(D)** 843.

TABLE 8–3. *Per lesion score table for Agatston coronary-calcium scoring*

Per lesion score	Maximum CT number per lesion	
	Greater than	Less than
1	130	199
2	200	299
3	300	399
4	400	No limit

Epidemiology of Coronary Calcium

Data from autopsy, intravascular ultrasound, and other imaging studies of the coronary arteries suggest that atherosclerotic plaque, with or without calcium, is present in 50% of individuals between the ages of 20 and 29, rising to 80% between the ages of 30 and 39. Atherosclerotic calcification is present in 50% of individuals between the ages of 40 and 49, rising to 80% between the ages of 60 and 69. Therefore, coronary calcium appears later in life than atherosclerotic plaque, and both calcium and plaque increase in prevalence with age. Since clinically significant stenosis appears in only 30% of individuals between the ages 60 and 69, most patients with coronary calcium do not develop clinically significant stenosis or experience symptomatic CAD (58).

The two most important risk factors for coronary calcium are age and gender. Hoff et al. published the percentiles of Agatston scores, stratified by age and sex, of 35,246 self-referred asymptomatic individuals who underwent EBCT for calcium screening. These data, plotted in Figure 8-10, form the epidemiological baseline of coronary calcium in the general population. There is a sizable variation of calcium scores within each age group, although their calcium scores consistently increased with age. For each age group, the calcium scores for men are substantially higher than those for women. Other risk factors suggested for coronary calcium include elevated plasma-cholesterol level, cigarette smoking, elevated blood pressure, diabetes, obesity, and elevated triglyceride level—all of which are risk factors associated with CAD.

Studies also suggest a correlation between calcium score and CAD-related symptoms and coronary findings. In a group of 1172 initially asymptomatic patients (baseline age 53 years ± 11 years, 71% men) followed for an average of 3.6 years, 39 either died or had coronary-related events, with some requiring interventional procedures. For an initial calcium score of more than 160, the odds ratio for predicting all coronary events was 15.8 and the odds ratio for predicting myocardial infarction and death was 22.2 (59). Therefore, while most asymptomatic individuals do not develop coronary symptoms, those with a moderate or higher calcium score are at substantially increased risk. In a group of 1764 symptomatic patients (baseline age 56 years ± 14 years for men and 60 years ± 16 years for women, 69% men) who underwent both EBCT calcium scoring and coronary cathe-

terization, a calcium score of 100 had positive predictive values of 76% and 71% for any coronary stenosis greater than 50% and 75%, respectively. Thus, a substantial fraction of symptomatic patients who have moderate calcium scores do harbor a significant coronary stenosis. In the same population, a calcium score of 0 had a negative predictive value of 97%. Thus, symptomatic patients who have no detectable coronary calcium are very unlikely to have CAD as the cause of their symptoms. Qualitatively similar results were found by other investigators (60,61).

Clinical Indications

In the year 2000, based on available epidemiological data, clinical trials, and pathophysiological evidence, the American College of Cardiology, jointly with the American Heart Association, produced an expert consensus document on EBCT for the diagnosis and prognosis of CAD (62). Their findings are summarized below:

i. A zero calcium score makes the presence of atherosclerotic plaque and significant coronary-obstructive lesion unlikely.
ii. A nonzero calcium score confirms the presence of CAD.
iii. The greater the amount of calcium, the greater the likelihood of occlusive CAD.
iv. A high calcium score may be consistent with moderate-to-high risk of a cardiovascular event within the subsequent 2 years to 5 years.

Based on these findings, the following clinical indications have been proposed.

Evaluation of Atypical Chest Pain

Patients presenting with atypical chest pain, such as those without a history of CAD and with indeterminate labo-

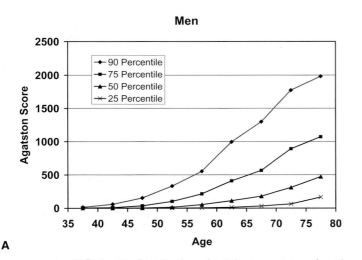
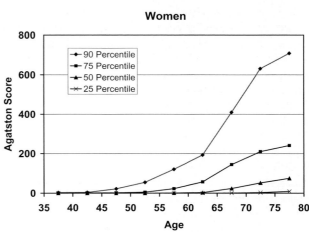

FIG. 8–10. Distribution of calcium score as a function of age. Plots show results for **(A)** 25,251 asymptomatic men and **(B)** 9995 asymptomatic women. The calcium scores for men are two to four times higher than for women of the same age.

ratory tests, including ECG, may benefit from coronary-calcium evaluation. This group of patients comprises a significant portion of ambulatory care, including emergency room visits. In EBCT studies examining this population, an absence of coronary calcium has more than 95% negative predictive value of excluding CAD as the cause of chest pain (63,64). The rare instances of false-negative results could be caused by rupture of noncalcific plaques in early disease found in younger patients or women.

Risk Assessment in Asymptomatic Patients

While it has been established that the calcium score correlates with symptomatic CAD and predicts risk of cardiac events, the incremental value of calcium score over "traditional" multivariate risk-assessment models, such as the Framingham risk-factor score, is not as well defined. Using multiple logistic-regression analyses, Raggi et al. demonstrated in a group of 676 asymptomatic patients that age- and sex-specific percentiles of EBCT calcium score provided incremental prognostic value to traditional risk factors for CAD (65). However, Detrano et al. reported no incremental value of calcium score in 1196 asymptomatic subjects. More definitive answers will be provided by the Multi-Ethnic Study of Atherosclerosis (MESA) trial sponsored by the National Heart, Lung, and Blood Institute of the National Institutes of Health. This study is intended to determine which comparative measures are additive to traditional coronary-risk-factor models. Until then, the use of coronary-calcium score in selected asymptomatic patients may be justified when traditional risk assessment is considered insufficient by the physician to direct further therapy plans.

Assessment of Therapeutic Response

Since coronary-calcium score correlates with atherosclerosis, serial calcium scores may be used to monitor the effectiveness of a particular therapy, such as lipid-lowering drug treatment. Furthermore, changes in serial calcium scores may guide the intensity of the therapy. In a study of 149 asymptomatic hyperlipidemic patients, 105 were randomized to treatment with a statin medication and 44 to no treatment (66). The average increases in EBCT-measured calcium volume after one year were 5% ± 28% and 52% ± 36% for the treated and untreated groups, respectively. The difference between the two groups was statistically significant ($P < 0.001$). Within the treated group, those who achieved a low-density lipid (LDL) level less than 120 mg/dL showed an average regression of 7% ± 23%, while those who achieved an LDL level above 120 mg/dL showed a progression of 25% ± 22%. Thus, it appears that the intensity of statin therapy has an impact on the progression of coronary calcium. While these results are encouraging, larger studies are needed to confirm these conclusions, establish the normal range, and determine if these changes translate to a reduction of cardiac events and deaths.

Coronary Angiography

For half a century, fluoroscopic coronary angiography has been the standard test for detection of stenotic lesions in coronary arteries and staging of CAD. Performed with modern fluoroscopic equipment, coronary angiography has spatial and temporal resolution unsurpassed by any other imaging modality. Endovascular interventional therapies, such as angioplasty and stent deployment, can be executed in the same setting when necessary. The enthusiasm for its use, however, is tempered greatly by potential complications associated with arterial catheterization, including stroke, dissection, and death. Although the risk of a major complication in current practice is generally less than 1%, this risk is justified only if the cardiac disease is life threatening or symptom limiting, and if the outcome of the angiogram would affect treatment options (67). Fluoroscopic coronary angiography plays no role in screening. For these reasons, there is a great desire to develop an alternative imaging test that is safer and more accessible to patients. Both MRI (68) and EBCT (69–71) have attempted to image coronary arteries, but neither modalities have gained acceptance in routine clinical practice. Magnetic-resonance imaging is limited by low signal-to-noise ratio, whereas EBCT is limited by poor spatial resolution. Multidetector CT overcomes both of these limitations and has shown promise in early clinical studies.

Imaging Considerations

In a typical MDCT coronary angiography protocol, images are scanned, using the thinnest slice thickness available, from the root of the aorta to the inferior surface of the heart during first pass of the contrast bolus. Retrospective gating is preferred because the cardiac phase for image reconstruction can be adjusted retrospectively to minimize motion artifacts. Studies have shown that the optimal cardiac phase for the right coronary artery, typically 40% to 50% of the interval between R-waves, occurs earlier than that for the left anterior descending artery and the left circumflex artery, typically 60% to 70% of the interval between R-waves (17,18). In practice, multiple cardiac phases are reconstructed at small intervals during diastole and images from each cardiac phase are inspected for image quality. The cardiac phase with the best visualization for a coronary artery segment is chosen for diagnostic evaluation of that segment.

To evaluate stenosis accurately, the lumen of a coronary vessel should be delineated clearly from the vessel wall. The quality of this delineation is affected by lumen size, degree of contrast opacification, motion artifacts, and artifacts from radiographically dense materials. With currently available submillimeter MDCT scanners, visualization of vessel lumen as small as 1.5 mm is feasible. The density of contrast opacification depends on the iodine density in the contrast material, the rate of contrast injection, and physiologic factors such as cardiac output. The degree of motion artifact is affected by heart rate and the magnitude of wall motion.

Dense materials that can create artifacts include coronary calcium, metallic stents, surgical clips, pacemaker wires, and dense contrast material mixing in the right atrium. The latter could confound visualization of the right coronary artery.

Several studies have demonstrated an inverse relationship between image quality of the coronary arteries and heart rate. Using a 4-slice MDCT scanner imaging at 1-mm detector width, Nieman et al. performed MDCT coronary angiography in 78 patients and found that sensitivity for detecting significant coronary stenosis dropped from 81% at an average heart rate of 56 beats per minute to 32% at an average heart rate of 82 beats per minute (26). Using a similar MDCT protocol, Giesler et al. reported comparable findings in a group of 100 patients. The sensitivity for stenosis dropped from 62% for those with heart rate less than 70 beats per minute to 33% for those with heart rate greater than 70 beats per minute (25). These results motivated the use of β_1 receptor antagonist to slow down the patient's heart rate during the MDCT scan.

In 126 patients who underwent MDCT coronary angiography, Gerber et al. not only confirmed the influence of heart rate on image quality, but also revealed the adverse effect of coronary calcium on vessel assessment (24). When the Agatston score for coronary calcium fell below 100, only 1% of the vessel segments were not visualized well enough to assess stenosis. In contrast, when the Agatston score rose above 100, 33% of the vessel segments could not be assessed. The poor luminal delineation was caused in part by the blooming effect of the in-plane image-reconstruction kernel, and in part by the poor spatial resolution in the slice direction. Coronary stents cause a similar problem. The newer generation of submillimeter scanners improve visualization within stents and light calcifications, especially in conjunction with transluminal image reformation (Figure 8-11). However, visualization of the lumen within heavily calcified walls likely will remain problematic.

Normal Coronary Arterial Anatomy

Since MDCT coronary angiography reveals coronary arteries and veins equally well, a thorough understanding of the normal and variant anatomy of the coronary vessels is crucial to avoid confusion between the two systems (72). An overview of the coronary arteries is presented below. A discussion of the coronary venous anatomy will be deferred to in the next section.

In 85% of the population, the coronary circulation is found to be right dominant, that is, the right coronary artery (RCA) supplies the inferoseptal and inferior walls of the left ventricle by giving rise to both the posterior descending artery (PDA) and the posterior left ventricular (PLV) branches (Figure 8-12). In 8% of the population, the coronary circulation is left dominant, where the PDA and PLV branches are both supplied by the left circumflex artery (LCx). In the remaining 7%, the coronary circulation is balanced dominant, where the RCA supplies the PDA while the LCx supplies the PLV branches.

The RCA normally originates from the right aortic sinus of Valsalva and courses anteriorly into the right atrioventricular groove (Figure 8-12). A conal artery may arise as the first branch of the RCA, although 50% of the time it arises from the aorta directly above the RCA. This conal artery supplies the myocardium at the right ventricular outflow tract. A sinoatrial nodal artery may arise from the proximal RCA or from the LCx in roughly equal frequency (Figure 8-13). The middle portion of the RCA usually gives rise to one or more acute marginal branches supplying the free wall of the right ventricle. The distal portion of the RCA wraps around the inferior surface of the heart. At the intersection of the interventricular septum and the atrioventricular groove, known as the crux, the RCA forms an inverse U, and at the apex of this U bend, the atrioventricular nodal branches commonly arise (Figure 8-14). In a right-dominant circula-

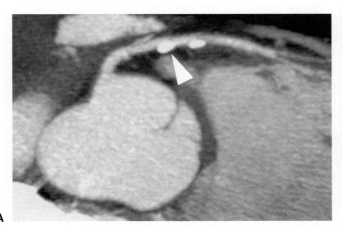
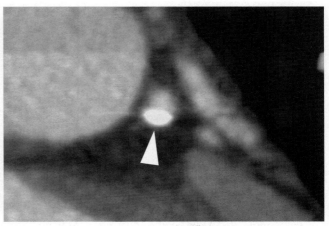

FIG. 8–11. Longitudinal and transluminal views of a left anterior descending artery. **A:** The longitudinal view shows two eccentric calcifications that seem to constrict the lumen. **B:** A transluminal view of the first calcification (*arrowhead*) clarifies that the contrast-filled lumen is narrowed only mildly.

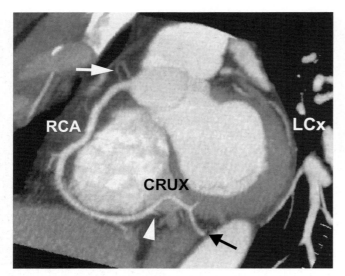

FIG. 8–12. Right coronary artery in a right-dominant circulation. In this short-axis view, a conal artery (*arrow*) originates from the aorta just above the RCA. The RCA follows the right atrioventricular groove and passes the inferior wall at the septum, called the crux, to the inferior surface of the left ventricle. The posterior descending artery (*arrowhead*) and the posterior left ventricular arteries (*black arrow*) branch from the distal RCA. A segment of the LCx is seen in the left atrioventricular groove.

tion, the RCA gives rise to the PDA before the crux and one or more PLV branches after the crux. The PDA has small perforator branches that supply the inferior septal wall.

The left main coronary artery (LMCA) originates from the left aortic sinus of Valsalva and courses to the left for a short distance. It bifurcates into the left anterior descending artery (LAD) and the LCx. In some patients, there is a third branch of the LMCA, called the ramus medianus, that bisects the angle between the LAD and the LCx (Figure 8-15). The

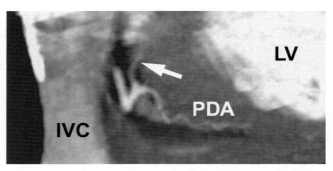

FIG. 8–14. Atrioventricular-node artery. In this magnified, sagittal reformatted view, the atrioventricular node artery (*arrow*) arises from the inverted U bend of the RCA, which also supplies the PDA. Labels are inferior vena cava (*IVC*) and left ventricle (*LV*).

ramus medianus functions like a diagonal branch and supplies the anterolateral wall of the left ventricle. The LAD gives rise to a number of perforator branches that dive deep into the interventricular septum. The LAD also gives rise to a number of surface branches, called the diagonal branches, that supply the anterolateral wall of the left ventricle. The distal LAD typically wraps around the apex and supplies its inferior portion. The LCx may give off a sinoatrial nodal branch (Figure 8-13B) before the LCx enters the left atrioventricular groove. There, the LCx gives rise to a number of obtuse marginal branches (OM) that supply the lateral wall of the left ventricle. In a left-dominant or balanced-dominant circulation, the LCx continues to the posterior and inferior walls, giving rise to the PLV branches; in a left-dominant circulation, the LCx supplies the PDA (Figure 8-16).

Clinical Results

Coronary artery disease can produce both stenotic and aneurysmal lesions of the coronary arteries, as shown in

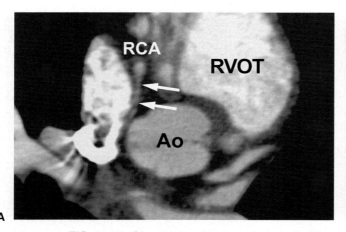

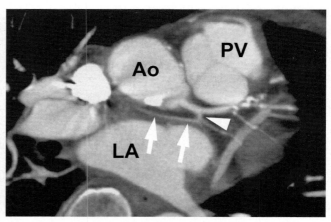

FIG. 8–13. Sinoatrial node artery. **A:** In half of the cases, the sinoatrial node artery (*arrows*) arises from the RCA, as seen on this axial view. **B:** In the other half, it originates from the LCx (*arrowhead*) just after it branches from the left main coronary artery, as seen on this oblique axial view. Labels are aorta (*Ao*), right ventricular outflow tract (*RVOT*), left atrium (*LA*), and pulmonary valve (*PV*).

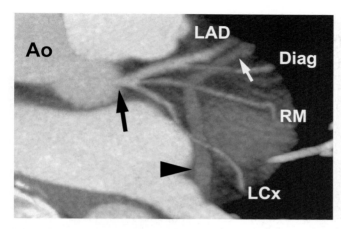

FIG. 8–15. Major branches of the left main coronary artery. Arising from the aorta (*Ao*), a short left main coronary artery (*black arrow*) trifurcates into a LAD, a ramus medianus artery (RM), and a LCx in this oblique axial view. The LAD gives rise to a diagonal branch (Diag). The greater cardiac vein (*black arrowhead*) is the companion vein of the LCx, while the anterior interventricular vein (AIV) (*white arrow*) is the companion vein of the LAD. The LAD, LCx, and AIV form a triangular area called the trigone of Brocq and Mouchet.

Figures 8–17 and 8–18, respectively. The stenotic lesions may limit blood flow sufficiently to produce myocardial ischemia. In the case of total occlusion (Figure 8-19), the result is myocardial infarction. A number of clinical trials have been conducted to evaluate the sensitivity and specificity of MDCT coronary angiography against fluoroscopic coronary angiography in the detection of significant coronary stenosis. Most of these trials employ a 4-slice MDCT technology with a 1-mm detector width. Results from newer MDCT technol-

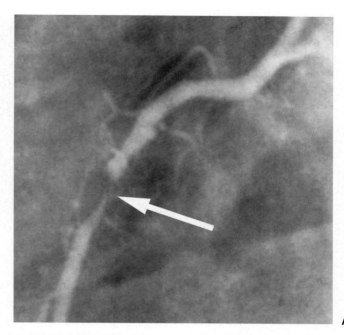

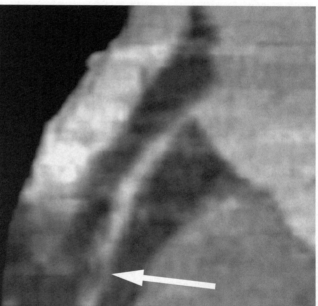

FIG. 8–17. Coronary stenosis. **A:** A fluoroscopic coronary angiogram reveals a tight stenosis in the RCA (*arrow*). **B:** The same lesion is seen on a reformatted planar view of a MDCT coronary angiogram (*arrow*).

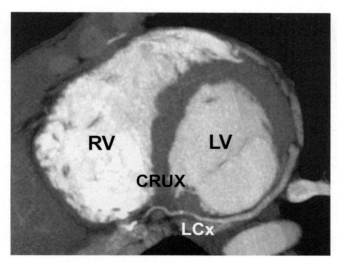

FIG. 8–16. Left circumflex artery in a left-dominant circulation. In this short-axis view, the LCx passes over the crux of the heart to supply the inferior wall of the right ventricle. Labels are right ventricle (*RV*) and left ventricle (*LV*).

ogy capable of submillimeter slice thickness are just beginning to appear in the literature.

From 2001 to 2003, eight clinical studies, summarized in Table 8.4, compared MDCT and fluoroscopic coronary angiography. Six of these studies employed 4-slice MDCT scanners at 1 mm detector width and a gantry rotation period of 0.5 second (8,24,25,73–75). The number of subjects varied between 25 and 105. Most of these studies excluded vessel diameter less than 2 mm. Of the vessel segments eval-

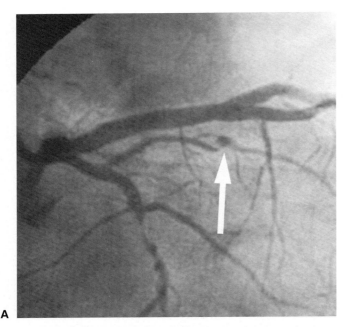

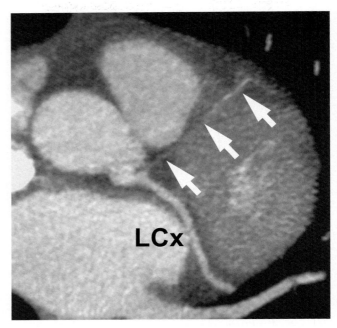

FIG. 8–19. Occlusion of a left anterior descending artery. Compared to the normal LCx, the LAD (*arrows*) is threadlike and has no contrast filling in this oblique axial view. This patient's LAD was dissected during pregnancy, resulting in an anterior-wall myocardial infarction.

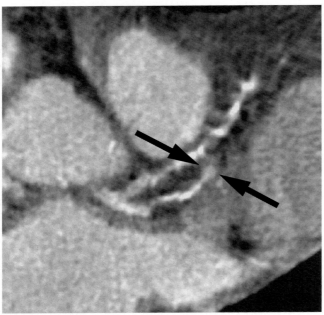

FIG. 8–18. Coronary aneurysm. **A:** A fluoroscopic coronary angiogram shows extensive CAD in this patient. A small aneurysm (*white arrow*) is identified in an OM. **B:** The same aneurysm (*black arrows*) is seen on an oblique axial view of a MDCT coronary angiogram.

uated, typically 75% (range 68%–95%) of these segments are visualized well enough to diagnose stenosis. Of the 25% nondiagnostic segments, the commonly cited reasons are heart rate greater than 60 beats per minute, Agatston score greater than 100, vessel diameter less than 2 mm, and poor contrast opacification (24). Of the 75% diagnostic segments, the sensitivity for detecting stenoses greater than 50% ranged from 81% to 93%, while the specificity ranged from 90%

to 97%. The sensitivity for detecting stenoses greater than 70% ranged from 82% to 91%, and the specificity ranged from 84% to 96%. Two studies examined 77 and 59 patients using a newer generation of MDCT that supports 12-detector rows at 0.75-mm detector width and a rotation period of 0.42 second (39,76). One study excluded vessel diameter smaller than 2.0 mm, and the other excluded vessels smaller than 1.5 mm. Compared with earlier scanners, the fraction of diagnostic coronary segments increased to 88% and 98%, respectively. Of these segments, the sensitivity for detecting greater than 50% stenoses ranged from 92% to 95%, while the specificity ranged from 86% to 93%. These initial results support the notion that submillimeter scanners improve visualization of coronary arteries and determination of stenosis. Although these results are encouraging, confirmation by larger clinical trials is needed.

Coronary Plaque Imaging

Cardiac MDCT has the ability to visualize directly abnormally thickened walls of the coronary arteries, a feat not possible with fluoroscopic angiography. If the wall thickness is known, the true extent of vessel narrowing can be estimated better (77). Furthermore, different constituents of atherosclerotic plaques, such as calcium, fibrous tissue, and lipid, have different radiographic densities (78). By quantifying the radiographic density of a plaque, it may be possible to characterize the composition of that plaque. The amount of lipid in a plaque and the thickness of the fibrous capsule

TABLE 8–4. *MDCT coronary-angiography clinical trials*

Author	Date	Detector	Subjects	β-blocker	Stenosis Definition	Vessels Diagnostic	Sensitivity	Specificity
Roper (39)*	2/2003	12 × 0.75 mm	77	Yes	50%	88%	92%	93%
Nieman (76)	10/2002	12 × 0.75 mm	59	Yes	50%	98%	95%	86%
Gerber (24)	1/2003	4 × 1.0 mm	25	Yes	70%	70%	82%	96%
Nieman (75)	11/2002	4 × 1.0 mm	78	No	50%	68%	81%	95%
Kopp (8)	11/2002	4 × 1.0 mm	102	No	50%	82%	93%	97%
Giesler (25)	10/2002	4 × 1.0 mm	100	Yes	70%	71%	91%	89%
Becker (74)	9/2002	4 × 1.0 mm	28	Yes	50%	95%	81%	90%
Achenbach (73)	5/2001	4 × 1.0 mm	64	No	70%	68%	91%	84%

* Reference number.

may prognosticate a vulnerable plaque at risk of catastrophic rupture (79). Thus, the imaging and characterization of coronary plaques are of considerable clinical significance.

Differentiation between calcific and noncalcific plaques usually is straightforward, since densities of the two plaques are substantially different (Figure 8-20). The separation between lipid-laden plaque and fibrous plaque is less clear. Schroeder et al. performed a preliminary study of 15 patients who underwent MDCT coronary angiography using a 4-slice scanner at 1-mm detector width (80). Patients were pretreated with sublingual nitroglycerin. Computed-tomography plaque density was characterized by averaging 16 random samples taken within visually well-defined coronary plaques. The patients also underwent intravascular ultra-

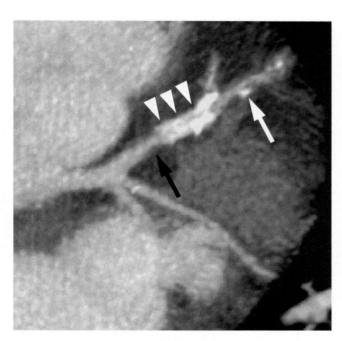

FIG. 8–20. Soft plaque, calcific plaque, and stent. Seen in this oblique axial view, a stent (*arrowheads*) has been laid across a left anterior descending artery stenosis. A significant amount of concentric low-density soft plaque (*black arrow*) is seen proximal to the stent. In addition, there are high-density calcific plaques (*white arrow*) along the LAD.

sound (IVUS) as the standard of reference for plaque characterization. Based on echogenicity, the plaques were classified as soft plaques (low echogenicity), intermediate plaques (high echogenicity without echo shadowing), and calcific plaques (echo shadowing). The different echogenicity of the soft plaques and intermediate plaques was due presumably to a larger lipid content of the former and a greater fibrous content of the latter. Correlation between IVUS classification and MDCT plaque-density measurements showed that the radiographic density of sonographically determined soft plaques was 14 HU ± 26 HU (range − 42 HU to + 47 HU), the density of intermediate plaques was 91 HU ± 21 HU (range 61 HU to 112 HU), and the density of calcific plaques was 419 HU ± 194 HU (range 126 HU to 736 HU). As expected, the density of soft plaques tended to be lower than that of intermediate plaques, suggesting a greater lipid content in the former.

The success of coronary plaque characterization depends greatly on image quality and spatial resolution. Quantitative density measurement is sensitive to partial volume effect, changes in contrast density within the lumen, and sharpness of the image-reconstruction kernel. Multidetector CT plaque characterization, although in its infancy, shows promise. However, further clinical trials will be needed to demonstrate its ultimate usefulness as a risk-stratification tool.

CORONARY-VEIN MAPPING

A number of endovascular therapies have been developed to treat various heart diseases that require cannulation of the coronary sinus (CS) and access to the coronary venous system. These therapies include retrograde perfusion of ischemic myocardium (81), radiofrequency ablation of accessory-conduction pathways (82), and experimental percutaneous *in-situ* coronary venous bypass (83). The most important therapy to date is the implantation of biventricular pacemakers and defibrillators for cardiac resynchronization, which has been shown to improve heart-failure symptoms, exercise tolerance, and left ventricular ejection fraction (84), and to reduce hospitalization and mortality in patients who suffer from severe heart failure (85). This procedure depends on

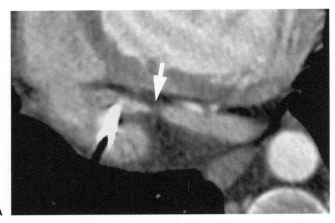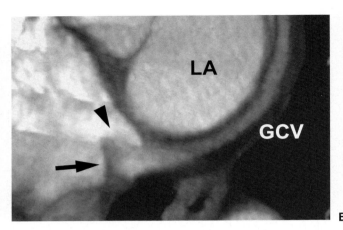

FIG. 8–21. Coronary sinus anomalies. **A:** In an axial view, a tight stenosis (*white arrow*) in the coronary sinus blocks access to the coronary venous system. **B:** In a short-axis view, a prominent Thebesian valve (*black arrow*) shields the entrance to the CS (*black arrowhead*). Labels are left atrium (*LA*) and greater cardiac vein (*GCV*).

the successful placement of a pacemaker lead into a coronary venous branch on the posterolateral surface of the left ventricle. Failure of cannulation occurs in a small but significant number of patients, reported at 8% (86). Causes of failure include abnormal origin of the CS, a CS covered by a large Thebesian valve, lack of accessible coronary veins on the left ventricular wall, and unanticipated venous stenosis. Some of these obstacles are illustrated in Figure 8-21. Coronary venous stenosis has been treated with angioplasty (87). Even for cases where pacemaker implantation ultimately was successful, the procedure time might be prolonged unnecessarily due to lack of a road map of the coronary veins. Preprocedure coronary vein mapping may prove useful for treatment planning. Coronary-vein mapping has been demonstrated with EBCT (88,89) and also can be achieved with cardiac MDCT.

Normal Coronary Venous Anatomy

Compared to coronary arterial anatomy, the coronary venous anatomy is even more variable (90). The major coronary veins are described best by their associations with companion arteries on the cardiac surface, as illustrated in Figure 8-22. In general, the coronary veins are larger in caliber and more visible than their companion arteries. Therefore, care must be taken not to confuse the two, especially in situations where an artery is occluded and only the vein remains visible.

The companion vein of the LAD is called the anterior interventricular vein (AIV). In most instances, the AIV situates to the left of the LAD over the interventricular septum, although in 12% of the cases the two veins cross each other (91). As the AIV courses toward the bifurcation of the LMCA, AIV turns away from the LAD and travels with the LCx in the left atrioventricular groove. The segment of vein within the left atrioventricular groove is called the greater

cardiac vein (GCV). The triangle bordered by the LCx, the LAD, and the AIV is called the trigone of Brocq and Mouchet, also depicted in Figures 8–15 and 8–22. The LMCA does not have a companion vein. The GCV accompanies the LCx along the left atrioventricular groove to the inferior surface of the heart. The GCV may cross the LCx within the atrioventricular groove. The greater cardiac vein receives venous drainage from a number of left marginal veins (LMV). The LMV situated over the posterolateral wall is the desired target for insertion of a left ventricular lead. The middle cardiac vein (MCV) pairs with the PDA and drains into the GCV. The confluence of GCV and MCV forms the CS, which travels only 1 cm or 2 cm before emptying into the right atrium. The entrance of the CS into the right atrium may be guarded by a Thebesian valve of variable prominence. In a small percentage of patients, a small cardiac vein (SCV) can be identified along with the RCA and drains into the CS. Additional small Thebesian veins may drain the right-side heart directly into the right atrium.

Imaging Considerations

A protocol for cardiac vein imaging is given in Table 8.2. The coronary veins are opacified most intensely after contrast passage through the myocardium, which can be achieved after steady infusion of contrast for a sufficiently long period. Bolus timing is not necessary. Because definition of the CS is crucial in this application, it is imaged first by scanning from the bottom to the top of the heart.

VALVULAR HEART DISEASE

Imaging of the heart valves to assess clinically significant diseases requires high temporal resolution to resolve rapidly moving parts. In addition, evaluation of physiological parameters, such as valvular-pressure gradients and re-

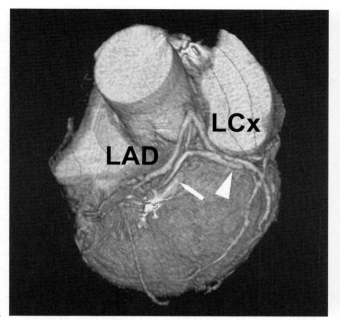

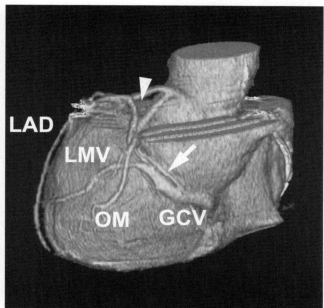

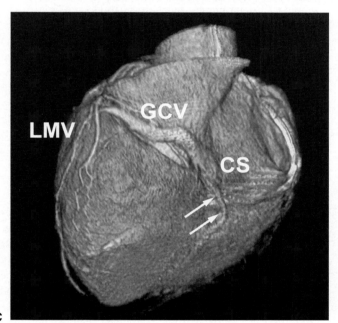

FIG. 8–22. Coronary venous system. The venous system can be traced on the surface of a virtual-rendered heart. **A:** Viewing at the anterior wall of the left ventricle, the AIV (*arrow*) accompanies the LAD. The AIV turns into the GCV (*arrowhead*), which accompanies the LCx. **B:** Viewing at the lateral wall, the GCV continues in the atrioventricular groove. A LMV, after crossing an obtuse marginal artery, joins the GCV. The GCV, in turn, crosses the LCx (*arrow*). The trigone of Brocq and Mouchet is seen at the upper margin (*arrowhead*). **C:** Viewing at the posterior wall, the GCV joins the MCV (*arrows*) to form a short-segment CS, which drains into the right atrium.

gurgitant flows, are important in the management of valvular stenosis and valvular regurgitation, respectively. These requirements are fulfilled by echocardiography and, to a lesser extent, by MRI and cardiac catheterization. The role of cardiac MDCT for the assessment of valvular heart disease is limited, given its relatively poor temporal resolution. In addition, using first-pass contrast technique, the tricuspid valve often is obscured by contrast-mixing artifacts in the right atrium. A short interval delayed scan is needed to image this valve. Despite these limitations, cardiac MDCT can image structures and small lesions of the valves at higher spatial resolution than other modalities.

Using a contrast-enhanced, retrospectively gated MDCT protocol, Willmann et al. demonstrated good correlation among MDCT, echocardiography, and surgical findings for mitral valve thickening, mitral valve calcification, and mitral-annulus calcification in 20 patients (92). The same investigators also reported good correlation for aortic valve morphology, aortic-annulus diameter, and aortic valve calcification in 25 patients (93). These measurements are useful for surgical planning of valve replacement.

Computed tomography can detect small calcific lesions of the aortic valve. Causes of aortic valve calcification include rheumatic heart disease, congenital bicuspid valve, and age-related degeneration. It has long been known that aortic-valve calcifications large enough to been seen on chest radiographs or fluoroscopy are associated strongly with valvular aortic stenosis. However, the relationship between a small amount of calcium detected by CT and aortic stenosis is not as well established. Lippert et al. reviewed 109 patients who underwent both routine chest CT and echocardiography (94). Aortic valve calcifications were found in 30% of the patients. Of these patients, only 15% showed an abnormal valvular pressure gradient of 25 mmHg or above, as estimated by echocardiography. Risk factors for aortic valvular stenosis include: amount of calcium, young age, and female gender. Attempts have been made to quantify aortic valve calcification to stratify the risk of aortic stenosis and guide preventive therapies in much the same way as coronary calcium scoring (95). Given that echocardiography can estimate the pressure gradient across a stenotic valve, echocardiography likely will remain the primary imaging tool for aortic stenosis. However, when a significant amount of aortic-valve calcification is discovered incidentally, especially in young or female patients, the possibility of aortic stenosis can be raised.

Cardiac MDCT is useful in the detection of valvular vegetations for endocarditis, as demonstrated in Figure 8-23. Although transesophageal echocardiography is the current imaging modality of choice for endocarditis (96), cardiac MDCT is less invasive. Multidetector CT provides better visualization of pulmonary valve lesions than echocardiography. Furthermore, MDCT is superior in detection and characterization of perivalvular abscess, a complication of endocarditis. The effectiveness of cardiac MDCT for this application will require further study.

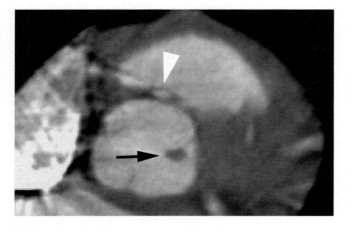

FIG. 8–23. Valvular vegetation. In this axial view, a small filling defect (*black arrow*) is seen attached to an aortic valve leaflet. This patient had endocarditis, and the filling defect was a surgically proven vegetation. This patient also had a supracristal ventricular septal defect (*white arrowhead*) that communicates between the left and right ventricular outflow tracts.

CARDIAC FUNCTION

Retrospectively gated cardiac MDCT studies can be reconstructed to produce a movie of the contracting ventricles. By reconstructing images at peak systole and end diastole, it is possible to quantify the minimum and maximum left and right ventricular volumes. From these volumes, global indices of systolic function, such as stroke volumes and ejection fractions, can be calculated. In addition, by measuring the left ventricular myocardial volume, the left ventricular mass can be derived. In current clinical practice, ventricular functions are evaluated in a number of ways, including echocardiography, fluoroscopic ventriculography, and nuclear scintigraphy. The most accurate method currently available is magnetic resonance cine imaging. Magnetic-resonance imaging has good spatial resolution and good endocardial delineation that allow accurate segmentation of the ventricles. Cardiac MDCT produces images of comparable or better spatial resolution and contrast at the endocardium, although at a significantly lower temporal resolution. Comparison between MDCT and biplane fluoroscopic ventriculography has shown good correlation (97), but trials comparing MDCT and MRI are ongoing. Currently, there are two roles for MDCT in cardiac-function imaging. First, whenever a retrospectively gated MDCT scan is performed—for example coronary angiography—the functional information already has been recorded and should be exploited and interpreted. Second, MDCT is a useful substitute when MRI is contraindicated. This happens most frequently when the patient has an implanted pacemaker, as illustrated in Figure 8-24.

Imaging Considerations

Contrast enhancement of the left and right ventricles should be maintained throughout the scan to optimize delineation of the endocardium. Images are reconstructed across the entire cardiac cycle, typically at 10% increments. By inspecting ventricular size, peak systole is identified as the cardiac phase when the ventricles are smallest, whereas end diastole is identified as the cardiac phase when the ventricles are largest. These two cardiac phases are selected, and their axial images are reformatted into short-axis views, typically at 5-mm to 10-mm thickness. The endocardium and epicardium of the left and right ventricles are traced manually or segmented automatically with a computer program to generate ventricular volumes and masses. Care must be taken to observe the ventricular boundaries at the valves. Computer workstations with specialized software are available commercially to assist with these measurements.

CONGENITAL HEART DISEASE

Congenital heart disease represents abnormalities in cardiovascular structure or function present at birth, although symptoms may not appear until later in life. About 0.8% of

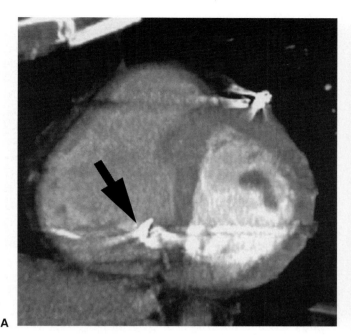
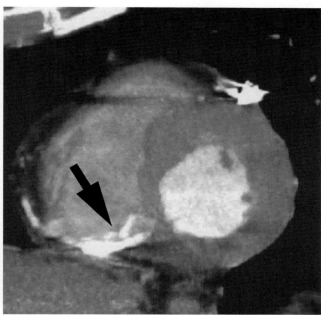

FIG. 8–24. Functional imaging of the heart. The axial MDCT images of the heart are reformatted into a stack of short-axis views. The ventricles then are segmented out and their volumes measured at **(A)** peak systole and **(B)** end diastole. A pacemaker lead (*arrow*) is seen in the right ventricle, which prevented this patient from undergoing an MRI study.

live births are complicated by a clinically significant cardiovascular malformation (98). Some common derangements are shunts, such as atrial and ventricular septal defects; abnormal chamber connections, such as tetralogy of Fallot and transposition of the great arteries; and extracardiac abnormalities, such as aberrant coronary arteries and aortic coarctation. A comprehensive discussion of imaging for congenital heart disease is beyond the scope of this chapter. In general, the goal of imaging is to determine both the structural abnormalities and their physiological consequences. The latter are measured by hemodynamic parameters including pressure, flow, velocity, and blood oxygenation. Echocardiography is the workhorse for the screening and diagnosis of congenital heart disease, especially in infants and young children. Advantages of echocardiography include its availability, safety, temporal resolution, and ability to quantify velocity and estimate pressure gradients. Both cardiac catheterization and MRI are second-line imaging modalities that provide additional diagnostic information.

With its superior spatial resolution and 3D imaging, cardiac MDCT is excellent for demonstrating anatomic structures and their spatial relationships, even in small infants. Cardiac MDCT particularly is useful for imaging regions not visualized well by echocardiography, such as the cardiac great vessels. Although cardiac MDCT development for congenital heart disease is still in its infancy, initial applications likely will parallel those attempted by conventional spiral CT for the evaluation of extracardiac vessels (99,100) and EBCT for assessment of aberrant coronary arteries

(101), surgical shunts (102), and intracardiac abnormalities (103–106).

Imaging Considerations

Because suspended respiration is necessary during MDCT, pediatric patients who cannot follow respiratory instructions should undergo general anesthesia. The goal should be reliable apnea for 30 seconds or less during the scan. Coordination with interested anesthesiologists is crucial for the timing of contrast injection, induction of apnea, and scanning. The scanning protocol is similar to cardiac function, in that 1-mm detector width usually suffices, although finer detector width could be used for small patients or small lesions. For children, radiation exposure should be adjusted to body weight and kept to a minimum. Because the contrast dose is scaled to body weight, the total volume of contrast for small children may be insufficient to provide for the timing bolus. In this situation, bolus tracking technique is helpful. If this is unavailable, scan delay after contrast injection is performed empirically based on estimated cardiac output. Lastly, since heart rate for infants is high, multisector reconstruction should be used.

Aberrant Coronary Arteries

Congenital coronary artery anomalies are uncommon disorders that are divided into four different forms: abnormal origin of the coronary arteries from the aorta, abnormal origin of a coronary artery from the pulmonary artery, coronary artery fistula, and abnormal coronary arrangements associated with congenital heart disease (107). Traditionally, these entities are screened by echocardiography. However, echocardiography is not completely accurate, and its success depends greatly on the skill of the operator. Definitive diagnosis requires coronary catheterization. Since most of these anomalies affect proximal large-caliber coronary arteries, they can be visualized reliably by noninvasive coronary angiography, which includes MRI and cardiac MDCT. Multidetector CT has the advantage of being a simpler, faster examination, an important benefit for patients requiring general anesthesia. Magnetic resonance coronary angiography has the advantage of not exposing patients to ionizing radiation, but requires special pulse sequences and skilled operators.

There are a number of different aberrant coronary arteries from the aortic sinuses, but only two configurations appear to be important clinically. The first configuration is an LMCA that arises from the RCA and passes between the aortic root and right ventricular outflow tract before bifurcating into an LAD and LCx. This type of aberrant left coronary artery is associated with sudden death, often during or immediately after vigorous exertion. This may be caused by ischemia induced by the dynamic compression of the LMCA between the cardiac great vessels. At baseline, these patients often are asymptomatic, with unrevealing physical examination and normal resting electrocardiogram, thereby making diagnosis difficult. Symptoms may include chest pain, unexplained dyspnea, and exertional syncope. The second configuration is an RCA that arises from the left aortic sinus of Valsalva and passes between the aortic root and right ventricular outflow tract before entering the right atrioventricular groove, as demonstrated in Figure 8-25. This configuration also may be responsible for sudden death and

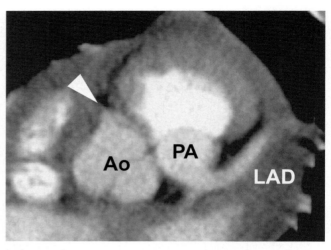

FIG. 8–26. Left coronary artery from the pulmonary artery. In this axial view, the left main coronary artery is seen arising from the pulmonary artery (PA). It supplies the LAD and the LCx. Blood in the left coronary circulation is desaturated and flows under low pressure, leading to ischemia or infarction of the myocardium. The right coronary artery (*arrowhead*) originates normally from the aorta (*Ao*).

myocardial ischemia, although the level of risk may be less than that with an aberrant LMCA.

In rare instances, the LMCA may arise from the pulmonary artery, as shown in Figure 8-26. This entity, the Bland–White–Garland syndrome, presents with myocardial ischemia and heart failure during infancy. The one-year mortality rate can be as high as 65% to 90%. In 10% to 15% of these patients, there are no significant cardiac symptoms until adulthood, when they present with exertional angina, dyspnea, palpitations, or even sudden death. These patients may have better developed collateral vessels from the RCA to the left coronary circulation that minimized the ischemic stress during their youth.

A coronary artery fistula is a communication between a coronary artery and another portion of the heart. If the coronary artery communicates with the right ventricle or the right atrium, there is a left-to-right shunt. If the communicates are large, there can be a volume overload of the right-side heart.

Certain congenital heart disease, such as tetralogy of Fallot, D-transposition of the great arteries, and pulmonary atresia with an intact ventricular septum, can develop anomalous coronary arteries. Knowledge of the exact locations of these vessels is critical for surgical planning to avoid injury to an unexpected coronary artery. Traditionally, these coronary arteries are mapped with fluoroscopic coronary angiography. However, cardiac MDCT has the advantage of showing not only the coronary arteries, but also their relationship to adjacent anatomic structures. This is demonstrated in Figure 8-27 for a patient with a D-transposition of the great arteries. An anomalous common trunk is seen originating from the anterior aortic root and bifurcating into an RCA

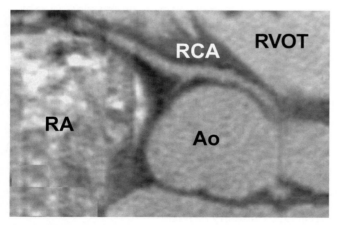

FIG. 8–25. Aberrant right coronary artery. In this image, an aberrant RCA travels between the aortic root (*Ao*) and the right ventricular outflow tract (RVOT) before it enters the right atrioventricular groove.

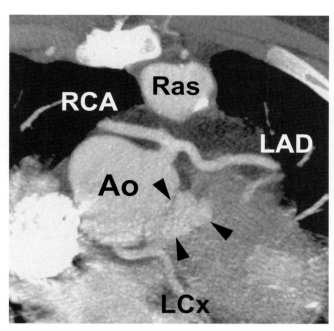

FIG. 8–27. D-transposition of the great arteries. In D-transposition, the pulmonary artery (PA) (*arrowheads*) is centered to the heart. The aorta is anterior and to the right of the pulmonary artery. In this patient, the PA (*black arrowheads*) is stenotic and his pulmonary trunk has been reconstructed with a Rastelli conduit (*Ras*), seen just behind the sternum. The coronary anatomy is anomalous in that the RCA and the LAD originate from a common trunk from an anterior aortic sinus, while the LCx originates from a posterior aortic sinus.

and LAD. This common trunk is in close proximity to a Rastelli conduit, which in turn lies immediately behind the sternum. This MDCT image helps guide the optimal surgical approach to this complex anatomic area.

Intracardiac Anomalies

Most intracardiac anomalies, such as atrial septal defect (ASD) and ventricular septal defect (VSD), are screened adequately and evaluated with echocardiography and, if hemodynamic measurements are necessary, cardiac catheterization. Still, these anomalies can be discovered as incidental findings in a routine MDCT scan and should be reported. Two examples are the muscular VSD shown in Figure 8-28 and the supracristal VSD shown in Figure 8-23. Cardiac MDCT is indicated for the work up of a sinus venosus ASD. This type of ASD, as shown in Figure 8-29, occurs high in the right atrium at the entrance of the superior vena cava. Although only 10% of all ASD belong to the sinus venosus type, it has a 90% association with partial anomalous pulmonary-venous return (PAPVR) of the right superior pulmonary veins. Because these veins lie within the right lung, they cannot be seen well by echocardiography. Cardiac MDCT readily localizes these vessels for surgical reconnection to the left atrium.

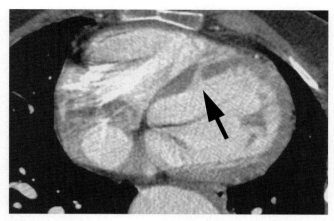

FIG. 8–28. Small muscular ventricular septal defect. An incidental ventricular septal defect (*arrow*) is found in the muscular septal of the ventricles in this patient with Marfan's syndrome.

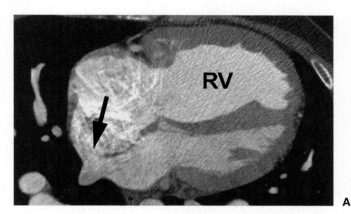

A

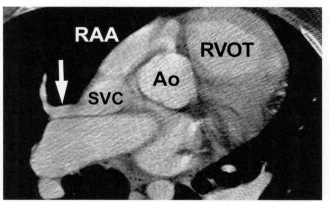

B

FIG. 8–29. Sinus venosus atrial septal defect. **A:** In this horizontal long-axis view, a pulmonary vein is seen entering the atria overriding the atrial septum. An atrial septal defect (ASD) (*arrow*) at this position allows pulmonary venous return to enter the right-side heart. Note that the right ventricle (*RV*) is dilated, its myocardium hypertrophic, and its septum bulges into the left ventricle, suggesting a component of pulmonary hypertension. **B:** In this axial view, the right superior pulmonary vein drains into the superior vena cava (*SVC*). Sinus venosus ASD is associated strongly with anomalous pulmonary venous return. Other labels are right atrial appendage (*RAA*), aorta (*Ao*), and right ventricular outflow tract (*RVOT*).

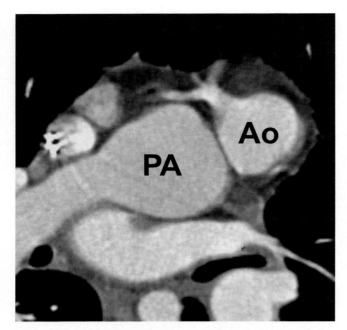

FIG. 8–30. L-transposition of the great arteries. In L-transposition, the PA is centered to the heart. The Ao is anterior and to the left of the pulmonary artery.

Cardiac MDCT, combined with 3D reconstruction, can demonstrate complex chamber arrangements elegantly, sometimes in views not available with echocardiography or cardiac catheterization. Therefore, cardiac MDCT is a useful adjunctive tool in the formal segmental analysis of congenital cardiac lesions, especially in complex cases. To illustrate, Figures 8–27 and 8–30 show the abnormal relationship between the aorta and the pulmonary artery in two types of transposition of the great arteries (TGA): D-TGA and L-TGA, respectively. D-TGA is associated with uncorrected transposition while L-TGA is associated with corrected transposition. In D-TGA, the aorta is situated in front and to the right of the pulmonary artery, hence the prefix D or dextro. In L-TGA, the aorta is situated in front and to the left of the pulmonary artery, hence the prefix L or levo. Figure 8-31 shows the four anomalies of tetralogy of Fallot: overriding aorta, VSD, right ventricular hypertrophy, and pulmonary stenosis. Figure 8-32 shows a more complex disorder of tricuspid atresia, which also includes an ASD, VSD, hypoplastic right ventricle, and muscular pulmonary atresia. In addition, cardiac MDCT can help treatment planning. For example, in cases with unequal ventricular sizes, measurements of chamber volumes help guide the decision between single-ventricle repair and two-ventricle restoration. Volumetric measurements can be accomplished with cardiac MDCT in the same manner as the evaluation of cardiac function.

Extracardiac Anomalies

Cardiac MDCT provides excellent noninvasive evaluations of extracardiac vascular anomalies, as has been seen in the example of PAPVR in Figure 8-29B. Contrast-enhanced CT angiography now replaces many invasive vascular studies carried out in the past by fluoroscopic angiography. Cardiac-gated MDCT further improves image quality by removing the arterial-pulsation artifacts seen in conventional CT angiography of the chest. Cardiac MDCT has proven useful in the detection and characterization of structural anomalies of the aorta, pulmonary arteries, vena cavae, and pulmonary veins.

Among congenital anomalies of the aorta, coarctation is the most common, representing 6.8% of significant congenital cardiac malformations at birth. It is associated with bicuspid aortic valve, circle of Willis aneurysm, VSD, subaortic obstruction, and mitral valve anomalies. Coarctation is associated with Turner Syndrome and Shone Syndrome.

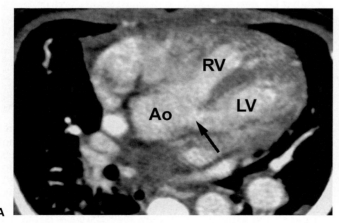

A

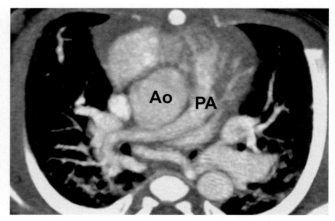

B

FIG. 8–31. Tetralogy of Fallot. This patient is a 1-month-old girl with tetralogy of Fallot. **A:** An axial view shows a ventricular septal defect (*arrow*), an aortic root overriding the septum, and right ventricular hypertrophy. **B:** In a higher axial view, a diffusely stenotic pulmonary artery (*PA*) is seen compared with the Ao. The left pulmonary artery is not included in this view.

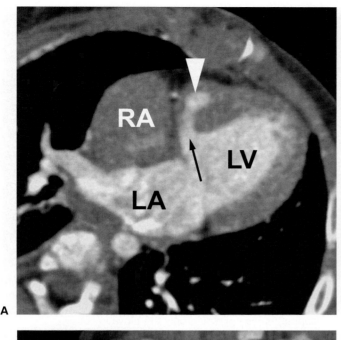

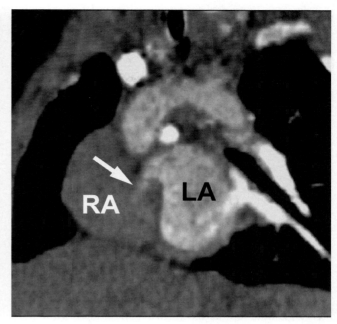

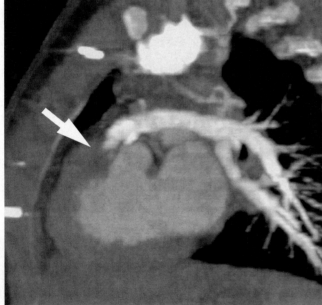

FIG. 8–32. Tricuspid atresia. The patient is a 1-year-old boy with tricuspid atresia treated with a bidirectional Glenn shunt. **A:** A four-chamber view shows a hypoplastic right ventricle (*arrowhead*) that is separated from the right atrium (*RA*), hence, tricuspid atresia. The right ventricle receives blood through a ventricular septal defect (*thin arrow*) from the left atrium (*LA*) and the left ventricle (*LV*). **B:** A short-axis view shows a trickle of contrast material (*arrow*) refluxing from the LA into the RA through an atrial septal defect. **C:** An oblique sagittal view shows a pulmonary atresia (*arrow*) where a contrast-filled pulmonary trunk is disconnected from the right ventricle.

The role of imaging is to determine the location of the coarctation, the degree and length of stenosis, the existence of collateral arteries, and other abnormalities of the aortic arch. Coarctation can be preductal where the stenosis is proximal to the origin of the left subclavian artery. This lesion produces arterial pressure difference between the left and right arms. More commonly, coarctation is juxtaductal as shown in Figure 8-33, where the stenosis is distal to the origin of the left subclavian artery. This stenosis produces an arterial-pressure difference between the upper and lower extremities. Patients may suffer from chronic hypertension, left ventricular hypertrophy, and eventually heart failure. Left unre-

paired, there is an increased risk for cerebral vascular accident.

Abnormal development of the embryological aortic arches may cause constriction of the trachea and esophagus. One form of vascular ring is a right aortic arch with an aberrant left subclavian artery that is retroesophageal. A left ligamentum arteriosum that connects between the left subclavian artery and left pulmonary artery completes the ring. This ring typically is loose and usually asymptomatic. In contrast, the rare double aortic arch forms a ring that compresses the trachea and esophagus and produces symptoms. In a double-aortic arch, the right arch usually is larger and

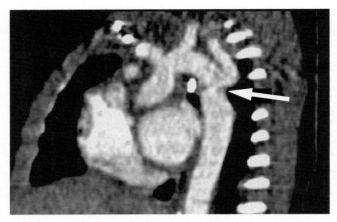

FIG. 8–33. Aortic coarctation. In this oblique sagittal view, a weblike aortic stenosis (*arrow*) is seen after the origin of the left subclavian artery. A patent ductus arteriosus ligation clip conveniently identifies the location of the ductus.

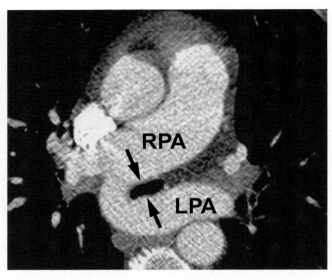

FIG. 8–35. Pulmonary sling. An axial view shows a left pulmonary artery (*LPA*) originating from a right pulmonary artery (*RPA*). The LPA travels behind the trachea but in front of the esophagus, compressing only the airway (*arrows*).

higher than the left, as shown in Figure 8-34. A third constrictive lesion is the pulmonary sling, where a left pulmonary artery arises from the right pulmonary artery and courses behind the trachea and in front of the esophagus, as shown in Figure 8-35. The trachea is compressed in front by the right pulmonary artery and behind by the left pulmonary artery. The esophagus is not constricted.

A number of congenital extracardiac shunts can produce unbalanced cardiac outputs from the aorta and pulmonary arteries. In most of these shunts, blood initially is driven from the systemic circulation into the pulmonary circulation.

If the shunt is large, the pulmonary arteries experience overcirculation, which over time will produce vascular fibrosis and pulmonary hypertension. In later stages, there may even be a paradoxical right-to-left shunt driven by the suprasystemic pulmonary pressure, called Eisenmenger's physiology. The most common congenital extracardiac shunt is patent ductus arteriosus. This embryological structure normally shunts blood from the pulmonary trunk to the descending aorta in utero. It closes soon after birth to establish separate aortic and pulmonary arterial flows. If the ductus arteriosus remains open, as shown in Figure 8-36, blood is shunted

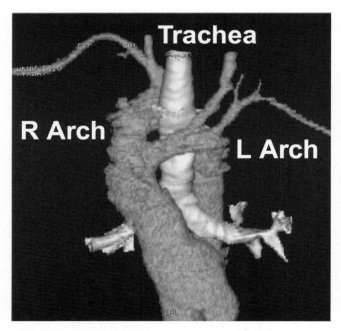

FIG. 8–34. Double aortic arch. A virtual rendering shows a double aortic arch encircling the trachea. Commonly, the right arch is higher and larger than the left.

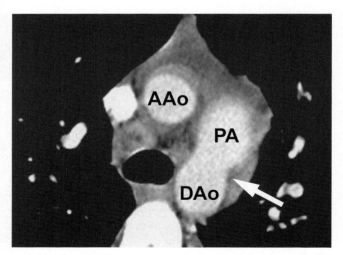

FIG. 8–36. Patent ductus arteriosus. An axial view shows the ascending aorta (*AAo*) and the descending aorta (*DAo*). The DAo communicates with the main pulmonary artery (*PA*) through a large patent ductus arteriosus (*arrow*).

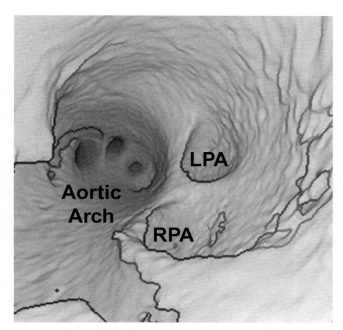

FIG. 8–37. Aortopulmonary window. An endoscopic view looking superiorly from the pulmonary trunk. The left pulmonary artery (*LPA*) and the right pulmonary artery (*RPA*) are seen. Through an aortopulmonary window, the aortic arch also can be seen, where the three cervical great vessels originate.

from the aorta to the pulmonary circulation. Truncus arteriosus and aortopulmonary windows are rare forms of shunt caused by incomplete septation between the aortic and pulmonary roots. The arterioventricular valves are normal in aortopulmonary windows, but malformed in truncus arteriosus. Figure 8-37 shows an endoscopic view of the septal defect in an aortopulmonary window that allows communication between the aorta and pulmonary trunk.

Cardiac MDCT has an important role in the detection of major aortopulmonary collateral shunts (MAPCS). These collateral vessels develop in the presence of pulmonary-artery stenosis associated with tetralogy of Fallot and pulmonary stenosis with an intact ventricular septum. A surgical procedure called unifocalization collects these collateral shunts and the stenotic pulmonary arteries to reconstruct patent central pulmonary arteries (108). The role of cardiac MDCT is to identify the anatomical locations and sizes of the major shunts, the lung regions they supply, and if possible, any competitive circuits among shunts and native pulmonary arteries. Figure 8-38 shows the atretic left and right main pulmonary arteries and innumerable MAPCS developed in a patient with tetralogy of Fallot.

CONCLUSION

In the short period of time since its introduction, cardiac MDCT has generated great excitement and fascination from the diagnostic imaging community. This enthusiasm is driven by the need for better and less invasive imaging tools to evaluate common yet important cardiovascular diseases. Currently, development and applications of this technology are focused on coronary artery disease, the most common cardiovascular disease in adults. Cardiac MDCT has shown its ability to image and quantify coronary calcium, an indicator of atherosclerotic burden in the coronary arteries, and to characterize soft plaques, revealing potentially unstable lesions at risk of rupture. More importantly, cardiac MDCT has demonstrated its ability to detect coronary stenosis with contrast-enhanced CT angiography, although it is not yet accurate enough to replace fluoroscopic coronary angiography. At this early stage, assessment of coronary stenosis with CT coronary angiography is limited by a number of factors, including low temporal resolution and artifacts from dense coronary calcium. However, with improvements in technol-

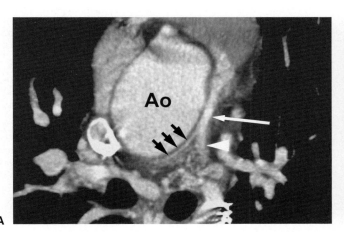
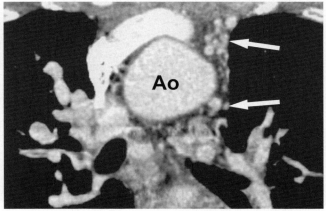

FIG. 8–38. Multiple aortopulmonary collateral shunts. In this adult patient with unrepaired tetralogy of Fallot, **(A)** an axial view shows a thin stenotic pulmonary trunk (*white arrow*) bifurcating into small right pulmonary artery (*black arrows*) and left pulmonary artery (*white arrowhead*). **B:** A higher axial view shows innumerable wormlike vascular channels that are aortopulmonary collateral shunts (*arrows*).

ogy, CT coronary angiography may parallel the clinical success seen in CT pulmonary angiography for the detection of pulmonary embolus. Cardiac MDCT also is useful in mapping coronary veins for endovascular treatment planning, in detecting morphologic abnormalities of the valves, in assessing cardiac function, and in evaluating the structural anomalies of congenital heart disease. The number of clinical applications likely will continue to grow in the near future.

REFERENCES

1. Moore SC, Judy PF, Garnic JD, et al. Prospectively gated cardiac computed tomography. *Med Phys* 1983;10:846–855.
2. Morehouse CC, Brody WR, Guthaner DF, et al. Gated cardiac computed tomography with a motion phantom. *Radiology* 1980; 134:213–217.
3. Becker CR, Ohnesorge BM, Schoepf UJ, et al. Current development of cardiac imaging with multidetector-row CT. *Eur J Radiol* 2000; 36:97–103.
4. Janowitz WR. Current status of mechanical computed tomography in cardiac imaging. *Am J Cardiol* 2001;88:35E–38E.
5. Gould R. Principles of ultrafast computed tomography: historical aspects, mechanisms of action, and scanner characteristics. Stanford W, Rumberger J, eds. *Ultrafast computed tomography in cardiac imaging: Principles and practice.* Mount Kisco, NY: Futura, 1992;1–15.
6. Stanford W, Rumberger J, eds. *Ultrafast computed tomography in cardiac imaging: Principles and practice.* Mount Kisco, NY: Futura, 1992.
7. Carr JJ, Danitschek JA, Goff DC, et al. Coronary artery calcium quantification with retrospectively gated helical CT: protocols and techniques. *Int J Cardiovasc Imaging* 2001;17:213–220.
8. Kopp AF, Schroeder S, Kuettner A, et al. Non-invasive coronary angiography with high resolution multidetector-row computed tomography. Results in 102 patients. *Eur Heart J* 2002;23:1714–1725.
9. Fayad ZA, Fuster V, Nikolaou K, et al. Computed tomography and magnetic resonance imaging for noninvasive coronary angiography and plaque imaging: current and potential future concepts. *Circulation* 2002;106:2026–2034.
10. Morgan-Hughes GJ, Roobottom CA, Marshall AJ. Aortic valve imaging with computed tomography: a review. *J Heart Valve Dis* 2002; 11:604–611.
11. Gerber TC, Sheedy PF, Bell MR, et al. Evaluation of the coronary venous system using electron beam computed tomography. *Int J Cardiovasc Imaging* 2001;17:65–75.
12. Juergens KU, Grude M, Fallenberg EM, et al. Using ECG-gated multidetector CT to evaluate global left ventricular myocardial function in patients with coronary artery disease. *AJR Am J Roentgenol* 2002; 179:1545–1550.
13. Kawano T, Ishii M, Takagi J, et al. Three-dimensional helical computed tomographic angiography in neonates and infants with complex congenital heart disease. *Am Heart J* 2000;139:654–660.
14. Lee JJ, Kang D. Feasibility of electron beam tomography in diagnosis of congenital heart disease: comparison with echocardiography. *Eur J Radiol* 2001;38:185–190.
15. Fuchs TO, Kachelriess M, Kalender WA. System performance of multislice spiral computed tomography. *IEEE Eng Med Biol Mag* 2000;19:63–70.
16. Kachelriess M, Ulzheimer S, Kalender WA. ECG-correlated image reconstruction from subsecond multi-slice spiral CT scans of the heart. *Med Phys* 2000;27:1881–1902.
17. Hong C, Becker CR, Huber A, et al. ECG-gated reconstructed multidetector row CT coronary angiography: effect of varying trigger delay on image quality. *Radiology* 2001;220:712–717.
18. Kopp AF, Schroeder S, Kuettner A, et al. Coronary arteries: retrospectively ECG-gated multi-detector row CT angiography with selective optimization of the image reconstruction window. *Radiology* 2001; 221:683–688.
19. Morin RL, Gerber TC, McCollough CH. Radiation dose in computed tomography of the heart. *Circulation* 2003;107:917–922.
20. Kachelriess M, Ulzheimer S, Kalender WA. ECG-correlated image reconstruction from subsecond multi-slice spiral CT scans of the heart. *Med Phys* 2000;27:1881–1902.
21. Ritchie CJ, Godwin JD, Crawford CR, et al. Minimum scan speeds for suppression of motion artifacts in CT. *Radiology* 1992;185:37–42.
22. Flohr T, Bruder H, Stierstorfer K, et al. New technical developments in multislice CT, part 2: sub-millimeter 16-slice scanning and increased gantry rotation speed for cardiac imaging. *Rofo Fortschr Geb Rontgenstr Neuen Bildgeb Verfahr* 2002;174:1022–1027.
23. Flohr T, Ohnesorge B. Heart rate adaptive optimization of spatial and temporal resolution for electrocardiogram-gated multislice spiral CT of the heart. *J Comput Assist Tomogr* 2001;25:907–923.
24. Gerber TC, Kuzo RS, Lane GE, et al. Image quality in a standardized algorithm for minimally invasive coronary angiography with multislice spiral computed tomography. *J Comput Assist Tomogr* 2003; 27:62–69.
25. Giesler T, Baum U, Ropers D, et al. Noninvasive visualization of coronary arteries using contrast-enhanced multidetector CT: influence of heart rate on image quality and stenosis detection. *AJR Am J Roentgenol* 2002;179:911–916.
26. Nieman K, Rensing BJ, van Geuns RJ, et al. Non-invasive coronary angiography with multislice spiral computed tomography: impact of heart rate. *Heart* 2002;88:470–474.
27. Mahesh M. Search for isotropic resolution in CT from conventional through multiple-row detector. *Radiographics* 2002;22:949–962.
28. Hunold P, Vogt FM, Schmermund A, et al. Radiation exposure during cardiac CT: effective doses at multi-detector row CT and electron-beam CT. *Radiology* 2003;226:145–152.
29. Becker C, Schatzl M, Feist H, et al. Assessment of the effective dose for routine protocols in conventional CT, electron beam CT and coronary angiography. *Rofo Fortschr Geb Rontgenstr Neuen Bildgeb Verfahr* 1999;170:99–104.
30. Cohnen M, Poll L, Puttmann C, et al. Radiation exposure in multislice CT of the heart. *Rofo Fortschr Geb Rontgenstr Neuen Bildgeb Verfahr* 2001;173:295–299.
31. Morin RL, Gerber TC, McCollough CH. Radiation dose in computed tomography of the heart. *Circulation* 2003;107:917–922.
32. Hunold P, Vogt FM, Schmermund A, et al. Radiation exposure during cardiac CT: effective doses at multi-detector row CT and electron-beam CT. *Radiology* 2003;226:145–152.
33. Morin RL, Gerber TC, McCollough CH. Radiation dose in computed tomography of the heart. *Circulation* 2003;107:917–922.
34. Becker C, Schatzl M, Feist H, et al. Assessment of the effective dose for routine protocols in conventional CT, electron beam CT and coronary angiography. *Rofo Fortschr Geb Rontgenstr Neuen Bildgeb Verfahr* 1999;170:99–104.
35. Morin RL, Gerber TC, McCollough CH. Radiation dose in computed tomography of the heart. *Circulation* 2003;107:917–922.
36. Kalender WA, Wolf H, Suess C. Dose reduction in CT by anatomically adapted tube current modulation. II. Phantom measurements. *Med Phys* 1999;26:2248–2253.
37. Jakobs TF, Becker CR, Ohnesorge B, et al. Multislice helical CT of the heart with retrospective ECG gating: reduction of radiation exposure by ECG-controlled tube current modulation. *Eur Radiol* 2002; 12:1081–1086.
38. Tamm EP, Thompson S, Venable SL, et al. Impact of multislice CT on PACS resources. *J Digit Imaging* 2002;15 Suppl 1:96–101.
39. Ropers D, Baum U, Pohle K, et al. Detection of coronary artery stenoses with thin-slice multi-detector row spiral computed tomography and multiplanar reconstruction. *Circulation* 2003;107:664–666.
40. Achenbach S, Moshage W, Ropers D, et al. Curved multiplanar reconstructions for the evaluation of contrast-enhanced electron beam CT of the coronary arteries. *AJR Am J Roentgenol* 1998;170:895–899.
41. Gulbins H, Reichenspurner H, Becker C, et al. Preoperative 3D-reconstructions of ultrafast-CT images for the planning of minimally invasive direct coronary artery bypass operation (MIDCAB). *Heart Surg Forum* 1998;1:111–115.
42. Saito K, Saito M, Komatu S, et al. Real-time dour-dimensional imaging of the heart with multi-detector row CT. *Radiographics* 2003;23: E8.
43. Mochizuki T, Murase K, Higashino H, et al. Two- and three-dimensional CT ventriculography: a new application of helical CT. *AJR Am J Roentgenol* 2000;174:203–208.
44. *American Heart Association: Heart and Stroke Facts: 1996, Statistical Supplement.* Dallas: American Heart Association, 2003.

45. Ross R, Glomset JA. The pathogenesis of atherosclerosis (second of two parts). *N Engl J Med* 1976;295:420–425.
46. Davies MJ, Thomas AC. Plaque fissuring—the cause of acute myocardial infarction, sudden ischaemic death, and crescendo angina. *Br Heart J* 1985;53:363–373.
47. Davies MJ. The composition of coronary-artery plaques. *N Engl J Med* 1997;336:1312–1314.
48. Wexler L, Brundage B, Crouse J, et al. Coronary artery calcification: pathophysiology, epidemiology, imaging methods, and clinical implications. A statement for health professionals from the American Heart Association writing Group. *Circulation* 1996;94:1175–1192.
49. Becker CR, Schoepf UJ, Reiser MF. Methods for quantification of coronary artery calcifications with electron beam and conventional CT and pushing the spiral CT envelope: new cardiac applications. *Int J Cardiovasc Imaging* 2001;17:203–211.
50. Horiguchi J, Nakanishi T, Ito K. Quantification of coronary artery calcium using multidetector CT and a retrospective ECG-gating reconstruction algorithm. *AJR Am J Roentgenol* 2001;177:1429–1435.
51. Ohnesorge B, Flohr T, Fischbach R, et al. Reproducibility of coronary calcium quantification in repeat examinations with retrospectively ECG-gated multisection spiral CT. *Eur Radiol* 2002;12:1532–1540.
52. Hong C, Becker CR, Schoepf UJ, et al. Coronary artery calcium: absolute quantification in nonenhanced and contrast-enhanced multidetector row CT studies. *Radiology* 2002;223:474–480.
53. Agatston AS, Janowitz WR, Hildner FJ, et al. Quantification of coronary artery calcium using ultrafast computed tomography. *J Am Coll Cardiol* 1990;15:827–832.
54. Becker CR, Kleffel T, Crispin A, et al. Coronary artery calcium measurement: agreement of multirow detector and electron beam CT. *AJR Am J Roentgenol* 2001;176:1295–1298.
55. Horiguchi J, Nakanishi T, Ito K. Quantification of coronary artery calcium using multidetector CT and a retrospective ECG-gating reconstruction algorithm. *AJR Am J Roentgenol* 2001;177:1429–1435.
56. Becker CR, Kleffel T, Crispin A, et al. Coronary artery calcium measurement: agreement of multirow detector and electron beam CT. *AJR Am J Roentgenol* 2001;176:1295–1298.
57. Yoon HC, Greaser LE, III, Mather R, et al. Coronary artery calcium: alternate methods for accurate and reproducible quantitation. *Acad Radiol* 1997;4:666–673.
58. Wexler L, Brundage B, Crouse J, et al. Coronary artery calcification: pathophysiology, epidemiology, imaging methods, and clinical implications. A statement for health professionals from the American Heart Association. Writing Group. *Circulation* 1996;94:1175–1192.
59. Arad Y, Spadaro LA, Goodman K, et al. Prediction of coronary events with electron beam computed tomography. *J Am Coll Cardiol* 2000;36:1253–1260.
60. Budoff MJ, Georgiou D, Brody A, et al. Ultrafast computed tomography as a diagnostic modality in the detection of coronary artery disease: a multicenter study. *Circulation* 1996;93:898–904.
61. Keelan PC, Bielak LF, Ashai K, et al. Long-term prognostic value of coronary calcification detected by electron-beam computed tomography in patients undergoing coronary angiography. *Circulation* 2001;104:412–417.
62. O'Rourke RA, Brundage BH, Froelicher VF, et al. American College of Cardiology/American Heart Association Expert Consensus document on electron-beam computed tomography for the diagnosis and prognosis of coronary artery disease. *Circulation* 2000;102:126–140.
63. Georgiou D, Budoff MJ, Kaufer E, et al. Screening patients with chest pain in the emergency department using electron beam tomography: a follow-up study. *J Am Coll Cardiol* 2001;38:105–110.
64. Laudon DA, Vukov LF, Breen JF, et al. Use of electron-beam computed tomography in the evaluation of chest pain patients in the emergency department. *Ann Emerg Med* 1999;33:15–21.
65. Raggi P, Cooil B, Callister TQ. Use of electron beam tomography data to develop models for prediction of hard coronary events. *Am Heart J* 2001;141:375–382.
66. Callister TQ, Raggi P, Cooil B, et al. Effect of HMG-CoA reductase inhibitors on coronary artery disease as assessed by electron-beam computed tomography. *N Engl J Med* 1998;339:1972–1978.
67. Baim DS, Grossman W. Complications of cardiac catheterization. In: Baim DS, Grossman W, eds. *Cardiac catheterization, angiography, and intervention*, 5th ed. Baltimore: Williams & Wilkins, 1996:17–38.
68. Kim WY, Danias PG, Stuber M, et al. Coronary magnetic resonance angiography for the detection of coronary stenoses. *N Engl J Med* 2001;345:1863–1869.
69. Achenbach S, Moshage W, Ropers D, et al. Curved multiplanar reconstructions for the evaluation of contrast-enhanced electron beam CT of the coronary arteries. *AJR Am J Roentgenol* 1998;170:895–899.
70. Nakanishi T, Ito K, Imazu M, et al. Evaluation of coronary artery stenoses using electron-beam CT and multiplanar reformation. *J Comput Assist Tomogr* 1997;21:121–127.
71. Nikolaou K, Huber A, Knez A, et al. Intraindividual comparison of contrast-enhanced electron-beam computed tomography and navigator-echo-based magnetic resonance imaging for noninvasive coronary artery angiography. *Eur Radiol* 2002;12:1663–1671.
72. Waller BF, Orr CM, Slack JD, et al. Anatomy, histology, and pathology of coronary arteries: a review relevant to new interventional and imaging techniques—Part I. *Clin Cardiol* 1992;15:451–457.
73. Achenbach S, Giesler T, Ropers D, et al. Detection of coronary artery stenoses by contrast-enhanced, retrospectively electrocardiographically-gated, multislice spiral computed tomography. *Circulation* 2001;103:2535–2538.
74. Becker CR, Knez A, Leber A, et al. Detection of coronary artery stenoses with multislice helical CT angiography. *J Comput Assist Tomogr* 2002;26:750–755.
75. Nieman K, Rensing BJ, van Geuns RJ, et al. Non-invasive coronary angiography with multislice spiral computed tomography: impact of heart rate. *Heart* 2002;88:470–474.
76. Nieman K, Cademartiri F, Lemos PA, et al. Reliable noninvasive coronary angiography with fast submillimeter multislice spiral computed tomography. *Circulation* 2002;106:2051–2054.
77. Schroeder S, Kopp AF, Baumbach A, et al. Noninvasive detection of coronary lesions by multislice computed tomography: results of the New Age pilot trial. *Catheter Cardiovasc Interv* 2001;53:352–358.
78. Davies MJ. The composition of coronary-artery plaques. *N Engl J Med* 1997;336:1312–1314.
79. Davies MJ, Thomas AC. Plaque fissuring—the cause of acute myocardial infarction, sudden ischaemic death, and crescendo angina. *Br Heart J* 1985;53:363–373.
80. Schroeder S, Kopp AF, Baumbach A, et al. Noninvasive detection and evaluation of atherosclerotic coronary plaques with multislice computed tomography. *J Am Coll Cardiol* 2001;37:1430–1435.
81. Kar S, Nordlander R. Coronary veins: an alternate route to ischemic myocardium. *Heart Lung* 1992;21:148–157.
82. Wen MS, Yeh SJ, Wang CC, et al. Radiofrequency ablation therapy of the posteroseptal accessory pathway. *Am Heart J* 1996;132:612–620.
83. Oesterle SN, Reifart N, Hauptmann E, et al. Percutaneous in situ coronary venous arterialization: report of the first human catheter-based coronary artery bypass. *Circulation* 2001;103:2539–2543.
84. Abraham WT, Fisher WG, Smith AL, et al. Cardiac resynchronization in chronic heart failure. *N Engl J Med* 2002;346:1845–1853.
85. Salukhe TV, Francis DP, Sutton R. Comparison of medical therapy, pacing and defibrillation in heart failure (COMPANION) trial terminated early; combined biventricular pacemaker-defibrillators reduce all-cause mortality and hospitalization. *Int J Cardiol* 2003;87:119–120.
86. Abraham WT, Fisher WG, Smith AL, et al. Cardiac resynchronization in chronic heart failure. *N Engl J Med* 2002;346:1845–1853.
87. Sandler DA, Feigenblum DY, Bernstein NE, et al. Cardiac vein angioplasty for biventricular pacing. *Pacing Clin Electrophysiol* 2002;25:1788–1789.
88. Gerber TC, Sheedy PF, Bell MR, et al. Evaluation of the coronary venous system using electron beam computed tomography. *Int J Cardiovasc Imaging* 2001;17:65–75.
89. Schaffler GJ, Groell R, Peichel KH, et al. Imaging the coronary venous drainage system using electron-beam CT. *Surg Radiol Anat* 2000;22:35–39.
90. Ortale JR, Gabriel EA, Iost C, et al. The anatomy of the coronary sinus and its tributaries. *Surg Radiol Anat* 2001;23:15–21.
91. Gerber TC, Sheedy PF, Bell MR, et al. Evaluation of the coronary venous system using electron beam computed tomography. *Int J Cardiovasc Imaging* 2001;17:65–75.
92. Willmann JK, Kobza R, Roos JE, et al. ECG-gated multi-detector row CT for assessment of mitral valve disease: initial experience. *Eur Radiol* 2002;12:2662–2669.
93. Willmann JK, Weishaupt D, Lachat M, et al. Electrocardiographically

gated multi-detector row CT for assessment of valvular morphology and calcification in aortic stenosis. *Radiology* 2002;225:120–128.

94. Lippert JA, White CS, Mason AC, et al. Calcification of aortic valve detected incidentally on CT scans: prevalence and clinical significance. *AJR Am J Roentgenol* 1995;164:73–77.

95. Morgan-Hughes GJ, Roobottom CA, Marshall AJ. Aortic valve imaging with computed tomography: a review. *J Heart Valve Dis* 2002; 11:604–611.

96. Sachdev M, Peterson GE, Jollis JG. Imaging techniques for diagnosis of infective endocarditis. *Infect Dis Clin North Am* 2002;16:319–337, ix.

97. Juergens KU, Grude M, Fallenberg EM, et al. Using ECG-gated multi-detector CT to evaluate global left ventricular myocardial function in patients with coronary artery disease. *AJR Am J Roentgenol* 2002; 179:1545–1550.

98. Friedman WF. Congenital Heart Disease in Infancy and Childhood. In: Braunwald E, ed. *Heart disease, a textbook of cardiovascular medicine*, 5th ed. Philadelphia: WB Saunders, 1997:877–962.

99. Kawano T, Ishii M, Takagi J, et al. Three-dimensional helical computed tomographic angiography in neonates and infants with complex congenital heart disease. *Am Heart J* 2000;139:654–660.

100. Westra SJ, Hill JA, Alejos JC, et al. Three-dimensional helical CT of pulmonary arteries in infants and children with congenital heart disease. *AJR Am J Roentgenol* 1999;173:109–115.

101. Ropers D, Moshage W, Daniel WG, et al. Visualization of coronary artery anomalies and their anatomic course by contrast-enhanced electron beam tomography and three-dimensional reconstruction. *Am J Cardiol* 2001;87:193–197.

102. Funabashi N, Rubin GD. Direct identification of patency achieved by a bi-directional Glenn shunt procedure: images by volume rendering using electron-beam computed tomography. *Jpn Circ J* 2001; 65:457–461.

103. Chen SJ, Li YW, Wang JK, et al. Three-dimensional reconstruction of abnormal ventriculoarterial relationship by electron beam CT. *J Comput Assist Tomogr* 1998;22:560–568.

104. Chen SJ, Li YW, Wang JK, et al. Usefulness of electron beam computed tomography in children with heterotaxy syndrome. *Am J Cardiol* 1998;81:188–194.

105. Funabashi N, Rubin GD. Qualitative blood flow differentiation: depiction of a left to right cardiac shunt across a ventricular septal defect using electron-beam computed tomography. *Jpn Circ J* 2000; 64:901–903.

106. Lee JJ, Kang D. Feasibility of electron beam tomography in diagnosis of congenital heart disease: comparison with echocardiography. *Eur J Radiol* 2001;38:185–190.

107. Gersony WM, Rosenbaum MS. Chapter 9: Congenital anomalies of the coronary circulation. In: *Congenital heart disease in the adult*. New York: McGraw–Hill, 2002:125–142.

108. McElhinney DB, Reddy VM, Hanley FL. Tetralogy of Fallot with major aortopulmonary collaterals: early total repair. *Pediatr Cardiol* 1998;19:289–296.

CHAPTER 9

Pediatric Chest Applications

Marilyn J. Siegel

INTRODUCTION

With the introduction of helical (spiral) computed tomography (CT) in the late 1980s, the applications of CT in the pediatric thorax expanded dramatically (1–3). The introduction of multidetector computed tomography (MDCT) again has created a wealth of new imaging opportunities (4–6). The ability to acquire multiple projections of raw data with each gantry rotation permits thinner slices, shorter scanning times, and greater volume coverage. These advantages have dramatically expanded the applications of CT in the pediatric chest. This chapter discusses the expanded role of MDCT in the pediatric chest, as well as the basic techniques for optimizing the examination.

PATIENT PREPARATION/TECHNIQUE

Pediatric patients have several inherent problems that are not present in adults, in particular patient motion, small body size, and lack of perivisceral fat. These problems can be minimized or eliminated by the appropriate use of sedation and intravenous (IV) contrast.

Sedation

Initial reports have suggested that the use of MDCT has reduced the frequency of sedation in infants and children 5 years of age and younger. The sedation rate for single-detector CT is reported to be approximately 30% (7). Early experience has suggested that the sedation rate for young children undergoing MDCT is less than 5% (8). The data on MDCT have included only small groups of patients; therefore, further experience will be required to determine the precise sedation rate in younger children. Sedation still will be required for very uncooperative children. In general, children older than 5 years of age will cooperate after verbal reassurance and explanation of the procedure.

Conscious sedation is used nearly always for imaging examinations, rather than general anesthesia. Conscious sedation is defined as a minimally depressed level of consciousness that retains the patient's abilities to maintain a patent airway, independently and continuously, and respond appropriately to physical stimulation and/or verbal command.

The drugs most frequently used for sedation are oral chloral hydrate and IV pentobarbital sodium. Oral chloral hydrate, 50 mg/kg to 100 mg/kg, with a maximum dosage of 2000 mg, is the drug of choice for children younger than 18 months. Intravenous pentobarbital sodium, 6 mg/kg with a maximum dose of 200 mg, is advocated in children older than 18 months. Pentobarbital sodium is injected slowly, in fractions of one-fourth the total dose, and is titrated against the patient's response. This is an effective form of sedation with a failure rate of less than 5%. Regardless of the choice of drug, the use of parenteral sedation requires trained personnel and adequate equipment to resusatate and maintain adequate cardiorespiratory support during and after the examination (9,10).

Patients who are to receive parenteral sedation should have no liquids by mouth for 3 hours, and no solid foods for 6 hours prior to the examination. Patients who are not sedated, but are to receive IV contrast should be NPO (nothing per mouth) for 3 hours prior to examination to minimize the likelihood of nausea or vomiting with possible aspiration during a bolus injection of IV contrast.

After being sedated, the infant or child is placed on a blanket on the CT table. When possible, the arms are extended above the head to avoid streak artifacts and to provide an easily accessible route for IV injection.

Special Technical Considerations

Intravenous Contrast Medium

With the exception of thoracic CT for pulmonary nodules and interstitial lung disease, nearly all CT examinations of the chest are performed with the administration of IV contrast material. Intravenous contrast medium is helpful to confirm a lesion thought to be of vascular origin, establish the relationship of a mass to vascular structures, and improve differentiation between normal and pathologic parenchyma.

If IV contrast is to be administered, it is helpful to have the IV line in place when the child arrives in the CT suite. This reduces patient agitation that otherwise would be associated with a venipuncture performed immediately prior to administration of contrast materal and this increases patient cooperation. The largest gauge cannula that can be placed is recommended.

The contrast dose is 2 mL/kg (not to exceed 4 mL/kg or 125 mL). A nonionic contrast medium should be used. The advantages of nonionic agents over ionic agents are less discomfort at the injection site, fewer side effects such as nausea and vomiting, and decreased patient motion during contrast administration (11,12).

Contrast can be administered by mechanical or hand injection (13). Power injectors are used when a 22-gauge or larger cannula can be placed in an antecubital vein. The contrast injection rate is determined by the caliber of the IV catheter. Suggested flow rates are 1.5 mL/sec to 2.0 mL/sec for a 22-gauge catheter and 2.0 mL/sec to 3.0 mL/sec for a 20-gauge catheter. The site of injection is monitored closely during the initial injection of contrast in order to minimize the risk of contrast extravasation. A power injector also can be used to administer contrast media via a central venous catheter or 24-gauge catheter if the rate of injection is slow (1 mL/sec). The benefit of power injection is the uniformity of contrast delivery, which allows for maximal enhancement. A manual injection is used if IV access is through a peripheral access line in the dorsum of the hand or foot. The complication rates for manual and power injections are similar (<0.4%), provided that the catheter is positioned properly and functions well (13).

Scan-Delay Times

The scan-delay time is the time between the start of the contrast administration and the start of the scan-data acquisition. In our experience, either an empiric delay based on the age of the patient and the area scanned or an automated tracking system was used.

For routine chest CT examinations (i.e., screening for metastases, tumor staging, evaluation of a mediastinal mass, or congenital lung anomaly), the scan delay after the start of contrast administration is set at 20 seconds to 30 seconds. Shorter delay (20 seconds) is used in neonates and infants (less than 2 years of age) who have higher cardiac output, with longer delay times used in older children and adolescents.

When assessment of vascular anatomy is the primary indication for the CT, a 12-second to 15-second delay after the start of IV contrast administration produces good vascular enhancement in patients under 2 years of age. A 20-second to 25-second delay is used in older children and adolescents.

Alternatively, an automated tracking method can be used in children and adolescents to trigger scan initiation. This allows customization of contrast enhancement for each individual patient, taking into account factors such as cardiac output and circulation time. The bolus tracking method uses continuous monitoring of the attenuation value within a large target vessel (e.g., aorta or pulmonary artery) by use of a series of low-dose axial images. A cursor is placed within a range of interest in the target vessel. When a predetermined level of contrast enhancement (usually 100 HU) is reached, the low-dose scanning is terminated and the diagnostic examination is initiated automatically. A default delay can be

TABLE 9–1. *Protocol 1*

Indication	Standard lung/mediastinum (Oncologic staging, detection of metastases, characterization of mediastinal or pulmonary mass, evaluation of trauma)
Extent	Lung apices to caudal bases
Scanner settings:	kVp: 80 for patients weighing <50 kg; higher kVp for larger patient.
Detector collimation	2.5 mm for 4-row scanner
	mA: lowest possible based on patient weight
	1.5 mm for 16-row scanner
Table speed	15–20 mm/rotation for 4-row scanner
	24–36 mm/rotation for 16-row scanner
Slice thickness	3–5 mm for 4-row scanner
	2–5 mm for 16-row scanner
IV contrast	Nonionic 280–320 mg iodine/mL
Contrast volume	2 mL/kg (maximum of 4 mL/kg or 125 mL, whichever is lower)
Contrast injection rate**	Hand injection: rapid push bolus
	Power injector:
	22 gauge: 1.5–2.0 mL/sec
	20 gauge: 2.0–3.0 mL/sec
Scan delay	20 to 30 sec
Miscellaneous	1. If the child is sedated or uncooperative, CT scans obtained at quiet breathing.
	2. Contrast medium used at discretion of radiologist in the evaluation of metastases. Routinely given for evaluation of mediastinal and pulmonary masses and trauma
	3. Use a standard reconstruction algorithm.

TABLE 9–2. *Protocol 2*

Indication	CT angiography (Cardiovascular anomalies, dissection, aneurysm, postoperative shunts)
Extent	Lung apices to caudal bases
Scanner settings:	kVp: 80 for patients weighing <50 kg; higher kVp for larger patient.
	mA: lowest possible based on patient weight
Detector collimation	2.5 mm for 4-row scanner
	1.5 mm for 16-row scanner
Table speed	15–20 mm/rotation for 4-row scanner
	24–36 mm/rotation for 16-row scanner
Slice thickness	3–5 mm for 4 row scanner
	2–5 mm for 16 row scanner
IV contrast	Nonionic 280–320 mg iodine/mL
Contrast volume	2 mL/kg (maximum of 4 mL/kg or 150 mL, whichever is lower)
Contrast injection rate	Hand injection: rapid push bolus
	Power injector:
	22 gauge: 1.5–2.0 mL/sec
	20 gauge: 2.0–3.0 mL/sec
Scan delay	Patient weight < 15 kg: 12 to 15 sec
	Patient weight > 15 kg: 20 to 25 sec
Miscellaneous	1. If the child is sedated or uncooperative, CT scans are obtained at quite breathing.
	2. If sequestration is suspected, scanning should extend through the upper abdominal aorta.
	3. Precontrast images are not needed for most examinations, but they are used in the evaluation of endovascular stents.
	4. Use standard reconstruction algorithm.

programmed in case the desired threshold is not achieved. This technology has proven particularly useful in CT angiography.

Precontrast scans are not obtained routinely for CT angiography in children. The exceptions are the evaluation of endoluminal stents, usually for repair of coarctation, and dissections. In these patients, calcification around the graft, which can mimic an endoleak on the contrast-enhanced scans, will be seen best on unenhanced scans. In patients with possible dissection, unenhanced scans are useful for localizing high-attenuation hematomas in the false lumen.

Technical Parameters for Thoracic Imaging

General principles for optimizing MDCT techniques are discussed below. Specific parameters for the most common types of thoracic CT examination in children are shown in Tables 9–1 through 9–4.

TABLE 9–3. *Protocol 3*

Indication	Tracheobronchial tree (Congenital anomalies, stricture, tumor, tracheomalacia)
Extent	Vocal cords to mainstream bronchi, just below carina
Scanneter settings:	kVp: 80 for patients weighing <50 kg; higher kVp for larger patient.
	mA: lowest possible based on patient weight
Detector collimation	2.5 mm for 4-row scanner
	1.5 mm for 16-row scanner
Table speed	15–20 mm/rotation for 4-row scanner
	24–36 mm/rotation for 16-row scanner
Slice thickness	3–5 mm for 4-row scanner
	2–5 mm for 16-row scanner
Patient instructions	Suspended inspiration
Contrast type	None
Comments	1. Aim for a single breath hold. Select pitch so that the area of interest can be scanned in a single breath hold in cooperative patients.
	2. Use high spatial resolution reconstruction (bone) algorithm
	3. Multiplanar and 3D reconstructions are useful to provide an overview of anatomy for surgical planning.
	4. If small airway obstruction or tracheomalacia is suspected, obtain scans in inspiration and expiration
	5. If the child sedated or uncooperative, CT scans obtained at quiet breathing.

TABLE 9–4. *Protocol 4*

Indication	Diffuse lung disease
Extent	Lung apices to caudal bases
Scanner settings:	kVp: 80 for patients weighing <50 kg; higher kVp for larger patient.
	mA: lowest possible based on patient weight
Detector collimation	1 mm
Table speed	10–20 mm
Slice thickness	3–5 mm for initial surveys; 1.25 mm for high-resolution CT
Patient instructions	Suspended inspiration
IV contrast	None
Miscellaneous	1. Expiration imaging can be useful to evaluate suspected areas of air trapping.
	2. If the child sedated or uncooperative, CT scans obtained at quiet breathing.

The imaging techniques described below reflect experience with a Plus 4 Volume Zoom and Sensation 16 scanners (Siemens, Iselin, NJ) with a 0.5 second rotation time. The techniques for evaluation of thoracic tumors, vascular lesions, and airway are similar. On a 4-row detector, most CT examinations are performed with a 2.5 mm slice collimation and a table speed of 15 to 20 mm per rotation. The scans are reconstructed at 2.5 to 5.0 mm. For detailed assessment of small stuctures, such as a patent ductus arteriosus or subsegmental pulmonary artery, a 1.0 mm collimation and a 2 mm reconstruction thickness should be considered. On a 16 row detector, the collimation is 1.5 mm with a table speed of 36 mm per rotation.

For the evaluation of diffuse lung diseases, CT scans are obtained with 1-mm slice acquisition thickness and table speed of 10 to 20 mm/rotation. Scans are obtained in inspiration and expiration if air trapping is suspected.

The field of view is chosen to cover the area of interest. A standard reconstruction algorithm usually suffices for routine studies and CT angiograms. A high-resolution algorithm is used for three-dimensional (3D) reconstructions of the airways.

Computed tomography (CT) examinations are performed with breath-holding at suspended inspiration in cooperative patients, usually children over 5 years to 6 years of age. Scans are obtained during quiet respiration in children who are unable to cooperate with breath-holding instructions and in patients who are sedated.

IMAGE-PROCESSING TECHNIQUES

Image-processing techniques include methods such as multiplanar reformation, shaded surface displays, maximum- and minimum-intensity projections, variable-thickness viewing (sliding slabs), and volume-rendering displays (14–17). The various reconstruction techniques have been described in detail elsewhere in this textbook. For the purpose of this chapter, a brief review of those techniques that have proven most useful in the pediatric chest is presented below.

Multiplanar Reformatting

Multiplanar reformatting, which is the simplest reformation technique, is used to assess the extent of disease

processes in the craniocaudal direction (Figure 9-1). Its advantages include rapid display and ease of generation of the images at the CT scanner and that it uses all of the attentuations in the dataset, presenting them in off-axis views (14). The major disadvantage of this technique is that it provides only a two-dimensional (2D) display of data; thus, it lacks depth cues.

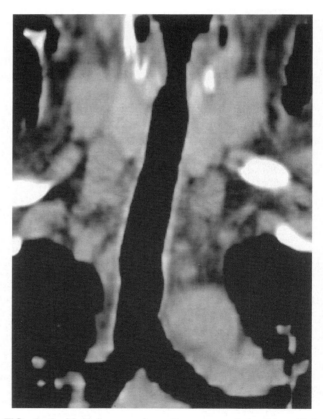

FIG. 9–1. Multiplanar reformation, normal trachea. Data acquired with 2.5-mm collimation and 15-mm table feed/rotation; axial images reconstructed at 3-mm increments with 2-mm reconstruction intervals. In the evaluation of tracheal abnormalities, multiplanar reformations can improve assessment of the extent of disease in the craniocaudal direction.

Variable-thickness Maximum- and Minimum-Intensity Projections

Small peripheral vessels and airways often are seen better as an assimilation of sections in a volume slab rather than in individual sections of equivalent thickness. In this technique, images are combined in multiples or "slabs" to create a thicker image (14). The volume slab technique can be used with either maximum-intensity projections (MIP), which display data based on the maximum-attenuation value, or minimum-intensity projections (MinIP), which display data based on the minimum-attenuation value. The former has been applied to the examination of pulmonary vessels, whereas the latter technique can be used to enhance evaluation of the airways.

Shaded-surface Display

The shaded-surface representation displays data in a 3D format based on an assigned threshold. All structures within the threshold range are displayed, whereas other tissues are deleted. The principle application of the shaded-surface display is the evaluation of osseous structures of the thorax.

3D Volume Rendering

Volume rendering largely has replaced other 3D reformatting techniques in evaluating airway and vascular pathology. Whereas the shaded-surface display and the MIP and MinIP reconstructions use only a portion of the attenuation values and their spatial relationships, volume rendering uses the entire attenuation composition and spatial relationships in the data set. The data can be manipulated so that the width, opacity, brightness, and color of the image can be altered. Depth cues also are used, unlike the other display techniques (Figure 9-2) (see color plate). Such post processing permits the data to be displayed from an external or internal perspective (i.e., "virtual bronchoscopy"). When 3D imaging is contemplated, the 2.5-mm-thick volumetric data are reconstructed with a section thickness of 3 mm and a reconstruction interval of 1 mm to 2 mm. The 1.55-mm thick data are reconstructed at a thickness of 2 mm.

RADIATION DOSE IN PEDIATRIC MDCT

Multidetector CT results in increased radiation dose compared to single-slice helical CT due to the larger aperture of its collimators. Techniques that minimize radiation dose are mandatory for CT examinations in children. These techniques include the use of low milliamperage setting, low kilovoltage settings, appropriate slice thickness, and higher pitches (18–25). Additionally, multiphasic studies should be performed only when necessary, rather than as a routine protocol.

The lowest possible MAs and kV should be used for CT in children. The tube currents recommended for thoracic CT examinations in children are shown in Table 9–5. In patients with smaller body habitus, all protocols can be per-

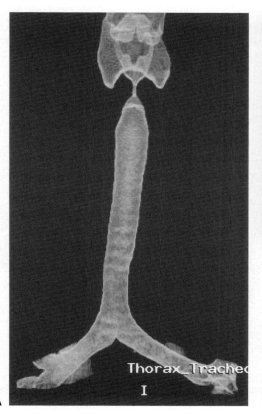

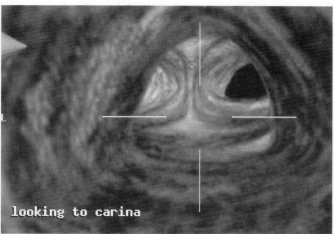

FIG. 9–2. Volume rendering, normal trachea. **A:** Coronal external volume-rendered image of normal trachea and right and left mainstem bronchi. Data acquired with 2.5-mm collimation and 15-mm table feed/rotation; axial images reconstructed at 3-mm increments and 2-mm intervals. **B:** Internal volume-rendered display (virtual bronchoscopy). Same data set as in **(A)**. View from above looking towards carina. (See Color Fig. 9–2B)

TABLE 9–5. *Milliamperage and kilovoltage settings versus patient weight*

Weight (Kg)	mA	kV
<15	25	80
15–24	30	80
25–34	45	80
35–44	75	80
45–54	100	80–120
>54	120–140	100–120

formed with 80 kV. The 80 kV approach lowers the dose to the patient by approximately 30% (compared with the standard 120 kV protocols) with better contrast visualization (25). A higher kilovolt will be needed in patients with large body habitus. All protocols are done with a pitch of 6 to 8.

The collimation determines the nominal or effective section thickness, which can be changed after the patient has left the department provided that the raw data have been saved. For example, if the chest is scanned with a 5 mm detector configuration, the minimum slice thickness is 5 mm. If the chest is scanned with a 1.0 mm detector configuration, the raw data can be reconstructed at 1.0, 2.5, 3.75, or 5.0 mm contiguous sections. Although 1.0 mm thick slices may improve resolution, they are not routinely used in children because they increase the radiation dose. As thinner sections are acquired, the radiation dose is necessarily increased to maintain photon flux, so long as image noise is held constant.

Pitch, which is defined as the table increment per gantry rotation divided by the thickness of the data slice, has an impact on resolution and radiation dose. Larger pitches increase temporal resolution and decrease radiation dose. It is recommended that a pitch greater than 1.5 be used for multidetector CT scanning in children.

CLINICAL APPLICATIONS

The most common clinical applications for CT of the pediatric chest are: i) evaluation of lung metastases, ii) evaluation of the character and extent of a mediastinal mass, iii) characterization of congenital pulmonary anomalies, iv) assessment of cardiovascular anomalies (CT angiography), iv) assessment of airway narrowing or mass, v) evaluation of diffuse lung disease, and vi) evaluation of complex chest-wall abnormalities.

Evaluation of Pulmonary Metastases (Protocol 1)

Computed tomography is a valuable technique for detection of pulmonary metastases in patients with known malignancies with a high propensity for lung dissemination, such as Wilms' tumor, osteogenic sarcoma, and rhabdomyosarcoma. Detection of one or more pulmonary nodules in such patients, or documentation of additional nodules in a patient with an apparent solitary metastasis for whom surgery is planned, may be critical to treatment planning. In the first instance, such detection may lead to additional treat-

ment (surgery, chemotherapy, or radiation); in the latter setting, demonstration of several metastatic nodules may negate surgical plans.

The temporal and spatial resolution afforded by helical CT improves the detection and characterization of pulmonary nodules. Although data are limited in children, studies in adults have shown that helical CT is a sensitive method for detecting pulmonary nodules (26).

Pulmonary metastases typically are found in the peripheral and subpleural areas of the lungs. Most metastases are round or oval lesions and well marginated. When the nodules are larger than adjacent vascular structures in the same area, the diagnosis of metastatic disease can be made with confidence. If the nodular opacity is similar in size or smaller than adjacent vessels, especially when centrally located, the interpretation is more difficult. Careful scrutiny of adjacent scans may be helpful in equivocal cases. If the suspicious density is contiguous with a vascular structure or branches and courses through the parenchyma on sequential scans, the lesion is probably a vessel rather than metastasis. If no vascular structures course toward the suspicious lesion on adjacent sections, it most likely represents a metastasis. Repeating the scan after changing the position of the patient from supine to prone or decubitus may be helpful for further assessment of a suspicious nodule. A vessel changes size and shape, whereas the appearance of a metastasis is unchanged.

Other causes of pulmonary nodules, besides metastases, include granuloma, mycobacterial and fungal infections (Figure 9-3), lymphoproliferative disorders, and some congenital anomalies, such as bronchial atresia and arteriovenous malformation (AVM). For most of these diagnoses, axial images suffice. In cases of pulmonary AVM, 3D imaging may provide a more confident diagnosis and better definition of the architecture of this lesion (27) (see discussion

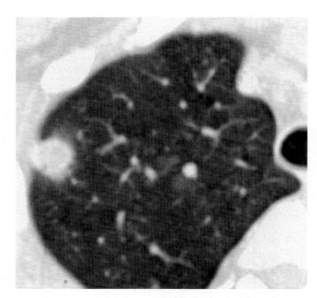

FIG. 9–3. Solitary nodule, invasive aspergillosis. A well-circumscribed nodule with a surrounding hazy infiltrate (*halo sign*) is demonstrated in the right upper lobe.

below). Primary lung neoplasms in children are rare and most are benign, usually papilloma or hamartoma.

Mediastinal Masses (Protocol 1)

Multidetector CT has several advantages in the evaluation of a widened mediastinum or mediastinal mass. Faster acquisition time improves spatial and temporal resolution and allows consistently high levels of vascular enhancement, which can facilitate characterization of mediastinal parenchymal lesions and definition of their extent. In general, axial images alone can provide sufficient information about the nature and extent of mediastinal masses. The ability to obtain multiplanar (coronal, sagittal, and oblique), and 3D images, can help in planning surgical or radiation therapy.

Anterior Mediastinal Masses

Lymphoma, thymic hyperplasia, teratoma, cystic hygroma, and thymic cysts are the most common anterior mediastinal masses in children (28–30). Rarer causes of anterior mediastinal masses include thymoma, enlarged thyroid, thymolipoma, and lipoblastoma.

Lymphoma

Lymphoma, including Hodgkin's disease and non-Hodgkin's lymphoma, is the most common cause of an anterior mediastinal mass (31,32). Nodular sclerosis is the most prevalent subtype of Hodgkin's disease and most commonly affects the neck and mediastinum. Mediastinal involvement occurs in more than 75% of pediatric patients with Hodgkin's disease, and involvement of superior mediastinal nodes or the thymus is seen in over 95% of cases. Intrathoracic

Hodgkin's disease usually assumes an orderly progression of disease along lymphatic chains, with rare instances of skip areas. Non-Hodgkin's lymphoma involves the mediastinum in about 50% of patients. In addition, the pattern of involvement is unpredictable, with skip areas common. In non-Hodgkin's lymphoma, superior mediastinal nodes are involved in slightly less than 75% of patients with intrathoracic lymphoma. Involvement of other nodal groups is more common.

On CT, nodal involvement in lymphoma ranges from mildly enlarged discrete nodes in a single area to large conglomerate masses in multiple regions. Typically, the enlarged nodes have discrete margins, are homogeneous, and show little enhancement after IV contrast administration.

Thymic involvement by lymphoma appears as an enlarged quadrilateral-shaped gland with convex lobulated margins (Figure 9-4) (33,34). The attenuation value of the lymphomatous organ is equal to that of soft tissue. Mean thickness of an infiltrated lobe ranges from 2.1 cm to 7.5 cm (normal, 0.4 cm to 2.1 cm). About 95% of patients have associated lymph-node disease elsewhere in the mediastinum. Calcifications can be seen in untreated lymphoma, but more often they are a post-treatment sequel. The calcifications are similar to those seen in granulomatous disease; however, in Hodgkin's disease, they are larger, more diffuse, and most often in the anterior mediastinum. Cystic areas due to ischemic necrosis also can be seen. Additional findings include mediastinal or hilar lymph node enlargement, airway narrowing, and compression of vascular structures.

Rebound Thymic Hyperplasia

Thymic hyperplasia, defined as greater than 50% increase in thymic volume over baseline, is another cause of

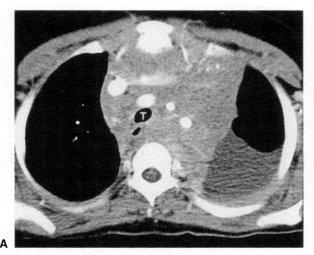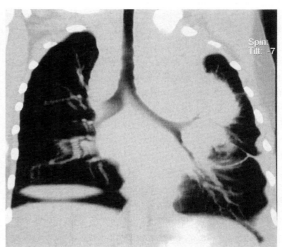

FIG. 9–4. Thymic Hodgkin's disease. **A:** Large predominantly soft-tissue-attenuation anterior mediastinal mass is seen in the expected position of the thymus. The mass compresses the trachea (*T*). A large left pleural effusion also is present. **B:** Multiplanar coronal reconstruction. Coronal reconstruction is superior to the axial plane for depicting tumor extent and tracheal compression.

thymic enlargement. It is a well-recognized effect of chemotherapy, especially when corticosteroids have been given as part of the treatment plan. The thymus usually decreases in volume after the start of chemotherapy. Several months after the initiation of chemotherapy, and usually between courses of chemotherapy, the thymus overgrows or rebounds in some patients.

Computed tomography features of hyperplasia are a diffusely enlarged gland, which usually maintains a normal configuration. The attenuation value of the hyperplastic thymus is similar to that of the normal organ and hence, is not helpful in differentiating tumor and hyperplasia. If there is absence of other active disease and the thymic enlargement correlates with the timing of chemotherapy, patients can be treated conservatively and followed with serial imaging studies. A decrease in size of the thymus on serial CT scans supports the diagnosis of rebound hyperplasia as the cause of thymic enlargement (33).

Germ-cell Tumors

Extragonadal germ-cell tumors are the most common cause of a fat-containing mediastinal lesion. Most are located in the anterior mediastinum, within or adjacent to the thymus. They arise from remnants of one or more primitive germ cell layers (ectoderm, endoderm, or mesoderm). Approximately 90% are benign, and histologically are either dermoid cysts (containing only ectodermal elements) or teratomas (containing tissues from all three germinal layers) (35). Benign germ cell tumors are cystic and contain sebaceous or gelatinous fluid. On CT, these tumors have well-circumscribed margins, thick walls, and an admixture of tissues: calcium, fat, and soft tissue (35–37). Although soft-tissue elements may be present, they are not a dominant element (Figure 9-5). A specific diagnosis of teratoma can be made with certainty by CT when calcifications and fat are demonstrated within an anterior mediastinal mass.

Malignant germ cell tumors, accounting for approximately 10% of all germ-cell tumors, include teratocarcinomas, seminomas, embryonal carcinomas, choriocarcinomas, and endodermal sinus (i.e., yolk sac) tumors. Compared with benign tumors, malignant germ cell neoplasms contain a predominance of soft-tissue-attenuation components (Figure 9-6). Central areas of cyst formation or necrosis are common, especially in the nonteratomatous tumors. Aggressive features, such as invasion of the mediastinal fat and chest wall, pulmonary metastases, and hepatic metastases also may be present.

Cystic Hygroma

Cystic hygromas are the most common cause of water-attenuation lesions in the anterior mediastinum. They usually are inferior extensions of cervical hygromas. On CT, they appear as nonenhancing thin-walled multiloculated masses with a near-water-attenuation value. The presence of contrast enhancement in the wall or internal septations suggests su-

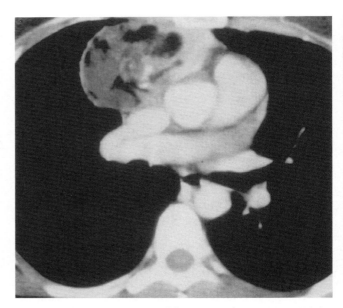

FIG. 9–5. Benign teratoma. A large complex mass containing fluid-filled cystic spaces, fat and calcification is seen anterior to the arch vessels. Computed tomography allows precise identification of fluid, fat, and calcium, which are classic features of a teratoma.

perimposed infection or a hemangiomatous component. Occasionally, marked dilatation of adjacent veins is noted.

Thymic Cysts

Thymic cysts are another cause of a water-attenuation lesion in the anterior mediastinum. Most are derived from persistence of the thymopharyngeal duct, but cysts in the thymus can be seen after trauma or thoracotomy, and in thymic involvement by lymphoma both before and following

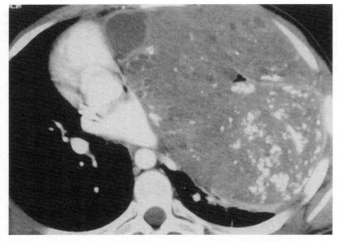

FIG. 9–6. Malignant teratoma. A large, predominantly soft-tissue-attenuation mass arises from the left lobe of the thymus. Some areas of fat and calcification also are seen. The large soft-tissue component (greater than 50% by volume) is characteristic of a malignant germ cell tumor.

treatment. Congenital cysts can be found in the neck and/or mediastinum or anywhere along the developmental pathway of the thymus. Multiple thymic cysts also have been described in association with HIV infection and Langerhans cell histiocytosis (38,39). On CT, benign thymic cysts are usually thin-walled homogeneous masses of near-water-attenuation value. They occasionally may have a higher attenuation value when the cyst's contents are proteinaceous or hemorrhagic. Cysts associated with neoplasms usually will have a prominent soft tissue component.

Middle Mediastinum

The common causes of middle mediastinal masses are lymphadenopathy and cysts of the embryonic foregut. Rare causes of middle mediastinal masses in children include aberrant subclavian artery, a dilated esophagus, and/or aneurysm of a patent ductus arteriosus.

Lymphadenopathy

Mediastinal or hilar lymph node enlargement in children usually is the result of granulomatous disease or lymphoma. The CT appearance of lymphadenopathy ranges from mildly enlarged discrete soft tissue masses to a single solid soft-tissue mass with poorly defined margins (Figure 9-7). Calcification within lymph nodes suggests old granulomatous disease, such as histoplasmosis or tuberculosis. Enlarged nodes with low attenuation may be seen in tuberculosis, lymphoma, and metastases from testicular carcinoma.

Mediastinal nodes with granulomatous disease usually undergo spontaneous resolution, often with calcification. Occasionally, healing is associated with extensive fibrosis of mediastinal or hilar soft tissues that may cause compression and occlusion of adjacent vessels or the tracheobronchial tree. This manifestation of histoplasmosis is termed fibrosing mediastinitis. Computed tomography findings include hilar, paratracheal, and/or subcarinal nodal masses (Figure 9-7), which often contain areas of calcification, venous obstruction, tracheobronchial narrowing, and pulmonary infiltrates due to venous obstruction or infarction.

Bronchopulmonary Foregut Cysts

Bronchopulmonary foregut malformations include bronchogenic, enteric, and neurenteric cysts. Bronchogenic cysts are the most common type of foregut cyst. They are lined by respiratory epithelium and are located most often in the subcarinal or right paratracheal regions. Enteric cysts, also known as esophageal duplications, are lined by gastrointestinal mucosa (40,41) and typically are located in the middle and/or mediastinum close to or within the wall of the esophagus. Neurenteric cysts are posterior mediastinal lesions that are connected to the meninges through a midline defect in one or more vertebral bodies and are lined by gastrointestinal epithelium.

Characteristic CT findings of foregut cysts include a nonenhancing round or tubular mass with well-defined margins, thin or imperceptible walls, and homogeneous near-water-attenuation value (Figure 9-8). However, some foregut cysts have higher attenuation values because the cyst fluid is proteinaceous or hemorrhagic, or contains calcium

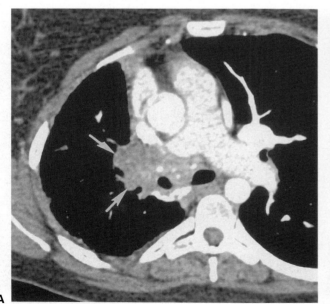
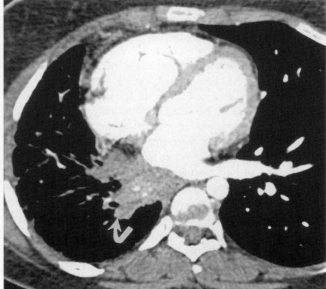

A   B

FIG. 9–7. Mediastinal lymphadenopathy in a patient with healed histoplasmosis and fibrosing mediastinitis. **A,B:** Computed tomography scans at the level of the main pulmonary artery and ventricles, respectively, demonstrate a right hilar (*arrows*) and a subcarinal (*curved arrow*) mass that narrows the right mainstem bronchus and occludes the right pulmonary artery.

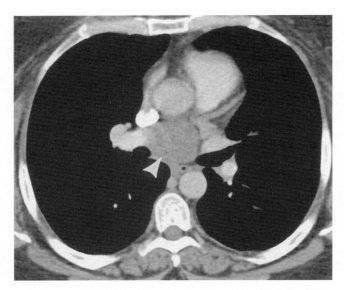

FIG. 9–8. Mediastinal bronchogenic cyst. A well-defined homogeneous water-attenuation mass (*arrowhead*) is seen in the subcarinal area.

carbonate or oxalate. Infected cysts may have a thickened wall. Additional findings include air or air–fluid levels and peripheral or central linear calcifications.

Posterior Mediastinum

Approximately 95% of posterior mediastinal masses in children are of neural origin. They can arise from sympathetic ganglia or from nerve sheaths. Ganglion cell tumors include neuroblastoma, ganglioneuroblastoma, or ganglioneuroma, while nerve sheath tumors usually are neurofibromas or schwannomas. Rare causes of posterior mediastinal masses include extralobar sequestration, Bochdalek hernia, hemangioma, lymphoma, extramedullary hematopoiesis, and lateral meningocele.

Ganglion cell tumors tend to have a fusiform or elongated shape and extend over the length of several vertebral bodies (Figure 9-9). They are of soft tissue attenuation and often contain areas of calcification. By comparison, nerve sheath tumors tend to be smaller, have a more spherical or oval shape, and occur near the junction of a vertebral body and an adjacent rib. They frequently have areas of low attenuation secondary to cystic degeneration, xanthomatous contents, or areas of hypocellularity. Both types of tumors may cause pressure erosion of a rib. Because of their origin from neural tissue, neurogenic tumors have a tendency to invade the spinal canal. Intraspinal extension is extradural in location, displacing and occasionally compressing the cord. Identification of intraspinal invasion is important clinically because affected patients require radiation therapy or a laminectomy prior to tumor debulking.

Congenital Pulmonary Masses

Congenital pulmonary anomalies encountered in childhood can be classified into two broad categories: anomalies with normal vasculature and anomalies with abnormal vasculature. Although not required for diagnosis, multiplanar reformations and 3D reconstructions may provide anatomic information that can aid in surgical planning.

Anomalies with Normal Vasculature (Protocol 1)

Congenital lobar emphysema, cystic adenomatoid malformation, and bronchial atresia are anomalies resulting from abnormal bronchial development. Chest radiography usually can suggest the diagnosis, and CT is performed to determine the extent of abnormality in patients in whom surgery is contemplated.

Congenital lobar emphysema or hyperinflation usually presents in the first six months of life with respiratory distress. Computed tomography shows an overinflated lobe with attenuated vascularity, compression of ipsilateral adjacent lobes, and mediastinal shift to the opposite side. Air trapping may be seen on expiratory scans. The sites of involvement in order of decreasing frequency are the left upper lobe (45% of cases), right middle lobe (30%), and right upper lobe (20%).

Cystic adenomatoid malformation is characterized by a proliferation of distal bronchioles that results in the formation of a cystic mass rather than normal alveoli. Patients usually present with respiratory distress soon after birth. Three types of cystic adenomatoid malformation have been described by pathologic examination. Type I contains a single cyst or multiple large cysts (>2 cm in diameter) and is the most common type. Type II contains multiple smaller cysts (1 mm–20 mm in diameter) and is the second most common type. Type III lesions appear as solid masses on visual inspection, but microscopically demonstrate tiny

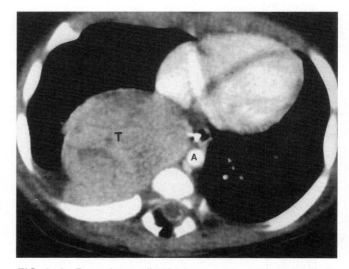

FIG. 9–9. Posterior mediastinal mass, neuroblastoma. Axial CT scan through the lower thorax shows a large soft tissue attenuation tumor (*T*) anterior to the lower thoracic spine. The tumor extends around the descending aorta (*A*). Also seen are bilateral pleural effusions.

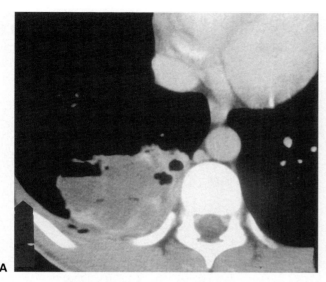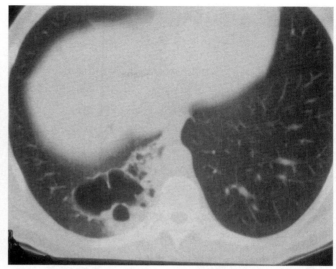

FIG. 9–10. Lung mass, cystic adenomatoid malformation. **A:** Axial image at mediastinal windows shows a predominantly fluid-filled mass in the right lower lobe. Some air-filled areas also are present. **B:** A scan at a more caudal level with lung windows shows a complex mass with several air-filled cysts.

cysts. This anomaly occurs with equal frequency in both lungs, although there is a slight upper lobe predominance. In neonates, the CT features are those of a complex mass containing single or multiple air-filled cysts surrounded by a well-defined wall. In children and adults, the cysts may contain fluid, air, or air–fluid levels (42) (Figure 9-10). Cystic adenomatoid malformation can occur in association with sequestration.

Bronchial atresia results from abnormal development of a segmental or subsegmental bronchus. It is usually asymptomatic and discovered on chest radiographs performed for other indications. The CT features of bronchial atresia include a hyperinflated lung surrounding the dilated mucoid-filled segmental or subsegmental bronchus, which usually is in close proximity to the hilum.

Anomalies with Abnormal Vasculature (Protocol 2)

Sequestration, hypogenetic lung syndrome, and arterovenous malformation (AVM) are congenital anomalies with abnormal vasculature. Bronchopulmonary sequestration is a congenital mass of pulmonary tissue that has no normal connection with the tracheobronchial tree and is supplied by an anomalous artery, usually arising from the aorta. Sequestrations in children may be extra- or intralobar. Extralobar sequestration is likely congenital in origin; it has its own pleura and drains to systemic veins (43–45). Intralobar sequestration most likely is an acquired abnormality related to infection; it is confined within the normal visceral pleura and has venous drainage to the pulmonary veins. The majority of sequestration occurs in the posterior basal segment of the left lower lobe.

The CT diagnosis is based on demonstration of enhancement of an anomalous systemic vessel, which usually arises from the aorta, however, upper abdominal vessels can be the source of arterial supply (Figure 9-11) (see color plate). The CT appearance of the pulmonary parenchyma depends on whether or not the sequestered lung is aerated. When the sequestration communicates with the remainder of the lung, usually after being infected, air or cystic areas may appear in the lesion. A sequestration that does not communicate appears as a homogeneous density. The lung adjacent to the sequestration can show decreased attenuation, likely due to air trapping.

The hypogenetic lung or scimitar syndrome is characterized by a small lung that is nearly always on the right, ipsilateral mediastinal displacement, a corresponding small or absent pulmonary artery, and anomalous pulmonary venous return (Figure 9-12) (see color plate). The anomalous return usually is into the inferior vena cava below the right hemidiaphragm, although it may enter the suprahepatic portion of the cava, hepatic vein, portal vein, azygous vein, or right atrium. Associated anomalies include systemic arterial supply to the hypogenetic lung and horseshoe lung. Horseshoe lung is a rare anomaly in which the posterobasal segments of both lungs are fused behind the pericardial sac (46).

Pulmonary AVM is characterized by a direct communication between a pulmonary artery and vein without an intervening capillary bed. This malformation can occur in isolation, can be multiple, or associated with AVM in the skin, mucous membranes, and other organs (Osler–Weber–Rendu syndrome). On CT, AVM appears as focal round or nodular masses with adjacent curvilinear opacities, representing the feeding artery and draining vein (Figure 9-13) (see color plate). Enhancement typically occurs during the same phase as the pulmonary artery or vein and before enhancement of the left atrium and left ventricle. Multislice CT with 3D volume renderings can provide a confident diag-

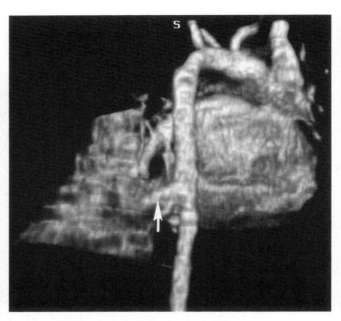

FIG. 9–11. Lung mass, intralobar pulmonary sequestration. **A:** Axial contrast-enhanced CT section demonstrates a vessel (*arrowheads*) arising laterally from the descending thoracic aorta (*A*) and extending to an area of left lower lobe opacity. **B:** 3D volume rendering viewed from behind shows the feeding artery (*arrow*) arising from the aorta and extending to the lower-lobe sequestration. Drainage was via a pulmonary vein, which entered the left atrium. The course of the artery and vein and their relationship to adjacent structures are seen better when the vascular structures, heart, and lung are viewed simultaneously. (See Color Fig. 9–11B)

nosis of pulmonary AVM and show the precise anatomy of the feeding arteries and draining veins, which is critical information for treatment planning (47,48).

Vascular Assessment (Protocol 2)

Computed tomography angiography has become a valuable technique for cardiovascular imaging and is challenging conventional angiography for assessing the thoracic vessels. Helical CT, particularly with multidetector capability, has advantages over conventional angiography. The volumetric acquisition of helical CT allows superior image resolution and clear delineation of the aorta and superior vena cava, as well as the pulmonary arteries and veins and their branches. The major vessels and their branches commonly overlap in conventional arteriography, obscuring their depiction. Other advantages of CT over angiography include shorter acquisition times, superior 3D renderings, and greater range of coverage, increasing conspicuity of vascular lesions. In addition, the radiation dose for CT angiography is at least two to three times less than the dose for angiography. In our experience, these advantages have resulted in CT replacing conventional arteriography for the assessment of many thoracic vascular abnormalities.

Computed tomography has also gained increasing acceptance as an alternative method to magnetic resonance (MR) imaging in the diagnosis of vascular anomalies. An important advantage of CT angiography over MR angiography is the shorter scan time for CT, which reduces the need for sedation, and the ability to scan extremely ill patients who cannot tolerate the long imaging times for MR examinations. There is the risk of radiation exposure in CT angiography, but in the critically ill patient, the risk of prolonged sedation may be greater than that of radiation.

Axial images usually are sufficient for diagnosis, but multiplanar or 3D reconstructions, particularly when viewed in a cine mode, provide better detail about anatomic relationships between the great vessels and tracheobronchial tree. Multiplanar and 3D reconstructions can also aid in the diagnosis of mild coarctations and improve the accuracy of determining the length of coarctation. In addition, these images can help in the planning of surgery or stent placement.

The number of vascular applications of MDCT continues to increase. Computed tomography angiographic techniques have been shown to be valuable in the evaluation of both congenital and acquired abnormalities of the thoracic aorta, systemic veins, and central pulmonary arteries and veins.

Aortic Lesions

The common anomalies of the thoracic aorta are the vascular rings and nonvalvular stenotic lesions (coarctation, interrupted arch, and supravalvular stenosis). Aneurysm formation and dissection can occur in children, although they are rare.

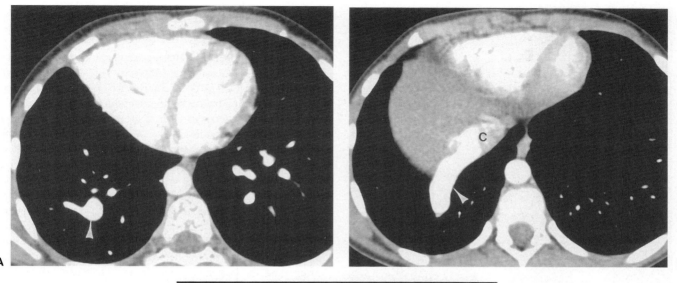

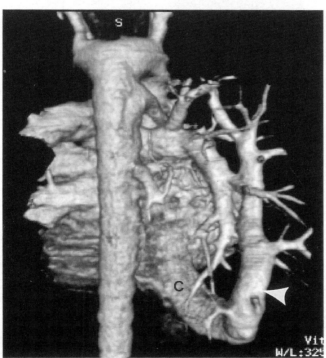

FIG. 9–12. Scimitar syndrome with partial anomalous venous return. **A:** Axial CT scan at the level of the ventricles shows part of the anomalous pulmonary vein. **B:** Several centimeters lower, the anomalous vessel enters the intrahepatic inferior vena cava. Note also the slightly smaller right hemithorax and the ipsilateral mediastinal shift. **C:** Volume-rendered 3D display. With this technique, it is possible to depict the entire course of the vessel on one image. *C*, inferior vena cava; *arrowhead*, anomalous vein. (See Color Fig. 9–12C)

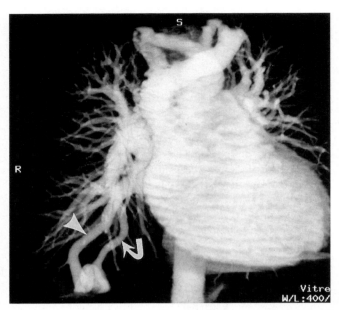

FIG. 9–13. Pulmonary AVM. 3D volume rendering in a young adult. The feeding artery (*arrow*) originates from the anterior segment artery of the right lower lobe. The draining vein (*arrowhead*) drains into the right inferior pulmonary vein. (See Color Fig. 9–13)

Vascular Rings

The diagnosis of a vascular ring usually can be suggested on conventional chest radiography. Additional imaging with CT can define further the anatomy for surgical planning (49,50). Patients with vascular rings may or may not have symptoms related to airway or esophageal compression.

The common symptomatic vascular rings are the double aortic arch and the right aortic arch with an aberrant left subclavian artery. The double aortic arch is characterized by two arches arising from a single ascending aorta, each giving rise to a subclavian and carotid artery before reuniting to form a single descending aorta. The right arch component tends to be larger and more cephalad than the left component (Figure 9-14) (see color plate). Both aortic arches may be patent or one, usually the left arch, may be atretic.

In the right aortic arch with an aberrant left subclavian artery, the aberrant subclavian artery arises as the last branch from the aortic arch and traverses the mediastinum behind the esophagus to reach the left arm (Figure 9-15). The left aortic arch is interrupted between the left common carotid artery and the left subclavian artery. The vascular ring is completed by the ligamentum arteriosum. Airway compression may be due to a tight ligamentum arteriosum, Kommerell's diverticulum, or a midline descending aorta. Compression due to diverticulum or ligament occurs at the level of the arch, whereas compression from a midline descending aorta occurs at the level of the carina or left mainstem bronchus (51). The right aortic arch with an aberrant left subclavian artery rarely is associated with congenital heart disease.

Aortic Coarctation

In patients with coarctation, a segment of the aorta is narrowed. The common site of constriction is immediately

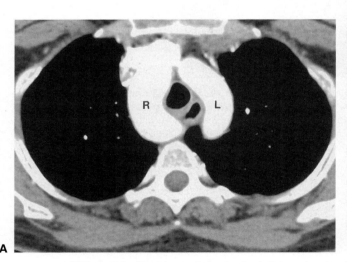

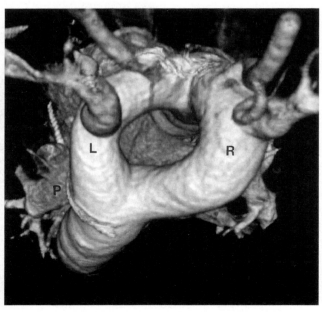

FIG. 9–14. Double aortic arch. **A:** Axial contrast-enhanced image shows a double aortic arch. **B:** Volume-rendered image (posterior view) in the same patient shows that the two arches unite just above the level of the pulmonary artery (*P*). *R*, right arch; *L*, left arch; *PA*, main pulmonary artery. (See Color Fig. 9–14B)

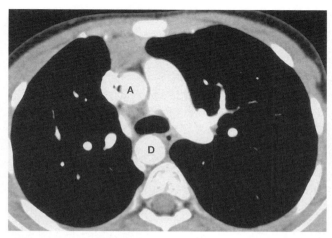

FIG. 9–15. Right aortic arch with aberrant left subclavian artery. Note the descending right arch (*D*). *A*, ascending aorta.

below the origin of the left subclavian artery at the insertion of the ductus arteriosus or ligamentum arteriosum, although the coarctation can occur anywhere along the course of the aorta. If the coarctation occurs between the left subclavian artery and the ductus arteriosus, it is termed preductal or

infantile coarctation. This type may be associated with aortic-arch hypoplasia. When the coarctation occurs distal to the ductus arteriosus, it is referred to as an adult coarctation. Collateral vessel formation is common in this form of coarctation (Figure 9-16) (see color plate).

The typical CT appearance of coarctation is a short segment area of luminal narrowing, with or without accompanying hypoplasia of the aortic arch or isthmus. Focal coarctations may be amenable to balloon dilatation, whereas long-segment coarctations often require surgical repair.

Collateral circulation is another finding of coarctation. The diagnosis of collateral blood-flow formation is based on the demonstration of anomalous vessels bridging the area of aortic stenosis and merging into the descending aorta. Identification of collateral flow is important for two reasons. First, if there are insufficient numbers of collateral vessels, crossclamping of the aorta during surgical repair may be contraindicated because it can result in spinal-cord ischemia. Second, the extent of collateral vessel formation can be an indicator of the severity of the narrowing. The larger the number of collaterals, the more likely it is that the coarctation is clinically significant. Following surgical repair or post-balloon angioplasty, CT can be used to demonstrate restenosis and aneurysm at the repair site.

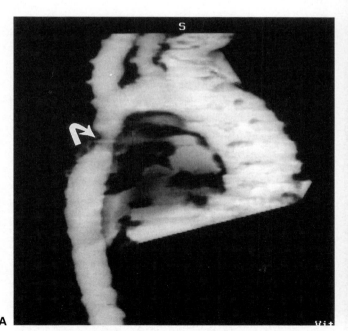
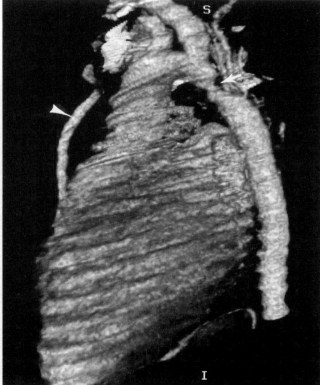

FIG. 9–16. Aortic coarctation. **A:** Preductal coarctation. Volume-rendered 3D reconstruction in an infant demonstrates focal narrowing (*curved arrow*) of the descending aorta just beyond the left subclavian artery. The irregularity of the vascular walls is caused by cardiac and respiratory motion. **B:** Post-ductal coarctation (*arrow*) in a young adult. Note the large mammary artery collateral vessel (*arrowhead*). (See Color Fig. 9–16B)

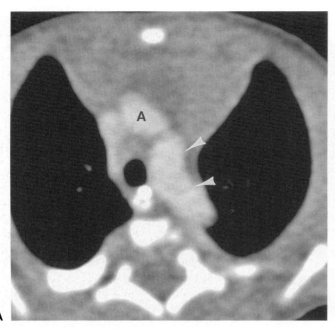
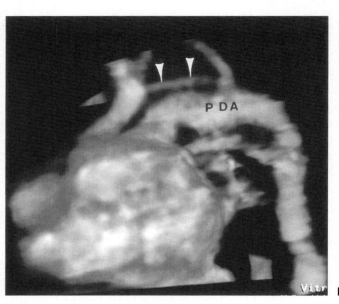

FIG. 9–17. Interrupted aortic arch. **A:** Axial CT section in a 2-kg neonate, acquired with 1.0-mm collimation and table speed of 15 mm per rotation, demonstrates a normal caliber ascending aorta (*A*). The vessel latter and inferior to the aorta is a dilated patent ductus arteriosus (*arrowheads*). **B:** Volume-rendered reconstruction shows a markedly hypoplastic transverse arch (*arrowheads*) and a large patent ductus arteriosus (PDA) that supplies the distal aorta. The volume-rendered reconstruction facilitates display of this complex anatomy. (See Color Fig. 9–17B)

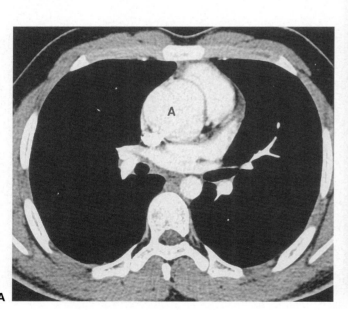
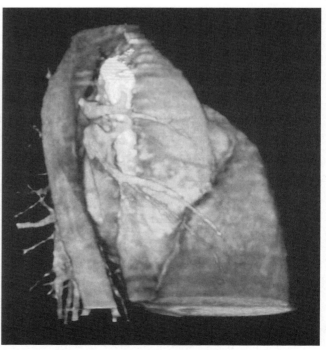

FIG. 9–18. Aortic aneurysm secondary to Marfan's disease. **A:** Axial contrast-enhanced CT shows a dilated ascending aorta (*A*) that compresses the adjacent main pulmonary artery. **B:** Oblique reconstruction reveals the full length of the aneurysm that extends from the aortic root to the transverse aorta. The oblique reconstruction shows better the extent of the aneurysm.

Interruption of the Aortic Arch

Interruption of the aortic arch is characterized by complete discontinuity between the ascending and the descending aorta. The three basic types of interrupted arch are, in descending order of frequency: Type A, interruption of the aortic arch distal to the left subclavian artery; Type B, interruption of the arch between the left common carotid artery and the left subclavian artery; and Type C, interruption of the arch proximal to the left carotid artery. The CT findings of arch interruption are absence of the transverse arch and a patent ductus arteriosus supplying the descending aorta (Figure 9-17) (see color plate). It is important not to confuse the patent ductus arteriosus with the transverse arch.

Other Causes of Nonvalvular Aortic Stenosis

Long-segment aortic narrowing has been associated with Takayasu's arteritis and William's syndrome. Takayasu's arteritis is a primary arteritis of unknown origin that affects the aorta and its major branches, as well as the pulmonary artery. William's syndrome is characterized by the combination of supravalvar aortic stenosis, peripheral pulmonary arterial stenosis, mental retardation, and "elfin facies." Computed tomography angiography can delineate the site and length of the aortic narrowing and the thickened arterial wall in Takayasu's arteritis (52).

Aortic Aneurysms and Dissections

Aortic aneurysms and dissections are rare in children. When they occur, they usually are associated with predisposing conditions, such as Turner's syndrome, coarctation of the aorta, Marfan's syndrome (Figure 9-18), Ehlers–Danlos syndrome, Kawasaki disease, prior surgery, or trauma. The CT findings of aortic aneurysm include dilatation of a variable segment of the aorta, intraluminal thrombus, and displacement of adjacent mediastinal structures. The diagnosis of aortic dilatation is made when the diameter of the aorta is greater than 50% of the normal diameter of the aorta, or when the diameter of the proximal descending aorta is 1.5 times the diameter of the descending thoracic aorta at the level of the diaphragm.

Computed-tomography features of acute aortic dissection are a false lumen and an intimal flap. Initial precontrast images of the thoracic aorta may be valuable to assist in the detection of high-attenuation hematoma in the false lumen. The entire thorax is then scanned during injection of IV contrast. The characteristic CT findings of dissection on contrast-enhanced images are contrast-filled true and false lumina separated by an intimal flap and delayed enhancement of the false lumen because of slower flow. Typically, the false lumen is on the outer curvature of the aorta (Figure 9-19).

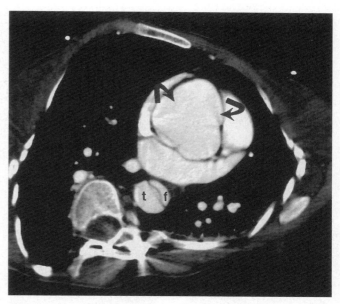

FIG. 9–19. Aortic dissection, Type B, as a complication of Marfan's' syndrome. Axial CT section at the level of the descending aorta shows an intimal flap separating the contrast-filled true (*t*) and false (*f*) lumina. Also note annuloaortic ectasia (*arrows*).

Pulmonary Arteries

The complex curving anatomy of the pulmonary arteries and veins also is suited well to MDCT angiography. Common anomalies of the pulmonary arteries are obstructive lesions of the right ventricular outflow tract (i.e., pulmonary artery atresia, hypoplasia, or stenosis), truncus arteriosus and its variants, and anomalous origin of the left pulmonary artery from the right pulmonary artery (pulmonary sling).

Obstructive Lesions

The role of CT angiography in patients with obstructive lesions of the pulmonary artery is to determine the presence, caliber, and confluence of the main pulmonary arteries and the presence of collateral vessels.

In the absence or hypoplasia of a main pulmonary artery, right-sided involvement is more common than left-sided involvement. The affected lung is decreased in size and hypoattenuating, and the vessels are systemic. There is no evidence of air trapping on expiration scans. Arterial supply may arise from a patent ductus arteriosus, aortopulmonary collateral arteries from the descending thoracic or upper abdominal aorta (Figure 9-20), direct origin of a pulmonary artery from the aorta, and other systemic arteries (53).

Truncus Arteriosus

In truncus arteriosus, a single vessel originates from the base of the heart and gives origin to the coronary, pulmo-

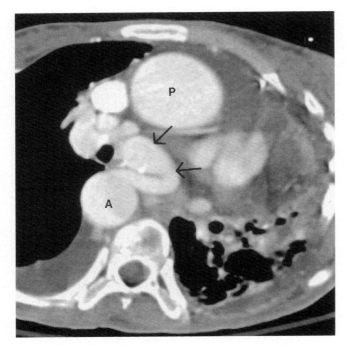

FIG. 9–20. Pulmonary atresia, collateral vessel formation. Axial image shows a dilated main pulmonary artery (*P*), a right descending aorta (*A*), and a hypertrophied collateral vessel (*arrows*) arising from the aorta. Bilateral pleural effusions also are present.

nary, and systemic arterial circulations. There is one semilunar valve. Truncus arteriosus needs to be differentiated from an aortopulmonary window, where there is an anomalous communication between the main pulmonary artery and the aorta and there are two semilunar valves. In hemitruncus, one of the pulmonary arteries, usually the right, originates from the ascending aorta.

Pulmonary Sling

In patients with pulmonary sling, the left pulmonary artery originates from the right pulmonary artery and crosses the mediastinum, extending between the trachea and esophagus to reach the left hilum. The abnormal anatomy is seen easily on axial CT angiography, although the relationship between the anomalous vessel and the esophagus and trachea may be seen better on reconstructions.

Pulmonary Veins

The common anomaly of the pulmonary veins is anomalous return, which occurs when a pulmonary vein enters the right heart or a systemic vein (54). Anomalous drainage of the pulmonary veins can occur in isolation or with the hypogenetic lung syndrome (Figure 9-12). The anomalous drainage results in a left-to-right shunt with pulmonary venous blood returning to the right side of the heart or to systemic veins. It may be partial or total; the latter requires a

right-to-left shunt via a septal defect or patent ductus arteriosus. The anomalous connection commonly involves the left superior and right inferior pulmonary veins. The anomalous left superior pulmonary vein drains into the left brachiocephalic vein, producing a vertical vein that courses lateral to the aortic arch and aortopulmonary window. The anomalous right inferior pulmonary vein drains cephalad into the azygous vein or caudal into the subdiaphragmatic inferior vena cava or portal vein.

Systemic Veins

The common systemic venous abnormalities include persistence of the left superior vena cava and interruption of the inferior vena cava with azygous or hemiazygous continuation. The persistent left superior vena cava drains the left jugular and subclavian veins, and in some cases, the left superior intercostal vein. It lies lateral to the left common carotid artery and anterior to the left subclavian artery, descends lateral to the main pulmonary artery, and drains into the coronary sinus posterior to the left ventricle.

In the interrupted inferior vena cava, the infrahepatic segment of the inferior vena cava between the liver and renal veins fails to develop, and either the hemiazygous or azygous veins act as collateral vessels to return blood from the renal veins to the heart. Azygous and hemiazygous continuation of the inferior vena cava can be an isolated abnormality, or it can coexist with congenital heart disease. Computed-tomography findings include dilatation of the azygos arch, the azygos vein, and the superior vena cava caudal to the azygos junction; enlargement of the azygos and hemiazygous veins in the paraspinal and retrocrural areas; and absence of the suprarenal and intrahepatic portions of the inferior vena cava (Figure 9-21). The hepatic veins drain into the right atrium via a common hepatic vein.

Congenital Heart Disease (Protocol 2)

Faster scan times coupled with the use of cardiac gating not only reduce artifacts, but also allow high-resolution imaging of intra- and extracardiac regions that previously were difficult to evaluate because of cardiac motion.

Most congenital cardiac lesions still are evaluated initially by echocardiography, but CT can be of use when echocardiography provides inadequate information. The major indications for CT in congenital cardiac anomalies include: i) evaluation of the size and patency of the pulmonary arteries in patients with cyanotic heart disease, such as pulmonary atresia and tetrology of Fallot; ii) detection of anomalous origin of the coronary artery; iii) determination of the extracardiac anatomy in patients with complex congenital heart disease (e.g., great vessel relationships, bronchial collateral vessels, and abdominal situs); iv) evaluation of surgically created systemic-to-pulmonary artery shunts in patients with complex anatomic heart diseases, such as truncus arteriosus, tetrology of Fallot, hemitruncus, and pulmonary atresia;

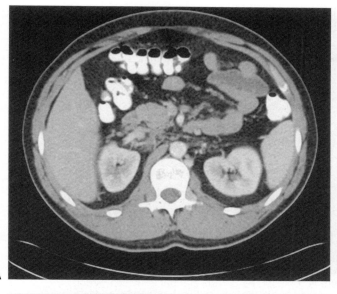

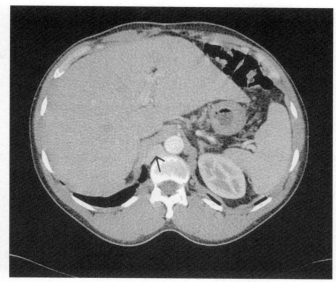

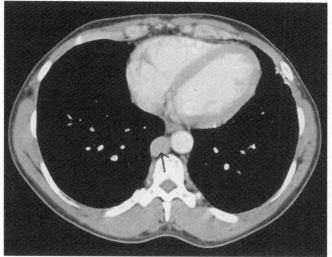

FIG. 9–21. Interrupted inferior vena cava with azygos continuation. **A:** Computed tomography scan at the level of the midpoles of the kidneys shows absence of an inferior vena cava. **B:** At the level of the hepatic hilus, an enlarged azygos vein (*arrow*) can be seen posterior to the crura. **C:** A more cephalad scan again shows the dilated azygos vein. At a higher level, it joined the superior vena cava.

and v) evaluation of the integrity of intracardiac baffles (Figure 9-22). Although CT angiography usually is not performed to evaluate intracardiac shunt lesions associated with septal defects, these lesions occasionally can be an incidental finding on an examination performed for other indications.

Evaluation of the Airway (Protocol 3)

Central-Airway Disease

The chest radiograph is usually the initial imaging study in patients with suspected airway abnormalities. However, evaluation of the airway may be difficult because of overlapping mediastinal structures. Multidetector CT with reformatted images can allow more precise depiction of tracheobronchial abnormalities (55–58). The faster scan times allow the acquisition of high-quality images in regions previously difficult to evaluate because of respiratory or cardiac motion.

Computed-tomography images of the airways are acquired in the axial plane and processed with both multiplanar reformations (in coronal, oblique, and sagittal planes) and volume rendering. (Figures 9–1 and 9–2).

Axial images are mandatory for assessing extraluminal disease, including the lung parenchyma and mediastinal structures. In selected cases, multiplanar reformations and 3D volume renderings can be helpful in showing mild stenoses and complex congenital airway abnormalities, such as abnormal origins of the bronchi or bronchoesophageal fistulas. They also can assist in demonstrating the relationship of the airway to surrounding vessels. Multiplanar reformations also can be used to study the extent of narrowing in the craniocaudal direction in patients with tracheomalacia. When tracheomalacia is suspected, scans are acquired at both end-inspiration and end-expiration and then reformatted in coronal and sagittal planes. This technique is limited to cooperative patients or patients who are on assisted venti-

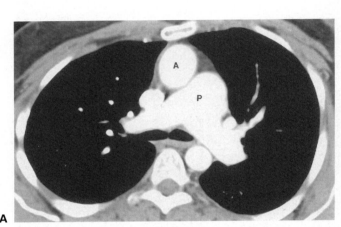
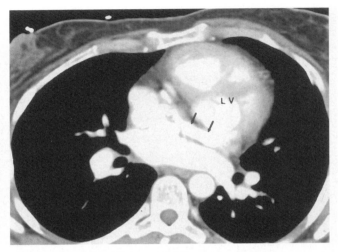

FIG. 9–22. Transposition of the great vessels and a mustard procedure. **A:** Axial CT scan shows the aorta (*A*) anterior to the pulmonary artery (*P*). **B:** A more caudal scan shows an artificial baffle (*arrows*). In the Mustard procedure, the native interatrial septum is replaced by an artificial baffle, which directs the pulmonary venous return to the right ventricle (*RV*) and the systemic venous blood to the left ventricle.

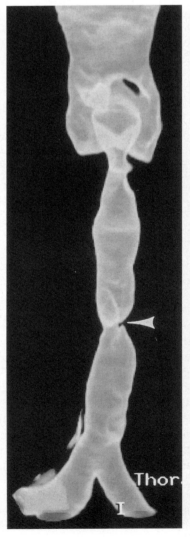
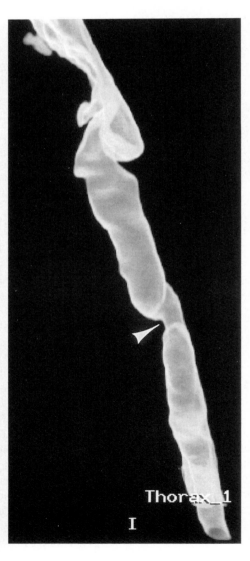

FIG. 9–23. Tracheal stricture secondary to prior intubation. **A** and **B:** Coronal and sagittal volume-rendered reconstructions show focal narrowing of the midtrachea (*arrowheads*). The entire length of the stricture is seen easily on the reconstructions.

lation. Virtual bronchoscopy has a rather limited application in the evaluation of the pediatric airway, but it can be helpful when there is a high-grade stenosis or large intraluminal tumor. This technique allows evaluation of the airways beyond the site of stenosis or neoplasm, which otherwise can be difficult to visualize by conventional bronchoscopy.

The tracheobronchial tree, including the trachea, carina and mainstem, lobar, and segmental bronchi are seen easily by CT with narrow collimation. The more common indications for CT of the airway are evaluation of congenital bronchial anomalies (e.g., tracheal or accessory bronchi, and bronchial hypoplasia or atresia) (59–60), assessment of tracheal narrowing due to stricture (61) or tumor, and detection or confirmation of tracheomalacia (62).

A tracheal or pig bronchus arises from the trachea above the carina, usually on the right side, and usually within 2 cm of the carina (53). The accessory cardiac bronchus nearly always arises from the inferior medial wall of the right main or intermediate bronchus. It usually ends blindly, although it occasionally may subtend a small amount of abnormal pulmonary parenchyma. Both the tracheal and accessory bronchus may serve as reservoirs for infectious organisms, leading to recurrent pneumonia (53).

Tracheal strictures are usually the sequela of intubation, tracheostomy placement, or surgical anastomoses. Short segmental narrowing is seen best on multiplanar or 3D reconstructions (Figure 9-23). Long-segment disease usually can be identified on axial, multiplanar, and 3D reconstructions.

In children, benign tracheobronchial tumors are more common than malignant neoplasms. Benign lesions usually are papillomas, hemangiomas, fibromas, and chondromas, with adenoid cystic carcinoma being the most common malignancy. Most tumors appear as smooth or irregular intraluminal masses with asymmetric narrowing of the tracheal lumen (Figure 9-24). Differentiation of benign and malignant tumors is difficult if the tumor is confined to the tracheal lumen. If there is extratracheal extension, a malignant lesion should be suspected.

Tracheomalacia refers to an abnormal weakness of the tracheal walls and supporting tissues, resulting in luminal collapse during expiration. Dynamic evaluation of airway caliber in the axial plane is possible with helical CT. The diagnosis of tracheomalacia can be made by CT when there is 50% or greater reduction in transluminal diameter during expiration (Figure 9-25) (62).

Small-Airway Disease

Bronchiolitis obliterans, also referred to as obliterative or constrictive bronchiolitis, is the most common indication for CT of the peripheral airways in children. Suspected bronchiectasis, although a common indication in adults, is a relatively uncommon indication for small airway CT in children. Bronchiolitis obliterans is characterized by small airway obstruction due to submucosal and peribronchiolar inflammation and fibrosis in the absence of diffuse parenchymal in-

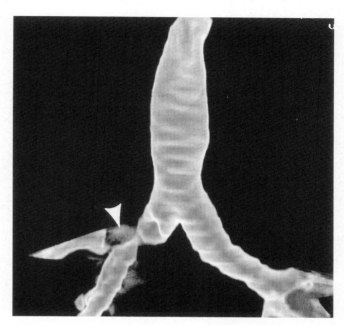

FIG. 9–24. Central airway tumor in a young adult following lung transplantation. Coronal 3D volume-rendered reconstruction shows a soft tissue mass arising from the lateral wall of the right mainstem bronchus and projecting into the bronchial lumen. The lumen of the airway at the level of the tumor is reduced. Final diagnosis was post-transplant lymphoproliferative disease. *Arrowhead*, tumor.

flammation. The disease primarily affects the terminal and respiratory bronchioles. Other findings include bronchiolectasia with inspissated secretions. Bronchiolitis obliterans may be caused by a variety of insults including bacterial, mycoplasmal, or viral infections, exposure to toxic gases, and/or drug therapy; it also may occur as a complication of lung or bone-marrow transplantation.

The high-resolution CT findings include areas of decreased lung attenuation, bronchiectasis, a tree-in-bud pattern, and poorly defined centrilobular nodules (63–66). The decreased attenuation represents a combination of oligemia and air trapping and often is termed mosaic perfusion. Air trapping can be confirmed by acquiring images during both inspiration and expiration (67,68). These images can be acquired at selected levels or through the entire lung volume. In the normal lung, attenuation values increase during expiration. Air trapping is seen as a paradoxical decrease in lung attenuation during expiration (Figure 9-26).

The tree-in-bud appearance is characterized by centrilobular branching or Y-shaped opacities. Centrilobular nodules appear as ill-defined centrilobular opacities. The use of volume slabs can aid in the diagnosis of both forms of centrilobular disease.

Diffuse Lung Disease (Protocol 4)

Chest radiography remains the imaging study of choice for evaluating most diffuse parenchymal lung disease. How-

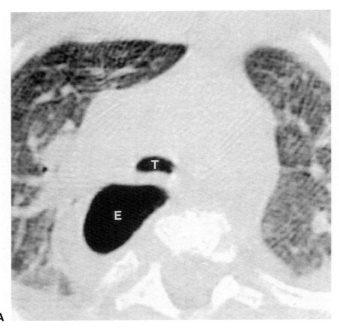
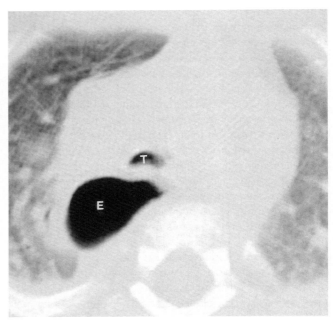

A   B

FIG. 9–25. Tracheomalacia in a 1-month-old girl who had undergone an esophageal pull through for repair of esophageal atresia and who had marked dyspnea on attempts to extubate. The patient was intubated during the CT scan, allowing images to be obtained in inspiration and expiration. **A:** Computed tomography scan during end inspiration, and **(B)** during end expiration, demonstrates a dilated esophagus (*E*) and marked collapse of the intrathoracic trachea (*T*), consistent with tracheomalacia, which was confirmed at fiberoptic bronchoscopy.

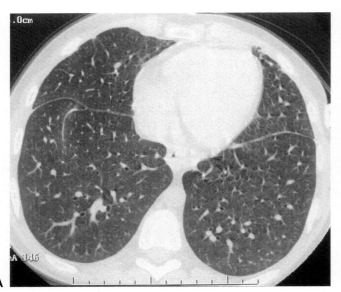
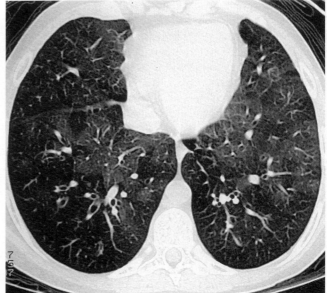

A   B

FIG. 9–26. Bronchiolitis obliterans in a 14-year-old girl after bilateral lung transplantation. **A:** Axial section at inspiration shows several areas of mild bronchial dilatation in the lower lobes. **B:** Scan during expiration shows mosaic attenuation. The lower-attenuation areas indicate air trapping and small airway obstruction. Mild bronchial dilatation is again noted.

ever, CT can be useful to better define and characterize an abnormality suspected on conventional chest radiography, especially when CT is performed with high-resolution technique using narrow (1 mm) collimation and a high spatial-frequency reconstruction algorithm. Indications for high-resolution CT of the lung parenchyma in children include: i) detection of disease in children who are at increased risk for lung disease (e.g., immunocompromised patients) and who have respiratory symptoms but a normal chest radiograph; ii) determination of the extent, distribution, and character of diffuse lung diseases; iii) localization of abnormal lung for biopsy; and iv) assessment of the response to treatment. Axial images suffice for diagnosis.

Recent reports have suggested that thin (1 mm) sections can be coupled with advanced image-processing techniques so that quantitative CT measurements of lung attenuation can be performed. Quantitative CT has been used to assess the regional distribution of emphysema, small-airway diseases, and pulmonary fibrosis (69,70).

Multiplanar and 3D Evaluation of the Chest Wall

Multiplanar and 3D surface-rendering techniques are ideal for displaying the complex osseous structures of the thorax. The ability to display chest-wall masses or thoracic-wall deformities in multiple projections can improve the understanding of anatomy and assist in planning complicated reconstructive surgery. In particular, CT can help to evaluate congenital and post-surgical changes (Figure 9-27) (see

color plate), assess the relationship of peripheral masses to the chest wall, and aid in surgical planning of pectus excavatum deformities.

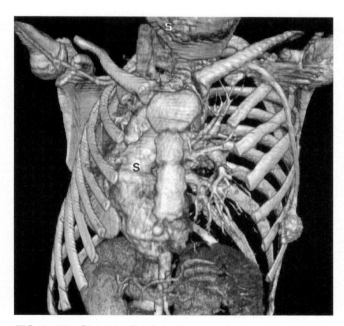

FIG. 9–27. Chest-wall deformity secondary to prior pneumonectomy. A preoperative CT scan was done to assess the volume of the right hemithorax prior to insertion of a chest prosthesis. Coronal volume-rendered image shows a small right hemithorax and dextroscoliosis of the thoracic spine (S). (See Color Fig. 9–27)

REFERENCES

1. Frush DP, Siegel MJ, Bisset GS. From the RSNA refresher courses: challenges of pediatric spiral CT. *Radiographics* 1997;17:939–959.
2. Siegel MJ. Techniques. In: Siegel MJ, ed. *Pediatric body CT*. Philadelphia: Lippincott Williams & Wilkins, 1999;1–41.
3. Siegel MJ, Luker GD. Pediatric applications of helical (spiral) CT. *Radiol Clin North Am* 1995;33:997–1022.
4. Donnelly LF, Frush DP, Nelson RC. Multislice helical CT to facilitate combined CT of the neck, chest, abdomen and pelvis in children. *AJR Am J Roentgenol* 2000;174:1620–1622.
5. Bhalla S, Siegel MJ. Multislice computed tomography in pediatrics. In: Silverman PM, ed. *Multislice computed tomography: a practical approach to clinical protocols.* Philedelphia: Lippincott Williams & Wilkins, 2002;231–282.
6. Siegel MJ. Multiplanar and 3D imaging with multidetector-row CT of the thoracic vessels and airways of the thoracic vessels and airways in a pediatric population. Accepted to *Radiology.*
7. Kaste SC, Young CW, Holmes TP, et al. *Effect of helical CT on the frequency of sedation in pediatric patients. AJR Am J Roentgenol* 1997;168:1001–1003.
8. Pappas JN, Donnelly LF, Frush DP. Reduced frequency of sedation of young children using new multi-slice helical CT. *Radiology* 2000;215:897–899.
9. Committee on Drugs. American Academy of Pediatrics: guidelines for monitoring and management of pediatric patients during and after sedation for diagnostic and therapeutic procedures. *Pediatrics* 1992;89:1110–1115.
10. American Society of Anesthesiologists Task Force. Practice guidelines for sedation and analgesia by non-anesthesiologist: a report by the American Society of Anesthesiologists Task Force on sedation and analgesia by non-anesthesiologists. *Anesthesiology* 1996;84:459–471.
11. Cohan RH, Ellis JH, Garner WL. Extravasation of radiographic contrast material: recognition, prevention and treatment. *Radiology* 1996;200:593–604.
12. Stockberger SM, Hickling JA, Liang Y, et al. Spiral CT with ionic and nonionic contrast material: evaluation of patient motion and scan quality. *Radiology* 1998;206:631–636.
13. Kaste SC, Young CW. Safe use of power injectors with central and peripheral venous access devices for pediatric CT. *Pediatr Radiol* 1995;26:499–501.
14. Cody DD. Image processing in CT. *Radiographics* 2002;2:1255–1268.
15. Lawler LP, Fishman EK. Multi-detector row CT of thoracic disease with emphasis on 3D volume rendering and CT angiography. *Radiographics* 2001;21:1257–1273.
16. Ravenel JG, McAdams HP, Remy-Jardin M, et al. Multidimensional imaging of the thorax. Practical applications. *J Thorac Imaging* 2001;16:279–281.
17. Ruben GD. Data explosion: the challenge of multidetector CT. *Eur J Radiol* 2000;36:74–81.
18. Donnelly LF, Emery KH, Brody AS, et al. Minimizing radiation dose for pediatric body applications for single-detector helical CT: strategies at a large children's hospital. *AJR Am J Roentgenol* 2001;176:303–306.
19. Frush DP, Slack CC, Hollingsworth CL, et al. Computer-simulated radiation dose reduction for abdominal multidetector CT of pediatric patients. *AJR Am J Roentgenol* 2002;179:1107–1113.
20. Haaga JR. Commentary. Radiation dose management weighing risk versus benefit. *AJR Am J Roentgenol* 2001;177:289–291.
21. Lucaya J, Piqeunas J, Garcia-Pena P, et al. Low-dose high resolution CT of the chest in children and young adults: dose, cooperation artifact, incidence and image quality. *AJR Am J Roentgenol* 2000;175:985–992.
22. Patterson A, Frush DP, Donnelly L. Helical CT of the body: setting adjusted for pediatric patients. *AJR Am J Roentgenol* 2001;176:297–301.
23. Rogalla P, Stover B, Scheer I, et al. Low-dose spiral CT: applicability to paediatric chest imaging. *Pediatr Radiol* 1999;29:565–569.

24. Slovis TL. The ALARA concept in pediatric CT: myth or reality. *Radiology* 2002;223:5–6.
25. Siegel MJ, Suess C, Schmidt B, Bradley D, Hildebolt C. Pediatric phantom sizes and shape variation: effect of multislice CT tube voltage on radiation dose and image. Submitted to *AJR*.
26. Remy-Jardin, Remy J, Giraud F, et al. Pulmonary nodules: detection with thick-section spiral CT versus conventional CT. *Radiology* 1993;187:513–520.
27. Remy J, Remy-Jardin M, Giraud F, et al. Angiotecture of pulmonary arteriovenous malformation: clinical utility of three-dimensional helical CT. *Radiology* 1994;191:657–664.
28. Bower RJ, Kiesewetter WB. Mediastinal masses in infants and children. *Arch Surg* 1996;112:1003–1009.
29. Merten DF. Diagnostic imaging of mediastinal masses in children. *AJR Am J Roentgenol* 1992;158:825–832
30. Meza MP, Benson M, Slovis TL. Imaging of mediastinal masses in children. *Radiol Clin North Am* 1993;31:583–604.
31. Hudson MM, Donaldson SS. Hodgkin's disease. In: Pizzo PA, Poplack DG, eds. *Principles and practice of pediatric oncology*, 3rd ed. Philadelphia: Lippincott Raven 1997;523–543.
32. Hammrick-Turner JE, Saif MF, Powers CI, et al. Imaging of childhood non-Hodgkin lymphoma: assessment by histologic subtype. *Radiographics* 1994;14:11–28.
33. Luker GD, Siegel MJ. Mediastinal Hodgkin disease in children: response to therapy. *Radiology* 1993;189:737–740.
34. Siegel MJ. Diseases of the thymus in children and adolescents. *Postgrad Radiol* 1993;13:106–132.
35. Quillin SP, Siegel MJ. CT features of benign and malignant teratomas in children. *J Comput Assist Tomogr* 1992;16:723–726.
36. Rosado-de-Christenson ML, Templeton PA, Moran CA. Mediastinal germ cell tumors: radiologic and pathologic correlation. *Radiographics* 1992;12:1013–1030.
37. Tecce PM, Fishman EK, Kuhlman JE. CT evaluation of the anterior mediastinum: spectrum of disease. *Radiographics* 1994;14:973–990.
38. Leonidas JC, Berdon WE, Valderrama E, et al. Human immunodeficiency virus infection and multilocular thymic cysts. *Radiology* 1996;198:377–379.
39. Mercado-Deane MG, Sabio H, Burton EM, et al. Cystic thymic hyperplasia in a child with HIV infection: imaging findings. *AJR Am J Roentgenol* 1996;166:171–172.
40. Haddon MJ, Bowen A. Bronchopulmonary and neurenteric forms of foregut anomalies. Imaging for diagnosis and management. *Radiol Clin North Am* 1991;29:241–254.
41. Reynolds M. Foregut cysts of the mediastinum in infants and children. In: Shields TW, ed. *Mediastinal surgery*. Philadelphia: Lea & Febiger, 1991;299–304.
42. Kim WS, Lee KS, Kim IO, et al. Congenital cystic adenomatoid malformation of the lung: CT-pathologic correlation. *AJR Am J Roentgenol* 1997;168:47–.
43. Frazier AA, Rosado de Christenson ML, Stocker JT, et al. Intralobar sequestration: radiologic–pathologic correlation. *Radiographics* 1997;17:725–745.
44. Gupta H, Mayo-Smith WW, Mainiero MB, et al. Helical CT of pulmonary vascular abnormalities. *AJR Am J Roentgenol* 2002;178:487–492.
45. Ko SF, Ng SH, Lee TY, et al. Noninvasive imaging of bronchopulmonary sequestration. *AJR Am J Roentgenol* 2000;175:1005–1012.
46. Woodring JH, Howard TA, Kanga JF. Congenital pulmonary venolobar syndrome revisited. *Radiographics* 1994;14:349–369.
47. Hoffman LV, Kuszyk BS, Mitchell SE, et al. Angioarchitecture of pulmonary AVM malformation characterization using volume-rendered 3D CT angiography. *Cardiovasc Intervent Radiol* 2000;23:165.
48. Lawler LP, Fishman EK. Arteriovenous malformations and systemic lung supply: evaluation by multidetector CT and three-dimensional volume rendering. *AJR Am J Roentgenol* 2002;178:493–494.
49. Katz M, Konen E, Rozenman, et al. Spiral CT and 3D image reconstruction of vascular rings and associated tracheobronchial anomalies. *J Comput Assist Tomogr* 1995;19:564–568.
50. Hopkins KL, Patrick LE, Simoneaux SF, et al. Pediatric great vessel anomalies: initial clinical experience with spiral CT angiography. *Radiology* 1996;200:811–815.
51. Donnelly LF, Fleck RJ, Pacharn P, et al. Aberrant subclavian arteries: cross-sectional imaging findings in infants and children referred for evaluation of extrinsic airway compression. *AJR Am J Roentgenol* 2002;178:1269–1274.
52. Yamada I, Nakagawa T, Himeno Y, et al. Takayasu arteritis: evaluation of the thoracic aorta with CT angiography. *Radiology* 1998;209:103–109.
53. Zylak CJ, Eyler WR, Spizarny DL, et al. Developmental lung anomalies in the adult: raidologic–pathologic correlation. *Radiographics* 2002;22:S25–S43.
54. Zwetsch B, Wicky S, Meuli R, et al. Three-dimensional image reconstruction of partial anomalous pulmonary venous return to the superior vena cava. *Chest* 1995;108:1743–1745.
55. Hoppe H, Walder B, Sonnenschein M, et al. Multidetector CT virtual bronchoscopy to grade tracheobronchial stenosis. *AJR Am J Roentgenol* 2002;178:1195–2000.
56. Remy-Jardin M, Remy J, Artaud D, et al. Tracheobronchial tree: assessment with volume rendering—technical aspects. *Radiology* 1998;208:393–398.
57. Remy-Jardin M, Remy J, Artaud D, et al. Volume rendering of the tracheobronchial tree: clinical evaluation of bronchographic images. *Radiology* 1998;208:761–770.
58. Sorantin E, Geiger B, Lindbichler F, et al. CT based virtual tracheobronchoscopy in children—comparison with axial CT and multiplanar reconstructions: preliminary results. *Pediatr Radiol* 2002;32:8–15.
59. McGuiness G, Naidich D, Garay S, et al. Accessory cardiac bronchus: CT features and clinical significance. *Radiology* 1993;189:563–566.
60. Al-Nakshabandi N, Lingawi S, Muller NL. Congenital bronchial atresia. *Can Assoc Radiol J* 2000;51:47–48.
61. Quint LE, Whyte RI, Kazerooni EA, et al. Stenosis of the central airways: evaluation by using helical CT with multiplanar reconstructions. *Radiology* 1995;194:871–877.
62. Gilkeson.RC, Ciancibello LM, Hejal RB, et al. Tracheobronchomalacia dynamic airway evaluation with multidetector CT. *AJR Am J Roentgenol* 2001;176:205–210.
63. Aquina SL, Gamsu G, Webb R, et al. Tree-in-bud pattern: frequency and significance on thin section CT. *J Comput Assist Tomogr* 1996;20:594–599.
64. Collins J, Blankenbaker, Stern EJ. CT patterns of bronchiolar disease: What is "tree-in-bud"? *AJR Am J Roentgenol* 1998;171:365–370.
65. Lau DM, Siegel MJ, Hildebolt CF, et al. Bronchiolitis obliterans syndrome: thin-section CT diagnosis of obstructive changes in infants and young children after lung transplantation. *Radiology* 1998;208:783–788.
66. Muller NL, Miller RR. Diseases of the bronchioles: CT and histopathologic findings. *Radiology* 1995;196:3–12.
67. Siegel MJ, Bhalla S, Gutierrez FR, et al. Post-lung transplantation bronchiolitis obliterans syndrome: usefulness of expiratory thin-section CT for diagnosis. *Radiology* 2001;220:455–462.
68. Stern EJ, Frank MS. Small airway disease of the lungs: findings at expiratory CT. *AJR Am J Roentgenol* 1994;163:37–41.
69. Bankier AA. Pulmonary emphysema: subjective visual grading vs. objective quantification with macroscopic morphometry and thin-section CT densitometry. *Radiology* 1999;211:851–858.
70. Genevois PA. Pulmonary emphysema: quantitative CT during expiration. *Radiology* 1996;199:825-829.

SECTION III

Gastrointestinal Applications

parenchymal phase (conventionally referred to as the portal venous phase, but more precisely the hepatic venous phase) occurs when there is visualization of contrast within the hepatic veins. This parenchymal venous phase is often the optimal time-to-image typical hypovascular metastasis, such as from gastrointestinal tract malignancies (Figure 10-1). Conversely, hypervascular lesions may go undetected if only a single parenchymal (hepatic venous phase) image is acquired. This occurs when "washout" of contrast from the highly vascular lesion coincides with increasing attenuation of the background normal liver. Thus, these lesions may become isoattenuating with the background hepatic parenchyma and go undetected.

Following the parenchymal phase of opacification, contrast diffuses into hypovascular tumors, and many lesions will demonstrate delayed enhancement. This phase of contrast enhancement has been referred to as the "equilibrium phase," and has been defined using time/density curves to plot the point at which the slope of the aortic and hepatic enhancement parenchymal curves become parallel. The equilibrium phase typically is about 90 seconds to 120 seconds after intravenous contrast injection. Hepatic imaging should be avoided during this phase due to the fact that the increasing attenuation of hepatic hypovascular lesions through contrast diffusion and the declining attenuation of the background hepatic parenchyma may result in intersecting curves of enhancement and obscure isoattenuating lesions. Very delayed scans, obtained at 7 minutes to 10 minutes after injection, may be useful for lesions that characteristically retain contrast (such as cholangiocarcinomas) when the rest of the liver has "washed out." However, few authorities advocate the routine use of these scans, although they are helpful in selected problematic cases.

Given the rapid acquisition of hepatic parenchymal scanning with MDCT (which, with currently available 16-slice scanners, may be accomplished in less than 10 seconds), it is possible to obtain hepatic scans at multiple phases of liver enhancement. However, due to radiation-dose limitations, a minimum number of scan acquisitions should be performed, tailored to the patient's known primary tumor and whether or not it is likely to be hyper- or hypovascular. Choices of phase of scan acquisition include unenhanced scans, early hepatic arterial phase (15 seconds to 25 seconds), late hepatic arterial phase or portal venous inflow phase (30 seconds to 55 seconds), hepatic parenchymal or hepatic venous phase (60 seconds to 80 seconds), and markedly delayed scans (7 minutes to 10 minutes following intravenous injection). Of course, the above times for each of these phases are relative and, in any given patient, may not be accurate, but serve as a rough guideline. The development of automated scan triggering based on hepatic temporal enhancement has reduced greatly the guesswork in obtaining hepatic-parenchymal venous-phase images (13–15). In general, scans are initiated after an attenuation value increases 40 HU over baseline unenhanced liver parenchyma. A similar strategy can be used to trigger automatically the onset of hepatic arterial-phase scanning if a CT angiogram is desired. Alternatively, a mini test bolus of 10 mL to 15 mL of contrast may be injected and serial scans obtained during the upper abdominal aorta to assess circulation time and choose the appropriate delay for scan acquisition of the arterial phase.

MDCT OF MALIGNANT HEPATIC LESIONS

Small Hypovascular Tumors

Traditionally, with dynamic incremental CT, only parenchymal phase (i.e., hepatic venous phase) images were performed to diagnose suspected hypovascular hepatic tumors. With the onset of single-slice spiral CT, scanning could be performed with a single breath hold and slice collimation was reduced from 10 mm (with dynamic incremental bolus CT) to 7 mm to 8 mm. Further modifications of spiral CT enabled back-to-back breath-held acquisition during arterial and venous phases. A few limited reports of single-slice spiral CT analyzing arterial phase images were disappointing and failed to demonstrate improved sensitivity for hypodense lesions (16). As we go forward in the era of 16-slice MDCT scanners with nearly volumetric scan acquisition, this issue may be worth revisiting, as arterial-phase images potentially may aid in characterization of subtle enhancement patterns of small hypodense lesions.

Small (less than 1.5 cm or 1 cm) hepatic lesions are quite common in day-to-day clinical practice, both in cancer patients and in the general population. Schwartz et al. noted small lesions less than 1 cm in 12.7% of 2.78 cancer patients (17). The authors retrospectively reviewed primarily venous-phase images obtained using dynamic incremental CT, and 82.8% of patients received intravenous contrast. Although the majority of these lesions showed no change on follow-up scans and therefore were felt to be benign, 11.6% of these lesions ultimately proved to be malignant.

Volk et al. have shown that benign hepatic tumors and tumor-like disorders (cysts, hemangiomas, adenomas, focal nodular hyperplasia, and biliary hematomas) may occur in up to a third of the general population without a known malignancy (18). In patients without a known primary malignancy, Jones et al. reported that these lesions are usually benign (19). The diagnosis is most difficult, therefore, in the cancer patient in whom a small hypodense lesion is encountered. The identification of hepatic metastases at an early stage potentially might be of considerable clinical value to initiate prompt surgery, ablative therapy, or chemotherapy.

Nino-Murcia et al. analyzed arterial phase enhancement patterns of hepatic tumors and emphasized the diagnostic value in identifying a peripheral continuous hypervascular rim (20). A thin peripheral area of rim enhancement proved relatively specific for either a metastasis or abscess (Figures 10–2 and 10–3). In addition, rim enhancement reliably excludes cysts or hemangiomas, which are the most common benign hypodense lesions in clinical practice. This finding greatly improved specificity in characterizing small hypo-

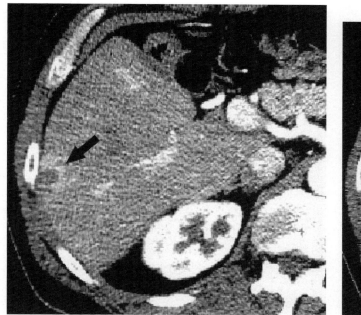
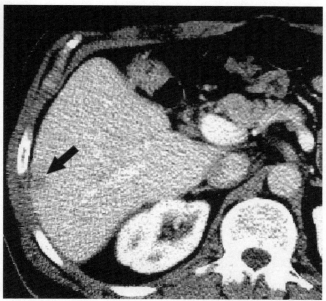

FIG. 10–2. A,B: Colon cancer metastasis. In **(A)**, note rim enhancement on arterial-phase image (*arrow*). On venous phase image, **(B)**, the lesion is inconspicuous and barely visible (*arrow*).

dense lesions. Although experience has shown that small abscesses also may demonstrate continuous peripheral rim enhancement, the clinical context often is quite different from patients with metastatic disease (Figure 10-4).

Multidetector CT potentially may aid in diagnosing small hypoattenuating lesions in several ways. The routine use of thinner collimation improves spatial resolution and facilitates lesion detection. Retrospective reconstruction is possible using thinner collimation and is an important advantage of MDCT to reduce partial volume effects. Most importantly, rapid scanning with a biphasic technique permits clear depiction of peripheral rim enhancement of epithelial metas-

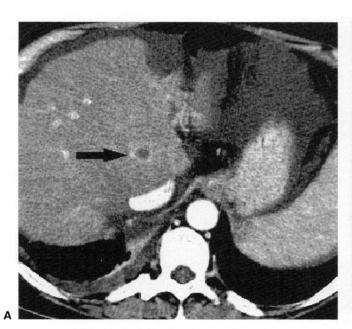
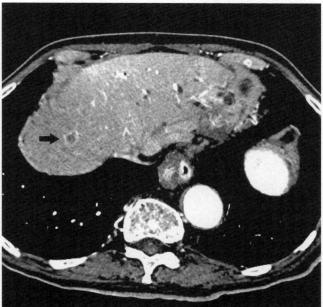

FIG. 10–3. A,B: Continuous rim enhancement of liver metastases in two different patients. **A:** A patient with lung cancer and rim enhancement from liver metastasis (*arrow*); **(B)** a patient with metastatic pancreatic cancer with rim enhancement.

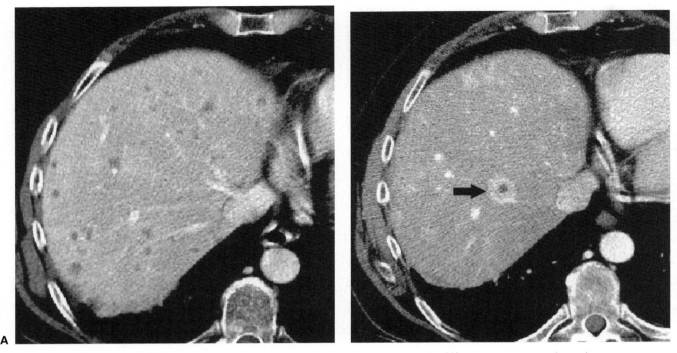

FIG. 10–4. A,B: Fungal microabscesses with rim enhancement. In (A), note numerous hypodense abscesses from candidiasis. Following treatment, in (B), note rim enhancement around lesion (*arrow*).

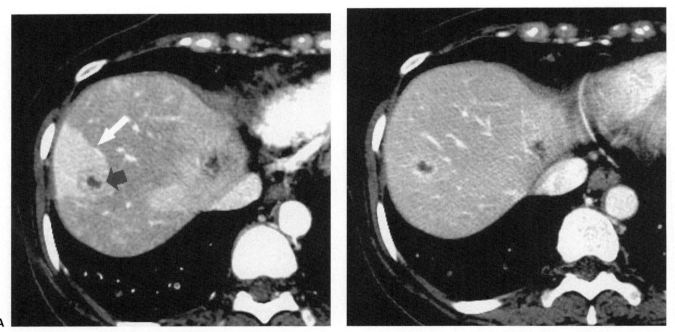

FIG. 10–5. A,B: Regional arterioportal shunting from liver metastases in two patients. A: An arterial phase image of the liver. Note wedge-shaped area of increased flow (*white arrow*) adjacent to hypodense liver metastasis from pancreatic cancer (*black arrow*). On venous-phase image (B), the arterioportal shunting is no longer evident. *(continued)*

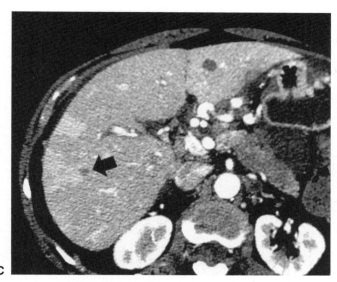

C

FIG. 10–5. C: *Continued.* In another patient **(C)**, note on arterial phase image the wedge-shaped area of increased attenuation distal to a small colon metastasis (*arrow*) due to arterioportal shunting.

to analyze more accurately the regional histogram around a small hypodense lesion that may facilitate detection of a subtle telltale ring of enhancement.

A second enhancement pattern associated with malignant hepatic lesions and seen almost exclusively on arterial-phase images is arterioportal shunting (21). Compression of portal or hepatic veins by focal lesions results in regional increased arterial flow to the affected segment (Figure 10-5). Hepatic artery to portal venous collaterals may develop through microscopic peribiliary channels. Arterial phase images aid in the detection of this transient flow phenomenon, which may disappear during the hepatic venous phase. Arterioportal shunting is not specific for malignancy and may be indicative of benign lesions, such as abscesses and small hemangiomas (21,22) (Figure 10-6). It is not uncommon, however, to visualize small arterioportal shunts in cirrhosis without an underlying mass. This finding is, therefore, most useful to diagnose metastatic disease in patients without cirrhosis. Hemangiomas may have associated arterioportal shunting, but usually can be diagnosed by their nodular discontinuous enhancement, and their propensity to track the degree of enhancement of the blood pool (22).

tases on arterial phase images. It seems likely that there will be renewed interest in analyzing arterial phase images with MDCT to improve early detection of hypovascular lesions such as colon cancer. While this approach may not necessarily improve sensitivity, it may increase specificity. In the near future, this may involve the use of software programs

Small Hypervascular Malignant Tumors

Much of the clinical research in this area has focused on the optimal scanning parameters to detect small HCCs (23–28). In addition, the diagnosis of small hypervascular metastases from carcinoids or neuroendocrine tumors occa-

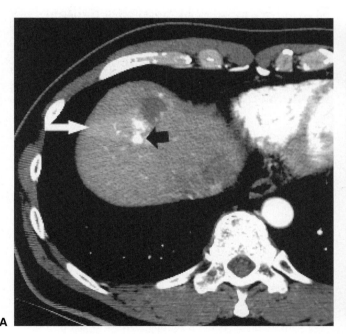

A

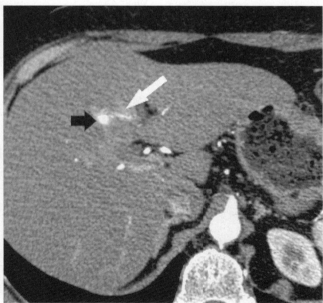

B

FIG. 10–6. A,B: Small hemangioma causing arterioportal shunting in two different patients. In **(A)**, note nodular areas of enhancement from the hemangioma on arterial phase image (*black arrow*). There is also adjacent wedge-shaped arterioportal shunting (*white arrow*). In another patient, **(B)**, a small "flash fill" hemangioma is seen on arterial phase image (*black arrow*) with adjacent arterioportal shunting (*white arrow*).

sionally may have important therapeutic significance in a clinical context where chemoembolization might be considered. More often, however, systemic chemotherapy rather than regional therapy or surgery is the main treatment option.

Given the widespread dissemination of hepatitis B, HCC is a major world-health issue. Mortality data show a direct association between lesion size and length of survival (29). Therefore, patients with cirrhosis are screened routinely for the development of HCC in order to detect lesions at an early, more curable stage. Patients with end-stage liver disease and small HCCs (solitary tumor less than 5 cm, 3 or fewer tumors less than 3 cm, and no vascular invasion) may undergo successfully liver transplantation with a 75% five-year survival rate (30). Due to cost considerations, ultrasound often is the screening and surveillance technique of choice to detect early HCCs, as it is impractical and too

expensive to perform either CT or MR in all patients with cirrhosis. However, once HCC is suspected, either on the basis of an abnormal ultrasound or elevated alpha-fetoprotein, imaging with CT or MR is mandatory to determine the size of the lesion or lesions and assess for vascular invasion (Figure 10-7).

With MDCT and a rapid intravenous bolus (4 mL/sec to 5 mL/sec), it is possible to obtain early and late arterial-phase images, at approximately 20 seconds and 40 seconds, respectively. While many authorities have noted the value of late arterial-phase images, the diagnostic utility of early arterial-phase images recently has been debated. The literature to date is unclear, with some authorities such as Kim et al. (25) demonstrating a clear benefit to the early arterial phase, and other authors such as Ichikawa et al. (26) showing no significant improvement in effectiveness with the double

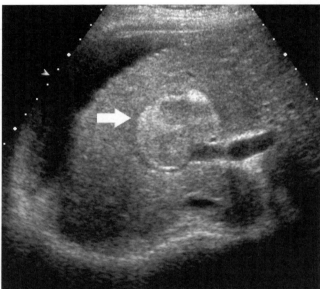

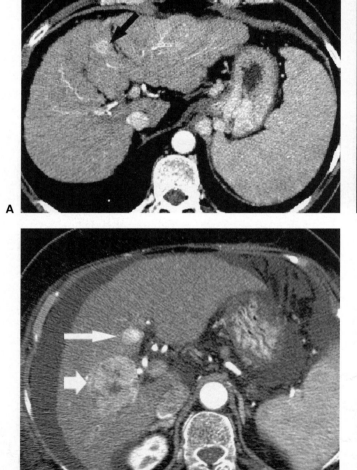

FIG. 10-7. A–C: Small hepatocellular carcinoma (HCC) seen only on late arterial phase images in two different patients. In **(A)**, note small hypervascular mass (*arrow*) in segment intravenous (IV) in a patient with cirrhosis. In another patient **(B)**, a screening-transverse sonogram demonstrates an echogenic 4-cm mass consistent with HCC (*arrow*). Arterial phase MDCT **(C)** demonstrates this hypervascular mass (*short arrow*) and an adjacent satellite nodule (*long arrow*) not seen on ultrasound.

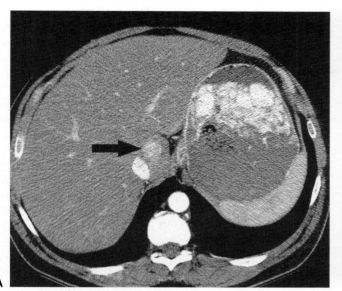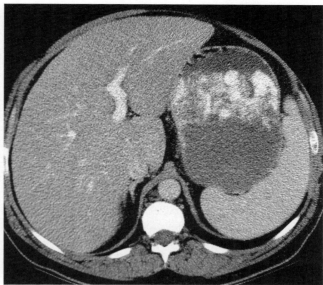

FIG. 10–8. A,B: Small HCC seen only on late arterial phase images. In **(A)**, which is late arterial phase, note small hyperdense mass (*arrow*). Venous phase **(B)** reveals no lesion.

arterial phase approach. These authors recommend only late arterial phase scans for detecting HCCs (Figures 10–7 and 10–8). However, a potential problem with late arterial-phase images is that the timing may not always be precise. Scans may be acquired during hepatic venous opacification, and small lesions may be obscured. Even using bolus-tracking methods, late arterial phase images in some patients may demonstrate a significant component of hepatic venous en-

hancement. Thus, late arterial phase images are not always reliable for detection of a small HCC.

Hepatic artery catheter MDCT, although an invasive study, has a limited but important role to play in the patient with known or suspected HCCs (31) (Figure 10-9). Lipiodol injection in the hepatic artery will show accumulation in small HCCs. This may be very important diagnostically, as many small lesions are not amenable to biopsy. In addition,

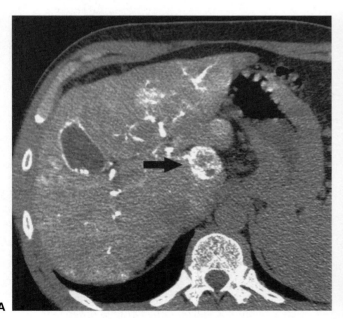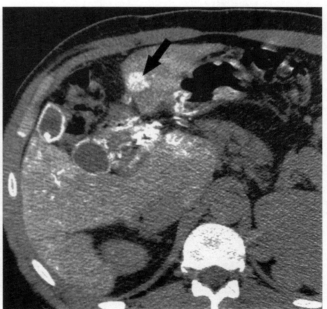

FIG. 10–9. A,B: Hepatic artery catheter CT in a patient with HCC. In **(A)** and **(B)**, additional HCC lesions were detected (*arrow*), not seen on intravenous MDCT biphasic study.

intraarterial enhancement may reveal small lesions not evident on intravenous-enhanced CT. The demonstration of additional hypervascular lesions not seen on intravenous studies may impact directly the decision to perform surgery, chemoinfusion, or chemoembolization (31).

MDCT of Small Benign Lesions

Scanning the liver with the high spatial and temporal resolution afforded by MDCT will inevitably increase detection of many more small (1.5 cm) hepatic lesions, both benign and malignant. Because of the relatively high prevalence of benign lesions (cysts, hemangiomas, FNH, etc.) in the general population, the real challenge for MDCT will be to differentiate between benign and malignant small hepatic lesions. As has been noted previously, in patients without risk factors for hepatic malignancy (i.e., known primary tumor or cirrhosis), the vast majority of incidentally discovered small lesions, whatever their enhancement pattern, can be followed expectantly without biopsy or intervention. In cancer patients and in patients with risk factors for HCC, however, an attempt must be made to arrive at a specific diagnosis. The single most important feature to consider when characterizing small lesions with MDCT is their pattern of enhancement following intravenous contrast.

Simple hepatic cysts have attenuation similar to water (less than 15 HU) and show no peripheral or internal enhancement on any phase of hepatic imaging. In addition, no "flow disturbance" generally is seen with these lesions, and there is no arterioportal shunting (Figure 10-10). Delayed images often are quite useful to demonstrate lack of "filling in" of the cyst. Retrospective reconstruction of MDCT images may improve the accuracy of attenuation values. Necrotic metastases rarely may mimic cysts, but there is usually

some degree of peripheral or internal enhancement, as well as regional flow disturbance with these lesions. Problematic lesions can be evaluated with tissue-harmonic sonography to demonstrate a thin echogenic wall and typical distal acoustic enhancement.

Differentiating small hemangiomas (less than 1.5 cm) from hypervascular tumors, such as HCCs, poses another challenge for MDCT. Hemangiomas occur in approximately 7.3% of the general population (32). Larger hemangiomas, often referred to as cavernous hemangiomas, rarely present diagnostic difficulty due to their characteristic enhancement pattern of nodular discontinuous puddling of contrast. This finding is less common, however, in small hemangiomas and was noted on only 62% to 68% of cases by Kim et al. (33) (Figure 10-11). Small hemangiomas may demonstrate diffuse homogeneous or heterogeneous enhancement, similar to small HCCs, in 17% to 30% of lesions. However, hemangiomas that "flash fill" tend to track the enhancement of the blood pool (Figure 10-6). Attenuation of these small hemangiomas is similar to the aorta on arterial phase images, and similar to the hepatic veins on the parenchymal or venous phase. Atypical hemangiomas occur in a very small percentage of lesions, typically 4% to 8%. There may be little or no enhancement demonstrated on either arterial or venous phase images within these hemangiomas, making them impossible to diagnose with confidence. Unlike hemangiomas, small HCCs typically demonstrate an enhancement pattern that does not track the blood pool. On arterial-phase images, HCC lesions are less dense than the aorta, and on venous phase images, they tend to have greater washout of contrast than hemangiomas, and they are typically hypodense compared to the hepatic veins.

As previously noted, arterioportal shunting occurs when a focal hepatic lesion exhibits mass effect and obstructs

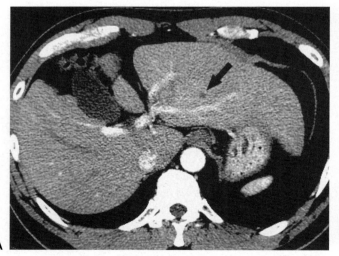
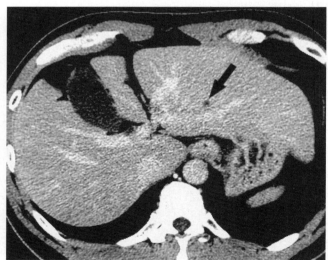

FIG. 10–10. A,B: Simple hepatic cyst. Biphasic MDCT with 2.5-mm collimation demonstrates 4-mm focal water-attenuation small lesion (*arrow*) on arterial **(A)** and venous phase **(B)**. Lack of enhancement or filling in establishes diagnosis of a simple cyst.

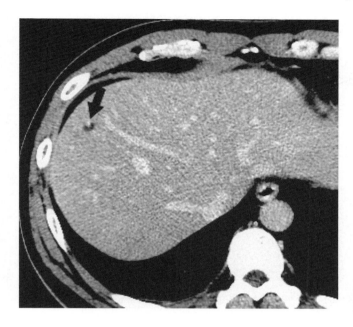

FIG. 10–11. Small hemangiomas with nodular peripheral enhancement on MDCT in two patients.

adjacent portal and hepatic veins (Figure 10-5). On arterial-phase images, a wedge-shaped or irregular area of increased attenuation is evident due to shunting of arterial blood to adjacent portal veins, probably through microscopic peribiliary collaterals. Because hemangiomas are "soft" lesions that represent histologically sinusoidal spaces filled with venous blood, they rarely demonstrate significant mass effect. Arterioportal shunting, however, has been reported with small hemangiomas (Figure 10-6). Kim et al. reported this finding in 28 of 109 hemangiomas (25.7%) on arterial phase images (22). Therefore, this finding cannot be used to exclude a small hemangioma.

Focal nodular hyperplasia (FNH) is a highly vascular lesion comprised of hepatocytes, bile ducts, blood vessels, Kupffer cells, and central fibrous tissue (34–37). Excluding cysts, it is second only to hemangiomas as the most common benign hepatic focal mass. Many pathologists consider FNH to be a vascular anomaly, rather than a hepatic "neoplasm." The hallmark of FNH on biphasic MDCT is its intense homogenous enhancement pattern on arterial phase images (34–37), and the rapid washout on venous phase images to become nearly isoattenuating with the normal liver (Figure 10-12). A central scar may or may not be present (30%–50% of cases show scar), and a central low-attenuation area is typical on arterial images (Figure 10-13) (37).

Patients with FNH typically have normal liver function, and the lesions typically are discovered incidentally. Given a lack of risk factors, the most important differential diagnostic possibility is fibrolamellar hepatocellular carcinoma (FHCC). Due to the fact the FHCC often is large and heterogeneous in enhancement and frequently contains calcifications, these two lesions often can be differentiated (38). In exceptional cases, scintigraphy or biopsy may be required for definitive diagnosis.

Hepatocellular adenomas are uncommon in clinical practice and most often are encountered in young women using oral contraceptives. Unfortunately, the imaging features with CT and MRI often are not specific enough to establish a specific diagnosis (39–41). Hepatocellular adenomas may regress significantly after patients discontinue oral contraceptive use. Large lesions often are resected due to their propensity to rupture and bleed and the small but finite risk of malignant degeneration (41). Multidetector CT may aid in the preoperative planning of these lesions by demonstrating aberrant hepatic vasculature (Figure 10-14).

On CT regenerative nodules often are isodense with hepatic parenchyma and only evident by their mass effect. Very rarely, they may appear as hypervascular nodules in Budd–Chiari syndrome or cirrhosis (42). In Budd–Chiari syndrome, hypoattenuating rings often are noted surrounding these regenerative nodules (Figure 10-15)(42).

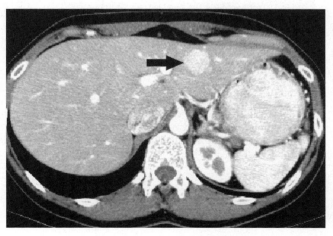

FIG. 10–12. Focal nodular hyperplasia. Note uniform hyperdense enhancement of left lobe lesion (*arrow*).

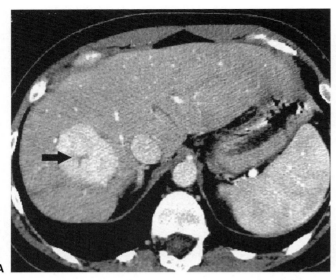

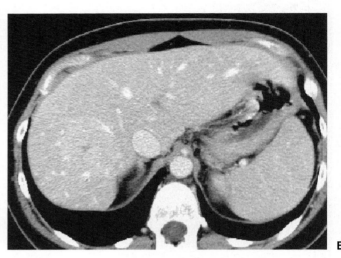

FIG. 10–13. A,B: Focal nodular hyperplasia on biphasic MDCT. In **(A)**, note hypervascular mass with low-attenuation central scar (*arrow*). On venous phase **(B)**, lesion is nearly isoattenuating with normal liver.

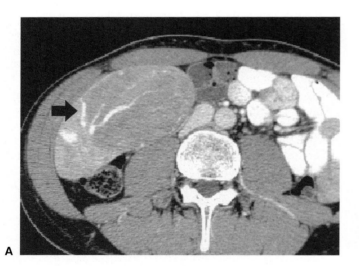

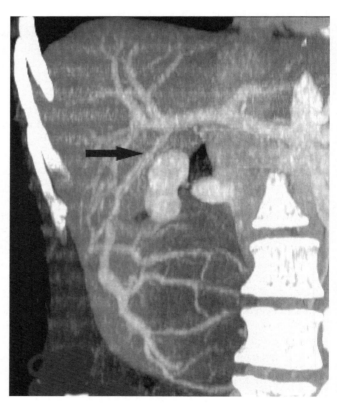

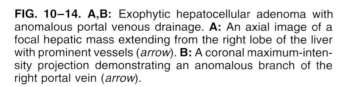

FIG. 10–14. A,B: Exophytic hepatocellular adenoma with anomalous portal venous drainage. **A:** An axial image of a focal hepatic mass extending from the right lobe of the liver with prominent vessels (*arrow*). **B:** A coronal maximum-intensity projection demonstrating an anomalous branch of the right portal vein (*arrow*).

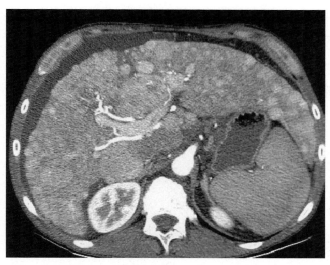

FIG. 10–15. Regenerative nodules in cirrhosis. Note innumerable hypervascular nodules, proven through biopsy to be benign regenerative nodules.

REFERENCES

1. Choi BI, Lee KH, Han JK, et al. Hepatic arterioportal shunts: dynamic CT and MR features. *Korean J Radiol* 2002;3(1):1–15.
2. Ji H, McTavish JD, Mortele KJ, et al. Hepatic imaging with multidetector CT. *Radiographics* 2001;21 Spec No:S71–S80.
3. Hu H, He HD, Foley WD, et al. Four multidetector–row helical CT: image quality and volume coverage speed. *Radiology* 2000; 215:55–62.
4. Costello P, Dupuy ED, Ecker CP, et al. Spiral CT of the thorax with reduced volume of contrast material: a comparative study. *Radiology* 1992;183:663–666.
5. Choi BI, Han JK, Cho JM, et al. Characterization of focal hepatic tumors. Value of two-phase scanning with spiral computed tomography. *Cancer* 1995;76(12):2434–2442.
6. Weg N, Scheer MR, Gabor MP. Liver lesions: improved detection with dual-detector-array CT and routine 2.5 mm thin collimation. *Radiology* 1998;209(2):417–426.
7. Wang G, Vannier MW. The effect of pitch in multislice spiral/helical CT. *Med Phys* 1999;26:2648–2653.
8. Kawata S, Murakami T, Kim T, et al. Multidetector CT: diagnostic impact of slice thickness on detection of hypervascular hepatocellular carcinoma. *AJR Am J Roentgenol* 2002;179(1):61–66.
9. Foley WD, Berland LL, Lawson TL, et al. Contrast enhancement technique for dynamic hepatic computed tomographic scanning. *Radiology* 1983;147:797–803.
10. Bader TR, Prokesch RW, Grabenwoger F. Timing of the hepatic arterial phase during contrast-enhanced computed tomography of the liver: assessment of normal values in 25 volunteers. *Invest Radiol* 2000;35(8): 486–492.
11. Frederick MG, McElaney BL, Singer A, et al. Timing of parenchymal enhancement on dual-phase dynamic helical CT of the liver: how long does the hepatic arterial phase predominate? *AJR Am J Roentgenol* 1996;166(6):1305–1310.
12. Foley WD, Mellisee TA, Hohenwalter MD, et al. Multiphase hepatic CT with a multirow detector CT scanner. *AJR Am J Roentgenol* 2000; 175(3):679–685.
13. Dinkel HP, Fieger M, Knupffer J, et al. Optimizing liver contrast in helical liver CT: value of a real-time bolus-triggering technique. *Eur Radiol* 1998;8(9):1608–1612.
14. Mehnert F, Pereira PL, Trubenbach J, et al. Biphasic spiral CT of the liver: automatic bolus tracking or time delay? *Eur Radiol* 2001;11(3): 427–431.
15. Kim T, Murakami T, Hori M, et al. Small hypervascular hepatocellular carcinoma revealed by double arterial phase CT performed with single breath-hold scanning and automatic bolus tracking. *AJR Am J Roentgenol* 2002;178(4):899–904.
16. Ch'en IY, Katz DS, Jeffrey RB Jr, et al. Do arterial phase helical CT images improve detection or characterization of colorectal liver metastases? *J Comput Assist Tomogr* 1997;21(3):391–397.
17. Schwartz LH, Gandras EJ, Colangelo SM, et al. Prevalence and importance of small hepatic lesions found at CT in patients with cancer. *Radiology* 1999;210(1):71–74.
18. Volk M, Strotzer M, Lenhart M, et al. Frequency of benign hepatic lesions incidentally detected with contrast-enhanced thin-section portal venous phase spiral CT. *Acta Radiol* 2001;42(2):172–175.
19. Jones EC, Chezmar JL, Nelson RC, et al. The frequency and significance of small (less than or equal to 15 mm) hepatic lesions detected by CT. *AJR Am J Roentgenol* 1992;158(3):535–539.
20. Nino-Murcia M, Olcott EW, Jeffrey RB Jr, et al. Focal liver lesions: pattern-based classification scheme for enhancement at arterial phase CT. *Radiology* 2000;215(3):746–751.
21. Quiroga S, Sebastia C, Pallisa E, et al. Improved diagnosis of hepatic perfusion disorders: value of hepatic arterial phase imaging during helical CT. *Radiographics* 2001;21(1):65–81, questionnaire 288–294.
22. Kim KW, Kim TK, Han JK, et al. Hepatic hemangiomas with arterioportal shunt: findings at two-phase CT. *Radiology* 2001; 219:707–711.
23. Hollett MD, Jeffrey RB Jr, Nino-Murcia M, et al. Dual-phase helical CT of the liver: value of arterial phase scans in the detection of small (< or = 1.5 cm) malignant hepatic neoplasms. *AJR Am J Roentgenol* 1995;164(4):879–884.
24. Murakami T, Kim T, Takamura M, et al. Hypervascular hepatocellular carcinoma: detection with double arterial phase multi-detector row helical CT. *Radiology* 2001;218(3):763–767.
25. Kim T, Murakami T, Hori M, et al. Small hypervascular hepatocellular carcinoma revealed by double arterial phase CT performed with single breath-hold scanning and automatic bolus tracking. *AJR Am J Roentgenol* 2002;178(4):899–904.
26. Ichikawa T, Kitamura T, Nakajima H, et al. Hypervascular hepatocellular carcinoma: can double arterial phase imaging with multidetector CT improve tumor depiction in the cirrhotic liver? *AJR Am J Roentgenol* 2002;179(3):751–758.
27. Paul SB, Gulati MS. Spectrum of hepatocellular carcinoma on triple phase helical CT: a pictorial essay. *Clin Imaging* 2002;26(4):270–279.
28. Sahani D, Saini S, Pena C, et al. Using multidetector CT for preoperative vascular evaluation of liver neoplasms: technique and results. *AJR Am J Roentgenol* 2002;179(1):53–59.
29. Wall WJ, Marotta PJ. Surgery and transplantation for hepatocellular cancer. *Liver Transpl* 2000;6(6 Suppl 2):S16–S22.
30. Cheng SJ, Pratt DS, Freeman RB Jr, et al. Living-donor versus cadaveric liver transplantation for non-resectable small hepatocellular carcinoma and compensated cirrhosis: a decision analysis. *Transplantation* 2001;72(5):861–868.
31. Sze DY, Razavi MK, So SK, et al. Impact of multidetector CT hepatic arteriography on the planning of chemoembolization treatment of hepatocellular carcinoma. *AJR Am J Roentgenol* 2001;177(6):1339–1345.
32. Hanafusa K, Ohashi I, Gomi N, et al. Differential diagnosis of early homogeneously enhancing hepatocellular carcinoma and hemangioma by two-phase CT. *J Comput Assist Tomogr* 1997;21(3):361–368.
33. Kim T, Federle MP, Baron RL, et al. Discrimination of small hepatic hemangiomas from hypervascular malignant tumors smaller than 3 cm with three-phase helical CT. *Radiology* 2001;219:699–706.
34. Brancatelli G, Federle MP, Grazioli L, et al. Focal nodular hyperplasia: CT findings with emphasis on multiphasic helical CT in 78 patients. *Radiology* 2001;219:61–68.
35. Mortele KJ, Praet M, Vlierberghe HV, et al. CT and MR imaging findings in focal nodular hyperplasia of the liver: radiologic–pathologic correlation. *AJR Am J Roentgenol* 2000;175:687–692.
36. Choi CS, Freeny PC. Triphasic helical CT of hepatic focal nodular hyperplasia: incidence of atypical findings. *AJR Am J Roentgenol* 1998; 170:391–395.
37. Carlson SK, Johnson CD, Bender CE, et al. CT of focal nodular hyperplasia of the liver. *AJR Am J Roentgenol* 2000;174:705–712.
38. Blachar A, Federle MP, Ferris JV, et al. Radiologists' performance in the diagnosis of liver tumors with central scars by using specific CT criteria. *Radiology* 2002;223:532–539.

39. Lim AK, Patel N, Gedroyc WM, et al. Hepatocellular adenoma: diagnostic difficulties and novel imaging techniques. *Br J Radiol* 2002; 75(896):695–699.
40. Coombs RJ, Woldenberg LS, Skeel RT, et al. Magnetic resonance imaging of hepatic adenoma. *Clin Imaging* 1990;14(1):44–47.
41. Chung KY, Mayo-Smith WW, Saini S, et al. Hepatocellular adenoma: MR imaging features with pathologic correlation. *AJR Am J Roentgenol* 1995;165(2):303–308.
42. Brancatelli G, Federle MP, Grazioli L, et al. Large regenerative nodules in Budd–Chiari syndrome and other vascular disorders of the liver: CT and MR imaging findings with clinicopathologic correlation. *AJR Am J Roentgenol* 2002;178(4):877–883.

CHAPTER 11

Multidetector CT of Parenchymal Liver Disease

Ihab R. Kamel, Elliot K. Fishman

INTRODUCTION

Computed tomography (CT) commonly is indicated for the evaluation of suspected liver pathology. The recent introduction of multidetector CT (MDCT) provides unique capabilities that especially are valuable in hepatic-volume acquisitions, combining short scan times, narrow collimation, and the ability to obtain multiphase data. These features result in improved lesion detection and characterization (1–3). Concomitant advances in computer-software programs have made three-dimensional (3D) applications practical for a range of hepatic-image analyses and displays. A variety of hepatic parenchymal diseases can be diagnosed accurately and characterized with MDCT. This chapter discusses the role of MDCT in the evaluation of parenchymal liver disease.

Imaging Technique

The main objective in scanning the liver using MDCT is to obtain accurately timed phases, each in a single breath hold. For routine scanning of the abdomen and pelvis, a detector configuration of 4 mm $\times$ 2.5 mm, table speed of 15 mm, and pitch of 6:1 allow for adequate coverage in a single breath hold of 20 seconds to 25 seconds. Image reconstruction of 5 mm, with optional 2.5-mm overlap, can be performed in such cases. Contrast enhancement typically is achieved using 120 mL to 150 mL (2 mL/kg) of nonionic contrast media injected intravenously with a power injector at a rate of 3 mL per second. Scan delay is 20 seconds to 25 seconds and 60 seconds to 65 seconds for arterial and portal venous phases, respectively. In patients undergoing dual-phase CT of the liver in addition to CT of the chest, abdomen, and pelvis, arterial-phase images of the liver should be obtained in the first breath hold at 25 seconds, followed by scans through the chest, abdomen, and pelvis in the second breath hold at 65 seconds.

For the evaluation of the hepatic vascular anatomy prior to hepatic resection, living-donor transplantation, or hepatic-

infusion pump insertion, a detector configuration of 4 mm $\times$ 1.25 mm with a pitch of 6:1 and 1-mm reconstructed slices will result in superior 3D image reconstruction and volume-rendering techniques. Positive oral contrast is not administered in such cases because it may degrade image reconstruction. In these cases, 750 mL of water is recommended as a negative contrast agent.

The indication for the study determines whether single-, dual-, or triple-phase scanning is performed. Noncontrast CT is unnecessary except for the detection of fat, such as in fatty infiltration or adenoma, calcification, such as in mucinous metastases, or hemorrhage. Dual-phase scanning generally is indicated in patients with cirrhosis and in the evaluation of hypervascular metastases. Recently, triple-phase scanning in the arterial phase, portal-vein-inflow phase, and portal-venous phase has been suggested (1,2,4–6). The first two phases typically are acquired in a single breath hold. The first phase is best for depicting small branches of the hepatic arteries without portal-venous enhancement. The second phase is best for depicting hypervascular metastases. The third acquisition is in the portal-venous phase and is best for hypovascular metastases. However, because of concerns about radiation dose, triple-phase scanning is not performed routinely.

Delayed CT images of the liver may be obtained 10 minutes to 15 minutes after the initiation of contrast injection and are useful for specific indications. Tumors with a large component of fibrosis demonstrate prolonged hyperdense enhancement of the stroma. This feature is characteristic of cholangiocarcinoma (7). Delayed images also can be obtained in cases of hepatic masses felt possibly to represent cavernous hemangioma, where progressive centripetal enhancement of the hemangioma is one of its characteristic features (8,9).

HEPATIC CIRRHOSIS

Cirrhosis is the end result of hepatic injury and may be due to chronic infection by hepatitis viruses, especially hepatitis C. It has been estimated that up to 50% of patients with hepatitis C eventually may develop cirrhosis (10). Other causes include alcoholic liver disease, primary biliary cirrhosis, primary sclerosing cholangitis, congestive heart failure (cardiac cirrhosis), and hemochromatosis.

Liver cirrhosis is a chronic and progressive disorder associated with architectural distortion, diffuse fibrosis, and regenerating nodules that result from liver-cell necrosis and degeneration. A spectrum of nodules, ranging from benign regenerating nodules to hepatocellular carcinoma (HCC) may be encountered (11). The incidence of HCC in the United States is rising due to the epidemic of chronic hepatitis-C infection. The relative risk of HCC in patients with cirrhosis due to hepatitis C is approximately 100 times the risk for patients with cirrhosis who are not infected, whereas patients with cirrhosis resulting from alcohol abuse or primary biliary cirrhosis have only a twofold to fivefold increased risk of HCC (12). Hepatitis C is responsible for 30% to 50% of current cases of HCC in the United States.

In early cirrhosis, the liver may appear normal in up to 25% of cases (13,14). With progression of the disease, nodularity of the liver surface and generalized heterogeneity of the hepatic parenchyma can be seen (Figure 11-1). Parenchymal nodules can be micro, macro, or mixed. Micronodular cirrhosis is characterized by regenerative nodules of relatively uniform small size (Figures 11–2 and 11–3). This pattern is seen in chronic alcoholic cirrhosis, hepatitis C, and biliary cirrhosis. In macronodular cirrhosis, the parenchymal nodules are larger, coarser, and more variable in size. The most common cause of macronodular cirrhosis is chronic hepatitis B. Nodular lesions commonly found in cirrhotic livers include regenerative nodules, which may progress to dysplastic nodules, and HCC. Detection of dysplastic nodules is difficult using MDCT because they may enhance in a fashion similar to surrounding liver parenchyma (15,16). Ferumoxide-enhanced magnetic resonance (MR), combined

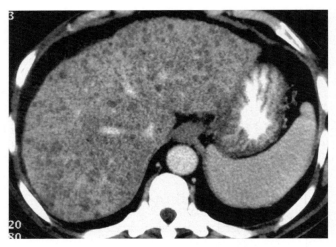

FIG. 11–2. Cirrhosis in a 53-year-old male. Notice the diffuse nodularity of the liver and mild splenomegaly.

with MDCT findings, may help in the differentiation of different nodules found in patients with cirrhosis (17,18). Hepatocellular carcinoma also has been shown to develop independent of regenerative or dysplastic nodules (19). With advanced cirrhosis, the volume of the right lobe and medial segment of the left lobe decreases, with increase in volume of the lateral segment of the left lobe (20,21).

Advanced cirrhosis is accompanied by alteration in hepatic blood flow. Periportal fibrosis and regenerative nodules cause extrinsic compression and tapering of the intrahepatic portal and venous branches. These changes result in altered hepatic perfusion, transsinusoidal arterioportal anastomoses, and portal hypertension (22–24). The portal vein

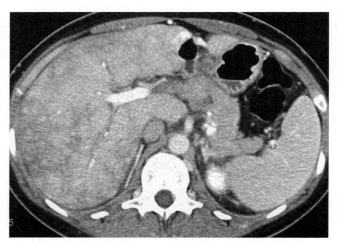

FIG. 11–1. Cirrhosis in a 30-year-old female. Computed tomography demonstrates nodular inhomogeneous parenchymal enhancement. This pattern of contrast enhancement is similar to that of patients with congestive heart failure.

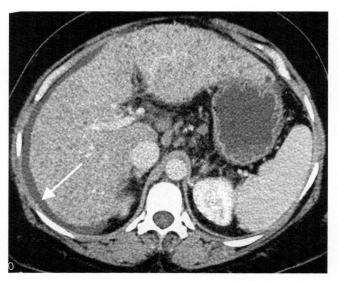

FIG. 11–3. Cirrhosis in a 48-year-old female. Innumerable small low-density contour-deforming nodules are seen scattered throughout the liver parenchyma. Biopsy showed mild active cirrhosis from chronic hepatitis C. Ascites also is identified (*arrow*).

(Figure 11-6), and it may be the major vascular supply to the hepatic parenchyma if portal-vein thrombosis is present. Patients with advanced cirrhosis and high arterial blood flow in the splenic artery are at increased risk of developing splenic-artery aneurysm, which is reported in up to 10% of patients (27). Following liver transplantation, decreased portal-vein pressure and increased splenic-artery flow may occur, resulting in increased risk of splenic-artery aneurysm rupture, especially if the aneurysm is larger than 1.5 cm (28,29).

The patterns of altered blood flow that result from cirrhosis are well depicted on MDCT because it allows for

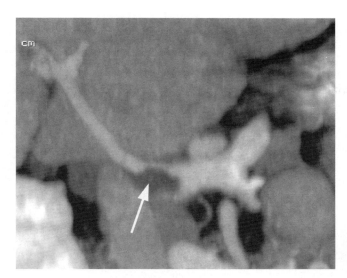

FIG. 11–4. Portal-vein thrombosis in a 56-year-old male. Maximum-intensity-projection image in the coronal plane reveals a clot in the superior mesenteric vein extending into the portal-vein confluence (*arrow*). Notice the small caliber of the portal vein due to decreased flow.

may become narrowed, and slow or retrograde flow may result in portal-vein thrombosis (Figure 11-4) and calcification (Figure 11-5). According to a recently reported study of 379 orthotopic liver transplants, portal-vein thrombosis or calcification was present in 39 patients (10.3%) (25). Preoperative knowledge of these findings is important because proper surgical planning (typically thrombectomy for nonocclusive thrombus, or bypass venous graft in occlusive thrombus) reduces the risk of rethrombosis. Compensatory hypertrophy of the hepatic artery often occurs in advanced cirrhosis (26). It becomes enlarged and beaded or tortuous

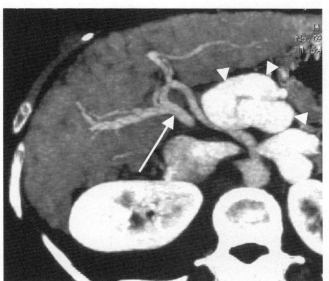

A

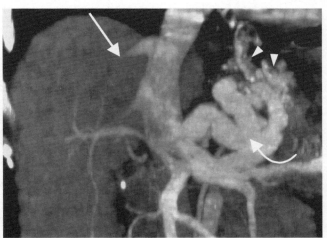

B

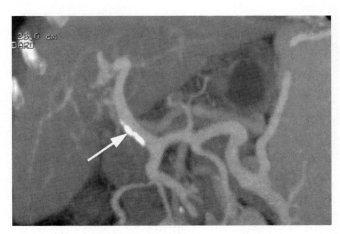

FIG. 11–5. Portal-vein calcification in a 47-year-old male. Maximum-intensity-projection image in the coronal plane shows linear calcification along the wall of the main portal vein (*arrow*).

FIG. 11–6. Cirrhosis in a 54-year-old female. **A:** Maximum-intensity-projection image of the arterial phase in the axial plane reveals marked nodularity of the liver parenchyma. Notice prominence of the hepatic artery (*arrow*) to compensate for portal hypertension. Large retroperitoneal collaterals (*arrowheads*) are present. **B:** Maximum-intensity-projection image of the PVP in the coronal plane reveals attenuation of the right hepatic vein (*arrow*), retroperitoneal collaterals (*curved arrow*), and gastroesophageal varices (*arrowheads*).

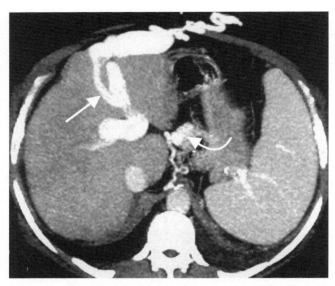

FIG. 11–7. Cirrhosis in a 57-year-old male. There is inhomogeneous parenchymal enhancement. Manifestations of portal hypertension include recanalization of the umbilical vein (*arrow*) towards the abdominal wall, as well as gastric varices (*curved arrow*). The spleen is mildly enlarged.

scanning during peak vascular enhancement. Hepatic enhancement is characteristically heterogeneous due to regenerating nodules, periportal fibrosis, and microcirculatory shunts that form between the portal-venous and hepatic-venous systems (30–32). Collateral vessels and varices secondary to portal hypertension appear as brightly enhancing structures on the portal-venous phase of MDCT. These commonly are seen in the distal esophagus, gastrohepatic ligament, and splenic hilum. Additionally, the paraumbilical

vein may be reanalyzed (Figure 11-7). Esophageal varices are the most clinically important collateral to demonstrate by MDCT. They are present in 65% of patients with advanced cirrhosis and are the cause of massive hematemesis and death in approximately half of these patients. Manifestations of portal hypertension may develop in patients with primary sclerosing cholangitis prior to overt CT signs of cirrhosis (33). Multiplanar reconstructions (MPR) with MDCT demonstrate these vascular channels in relationship to the liver and major vessels.

Dual-phase CT, in the hepatic-arterial (HAP) and portal-venous (PVP) phases, is necessary in evaluating the cirrhotic liver for HCC. Demonstration of a hypervascular mass on the HAP of a dual-phase CT scan is highly suggestive of HCC (Figures 11–8 and 11–9). Many investigators have shown that the HAP demonstrates significantly more HCC lesions than PVP or unenhanced images (34–36). Lesion conspicuity is increased in the HAP because most HCCs are hypervascular, and because the cirrhotic liver receives less portal-venous inflow due to portal hypertension. The HAP images also are useful in differentiating portal-tumor thrombus from portal-bland thrombus because the tumor thrombus enhances in the arterial phase. Portal-venous-phase scans are required for assessment of portal-vein patency and evaluation of extrahepatic abnormal organs. Occasionally, it may be difficult to differentiate abnormal-liver parenchyma of cirrhosis from diffuse or multifocal HCCs (Figure 11-10). Focal contour abnormality, vascular invasion or thrombosis, and mass effect on the hepatic vasculature are important clues to the diagnosis of an underlying tumor.

The accuracy of helical CT in detecting HCC in patients with cirrhosis recently has been reported in a large pretransplant patient population (34). In the surveillance of 430 cases

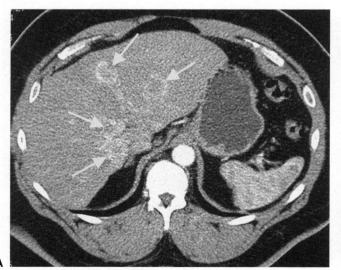

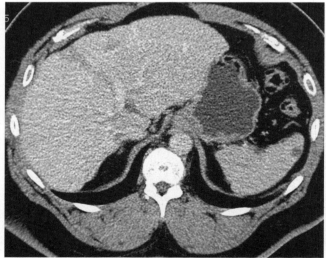

FIG. 11–8. Multifocal HCC in a 54-year-old male with cirrhosis. Computed tomography in arterial phase **(A)** shows four rim-enhancing masses (*arrows*). These are less conspicuous on portal-venous phase **(B)**.

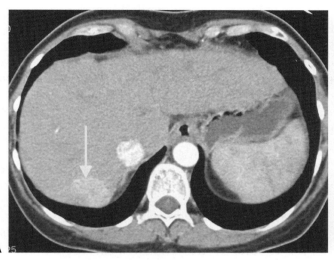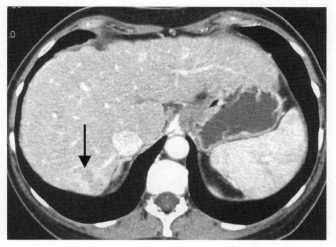

FIG. 11–9. HCC complicating cirrhosis in a 59-year-old male. The liver demonstrates nodular contour. Arterial **(A)** and portal-venous **(B)** phases demonstrate a hypervascular mass in the right lobe posteriorly (*arrow*), with early arterial enhancement. Note is made of splenomegaly.

of cirrhosis with no clinical suspicion of HCC, 320 underwent triphasic CT, 92 underwent noncontrast and portal-venous phase CT, and 18 underwent only noncontrast CT. At pathology, 59 patients (14%) had HCC. Helical CT detected HCC in only 26 patients, with a sensitivity of 44%. Multidetector CT is expected to improve sensitivity in detecting HCC in cirrhotic patients, particularly due to improved spatial resolution.

A heterogeneous pattern of parenchymal enhancement in cirrhosis should be distinguished from the transient hepatic-attenuation difference (THAD), which may result in false-positive lesions. Transient hepatic-attenuation difference often is identified as a focal peripheral wedge of increased enhancement, with no mass effect or distortion of

liver capsule (Figure 11-11). These lesions have a straight margin and contain normal vessels (37). They may be due to arterioportal shunts and are seen only on hepatic arterial-phase imaging (26). If CT findings of THAD are not characteristic, or if an associated focal lesion is suspected, iodized-oil-CT (Figure 11-12) or MR imaging should be performed to exclude HCC (22).

STORAGE AND METABOLIC DISORDERS

Fatty Infiltration

Fatty infiltration of the liver, or steatosis, is a potentially reversible process that can result from increased production

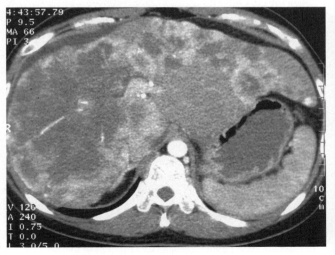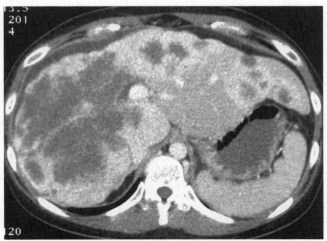

FIG. 11–10. Multifocal HCC in a 32-year-old female. Arterial **(A)** and portal-venous **(B)** phases demonstrate multiple hypervascular masses with central necrosis. Moderate compensatory hypertrophy of the left lobe also is seen.

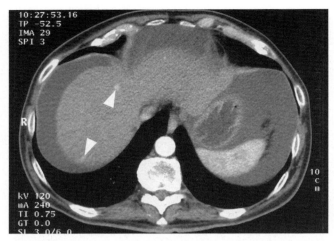

FIG. 11–11. Transient hepatic-attenuation difference in a 56-year-old male. Focal peripheral wedge-shaped areas of increased enhancement (*arrowheads*) are seen commonly in patients with cirrhosis.

or mobilization of fatty acids (e.g., hyperalimentation, starvation, obesity, steroid use, diabetes mellitus) or hepatocellular injury (e.g., alcoholic liver disease, hepatitis, or drug-induced injury) (38). Fatty infiltration of the liver in the absence of alcohol abuse is a cause of nonalcoholic steatohepatitis (NASH) (39,40). Most patients are obese women with diabetes mellitus, hypercholesterolemia, or hypertriglyceridemia. The histologic picture is indistinguishable from that of alcoholic hepatitis.

The distribution of steatosis can be focal, regional, or diffuse. On noncontrast CT, the attenuation value of the normal liver ranges between 45 HU and 65 HU, and is usually 8 HU to 10 HU greater than the spleen (41). Diffuse fatty infiltration results in decreased attenuation of the liver 10

HU to 20 HU less than that of the spleen (42). Attenuation of the liver parenchyma may, in severe cases, drop below the hepatic vessels (Figure 11-13). Diagnosis of fatty infiltration is less reliable on contrast-enhanced CT because of the variability of the relative attenuation of the liver and spleen (Figure 11-14).

Hepatic fatty infiltration can be focal, regional, or subtotal with focal sparing (43,44). Nonuniform involvement of the liver may be due to aberrant vascular supply to areas of fat deposition or areas that are spared in diffuse fatty infiltration (45–47). Typical locations of these areas include the medial segment of the left liver lobe, around the falciform ligament (Figure 11-15), the gallbladder fossa (Figure 11-16), the subcapsular region (Figure 11-17), and the porta hepatis (Figure 11-18). Clues that may help in identifying focal fatty infiltration or focal sparing include typical loca-

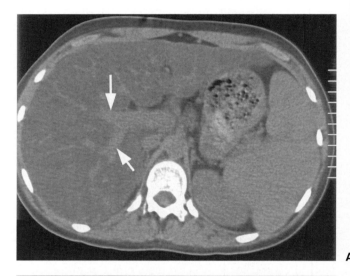

A

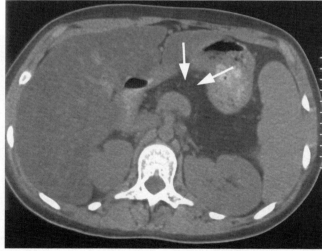

B

FIG. 11–13. Severe fatty infiltration of the liver in a 20-year-old female with cystic fibrosis. **A:** The liver is lower in density than the nonenhanced hepatic blood vessels (*arrows*). **B:** Axial image through the pancreas reveals marked fatty replacement of the entire pancreas (*arrows*).

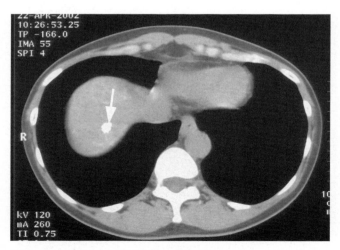

FIG. 11–12. Lipiodol CT in a 52-year-old male with history of hepatitis C and indeterminate liver nodule. Noncontrast CT 6 weeks after intraarterial administration of lipiodol reveals prolonged retention of lipiodol (*arrow*), suspicious for HCC.

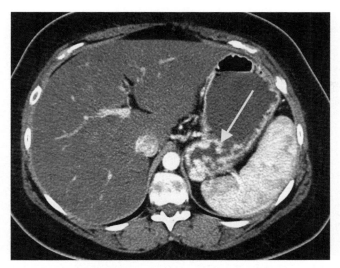

FIG. 11–14. Fatty infiltration of the liver in a 36-year-old female with history of hepatitis C. Gastric fundal varices are also present (*arrow*).

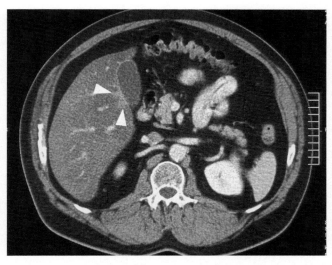

FIG. 11–16. Fatty infiltration in a 58-year-old male. There are areas of sparing near the gallbladder fossa (*arrowheads*).

tion and distribution, absence of mass effect, sharply angulated boundaries, and nonspherical shape. Scanning during peak vascular enhancement in the PVP can demonstrate readily normal caliber vessels coursing through the area of focal fatty infiltration. In spite of these clues, differentiation form primary or metastatic involvement of the liver occasionally can be difficult and may create diagnostic challenges for the radiologists. Additional imaging with MR or positron emission tomography may help in establishing the diagnosis (48).

Focal fatty sparing is most commonly an incidental benign finding seen in areas of aberrant vascularity near the gallbladder fossa or in the porta hepatis. It also may be seen following hepatic irradiation, or in the parenchyma, which

lacks portal-venous flow due to the occlusion from small tumors or thrombi.

Detecting fatty infiltration of the liver is of paramount importance in the preoperative evaluation of potential liver donors. Fatty infiltration is reported in approximately 10% of potential donors and could be a contraindication to transplantation (49,50). Fatty livers are less resistant to cold and warm ischemia, which may be induced at surgery, and may cause primary graft nonfunction after transplantation (51).

Hemochromatosis

The liver stores iron and may manifest with the consequences of iron overload. Primary hemochromatosis is an

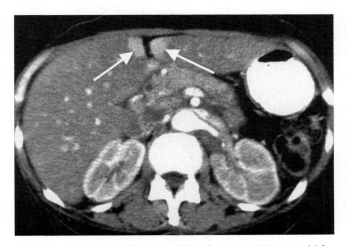

FIG. 11–15. Fatty infiltration of the liver in a 51-year-old female with history of colon cancer. Fatty sparing is seen on both sides of the falciform ligament (*arrows*).

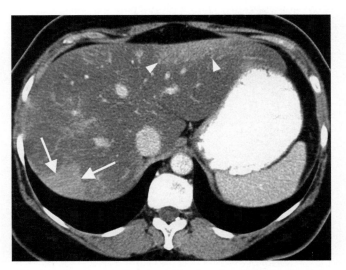

FIG. 11–17. Fatty infiltration of the liver in a 48-year-old male. Geographic regions of fatty sparing also are seen in the periphery (*arrows*). Normal vessels are seen coursing undisturbed through the liver parenchyma (*arrowheads*).

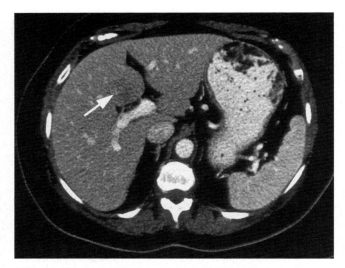

FIG. 11–18. Focal fat in a 61-year-old female. Low-attenuation "pseudolesion" near the porta hepatis (*arrow*) is a common location for focal fatty infiltration. This should not be mistaken for a mass.

autosomal-recessive disorder characterized by the abnormal absorption of iron from the bowel and its deposition into the hepatocytes, pancreatic-acinar cells, myocardium, joints, endocrine glands, and skin (52). Early symptoms include abnormal liver-function tests, diabetes, and arthritis. Advanced cases may lead to hepatic-cell necrosis, fibrosis, and cirrhosis. Hepatocellular carcinoma is reported in approximately 35% of advanced cases (53). Secondary hemochromatosis is the result of multiple blood transfusions and iron deposition in the reticuloendothelial system of the liver, spleen, and, less often, bone marrow.

On noncontrast CT, the liver has increased attenuation, typically measuring 70 HU and 130 HU. This finding, however, is nonspecific, and the differential diagnosis includes

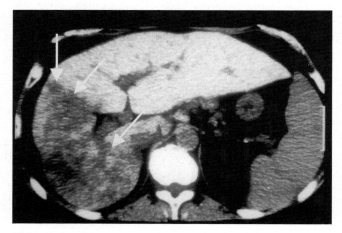

FIG. 11–19. Hemochromatosis in an elderly patient. Notice the high density of the liver parenchyma on the noncontrast CT. Areas of low density in the right lobe are due to HCC (*arrows*).

gold or Thorotrast deposition, Type-IV glycogen-storage disease, and following amiodarone administration (54). Performing dual-phase CT in patients with primary hemochromatosis is important to evaluate for HCC (Figures 11–19 and 11–20).

Amyloidosis

Amyloidosis is due to the deposition of protein–mucopolysaccharide complexes (55). Primary amyloidosis is associated with multiple myeloma and monoclonal gammopathy, while secondary amyloidosis is associated with chronic infection, rheumatoid arthritis, and malignant tumors. The other organs that may be involved include the spleen and

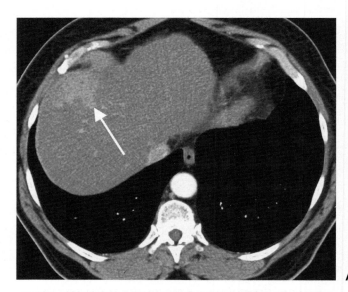

A

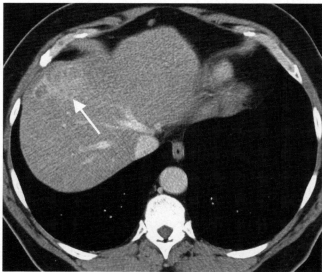

B

FIG. 11–20. Hepatocellular carcinoma in a 69-year-old male with history of hemochromatosis. Computed tomography in arterial **(A)** and portal-venous **(B)** phases shows lobulated hypervascular mass in the right lobe (*arrow*).

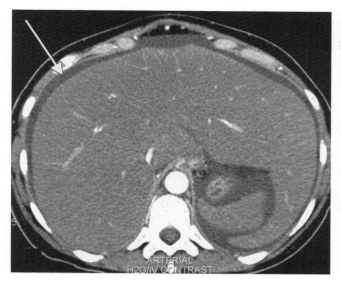

FIG. 11–21. Primary amyloidosis in a 62-year-old female. Notice the diffuse hepatic enlargement and the presence of small amount of ascites (*arrow*).

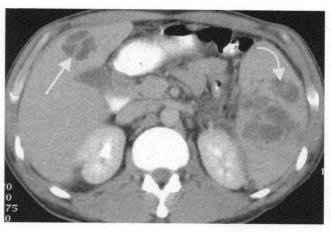

FIG. 11–22. Hepatic and splenic abscesses in a 34-year-old male. The patient has occupationally acquired melioidosis, an infectious disease caused by the bacterium *Burkholderia pseudomallei*. Notice the presence of splenomegaly and the multiloculated abscesses in the liver (*arrow*) and spleen (*curved arrow*).

kidney (56,57). Hepatic amyloidosis manifests as nonspecific diffuse hepatomegaly due to amyloid deposition (Figure 11-21). Spontaneous hepatic (58) and/or splenic (59) rupture may occur and is associated with high mortality rate. Diffuse calcification of the abdominal viscera has been reported, particularly involving the liver and spleen (60). It also can result in cholestasis and acute hepatic failure that require transplantation. When focal, CT also may demonstrate areas of low attenuation known as amyloid pseudotumors. These have delayed enhancement on contrast-enhanced CT (61).

INFECTIOUS AND INFLAMMATORY DISORDERS

Abscess

Pyogenic abscesses usually are caused by *Clostridium* or gram-negative bacteria. Mortality rate remains high, approximately 8% according to a recent study (62). Bacterial infection can spread to the liver through either direct spread from the biliary tree in patients with cholangitis or cholecystitis, or following percutaneous internal-biliary drainage (63). Hematogenous spread from the bowel by the portal vein also can occur. This may occur in patients with appendicitis, diverticulitis, or inflammatory-bowel disease. Initial treatment is intravenous antibiotics. Laparotomy or percutaneous drainage with subsequent laparotomy may be indicated, especially if there is unresolving jaundice, renal impairment, multiloculation, biliary communication, or rupture at presentation.

Multidetector CT is useful in detection, localization, and, if indicated, guidance for drainage. On contrast-enhanced CT, bacterial abscess has a central area of low attenuation due to necrosis, with a thick rim of peripheral enhance-

ment or a capsule. Multiple surrounding satellite abscesses also may be detected, resulting in the "cluster sign" (64,65) (Figures 11–22 and 11–23). Gas bubbles, reported in approximately 20% of cases (66) can be detected well by MDCT (Figures 11–24 and 11–25). Hepatic abscess and other inflammatory conditions can result in a high-attenuation area adjacent to the site of inflammation on arterial-phase images. This is due to hyperemia and increased arterial-blood flow, and disappears on PVP images. Normal vessels can be seen coursing through the area of high attenua-

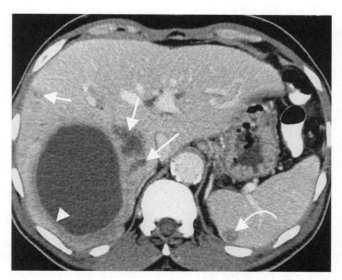

FIG. 11–23. Large hepatic abscess in a 62-year-old male. The collection has a thick enhancing rim (*arrowhead*). Smaller surrounding-satellite cavities also are identified (*arrows*). This appearance is indistinguishable from cystic or necrotic neoplasm. Note a small hemangioma in the spleen (*curved arrow*).

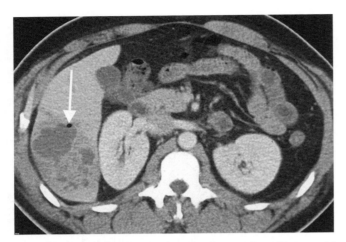

FIG. 11–24. Multiloculated hepatic abscess in a 43-year-old male. Note a small air bubble (*arrow*) within the collection.

tion, with no mass effect or vascular displacement. This transient segmental enhancement usually decreases or resolves following appropriate antibiotic therapy (67).

The CT appearance of hepatic abscess is nonspecific, and the differential diagnosis includes cystic or necrotic metastases. Careful clinical history usually helps in distinguishing these categories (66).

Hepatitis

The most common cause of hepatitis is viral infection. However, other causes include bacterial or fungal infections, autoimmune disorders, alcohol abuse, radiation therapy, or drugs. Hepatitis becomes chronic in three months to six months, and when severe, often leads to cirrhosis and liver failure.

In acute hepatitis, fulminant hepatic necrosis may occur. Multidetector CT may demonstrate hepatomegaly, periportal edema, gallbladder-wall thickening, and heterogeneous enhancement after contrast administration (Figure 11-26). Occasionally, CT may detect enlarged periportal lymph nodes. These findings are nonspecific and can be seen in patients with congestive heart failure, hepatic trauma, liver transplantation, cirrhosis, and malignancy. In chronic hepatitis, CT features are of those of cirrhosis and portal hypertension.

Radiation-induced hepatitis typically occurs 2 weeks to 6 weeks after the completion of radiotherapy. The threshold dose ranges between 30 Gy and 35 Gy, but higher doses may be tolerated if only part of the liver is irradiated (68). Clinical findings include jaundice, hepatomegaly, and ascites. Multidetector CT findings include a sharply defined geo-

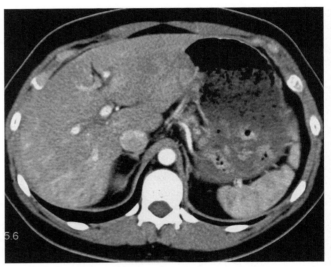

A

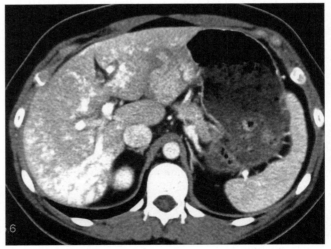

B

FIG. 11–26. Fulminant drug-induced (ecstasy) hepatitis in a 26-year-old female. Arterial **(A)** and portal-venous **(B)** phases demonstrate heterogeneous parenchymal enhancement, best seen on PVP images. Biopsy revealed severe panlobular hepatitis. Viral markers were negative.

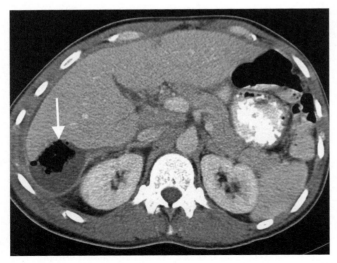

FIG. 11–25. Subcapsular hepatic abscess in a 48-year-old male. Notice the presence of air (*arrow*) within the fluid collection.

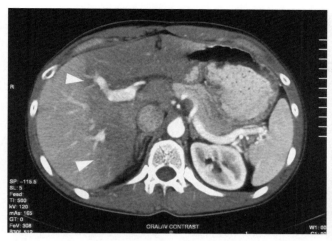

FIG. 11–27. Radiation-induced hepatitis in a 32-year-old female. Notice the sharp demarcation of the geographic region of low attenuation (*arrowheads*). Normal vessels are seen coursing through the liver parenchyma.

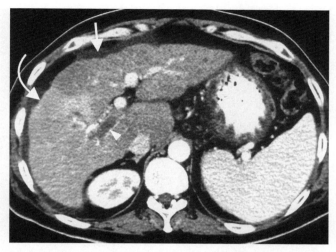

FIG. 11–28. Portal-vein-thrombosis complicating cirrhosis in a 56-year-old male. The liver demonstrates nodular contour. Note is made of ascites (*arrow*) and splenomegaly. There is a clot in the right portal vein (*arrowhead*) causing perfusion change in the right lobe (*curved arrow*).

graphic region of low attenuation on PVP images along the radiation port (69) (Figure 11-27). On delayed images, the hypodense area becomes hyperdense due to decreased vascular perfusion and venous stasis. Normal-caliber vessels can be seen coursing through the low-attenuation lesion. However, narrowing and irregularity of the hepatic vessels also may occur and probably are due to sinusoidal congestion and perisinusoidal edema (70). Over time, the irradiated area contracts, with compensatory hypertrophy of the remaining liver.

Candidiasis

Hepatic candidiasis results from systemic fungal infection with *Candida albicans*. The disease typically is seen in immunocompromised patients following the treatment of hematological malignancies (71). On CT, the liver contains multiple small hypodense lesions, with peripheral or rim enhancement following contrast administration. These findings are nonspecific. Differential diagnosis in such cases includes metastatic disease, lymphoma, and leukemia.

DIFFUSE HEPATIC VASCULAR DISEASE

Portal-Vein Thrombosis

Portal-vein thrombosis can occur in cirrhosis (Figure 11-28), infection, trauma, hypercoagulable states (Figure 11-29), extrinsic tumor compression, or direct invasion. The presence of arterial phase enhancement of the thrombus and expansion of the portal vein suggest tumor thrombus, and these findings help in distinguishing tumor thrombus from bland thrombus (72). Prolonged thrombosis results in cavernous transformation of the main portal vein, and the ap-

pearance of small dilated periportal collaterals. Alternatively, recanalization of thrombosed portal vein may occur.

On unenhanced CT, the attenuation of acute thrombus is approximately 60 HU to 70 HU (73). Following intravenous-contrast administration, the acute thrombus appears as a hypoattenuating-filling defect in the portal vein, with partial or complete occlusion. These findings are best seen on PVP images. Perivenous-fat stranding may be observed in patients with portal vein phlebitis (74).

Portal-vein thrombosis results in alteration of the hepatic-blood supply and a change in hepatic attenuation due to fatty infiltration. Altered perfusion also may result in THADs, which cause pseudolesions on late arterial-phase images (37). Multidetector CT in the PVP results in peak contrast opacification of the main portal vein, accurately depicting the site and extent of thrombosis. It also can detect small dilated periportal collaterals (Figure 11-30). Transient increased attenuation, best seen in the arterial phase, can be demonstrated in portions of the liver that are deprived of the portal-blood flow (75,76). In segmental-portal-vein thrombosis, the hyperattenuating lesions often are wedge shaped, with the base toward the liver capsule in the vascular territory involved. Focal alteration of hepatic enhancement also can be due to tumors. Typically, the responsible lesion is present at the apex of the perfusion abnormality. Therefore, it is critical to search for an underlying neoplasm when evaluating any wedge-shaped flow-related perfusion abnormality. If present, a tumor may be isoattenuating to the hyperattenuating surrounding liver parenchyma and may be difficult to detect on the arterial phase. In such cases, imaging in the PVP or delayed phase may be essential for lesion detection (77).

Thrombosis of the portal vein was considered at one

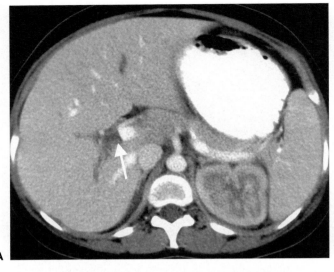

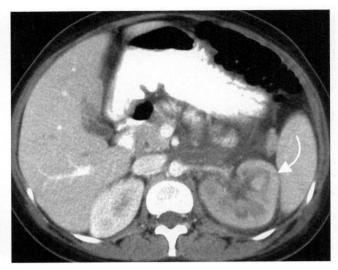

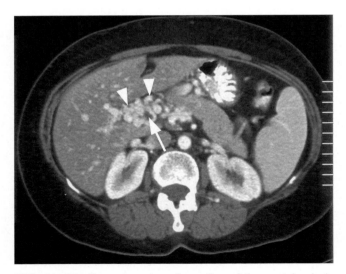

FIG. 11–29. Post-partum portal-vein thrombosis in a 22-year-old female. Computed tomography demonstrates an occlusive clot in the right portal vein [*arrow* in **(A)**]. The patient also has complete infarction of the left kidney [*curved arrow* in **(B)**] due to renal-vein thrombosis and pulmonary embolism [*arrowhead* in **(C)**].

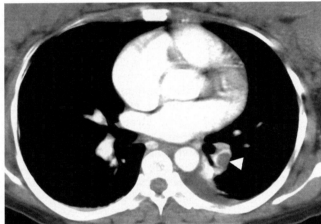

FIG. 11–30. Cavernous transformation of the portal vein in a 59-year-old female. Central thrombus is demonstrated in the portal vein (*arrow*), with dense opacification of several large periportal collaterals (*arrowheads*).

time an absolute contraindication to liver transplantation. However, several surgical techniques now are available for the management of such cases. Acute portal-vein thrombosis is treated by manual thrombectomy at the time of surgery. If chronic portal-vein thrombosis is present, the donor portal vein is anastomosed to the splenomesenteric confluence. Diffuse chronic thrombosis of the portal vein and the superior mesenteric vein remains a contraindication to liver transplantation (72).

Following liver transplantation, MDCT accurately can delineate the site of extrahepatic portal-vein anastomosis and any possible stenosis, narrowing or thrombosis. Portal-vein thrombosis or stenosis is reported in 1% to 3% of cases of orthotopic liver transplantation, and it results from vascular malalignment, difference in caliber of anastomosed vessels, previous portal-vein thrombosis or calcification, or hypercoagulable states (27). Clinical presentation includes symptoms of portal hypertension, liver failure, and ascites. Computed tomography can demonstrate filling defects within the portal vein or focal narrowing at the site of anastomosis. Treatment includes transluminal angioplasty, surgical

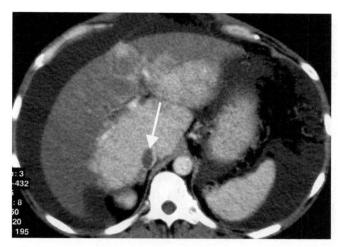

FIG. 11–31. Budd–Chiari syndrome in a 53-year-old male. Computed tomography demonstrates patchy peripheral-parenchymal enhancement with normal enhancement of the caudate lobe. The IVC is narrowed, with a nonocclusive clot seen within (*arrow*). The patient also has cirrhosis and ascites.

thrombectomy, placement of a venous graft, or retransplantation.

Budd–Chiari Syndrome

Budd–Chiari syndrome involves hepatic-venous-outflow obstruction, resulting in progressive hepatic failure, ascites, and portal hypertension (74). The syndrome most commonly is idiopathic. Other etiologies include hematologic and myeloproliferative diseases, hypercoagulable states, tumors, and infections.

Multidetector CT findings in patients with Budd–Chiari syndrome include the detection of hepatic vein or inferior vena cava (IVC) thrombosis (78). Narrowing or nonvisualization of the hepatic veins or IVC also may occur (Figure 11-31). Secondary changes include the development of intraparenchymal collaterals and dilatation of the azygos vein. Parenchymal-liver changes also can be observed due to venous obstruction (Figure 11-32). In an acute stage, the hepatic segments that are drained by the obstructed vein appear swollen due to stagnant venous flow. Wedge-shaped increased enhancement in the arterial phase can be seen similar to portal-vein thrombosis, but with the vertex of the wedge-shaped areas pointing to the IVC rather than the hepatic hilum (79). Heterogeneous enhancement persists in the PVP (37) and becomes homogeneous on delayed scans (80). Compensatory hypertrophy of the caudate lobe may occur due to a separate unaffected venous drainage directly into the IVC. Fibrosis and segmental volume loss may occur if the disease becomes chronic. Benign regenerative nodules also may occur. Caution must be used when making the diagnosis of Budd–Chiari syndrome on MDCT because nonopacification of the hepatic veins will occur if scanning is performed in the arterial phase or in patients with heart failure or poor cardiac output.

Passive Hepatic-venous Congestion

Severe right-sided heart failure due to congestive heart failure or pericardial tamponade may result in passive-hepatic congestion that manifests on contrast-enhanced cross-sectional-imaging studies as a heterogeneous mosaic-like enhancement with reflux of contrast from the right atrium into the IVC (74) (Figure 11-33). In early cases, linear regions of decreased enhancement are due to delayed enhance-

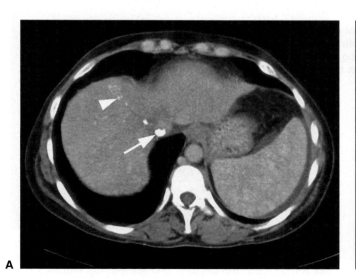

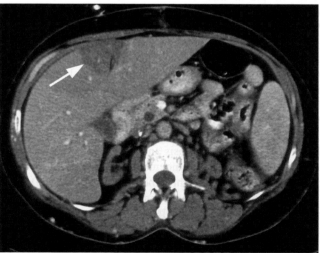

A   B

FIG. 11–32. Thrombosis and calcification of the IVC in a 41-year-old female. **A:** Dense calcification is identified along the IVC (*arrow*) and the middle hepatic vein (*arrowhead*). **B:** Wedge-shaped hypodense area near the falciform ligament (*arrow*), secondary to IVC occlusion. The kidneys are small due to chronic renal failure.

cularization surgery. Extrahepatic pseudoaneurysms usually develop at the site of anastomosis or as a complication to angioplasty. When ruptured, these can lead to massive intraperitoneal hemorrhage. Treatment includes surgical resection, embolization, or exclusion with stent placement (27).

DIFFUSE NEOPLASTIC DISEASES

Metastatic Disease

Hepatic metastasis, when diffuse, may be difficult to differentiate from parenchymal disease. Diffuse metastatic disease can occur with many primary tumors including melanoma, malignant islet-cell tumors, pancreatic adenocarcinoma, breast carcinoma, and colonic adenocarcinoma. Computed tomography appearances of diffuse hepatic metastases depend on the vascularity of the lesions compared to normal surrounding-liver parenchyma. Hypovascular lesions, such as metastases of colorectal adenocarcinoma, have lower attenuation compared with normal liver and are detected best on PVP images (86) (Figure 11-38). Hypervascular metastases, including islet-cell tumors, melanoma, sarcoma, renal-cell carcinoma, and certain subtypes of breast and lung carcinoma, enhance more rapidly than normal liver and are detected best on HAP images. Occasionally, diffuse metastatic involvement is very subtle and may present as diffuse parenchymal heterogeneity, vascular and architectural distortion, or alterations of the liver contour. Severe contour deformities result in "pseudocirrhosis" described in patients with treated breast cancer (87) (Figure 11-39).

Multidetector CT plays a critical role prior to surgery and intraarterial-chemotherapy-pump placement. It is valuable in delineating the relationship of tumor to adjacent vessels, providing accurate segmental localization. It can demonstrate accurately arterial vascular variants that could

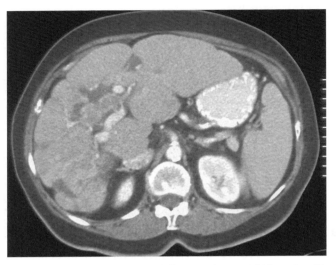

FIG. 11–39. "Pseudocirrhosis" in an 80-year-old female with treated breast metastasis. There is heterogeneous enhancement of the liver, with capsular retraction and large nodules.

impact pump placement and can provide important landmarks that can be followed during surgery using intraoperative ultrasound.

Lymphoma

Hepatic lymphoma can be primary or secondary. Primary lymphoma is rare and classically presents as a focal mass with rim enhancement (88,89). Mild hepatomegaly also may be present. Lymphadenopathy, splenomegaly, and bone-marrow involvement are rare in primary lymphoma (90). Secondary lymphoma is more common and occurs in both Hodgkin's and non-Hodgkin's lymphoma. In patients

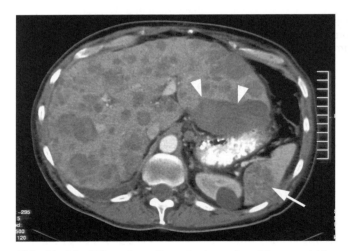

FIG. 11–38. Diffuse hepatic metastases in a 66-year-old female with history of lung cancer. A large subcapsular hematoma also is seen along the left lobe (*arrowheads*) after the patient received anticoagulation. Metastasis also involves the spleen (*arrow*).

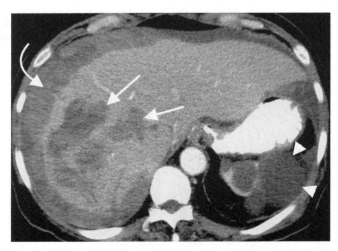

FIG. 11–40. Large-cell lymphoma in a 53-year-old male. The patient has parenchymal (*arrows*) and subcapsular (*curved arrow*) hematoma. The spleen is surgically absent. Multiple left-renal cysts also are seen (*arrowheads*).

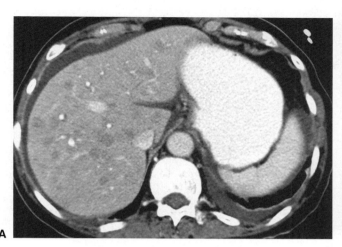

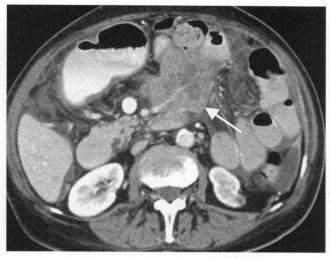

FIG. 11–41. Large-cell lymphoma in a 79-year-old female. Computed-tomography image through the liver **(A)** demonstrates innumerable hypodense lesions indicating extensive tumor infiltration. Axial image more inferiorly **(B)** reveals a large mass at the root of the mesentry (*arrow*), causing partial small-bowel obstruction.

with human-immunodeficiency-virus (HIV) infection, the incidence of non-Hodgkin's lymphoma is rising. It usually is aggressive and differentiated poorly. The liver is the second most common site of abdominal involvement after the gastrointestinal tract, with an incidence of up to 45% (91,92).

On CT, the liver parenchyma is infiltrated diffusely with neoplastic cells without significant architectural distortion, resulting in innumerable low-attenuation lesions scattered throughout the liver (Figures 11–40 and 11–41). A thin enhancing rim also may be present. Rarely, non-Hodgkin's lymphoma may present with periportal-infiltrating mass on CT (93). Computed tomography is important in detecting hepatic lymphoma, as well as staging of the disease by providing information about extrahepatic-organ involvement (94). The differential diagnosis for hepatic involvement includes infections such as atypical mycobacteria, fungal, biliary angiomatosis, and neoplasms such as Kaposi's sarcoma and metastases.

CONGENITAL DISEASES

Polycystic Liver Disease

Hepatic cysts are common and are present in 2.5% of the population (95) (Figure 11-42). In autosomal-dominant adult polycystic disease, hepatic cysts are multiple and are found in 40% of cases (Figure 11-43). Patients usually are asymptomatic, and hepatic dysfunction rarely occurs (96). Advanced disease can lead to hepatomegaly, liver failure, or Budd–Chiari Syndrome (97). Hepatic cysts are lined by an imperceptible wall of cuboidal epithelium and contain

serous fluid. On nonenhanced CT scans, the liver disease contains multiple homogeneous and hypodense cysts. No cyst wall, septal enhancement, or mural nodules are identified after administration of intravenous contrast (95). Large cysts may be amenable to laparoscopic deroofing or open fenestration (Figure 11-44). Percutaneous-alcohol ablation is an alternative treatment to reduce compression on surrounding liver parenchyma. For cases with diffuse hepatic involvement or recurrence after a deroofing procedure, partial resection or liver transplantation may be performed (98).

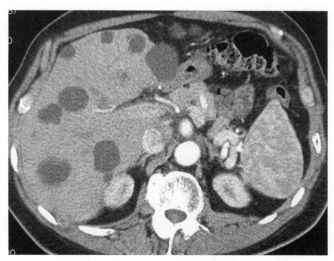

FIG. 11–42. Multiple incidental simple-liver cysts in a 50-year-old male. These are hypodense well-defined lesions with no enhancement, septations, or mural nodules.

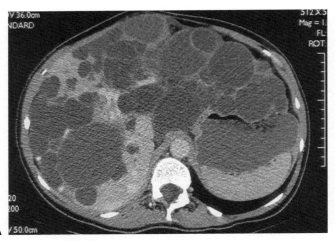 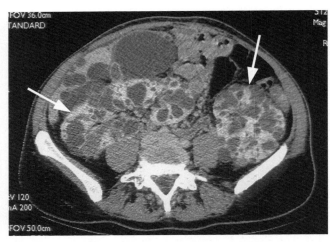

FIG. 11–43. Adult polycystic disease in a 30-year-old female. **A:** Diffuse hepatic involvement with minimal normal parenchyma remaining in the right lobe. **B:** Both kidneys are enlarged (*arrows*) and contain multiple cysts.

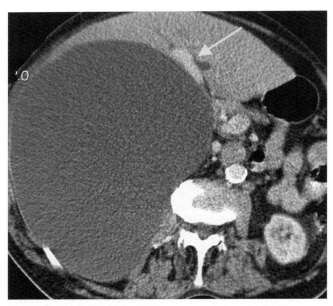

FIG. 11–44. Giant liver cyst in a 78-year-old male. Notice the mass effect on the left portal vein (*arrow*). The patient had abdominal pain and underwent deroofing procedure.

REFERENCES

1. Foley WD, Mallisee TA, Hohenwalter MD, et al. Multiphase hepatic CT with a multirow detector CT scanner. *AJR Am J Roentgenol* 2000; 175:679–685.
2. Ji H, McTavish JD, Mortele KJ, et al. Hepatic imaging with multidetector CT. *Radiographics* 2001;21 Spec No:S71–S80.
3. Hu H, He HD, Foley WD, et al. Four multidetector-row helical CT: image quality and volume coverage speed. *Radiology* 2000; 215:55–62.
4. Mitsuzaki K, Yamashita Y, Ogata I, et al. Multiple-phase helical CT of the liver for detecting small hepatomas in patients with liver cirrhosis: contrast-injection protocol and optimal timing. *AJR Am J Roentgenol* 1996;167:753–757.
5. Murakami T, Kim T, Takahashi S, et al Hepatocellular carcinoma: multidetector row helical CT. *Abdom Imaging* 2002;27:139–146.
6. Paulson EK, McDermott VG, Keogan MT, et al. Carcinoid metastases to the liver: role of triple-phase helical CT. *Radiology* 1998; 206:143–150.
7. Lacomis JM, Baron RL, Oliver JH 3rd, et al. Cholangiocarcinoma: delayed CT contrast enhancement patterns. *Radiology* 1997; 203:98–104.
8. Kim T, Federle MP, Baron RL, et al. Discrimination of small hepatic hemangiomas from hypervascular malignant tumors smaller than 3 cm with three-phase helical CT. *Radiology* 2001;219:699–706.
9. Leslie DF, Johnson CD, Johnson CM, et al. Distinction between cavernous hemangiomas of the liver and hepatic metastases on CT: value of contrast enhancement patterns. *AJR Am J Roentgenol* 1995; 164:625–629.
10. Genesca J, Esteban JI, Alter HJ. Blood-borne non-A, non-B hepatitis: hepatitis C. *Semin Liver Dis* 1991;11:147–164.
11. Brown JJ, Naylor MJ, Yagan N. Imaging of hepatic cirrhosis. *Radiology* 1997;202:1–16.
12. Ince N, Wands JR. The increasing incidence of hepatocellular carcinoma. *N Engl J Med* 1999;340:798–799.
13. Dodd GD 3rd, Baron RL, Oliver JH 3rd, et al. Spectrum of imaging findings of the liver in end-stage cirrhosis: Part II, focal abnormalities. *AJR Am J Roentgenol* 1999;173:1185–1192.
14. Dodd GD 3rd, Baron RL, Oliver JH 3rd, et al. Spectrum of imaging findings of the liver in end-stage cirrhosis: part I, gross morphology and diffuse abnormalities. *AJR Am J Roentgenol* 1999;173:1031–1036.
15. Choi BI. Hepatocellular carcinoma and precancerous lesions: advances in imaging. *Abdom Imaging* 2002;27:115–116.
16. Lim JH, Choi BI. Dysplastic nodules in liver cirrhosis: imaging. *Abdom Imaging* 2002;27:117–128.
17. Lim JH, Choi D, Cho SK, et al. Conspicuity of hepatocellular nodular lesions in cirrhotic livers at ferumoxides-enhanced MR imaging: importance of Kupffer cell number. *Radiology* 2001;220:669–676.
18. Imai Y, Murakami T, Yoshida S, et al. Superparamagnetic iron oxide-enhanced magnetic resonance images of hepatocellular carcinoma: correlation with histological grading. *Hepatology* 2000;32:205–212.
19. Kondo F, Ebara M, Sugiura N, et al. Histological features and clinical course of large regenerative nodules: evaluation of their precancerous potentiality. *Hepatology* 1990;12:592–598.
20. Fisher MR, Gore RM. Computed tomography in the evaluation of cirrhosis and portal hypertension. *J Clin Gastroenterol* 1985;7:173–181.
21. Harbin WP, Robert NJ, Ferrucci JT Jr. Diagnosis of cirrhosis based on regional changes in hepatic morphology: a radiological and pathological analysis. *Radiology* 1980;135:273–283.
22. Kim TK, Choi BI, Han JK, et al. Nontumorous arterioportal shunt mimicking hypervascular tumor in cirrhotic liver: two-phase spiral CT findings. *Radiology* 1998;208:597–603.
23. Quiroga S, Sebastia C, Pallisa E, et al. Improved diagnosis of hepatic

perfusion disorders: value of hepatic arterial phase imaging during helical CT. *Radiographics* 2001;21:65–81, questionnaire 288–294.

24. Yu JS, Kim KW, Sung KB, et al. Small arterial-portal venous shunts: a cause of pseudolesions at hepatic imaging. *Radiology* 1997; 203:737–742.

25. Brancatelli G, Federle MP, Pealer K, et al. Portal venous thrombosis or sclerosis in liver transplantation candidates: preoperative CT findings and correlation with surgical procedure. *Radiology* 2001; 220:321–328.

26. Itai Y, Matsui O. Blood flow and liver imaging. *Radiology* 1997; 202:306–314.

27. Quiroga S, Sebastia MC, Margarit C, et al. Complications of orthotopic liver transplantation: spectrum of findings with helical CT. *Radiographics* 2001;21:1085–1102.

28. Lee PC, Rhee RY, Gordon RY, et al. Management of splenic artery aneurysms: the significance of portal and essential hypertension. *J Am Coll Surg* 1999;189:483–490.

29. Robertson AJ, Rela M, Karani J, et al. Splenic artery aneurysm and orthotopic liver transplantation. *Transpl Int* 1999;12:68–70.

30. Mulhern CB Jr, Arger PH, Coleman BG, et al. Nonuniform attenuation in computed tomography study of the cirrhotic liver. *Radiology* 1979; 132:399–402.

31. Huet PM, Du Reau A, Marleau D. Arterial and portal blood supply in cirrhosis: a functional evaluation. *Gut* 1979;20:792–796.

32. Popper H. Pathologic aspects of cirrhosis. A review. *Am J Pathol* 1977; 87:228–264.

33. Blachar A, Federle MP, Brancatelli G. Primary biliary cirrhosis: clinical, pathologic, and helical CT findings in 53 patients. *Radiology* 2001; 220:329–336.

34. Peterson MS, Baron RL, Marsh JW Jr, et al. Pretransplantation surveillance for possible hepatocellular carcinoma in patients with cirrhosis: epidemiology and CT-based tumor detection rate in 430 cases with surgical pathologic correlation. *Radiology* 2000;217:743–749.

35. Kim T, Murakami T, Takahashi S, et al. Optimal phases of dynamic CT for detecting hepatocellular carcinoma: evaluation of unenhanced and triple-phase images. *Abdom Imaging* 1999;24:473–480.

36. Baron RL, Oliver JH 3rd, Dodd GD 3rd, et al. Hepatocellular carcinoma: evaluation with biphasic, contrast-enhanced, helical CT. *Radiology* 1996;199:505–511.

37. Chen WP, Chen JH, Hwang JI, et al. Spectrum of transient hepatic attenuation differences in biphasic helical CT. *AJR Am J Roentgenol* 1999;172:419–424.

38. Nomura F, Ohnishi K, Ochiai T, et al. Obesity-related nonalcoholic fatty liver: CT features and follow-up studies after low-calorie diet. *Radiology* 1987;162:845–847.

39. Reid AE. Nonalcoholic steatohepatitis. *Gastroenterology* 2001; 121:710–723.

40. Clark JM, Brancati FL, Diehl AM. Nonalcoholic fatty liver disease. *Gastroenterology* 2002;122:1649–1657.

41. Piekarski J, Goldberg HI, Royal SA, et al. Difference between liver and spleen CT numbers in the normal adult: its usefulness in predicting the presence of diffuse liver disease. *Radiology* 1980;137:727–729.

42. Bydder GM, Chapman RW, Harry D, et al. Computed tomography attenuation values in fatty liver. *J Comput Tomogr* 1981;5:33–35.

43. Kawamori Y, Matsui O, Takahashi S, et al. Focal hepatic fatty infiltration in the posterior edge of the medial segment associated with aberrant gastric venous drainage: CT, US, and MR findings. *J Comput Assist Tomogr* 1996;20:356–359.

44. White EM, Simeone JF, Mueller PR, et al. Focal periportal sparing in hepatic fatty infiltration: a cause of hepatic pseudomass on US. *Radiology* 1987;162:57–59.

45. Yoshikawa J, Matsui O, Takashima T, et al. Focal fatty change of the liver adjacent to the falciform ligament: CT and sonographic findings in five surgically confirmed cases. *AJR Am J Roentgenol* 1987; 149:491–494.

46. Kawashima A, Suehiro S, Murayama S, et al. Focal fatty infiltration of the liver mimicking a tumor: sonographic and CT features. *J Comput Assist Tomogr* 1986;10:329–331.

47. Adkins MC, Halvorsen RA Jr, duCret RP. CT evaluation of atypical hepatic fatty metamorphosis. *J Comput Assist Tomogr* 1990; 14:1013–1015.

48. Siegelman ES, Rosen MA. Imaging of hepatic steatosis. *Semin Liver Dis* 2001;21:71–80.

49. Kamel IR, Kruskal JB, Keogan MT, et al. Multidetector CT of potential right-lobe liver donors. *AJR Am J Roentgenol* 2001;177:645–651.

50. Kamel IR, Kruskal JB, Pomfret EA, et al. Impact of multidetector CT on donor selection and surgical planning before living adult right lobe liver transplantation. *AJR Am J Roentgenol* 2001;176:193–200.

51. Cheng YF, Chen CL, Lai CY, et al. Assessment of donor fatty livers for liver transplantation. *Transplantation* 2001;71:1221–1225.

52. McLaren GD, Muir WA, Kellermeyer RW. Iron overload disorders: natural history, pathogenesis, diagnosis, and therapy. *Crit Rev Clin Lab Sci* 1983;19:205–266.

53. Deugnier YM, Guyader D, Crantock L, et al. Primary liver cancer in genetic hemochromatosis: a clinical, pathological, and pathogenetic study of 54 cases. *Gastroenterology* 1993;104:228–234.

54. Guyader D, Gandon Y, Deugnier Y, et al. Evaluation of computed tomography in the assessment of liver iron overload. A study of 46 cases of idiopathic hemochromatosis. *Gastroenterology* 1989;97:737–743.

55. Mergo PJ, Ros PR. Imaging of diffuse liver disease. *Radiol Clin North Am* 1998;36:365–375.

56. Ros PR, Sobin LH. Amyloidosis: the same cat, with different stripes. *Radiology* 1994;190:14–15.

57. Gertz MA, Kyle RA. Hepatic amyloidosis: clinical appraisal in 77 patients. *Hepatology* 1997;25:118–121.

58. Bujanda L, Beguiristain A, Alberdi F, et al. Spontaneous rupture of the liver in amyloidosis. *Am J Gastroenterol* 1997;92:1385–1386.

59. Sandberg-Gertzen H, Ericzon BG, Blomberg B. Primary amyloidosis with spontaneous splenic rupture, cholestasis, and liver failure treated with emergency liver transplantation. *Am J Gastroenterol* 1998; 93:2254–2256.

60. Jacobs JE, Birnbaum BA, Furth EE. Abdominal visceral calcification in primary amyloidosis: CT findings. *Abdom Imaging* 1997;22:519–521.

61. Urban BA, Fishman EK, Goldman SM, et al. CT evaluation of amyloidosis: spectrum of disease. *Radiographics* 1993;13:1295–1308.

62. Barakate MS, Stephen MS, Waugh RC, et al. Pyogenic liver abscess: a review of 10 years' experience in management. *Aust N Z J Surg* 1999;69:205–209.

63. Pennington L, Kaufman S, Cameron JL. Intrahepatic abscess as a complication of long-term percutaneous internal biliary drainage. *Surgery* 1982;91:642–645.

64. Barreda R, Ros PR. Diagnostic imaging of liver abscess. *Crit Rev Diagn Imaging* 1992;33:29–58.

65. Murphy BJ, Casillas J, Ros PR, et al. The CT appearance of cystic masses of the liver. *Radiographics* 1989;9:307–322.

66. Halvorsen RA, Korobkin M, Foster WL, et al. The variable CT appearance of hepatic abscesses. *AJR Am J Roentgenol* 1984;142:941–946.

67. Gabata T, Kadoya M, Matsui O, et al. Dynamic CT of hepatic abscesses: significance of transient segmental enhancement. *AJR Am J Roentgenol* 2001;176:675–679.

68. Lawrence TS, Robertson JM, Anscher MS, et al. Hepatic toxicity resulting from cancer treatment. *Int J Radiat Oncol Biol Phys* 1995; 31:1237–1248.

69. Jeffrey RB Jr, Moss AA, Quivey JM, et al. CT of radiation-induced hepatic injury. *AJR Am J Roentgenol* 1980;135:445–448.

70. Willemart S, Nicaise N, Struyven J, et al. Acute radiation-induced hepatic injury: evaluation by triphasic contrast enhanced helical CT. *Br J Radiol* 2000;73:544–546.

71. Lewis JH, Patel HR, Zimmerman HJ. The spectrum of hepatic candidiasis. *Hepatology* 1982;2:479–487.

72. Pannu HK, Maley WR, Fishman EK. Liver transplantation: preoperative CT evaluation. *Radiographics* 2001;21 Spec No:S133–S146.

73. Haddad MC, Clark DC, Sharif HS, et al. MR, CT, and ultrasonography of splanchnic venous thrombosis. *Gastrointest Radiol* 1992;17:34–40.

74. Mitchell DG, Nazarian LN. Hepatic vascular diseases: CT and MRI. *Semin Ultrasound CT MR* 1995;16:49–68.

75. Mathieu D, Vasile N, Dibie C, et al. Portal cavernoma: dynamic CT features and transient differences in hepatic attenuation. *Radiology* 1985;154:743–748.

76. Mathieu D, Vasile N, Grenier P. Portal thrombosis: dynamic CT features and course. *Radiology* 1985;154:737–741.

77. Lee SJ, Lim JH, Lee WJ, et al. Transient subsegmental hepatic parenchymal enhancement on dynamic CT: a sign of postbiopsy arterioportal shunt. *J Comput Assist Tomogr* 1997;21:355–360.

78. Soyer P, Rabenandrasana A, Barge J, et al. MRI of Budd–Chiari syndrome. *Abdom Imaging* 1994;19:325–329.

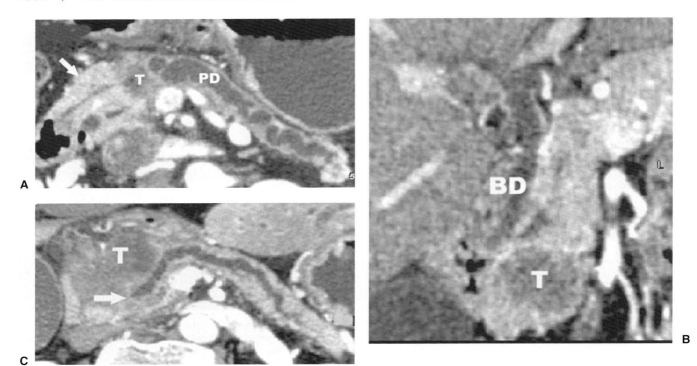

FIG. 12–5. A: A CPR of the pancreas demonstrating a hypoattenuating tumor (*T*) obstructing the pancreatic duct (*PD*). Note the normal enhancing head of the pancreas (*arrow*). **B:** A CPR through the bile duct (*BD*) demonstrating a well-defined hypoattenuating tumor (*T*) in the neck of the pancreas. **C:** Demonstrates a hypoattenuating tumor (*T*) obstructing the pancreatic duct (*arrow*).

a 35-second to 40-second delay. This late-arterial phase has been termed the pancreatic-parenchymal phase. The normal pancreas enhances avidly during the late-arterial phase of an intravenous contrast injection. Scanning at this time takes advantage of the fact that most ductal adenocarcinomas are hypovascular and will appear as low-attenuating masses compared to the intensely enhancing normal pancreas (Figure. 12–5). Hollett et al. have demonstrated a significant reduction in the pancreatic-parenchymal enhancement during the venous phase (60 seconds to 70 seconds following intravenous injection) (29). Therefore, most authorities feel that pancreatic phase scanning provides the greatest conspicuity for tumor identification (30,31). In addition to improving visualization of the tumor, the pancreatic phase facilitates visualization of major arterial structures to identify a critical finding of nonresectability: arterial encasement. Other lesions such as neuroendocrine tumors, which may mimic ductal adenocarcinoma, are characterized best in this late-arterial phase, as they are characteristically hypervascular. Scanning the entire liver during this phase will aid in the detection of hypervascular liver metastasis from malignant neuroendocrine tumors or depicting ring-like enhancement from metastatic adenocarcinoma of the pancreas.

Following scan acquisition during the late-arterial phase, the patient is instructed to breathe deeply and is repositioned to begin a second spiral acquisition at 70 seconds to 80 seconds following the initiation of contrast to scan the

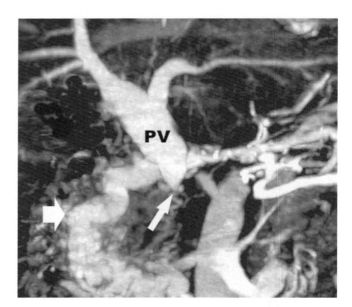

FIG. 12–6. Maximum-intensity projection demonstrating occlusion of portal venous system. Note focal area of occlusion of the main extrahepatic portal vein (*PV*) at the level of the junction of the superior mesenteric vein (*long arrow*). The *short arrow* indicates large collateral in the hepatoduodenal ligament.

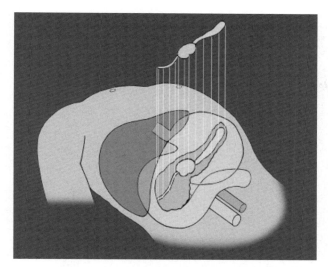

FIG. 12–7. Technique of CPR. In this schematic drawing, the pancreatic duct has been traced in its entirety in order to display focal dilatation of the distal duct by tumor in the mid-body of the pancreas.

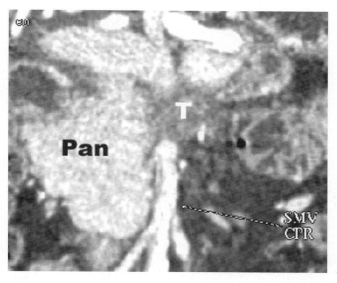

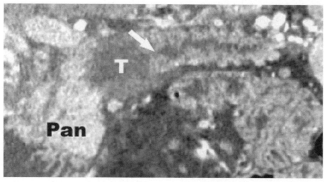

FIG. 12–9. Curved-planar reformation of locally invasive pancreatic carcinoma. **A:** A CPR of the root of the mesentery and superior mesenteric vein. Note hypodense tumor (*T*) adjacent to the superior mesenteric vein (*SMV*). This indicates root of the mesentery invasion. Normal enhancing pancreas is seen adjacent to the tumor (*PAN*). **B:** A CPR of the main pancreatic duct demonstrates the interrupted duct sign. Note obstruction and dilatation of the distal duct (*arrow*) by hypodense tumor (*T*). The normal enhancing pancreas is seen in the neck of the pancreas (PAN).

entire upper abdomen during the portal venous phase. Slice collimation for the venous phase is 2.5 mm to 5 mm depending upon the patient's body habitus. The portal-venous-phase acquisition is critical for the detection of hypovascular liver metastasis and the evaluation of tumor encasement of the portal venous system (Figure 12-6). Not infrequently, the depiction of collateral vessels from venous occlusion is an important secondary finding that is appreciated best during the portal-venous phase.

Both the pancreatic-parenchymal phase and the portal venous phase are reconstructed with overlapping reconstructions approximately one half the slice thickness of the scan acquisition in order to ensure optimal image display with 2D and 3D reformations (Figures 12–7 through 12–12).

IMAGING PROCESSING AND DISPLAY

One of the clear advantages of MDCT is the ability to obtain a volumetric dataset with near-isotropic voxels. These

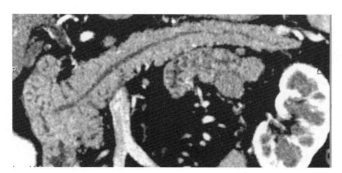

FIG. 12–8. Curved-planar reformation of the normal pancreatic duct. Note the pancreatic duct is 2 mm to 3 mm in its entirety without focal dilatation or evidence of a parenchymal mass.

datasets substantially improve the quality of 2D and 3D reformations. The evaluation of the peripancreatic vasculature often is the critical determinant in diagnosing locally advanced pancreatic carcinoma; thus, image displays that highlight tumor involvement of the major arteries and veins greatly facilitate diagnosis of locally advanced pancreatic carcinoma. While it is likely that in the near future there will be close integration of image display software to perform advanced visualization techniques, such as 2D and 3D reformations directly from the scanner, to date these reformations must be performed offline with a dedicated 3D workstation.

It certainly is true that for an experienced radiologist the axial images alone provide sufficient information to make an accurate diagnosis in the majority of patients. However, on occasion, the 2D and 3D displays provide unique informa-

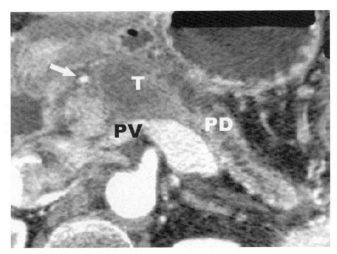

FIG. 12–10. Encasement of the gastric duodenal artery by pancreatic carcinoma. Note hypodense tumor (*T*) and dilated and obstructed pancreatic duct (*PD*). There is encasement of the gastric duodenal artery (*arrow*), as well as mass effect on the portal vein (*PV*) by the tumor.

tion regarding the extent of the tumor that may be difficult to appreciate on axial images alone. Perhaps the most significant contribution of these unique visualization displays is for our referring clinicians. A MDCT of the pancreas for staging of ductal adenocarcinoma may involve hundreds of images. A limited number of 2D and 3D displays often can display rapidly the salient features of the tumor that create a time-efficient review of the case for busy surgeons and gastroenterologists (32).

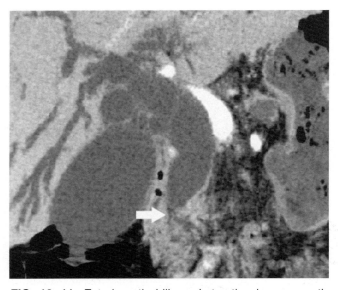

FIG. 12–11. Extrahepatic biliary obstruction by pancreatic carcinoma. Minimum-intensity projection of the biliary tree demonstrates abrupt termination of the distal duct due to an isodense pancreatic carcinoma (*arrow* indicates point of obstruction).

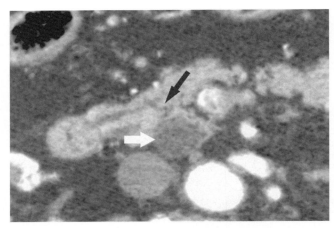

FIG. 12–12. Side-branch IPMT. Note cystic mass in the uncinate process on the MinIP (*arrow*, side-branch IPMT). The connection to the ductal system is noted by the *black arrow.*

One significant limitation of the requirement to perform offline-imaging processing is that it is somewhat time consuming, although attempts are being made to automate some types of image display (33). A complete depiction of all the peripancreatic vasculature with an array of 2D and 3D displays may take trained technologists 20 minutes to 30 minutes; thus this is not time efficient for most radiologists to perform the reformations themselves. The requirement for trained personnel to perform offline reformations has limited the extent of utilization of these image displays. It is clear that a closer integration of the display software with the CT-scan acquisition will enhance the applicability of these displays and lead to more widespread use in the radiologic community.

A number of important technical factors to achieving optimal 2D and 3D displays have been learned from prior experience with the processing of CT-angiography data. It is essential to perform overlapping reconstructions at one half the slice thickness of the scan acquisition in order to ensure optimal spatial resolution. In addition, the pancreatic-parenchymal-phase images are reconstructed with a 20-cm field of view focusing directly on the pancreas and peripancreatic vasculature. This focused reconstruction also aids in improving the quality of reformations.

There are a variety of image display and image processing options that may be used to delineate both the pancreatic tumor and its local involvement of the peripancreatic vasculature. These include curved planar reformations, minimum-intensity images, volume-rendered images, standard coronal and sagittal plane reformations, as well as coronal-oblique reformations along the splenic-portovenous confluence.

IMAGE DISPLAY OPTIONS

Curved Planar Reformations

Curved planar reformations (CPRs) display in 2D the 3D course of a tubular structure within the CT volumetric dataset (9,33). This type of display is understood easily by pancreatic surgeons and gastroenterologists, and thus has an important role in time-efficient display of complex anatomic relationships. Curved planar reformations are obtained by manually tracing the course of a tubular structure through a stacked volume of axial-sagittal-coronal images (Figure 12-7). The proscribed plane then is displayed in a 2D image, delineating the entire 3D course of the blood vessel or ductal structure. Curved planar reformations were obtained routinely in two orthogonal planes. Curved-transverse and curved-coronal reformations have been the most useful for our clinicians. Curved-planar reformations may be valuable for tracing the course of the common bile duct, common pancreatic duct, and peripancreatic arterial and venous structures (Figures 12–8 through 12–10). Because soft tissues are displayed at the same time as various ductal and vascular structures, they particularly are useful for determining vascular encasement and/or complete or partial obstruction of the common bile duct or pancreatic duct (9). Although it takes a modest degree of training to be able to trace accurately through a stack of images, the anatomic planes of the various pancreatic ductal and tubular structures, these reformations are performed routinely by technologists dedicated to the use of 3D workstations.

Minimum-intensity Projections

Minimum-intensity projections (MinIPs) are derived using a ray-projection technique, which records the minimum pixel value along the projection (34). The main value of MinIPs is to display low-attenuating structures such as the pancreatic and common bile ducts (Figures. 12–11 through 12–14). Minimum-intensity projections generally are performed on a slab of images 15 mm to 30 mm thick, depending upon the low-attenuation structures that are to be dis-

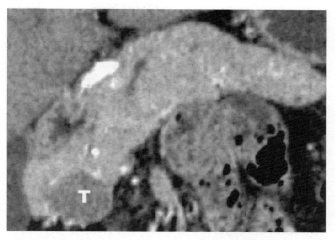

FIG. 12–14. Minimum-intensity projection display of carcinoma of the pancreas. Note hypoattenuating tumor (*T*) within the head of the pancreas.

played. Maximum-intensity images (recording the highest attenuation along the projection) may be useful to evaluate high-attenuation structures such as the peripancreatic vasculature (Figure 12-15).

Volume Rendering

Volume rendering interpolates all of the attenuation values along a pixel projection, assigning both color and opacity to each voxel (11,12). Different anatomic structures

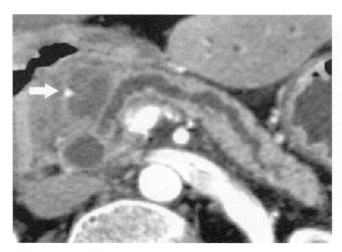

FIG. 12–13. Minimum-intensity projection demonstrating gastroduodenal artery encasement (*arrow*). Note surrounding hypoattenuating tumor and dilated pancreatic duct.

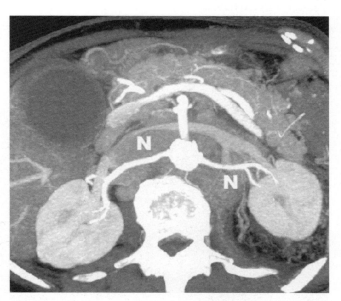

FIG. 12–15. Maximum-intensity projection of patient referred for suspicion of pancreatic carcinoma. Note excellent visualization of the abdominal vasculature from an inferior-to-superior view. There is bulky retroperitoneal lymphadenopathy from metastatic carcinoma of the lung surrounding the renal arteries (*N*, nodes).

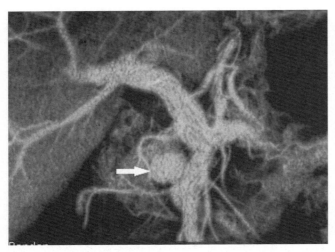

FIG. 12–16. Volume-rendered image of insulinoma. Note high-attenuation rounded focus in the neck of the pancreas immediately adjacent to the SMV (*arrow*). At surgery, this was proven to be an insulinoma.

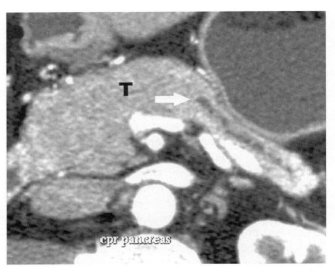

FIG. 12–18. Large isoattenuating pancreatic carcinoma. Note "interrupted duct" sign (*arrow*) by large isodense tumor (*T*).

can be highlighted depending upon their attenuation by varying the opacity and color curves (Figure 12-16). The main value of volume-rendered images is to delineate peripancreatic vessels and tumor encasement. Cut-plane volume-rendered images, which eliminate extraneous soft tissues, may be performed, and a series of images may be performed to rotate along a specific axis to provide unique spatial orientation of complex structures.

MDCT FINDINGS IN PANCREATIC DUCTAL ADENOCARCINOMA

The majority of ductal adenocarcinomas of the pancreas are hypovascular and will be most conspicuous during the pancreatic-parenchymal phase of a late-arterial intravenous (IV) injection. However, a small percentage (approximately

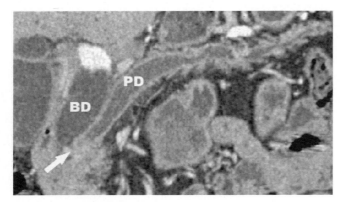

FIG. 12–17. Double duct sign from isodense pancreatic carcinoma. Note marked dilatation of the bile duct (*BD*) and main pancreatic duct (*PD*) by isoattenuating pancreatic carcinoma (*arrow*).

10%) of ductal adenocarcinomas are isodense, showing little attenuation-value difference from the normal enhancing pancreas (Figures 12–17 and 12–18). Although larger isodense pancreatic carcinomas will demonstrate an obvious contour abnormality of the pancreas with surrounding mass effect, smaller isodense tumors may not be detected easily unless it is recognized clearly that there is partial or complete obstruction of the pancreatic duct (the "interrupted duct" sign). In the absence of intraductal calcifications indicating chronic pancreatitis, dilatation of the main pancreatic duct always should be viewed with suspicion for an underlying pancreatic-parenchymal or intraductal mass. The same degree of ductal size should be apparent in all areas of the gland, including the head, body, and tail. Focal dilatation of the pancreatic duct in the body or the tail often is a key finding in a small isodense carcinoma. Thus, the interrupted duct sign is a critical finding in order not to miss a small isoattenuating lesion. Various 2D and 3D displays (CPR and MinIPs) often highlight areas of partial or complete pancreatic ductal obstruction, facilitating the diagnosis. Studies have demonstrated that isoattenuating lesions on both pancreatic-phase and venous phase images correlate with tumors of increased cellularity. In addition, lesions that initially are hypodense on the pancreatic-parenchymal phase that are noted to be hyperdense on later venous-phase images correlate with fibrotic changes within the tumor.

LOCAL STAGING OF PANCREATIC CARCINOMA

The main values of MDCT of the pancreas are: i) improved spatial resolution that accompanies the use of thinner collimation and ii) optimal contrast enhancement of the pancreas and surrounding vasculature during the late-arterial phase. Whether MDCT will have a major impact on local staging compared to single-slice CT is debatable, given the fact that approximately 70% of the patients presenting with adenocarcinoma already have obvious locally advanced or metastatic disease (13–15). Single-slice helical CT appears to be highly accurate (virtually 100%) for staging patients with locally advanced disease by virtue of detecting encasement of peripancreatic vessels or direct involvement of adjacent organs such as the stomach or spleen (15). In most instances, only lesions in the head of the pancreas are truly resectable for cure. Lesions of the body and tail usually have extrapancreatic perineural lymphatic invasion at the time of clinical presentation. The combination of CT, MRI, magnetic resonance cholangio pancreatography (MRCP), and endoscopic ultrasound has facilitated greatly the diagnosis of local staging.

The most commonly used criteria to diagnose locally advanced disease include tumor encasement or occlusion of major extrapancreatic blood vessels and direct invasion of contiguous solid or hollow organs (Figures 12–19 through 12–27). Although a few surgeons take the view that patients can undergo successfully reconstruction of the portal vein when encased by tumor, most authorities believe that venous encasement or invasion indicates a poor prognosis; thus, these patients are considered to have locally advanced disease not resectable for cure (Figures 12–19 and 12–20)(35).

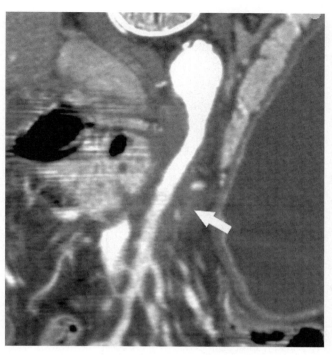

FIG. 12–20. Encasement of the SMA by pancreatic carcinoma on CPR. Note soft tissue infiltration along the length of the proximal SMA (*arrow*) indicating a lesion not resectable for cure.

It generally is accepted that if there is a clearly visible fat plane between the tumor and major peripancreatic vessels such as the superior mesenteric artery and vein, in the absence of peritoneal or hepatic metastases, pancreatic resection can be accomplished without positive margins. Surgical

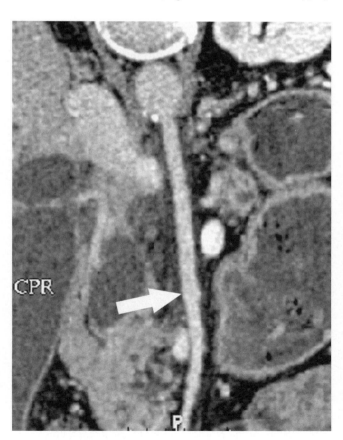

FIG. 12–19. Normal CPR of the superior mesenteric artery (SMA). Note the preserved fat at the root of the mesentery along the course of the SMA.

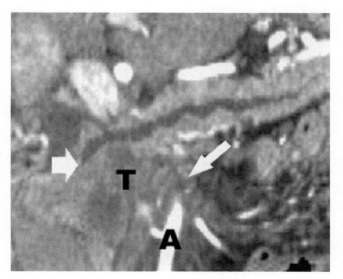

FIG. 12–21. Root of the mesentery and SMA encasement from pancreatic carcinoma. Note hypodense tumor (*T*) with involvement of the root of the mesentery (*long arrow*). Note the obstructed pancreatic duct (*arrow, A,* SMA).

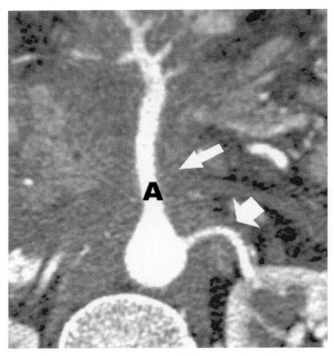

FIG. 12–22. Superior mesenteric artery and renal artery encasement from pancreatic carcinoma. Note extensive soft-tissue infiltration (*arrow*) around the SMA (*A*). *Short arrow* indicates encasement of an accessory left renal artery by tumor.

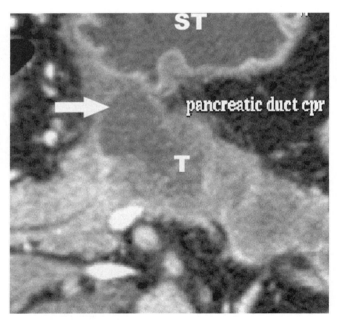

FIG. 12–23. Hollow viscous invasion from pancreatic carcinoma. Note hypodense tumor in the body of the pancreas extending through the lesser sac (*arrow*) to invade the serosa of the stomach (*ST*).

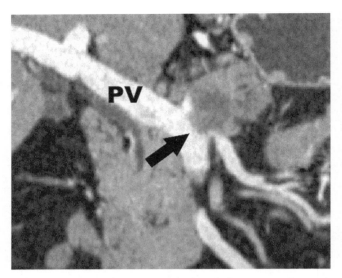

FIG. 12–24. Invasion of the splenic vein by pancreatic carcinoma. Note hypoattenuating tumor mass invading the splenic vein at its junction with the SMV (*arrow*). Main portal vein is free of tumor (*PV*).

margins following pancreatic resection are critical, as clinical pathologic studies have shown that there is no survival benefit to the surgery in patients with positive surgical margins. Contiguity of the tumor to the superior mesenteric artery and vein does not necessarily indicate adventitial invasion. If there is soft tissue infiltrating circumferentially around the artery, tumor encasement can be diagnosed with confidence. Some authorities have demonstrated that the degree of circumferential involvement at the vessel is highly predictive of vascular invasion. If 50% or more of the circumference of this superior mesenteric vein or artery infiltrated with tumor, there is a strong likelihood of vascular invasion, making the patient nonresectable for cure (31,36,37). In some patients, tumor infiltration of the superior mesenteric vein (SMV) results in a "teardrop" configuration rather than the normal rounded or oval appearance (Figures 12–26 and 12–27).

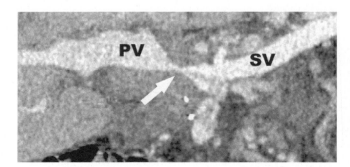

FIG. 12–25. Venous encasement by pancreatic carcinoma on CPR. Note a hypodense tumor narrowing the extrahepatic portal vein (*PV*) just proximal to its junction with the splenic vein (*arrow*; *SV*, splenic vein).

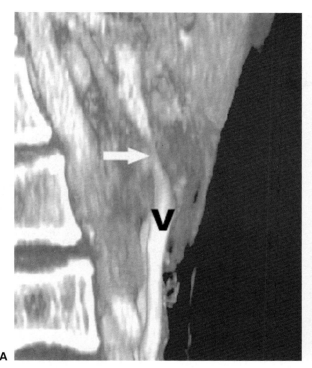
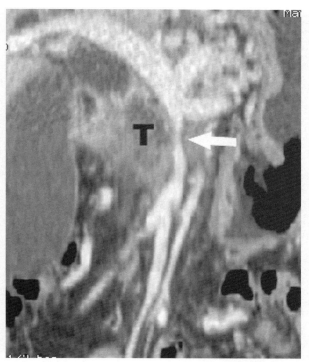

A   B

FIG. 12–26. Superior mesenteric vein encasement by pancreatic carcinoma. Sagittal view **(A)** demonstrates marked narrowing of the SMV by pancreatic carcinoma (V, vein). The tumor is less apparent on the volume-rendered view. In **(B)**, which is a CPR of the splenic portal venous system, note the good visualization of the hypoattenuating tumor (T) and the marked narrowing of the SMV (*arrow*).

PITFALLS IN THE DIAGNOSIS OF PANCREATIC ADENOCARCINOMA

Distinguishing focal pancreatitis from ductal adenocarcinoma has been an ongoing clinical and imaging problem. Enhancement patterns of the mass due to chronic inflammation and fibrosis may mimic that of carcinoma. In a clinical setting of chronic pancreatitis, the CT demonstration of generalized dilatation of the pancreatic duct with multiple intraductal concretions makes diagnosis of chronic pancreatitis very likely. In the absence of these findings, a focal hypodense mass may be either entity. Percutaneous-guided biopsy may be helpful in selected cases, as may PET scanning. More recently, MRCP is demonstrating that most inflammatory pancreatic masses have either a normal pancreatic duct or smooth tapering of the pancreatic duct (duct-penetrating sign), which may be the most useful finding to differentiate the two (38).

LESS COMMON PANCREATIC TUMORS

Multidetector CT has been of particular value in the detection of neuroendocrine tumors, both functional and nonfunctional. Both types of lesions are characteristically hypervascular, and therefore are imaged best during the pancreatic-parenchymal phase of the contrast injection. The newest MDCT scanners with both 8- and 16-slice options can image the entire liver with very thin collimation (1.25 mm) and thus detect even relatively small hypervascular metastasis from these lesions (Figure 12-28). The most common functioning neuroendocrine tumors encountered in clinical practice are insulinomas and gastronomas (39). Rare lesions include glucagonomas, somatostatinomas, carcinoid tumors, and tumors that secrete vasoactive intestinal peptide (VI-Poma). In general, nonfunctioning tumors often present clin-

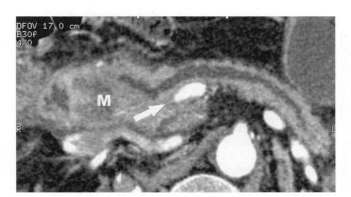

FIG. 12–27. Teardrop sign indicating invasion of the SMV by pancreatic carcinoma. Note hypoattenuating tumor mass (*M*) and abnormal configuration of the SMV, which has the appearance of a teardrop (*arrow*). This is due to infiltration of the adventitia of the SMV, making the patient not resectable for cure.

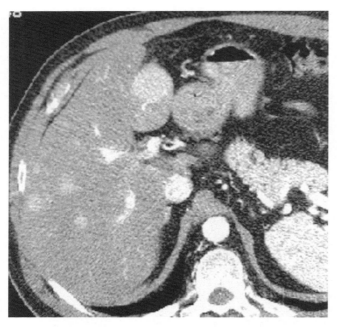

FIG. 12–28. Multiple hypervascular liver metastases from metastatic neuroendocrine tumor of the pancreas. Note numerous hyperattenuating foci in the liver.

ically due to the mass effect from their large size. Although they may produce small amounts of hormones, they are insufficient to cause clinically recognizable syndromes.

Until quite recently, functioning neuroendocrine tumors, particularly in patients with multiple endocrine-neoplasia syndromes, required invasive procedures for detection and localization of these lesions. Not infrequently, these lesions are small and multiple. In the past, arteriography and portal venous sampling were used frequently for diagnosis and localization. The combination of MDCT, MRI, and intraoperative ultrasound largely has supplanted invasive procedures (Figure 12-29) (40–42). Preoperatively, either dual-phase MDCT or MRI with gadolinium enhancement is obtained followed by careful evaluation of the pancreas and duodenum with intraoperative ultrasound. In experienced hands, this is a highly effective way to diagnose even small hypervascular lesions.

CYSTIC PANCREATIC NEOPLASMS

Cystic pancreatic tumors may be classified according to the cells of origin (acinar, centroacinar, or ductal cells) and their relationship to the main pancreatic ductal system (43,44). These lesions most often are epithelial in origin. Although relatively uncommon, the use of thin-collimation

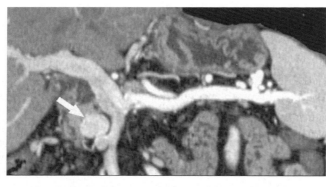

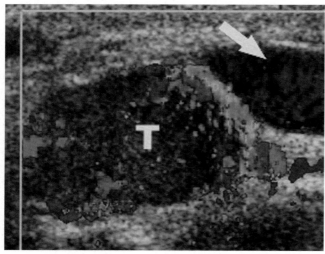

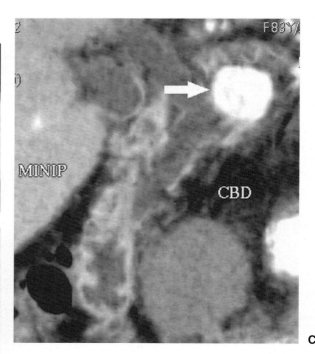

FIG. 12–29. Neuroendocrine tumor. **A:** A CPR of the portal-venous system demonstrates high-attenuating neuroendocrine tumor (*arrow*) in the neck of the pancreas. At surgery, this proved to be an insulinoma. In the same patient, **(B)** shows a hypervascular tumor nodule seen on intraoperative ultrasound (*T*, tumor, *arrow*, SMV). Minimum-intensity image in the same patient, **(C)**, demonstrates proximity of hypervascular tumor nodule (*arrow*) to common bile duct.

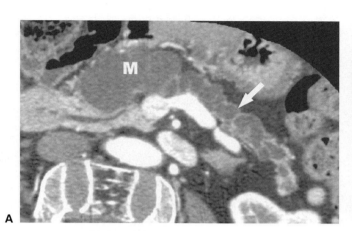

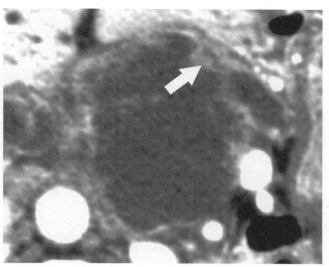

FIG. 12–30. Mucinous cystic lesions of the pancreas. Note in **(A)** a cystic mass in the neck of the pancreas (*M*) obstructing the distal pancreatic duct (*arrow*). Note marked parenchymal atrophy of the distal pancreas. There are no features to suggest a malignant neoplasm. This was a mucinous cystadenoma at surgery. **B:** A mucinous cystadenocarcinoma. Note cystic mass in the head of the pancreas containing mural nodularity along the wall. Surgery revealed frank adenocarcinoma within the cystic mass. *Arrow* indicates tumor nodule.

MDCT has improved substantially the detection of smaller lesions. Microcystic neoplasms are glycogen rich, benign lesions that in the past have been referred to as serous cystadenomas (43,44,44a,44b). Mucinous cystic neoplasms (in the past referred to as macrocystic adenomas or adenocarcinomas) all are considered to have malignant potential (Figure 12-30). Mucinous cystic tumors that arise from the ductal epithelium are referred to as intraductal papillary mucinous tumors (IPMT). Although IPMT lesions are somewhat more common in men, other types of cystic neoplasms have a striking predilection for women.

Mucinous cystic tumors, whether intrinsic to the ductal system or separate cystic masses, all have substantial malignant potential. They are morphologically and pathologically quite similar to mucinous cystic neoplasms of the ovary. Specific features of malignancy include thickened and irregular septations within the lesion, as well as mural nodules. Calcification, although relatively uncommon, occurs characteristically on the periphery of this lesion, as opposed to the central calcification that may be seen with microcystic adenomas (Figure 12-30). Therefore, the only lesions that can be followed safely are lesions that can be classified morphologically as microcystic neoplasms or very small side-branch IPMT lesions. Microcystic neoplasms characteristically have tiny, often microscopic, cystic elements separated by fibrous stroma (43). During the arterial phase of injection, the fibrous stroma enhance intensely, giving an almost-solid appearance to this lesion in many areas of the tumor (Figure 12-31). If this distinctive morphology can be recognized, a definitive diagnosis of microcystic adenoma can be established and the patient followed with serial-imaging studies.

On the other hand, in the absence of definitive morphology, surgery or cyst aspiration must be performed to achieve a more definitive diagnosis. Positron-emission-tomography scanning may play a role in assessing malignant lesions due to the hypermetabolic function of these tumors.

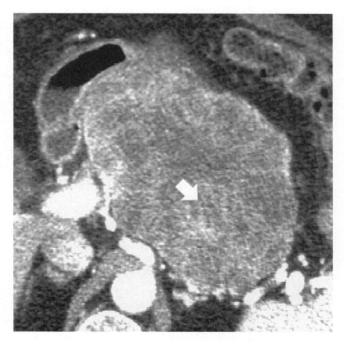

FIG. 12–31. Microcystic adenoma. Note linear enhancement of dense stromal tissue (*arrow*), diagnostic of microcystic adenoma.

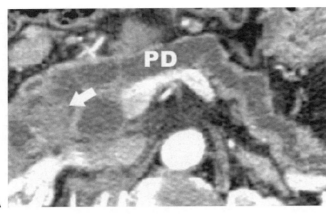
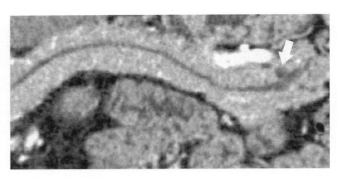

FIG. 12–32. A,B: Main duct-type intraductal papillary mucinous tumor (IPMT). Note marked dilatation of the main pancreatic duct (*PD*) and soft-tissue mass within the ductal system in the neck of the pancreas (*arrow*). At surgery, adenocarcinoma from the IPMT was detected. **B:** Demonstrates combined side-branch and main ductal form of IPMT. Note cystic outpouching of the distal pancreatic duct in its tail, with slight focal dilatation of the main duct adjacent to it. At surgery, a side-branch IPMT was detected with mucin involving the main pancreatic duct. Hyperplasia was noted without frank invasive carcinoma.

Intraductal papillary mucinous tumors may be classified according to the extent and anatomic degree of involvement of the main pancreatic-ductal system (44–48). These include main duct type, branch duct type, or combined lesions (Fig. 12-32). With main duct-type lesions, there may be marked generalized dilatation of the main pancreatic duct. In other examples, it may be more focal and segmental.

REFERENCES

1. Klein AP, Hruban RH, Brune KA, et al. Familial pancreatic cancer. *Cancer J* 2001;7(4):266–273.
2. Li D. Molecular epidemiology of pancreatic cancer. *Cancer J* 2001; 7(4):259–265.
3. Tsiotos GG, Farnell MB, Sarr MG. Are the results of pancreatectomy for pancreatic cancer improving? *World J Surg* 1999;23(9):913–919.
4. Cooperman AM. Pancreatic cancer: the bigger picture. *Surg Clin North Am* 2001;81(3):557–574.
5. Bathe OF, Caldera H, Hamilton KL, et al. Diminished benefit from resection of cancer of the head of the pancreas in patients of advanced age. *J Surg Oncol* 2001;77(2):115–122.
6. Brand R. The diagnosis of pancreatic cancer. *Cancer J* 2001;7(4): 287–297.
7. Johnson CD. Pancreatic carcinoma: developing a protocol for multidetector row CT. *Radiology* 2001;220(1):3–4.
8. Fishman EK, Horton KM, Urban BA. Multidetector CT angiography in the evaluation of pancreatic carcinoma: preliminary observations. *J Comp Assist Tomogr* 2000;24(6):849–853.
9. Nino-Murcia M, Jeffrey RB Jr, Beaulieu CF, et al. Multidetector CT of the pancreas and bile duct system: value of curved planar reformations. *AJR Am J Roentgenol* 2001;176(3):689–693.
10. Tamm E, Charnsangavej C. Panceatic cancer: current concepts in imaging for diagnosis and staging. *Cancer J* 2001;7(4):298–311.
11. Horton KM, Fishman EK. Multidetector CT angiography of pancreatic carcinoma: part 1, evaluation of arterial involvement. *AJR Am J Roentgenol* 2002;178(4):827–831.
12. Horton KM, Fishman EK. Multidetector CT angiography of pancreatic carcinoma: part 2, evaluation of venous involvement. *AJR Am J Roentgenol* 2002;178(4):833–836.
13. Tamm E, Charnsangavej C. Pancreatic cancer: current concepts in imaging for diagnosis and staging. *Cancer J* 2001;7(4):298–311.
14. Del Frate C, Zanardi R, Mortele K, et al. Advances in imaging for pancreatic disease. *Curr Gastroenterol Rep* 2002;4(2):140–148.
15. Freeny PC. Pancreatic carcinoma: imaging update 2001. *Dig Dis* 2001; 19(1):37–46.
16. Hanbidge AE. Cancer of the pancreas: the best image for early detection—CT, MRI, PET or US? *Cancer J Gastroenterol* 2002;16(2): 101–105.
17. Fischer U, Vosshenrich R, Horstmann O, et al. Preoperative local MRI-staging of patients with a suspected pancreatic mass. *Eur Radiol* 2002; 12(2):296–303.
18. Robinson PA. The role of MRI in pancreatic cancer. *Eur Radiol* 2002; 12(2):267–269.
19. Meining A, Dittler HJ, Wolf A, et al. You get what you expect? A critical appraisal of imaging methodology in endosonographic cancer staging. *Gut* 2002;50(5):599–603.
20. Levy MJ, Wiersema MJ. Endoscopic ultrasound in the diagnosis and staging of pancreatic cancer. *Oncology* 2002;16(1):29–38, 43; discussion 44, 47–49, 53–56.
21. Jadvar H, Fischman AJ. Evaluation of pancreatic carcinoma with FDG PET. *Abdom Imaging* 2001;26(3):254–259.
22. Sperti C, Pasquali C, Chierichetti F, et al. Value of 18-fluorodeoxyglucose positron emission tomography in the management of patients with cystic tumors of the pancreas. *Ann Surg* 2001;234(5):675–680.
23. Valls C, Andia E, Sanchez A, et al. Dual-phase helical CT of pancreatic adenocarcinoma: assessment of resectability before surgery. *AJR Am J Roentgenol* 2002;178(4):821–826.
24. Kedra B, Popiela T, Sierzega M, et al. Prognostic factors of long-term survival after resective procedures for pancreatic cancer. *Hepatogastroenterology* 2001;48:1762–1766.
25. Farnell MB, Nagorney DM, Sarr MG. The Mayo Clinic approach to the surgical treatment of adenocarcinoma of the pancreas. *Surg Clin North Am* 2001;81(3):611–623.
26. Lee JH, Whittington R, Williams NN, et al. Outcome of pancreaticodu-odenectomy and impact of adjuvant therapy for ampullary carcinomas. *Int J Radiat Oncol Biol Phys* 2000;47(4):945–953.
27. Toh SK, Davies N, Dolan P, et al. Good outcome from surgery for ampullary tumor. *Aust N Z J Surg* 1999;69(3):195–198.
28. Howe JR, Klimstra DS, Moccia RD, et al. Factors predictive of survival in ampullary carcinoma. *Ann Surg* 1998;228(1):87–94.
29. Hollett MD, Jorgensen MJ, Jeffrey RB Jr. Quantitative evaluation of pancreatic enhancement during dual-phase helical CT. *Radiology* 1995; 195(2):359–361.
30. Boland GW, O'Malley ME, Saez M, et al. Pancreatic-phase versus portal vein-phase helical CT of the pancreas: optimal temporal window

for evaluation of pancreatic adenocarcinoma. *AJR Am J Roentgenol* 1999;172(3):605–608.

31. Lu DSK, Vedantham S, Krasny RM, et al. Two-phase helical CT for pancreatic tumors: pancreatic versus hepatic phase enhancement of tumor, pancreas, and vascular structures. *Radiology* 1996;199(3): 697–701.

32. Rubin GD. Data explosion: the challenge of multidetector-row CT. *Eur J Radiol* 2000;36(2):74–80.

33. Raman R, Napel S, Beaulieu CF, et al. Automated generation of curved planar reformations from volume data: method and evaluation. *Radiology* 2002;223(1):275–280.

34. Raptopoulos V, Prassopoulos P, Chuttani R, et al. Multiplanar CT pancreatography and distal cholangiography with minimum intensity projections. *Radiology* 1998;207(2):317–324.

35. Tuech JJ, Pessaux P, Arnaud JP. Portal vein resection in pancreatic head carcinoma. Part 2: clinical significance. *Hepatogastroenterology* 2001;48(39):888–891.

36. Hough TJ, Raptopoulos V, Siewert B, et al. Teardrop superior mesenteric vein: CT sign for unresectable carcinoma of the pancreas. *AJR Am J Roentgenol* 1999;173(6):1509–1512.

37. O'Malley ME, Boland GW, Wood BJ, et al. Adenocarcinoma of the head of the pancreas: determination of surgical unresectability with thin-section pancreatic-phase helical CT. *AJR Am J Roentgenol* 1999; 173(6):1513–1518.

38. Ichikawa T, Sou H, Araki T, et al. Duct-penetrating sign at MRCP: usefulness for differentiating inflammatory pancreatic mass from pancreatic carcinoma. *Radiology* 2001;221(1):107–116.

39. Brentjens R, Saltz L. Islet cell tumors of the pancreas. *Surg Clin North Am* 2001;81(3):527–542.

40. Ichikawa T, Peterson MS, Federle MP, et al. Islet cell tumor of the pancreas: biphasic CT versus MR imaging in tumor detection. *Radiology* 2000;216(1):163–171.

41. Owen NJ, Sohaib SA, Peppercorn PD, et al. MRI of pancreatic neuroendocrine tumors. *Br J Radiol* 2001;74(886):968–973.

42. Hiramoto JS, Feldstein VA, LaBerge JM, et al. Intraoperative ultrasound and preoperative localization detects all occult insulinomas. *Arch Surg* 2001;136(9):1020–1025, discussion 1025–1026.

43. Curry CA, Eng J, Horton KM, et al. CT of primary cystic pancreatic neoplasms: can CT be used for patient triage and treatment? *AJR Am J Roentgenol* 2000;175(1):99–103.

44a. Megibow AJ, Lavelle MT, Rofsky NM. Cystic tumors of the pancreas: the radiologist. *Surg Clin North Am* 2001;81(3): 489–495.

44b. Taouli B, Vilgrain V, O'Toole D, et al. Intraductal papillary mucinous tumors of the pancreas: features with multimodality imaging. *J Comput Assist Tomogr* 2002;26(2):223–231.

45. Sugiura H, Kondo S, Islam HK, et al. Clinicopathologic features and outcomes of intraductal papillary-mucinous tumors of the pancreas. *Hepatogastroenterology* 2002;49(43):263–267.

46. Procacci C, Carbognin G, Biasiutti C, et al. Intraductal papillary mucinous tumors of the pancreas: spectrum of CT and MR findings with pathologic correlation. *Eur Radiol* 2001;11(10):1939–1951.

47. Silas AM, Morrin MM, Raptopoulos V, et al. Intraductal papillary mucinous tumors of the pancreas. *Am J Radiol* 2001;176(1):179–185.

48. Taouli B, Vilgrain V, Vullierme MP, et al. Intraductal papillary mucinous tumors of the pancreas: helical CT with histopathologic correlation. *Radiology* 2000;217(3):757–764.

CHAPTER 13

Multidetector CT Evaluation of Acute Pancreatitis and Its Complications

Elliot K. Fishman

INTRODUCTION

Multidetector computed-tomography (MDCT) scanners using 4-detector rows, and more recently, 16-detector rows, are the latest advancement in computed-tomography (CT) technology and quickly have become the gold standard for evaluation of pancreatic pathology. The usefulness of CT in detection and staging of pancreatic neoplasms has been addressed. This chapter will focus on the role of MDCT in evaluation of patients with known or suspected pancreatic inflammatory disease, with emphasis on the use of CT to guide patient therapy and determine surgical management versus medical management.

Acute Pancreatitis: An Overview

Acute pancreatitis is a complex inflammatory process involving the pancreatic gland. The pathological definition of acute pancreatitis is a nonbacterial inflammation of the pancreatic gland caused by the activation and digestion of the gland by its own enzymes. The pathophysiology of pancreatitis is a chain of events resulting from blockage of the pancreatic duct with subsequent release of pancreatic enzymes into the interstitium of the gland. In its early stage, pancreatitis is characterized by interstitial edema. Peripancreatic-fat necrosis results from more severe involvement. Involvement of the parenchymal acini of the gland also occurs, resulting in foci of hemorrhage, vascular necrosis, disruption of the pancreatic ducts, and eventually pancreatic necrosis. Mild acute pancreatitis is characterized clinically by minimal symptoms, which respond rapidly to conservative management, with few patients progressing to severe pancreatitis. Severe pancreatitis presents with more pronounced signs and symptoms and can progress to hemorrhagic or necrotizing pancreatitis. These patients may demonstrate multisystem organ failure, hypotension, and shock, as well as hypocalcemia and disseminated intravascular coagulation.

The most common etiology of acute pancreatitis is gallbladder disease (i.e., cholelithiasis), which accounts for over 40% of cases. Alcoholic pancreatitis is the cause in another 40% of patients. Other causes include hypercalcemic states, of which the most commonly recognized condition is hyperparathyroidism, as well as hyperlipidemia, familial pancreatitis, trauma including postprocedure trauma [i.e., endoscopic retrograde cholangiopancreatography (ERCP)], drug-induced pancreatitis (i.e., steroids, thiazide diuretics, and azathioprine), and rare causes such as a scorpion bite (1–5) (Figures 13–1, 13–2, and 13–3).

Role of MDCT in Pancreatitis

Most cases of acute pancreatitis are diagnosed clinically and do not rely on imaging (5). However, the history and presentation of the patient often may not be straightforward, and a reliable imaging modality is needed to establish the diagnosis (2–4,6). For nearly two decades, CT has been the imaging procedure of choice in the initial evaluation and follow up of patients with suspected pancreatitis. The sensitivity of helical CT for the diagnosis of acute pancreatitis is not known, especially in very mild cases, but it is reasonable to assume that a good quality contrast-enhanced helical-CT scan will demonstrate definite changes in the vast majority of patients with moderate-to-severe involvement. Helical CT depicts all but the mildest forms of acute pancreatitis, demonstrates most major complications, and can help guide percutaneous aspiration and drainage. Helical CT also is indicated when there is failure of clinical response to treatment. In addition, helical CT confidently can detect other causes of abdominal pain in patients initially thought to have

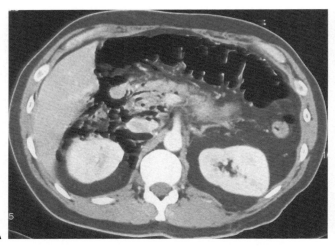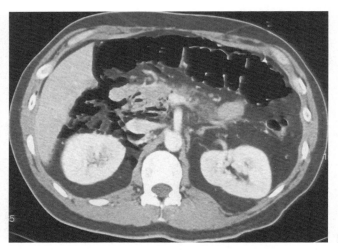

FIG. 13–1. Acute pancreatitis following ERCP. **A,B:** Computed tomography demonstrates air around pancreas, portal vein, and right kidney due to perforation of duodenum at time of sphincterotomy. Inflammation of pancreatic gland is shown as well.

symptoms of acute pancreatitis (Figures 13–4, 13–5, and 13–6).

Helical-CT Technique

Diagnostic evaluation of the pancreas, with either single- or multidetector-row helical CT, always has required careful attention to study technique and protocol. Dual-phase helical scanning during both the arterial- and portal-venous phases has several advantages when imaging the pancreas. The arterial phase is superior to the portal-venous phase for visualization of mesenteric and peripancreatic arteries. Opacification of the splenic-vein, superior mesenteric-vein, and portal-venous confluence is obtained better during the more delayed portal-venous phase. The pancreatic paren-

chyma is seen best in the parenchymal phase, approximately 50 seconds after the start of injection (7–8).

Although specific parameters will vary between scanners, several basic scanning concepts remain constant. Thin collimation scanning is essential. With single-detection helical CT, slice collimation typically was 3.0 mm to 5.0 mm, with a reconstruction interval of 2.0 mm to 5.0 mm. With the newest MDCT scanners, typical study parameters are 3.0-mm slice thickness and data reconstruction at 3 mm for routine studies. When complications are suspected, or when more detail is needed, 1.0-mm detectors can be used on a 4-slice scanner to obtain 1.25-mm slice thickness and reconstruct data at 1.0-mm intervals. On a 16-slice scanner, 0.75-mm detectors can be used to create 0.75-mm slice thickness and reconstruct data at 0.5-mm intervals. Typically, the en-

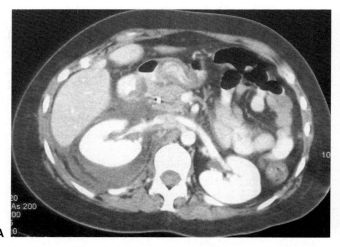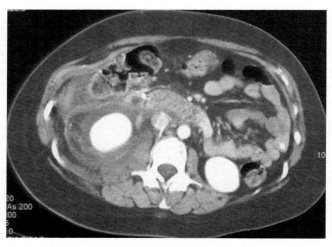

FIG. 13–2. Post-ERCP pancreatitis with extensive inflammation tracking to right perirenal and pararenal spaces. **A,B:** Computed tomography demonstrates inflammation of pancreas with fluid tracking to right lower quadrant, as is common in post-ERCP pancreatitis. Please note that this fluid within perirenal space can result in a Page kidney.

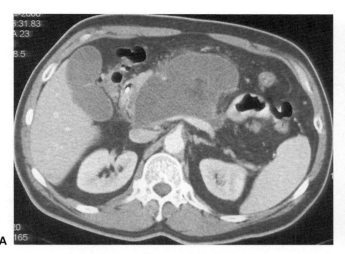
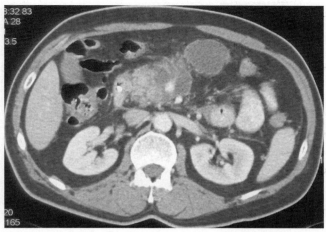

FIG. 13–3. Acute pancreatitis in patient with hypercalcemia felt to be due to parathyroid adenoma. **A,B:** Computed tomography demonstrates evidence of acute pancreatitis with fluid around pancreatic head and body. Mass effect on portal vein is noted.

tire abdomen and pelvis is scanned in order to evaluate fully the extent of pancreatic-fluid collections and ascites.

Bolus intravenous (IV)-contrast administration also is critical. The injection rate for evaluation of suspected pancreatitis is typically 2 mL to 3 mL per second, with the higher injection rate helpful for vascular and three-dimensional (3D) mapping. A total of 100 mL to 120 mL nonionic contrast agent is sufficient for most cases. Scans in the arterial phase begin 25 seconds to 30 seconds after the start of contrast injection, and at 50 seconds to 60 seconds for portal-phase imaging. Dual-phase studies combine both acquisi-

tions and are recommended in most patients, especially when there are clinical concerns of hemorrhage, pseudoaneurysm, or necrosis. In addition, initial noncontrast images of the pancreas can be helpful for depiction of acute hemorrhage.

In the past, positive oral contrast (750 mL–1000 mL) commonly was used for differentiating fluid collections from unopacified bowel. However, with the use of 4-slice and 16-slice MDCT, water now is used routinely as a negative contrast agent. When combined with bolus IV-contrast administration, water provides an alternative to positive contrast and is recommended when 3D imaging and vascular

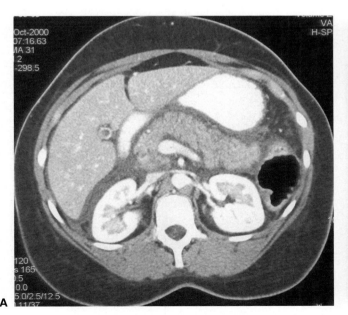
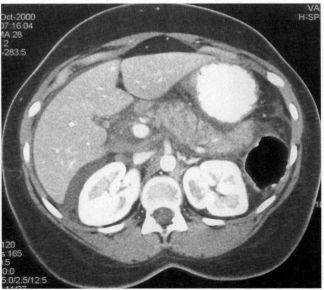

FIG. 13–4. Acute pancreatitis with glandular edema. **A,B:** MDCT demonstrates acute pancreatitis with diffuse edema of the pancreatic gland with minimal peripancreatic fluid. The gland enhances homogeneously. The patient was successfully treated with medical therapy.

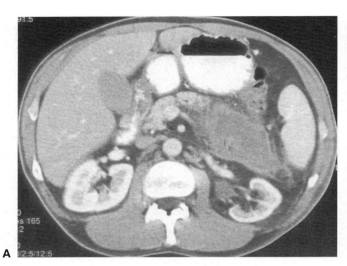
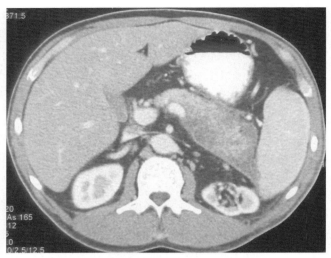

A **B**

FIG. 13–5. Acute pancreatitis with inflammation of the pancreatic tail and peripancreatic tissues. **A,B:** Inflammation of pancreatic tail with peripancreatic inflammation defined. Fluid tracts in left anterior pararenal space and extend towards the spleen.

mapping are desired. Prior to the study, 750 cc to 1000 cc of water is administered routinely over a 15-minute to 20-minute period.

With 16-slice MDCT, the pancreas now is imaged routinely in a volume mode rather than as routine axial images. The combination of multiplanar imaging (coronal, sagittal) combined with 3D volume rendering is ideal for defining the true extent of disease. Volume displays especially are valuable in defining the interrelationships between pseudocysts and adjacent organs, as well as in defining vascular complications ranging from pseudoaneurysms, venous thrombosis, and/or collateralization due to complications, including portal vein and/or splenic vein occlusion.

Grading of Pancreatitis with CT

The International Symposium on Acute Pancreatitis classified pancreatitis into two subgroups—mild acute pancreatitis and severe acute pancreatitis (2,5). Specifically, an attempt was made to create a classification system based on clinical and laboratory parameters and specific CT findings. Mild acute pancreatitis is a self-limiting disease and is the most common form of pancreatitis. Patients usually recover uneventfully without complications. On the other hand, severe acute pancreatitis is associated with a protracted course with a high incidence of complications and a defined mortality rate. Injury to the pancreatic parenchyma is a key finding,

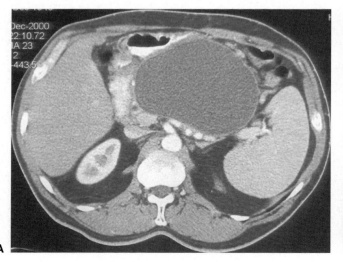
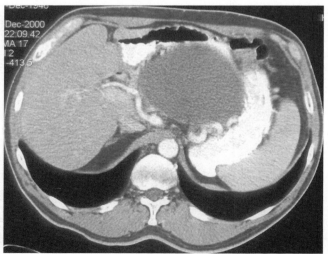

A **B**

FIG. 13–6. Pseudocyst in the lesser sac in a patient with a history of acute abdominal pain. **A,B:** Twelve-centimeter pseudocyst compresses the stomach and the mesenteric vessels. Most pseudocysts will resolve on their own, but this one eventually was drained with a cystgastostomy.

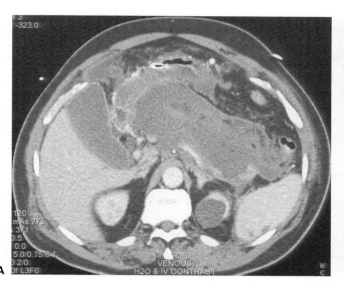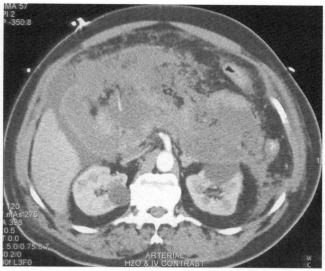

FIG. 13–7. Acute pancreatitis with early pancreatic necrosis. **A,B:** Multidetector CT in venous phase demonstrates early necrosis of portions of the pancreatic gland with diffuse fluid and induration in pancreas and peripancreatic zone. Fluid tracts into mesentery and pararenal spaces.

which explains why severe acute pancreatitis also is referred to commonly as necrotizing pancreatitis. The key to successful management of patients with pancreatitis is early detection of necrotizing pancreatitis, which has an associated mortality of up to 23% (9–12) (Figures 13–7 and 13–8).

Although clinical signs of severe pancreatitis do exist and include tachycardia, hypotension, shock, respiratory distress, and peritonitis, these often appear late in the course of the disease process. In fact, the clinical diagnosis of acute severe pancreatitis was missed in over 30% of cases in several large series (12–14). In the past, a few attempts were

made to correlate clinical signs with disease extent. The Ranson criteria for severity of acute pancreatitis was based on a series of 11 objective signs, such as patient age, white-blood-cell count, and calcium and serum glucose levels (5). An increasing number of positive findings corresponds to an increasing severity of disease and a higher mortality rate. With two or fewer signs, there generally is no mortality, but with six or more criteria, the mortality rate exceeds 50% (5).

The normal pancreas enhances avidly with IV contrast. Areas of nonenhancement correlate with pancreatic necrosis, and the extent of the necrosis is an excellent predictor of

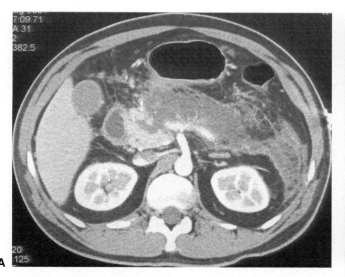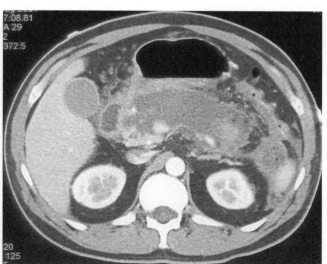

FIG. 13–8. Acute severe pancreatitis with peripancreatic fluid. **A,B:** Diffuse inflammation of pancreatic gland with area of pancreatic necrosis with involvement of left anterior pararenal space. The patient's pancreatitis was managed initially with intravenous antibiotics and parenteral nutrition. Subsequently, drainage of a pseudocyst was performed (4 months later).

TABLE 13–1. *Balthazar score*

Grade A: normal
Grade B: focal or diffuse enlargement of the pancreas
Grade C: pancreatic gland abnormalities associated with peripancreatic inflammation
Grade D: fluid collection in a single location
Grade E: two or more fluid collections and/or the presence of gas in or adjacent to the pancreas

TABLE 13–2. *Computed-tomography severity index (CTSI)*

CT grade based on Balthazar score plus pancreatic necrosis with a maximum score of 10 points

Grade A: 0 points
Grade B: 1 point
Grade C: 2 points
Grade D: 3 points
Grade E: 4 points

Points are given for necrosis with <30% being 2 points, 30% to 50% necrosis being 4 points, and >50% necrosis being 6 points.

outcome. Balthazar demonstrated that there was close correlation between the presence of necrosis and course of hospitalization, including morbidity and mortality (15). In addition, the extent of necrosis was correlated directly with the rate of morbidity and mortality. Based on this work, a CT severity index was developed that attempted to use CT as a numeric grading system for the radiological grading of pancreatitis (15). The system provides a score between 0 and 10, with higher morbidity and mortality correlated to higher scores. A severity score of 7 to 10 had a 92% complication rate and a 17% mortality rate, while a score of 0 or 1 had zero morbidity or mortality (Tables 13.1 and 13.2).

The extent of pancreatic enhancement will vary, based on a number of technical parameters and study-design features. Kim et al. found the optimal time for imaging for necrosis to be in the venous phase, or 50 seconds to 60 seconds after contrast injection (16). The injection rate should be in the 3-cc-per-second range. Pancreatic enhancement normally is in the 100-Hounsfield units (HU) to 150-HU range. Enhancement less than 30 HU is representative of decreased vascular perfusion of the gland and correlates well with necrosis. Caution in defining pancreatic necrosis is important, as areas of peripancreatic fluid can simulate areas of necrosis. Pancreatic necrosis is detected ideally on scans performed 48 hours to 72 hours after the onset of an attack of acute pancreatitis. Scans performed within the first 24 hours may be falsely negative or equivocal. Although scans commonly are done at time of admission, the need for a second study should be kept in mind for patients without initial rapid improvement (Figures 13–9 and 13–10).

Van den biezenbos et al. compared the success of the computed-tomography severity index (CTSI) with the Simplified Acute Physiology (SAP) score in predicting patient outcomes in a series of 45 patients (17). The authors found that, although CT scoring and the SAP score had no significant benefit in identifying patients with severe outcomes, the CTSI score was better in predicting a favorable outcome.

CT FINDINGS

Uncomplicated Acute Pancreatitis

Mild cases of acute pancreatitis reveal a minimal increase in the size of the pancreas, often involving the entire

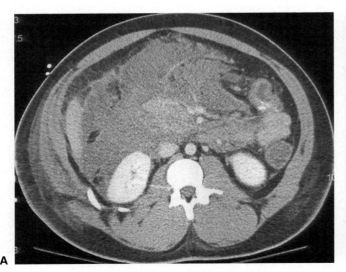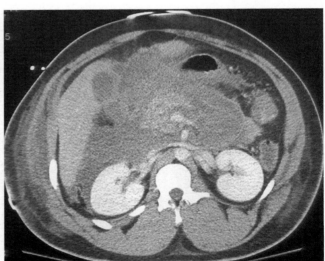

FIG. 13–9. Acute pancreatitis with extensive peripancreatic inflammation. **A,B:** A key finding in this case is the normal gland enhancement despite the extensive inflammatory response in and around the gland. The patient's pain worsened the morning after admission to the hospital.

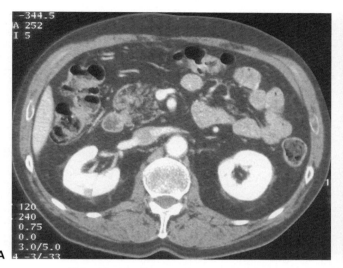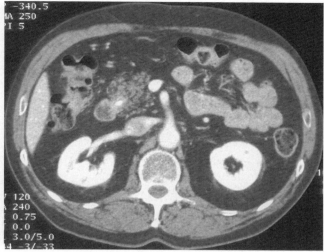

FIG. 13–10. Pancreatitis due to impacted common duct stone. **A,B:** Multidetector CT demonstrates impacted stone in distal common duct, which led to mild pancreatitis. Thin collimation allows routine determination of ductal system and detection of common duct stones as a cause of pancreatitis.

gland. The pancreatic contour becomes irregular with inflammatory changes, and peripancreatic-fat planes become blurred and appear thickened. Peripancreatic extension of the inflammatory process is relatively common because the pancreas does not have a capsule. Thickening of the mesentery, renal fascia, and lateroconal fascia is common. More severe forms of pancreatitis can result in moderate to marked increase in the size of the gland. The enlarged gland commonly shows edematous changes of the parenchyma, with typical measurements from 5 HU to 20 HU. There can be total obliteration of the peripancreatic fat by relatively high-attenuation inflammatory exudates, necrotic tissue, and blood (Figures 13–11 and 13–12).

Fluid Collections and Exudates

As pancreatitis progresses, small fluid collections can accumulate in and around the gland (18–20). Fluid collections lack a well-defined capsule and are confined by the anatomic space in which they arise. Many collections spontaneously resolve, but some will progress to pseudocyst formation and secondary infection or hemorrhage. The most common site of extrapancreatic fluid collection is the lesser sac, located directly anterior to the pancreas and posterior to the stomach. The next most common location is the left anterior pararenal space. Larger fluid collections can extend over the psoas muscles to enter the pelvis and groin. Exu-

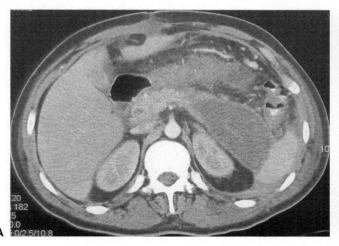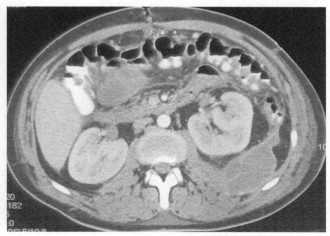

FIG. 13–11. Acute pancreatitis due to Depakote ingestion. **A,B:** Multidetector CT demonstrates acute pancreatitis with the most extensive inflammation in distal body and the tail of the pancreas. Extensive involvement of the left posterior pararenal space is seen.

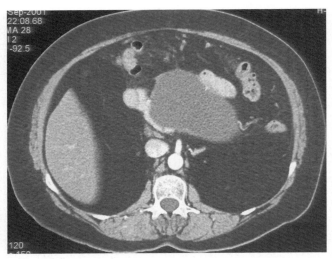

FIG. 13–12. Pseudocyst due to acute pancreatitis. **A,B:** Well-defined pseudocyst without discernible cyst wall is seen. No evidence of cyst capsule is noted. The pseudocyst resolved without medical or surgical intervention.

dates also can invade the posterior pararenal space, perirenal space, mesocolon, and mesentery. These fluid collections also can tract upward and present as posterior mediastinal masses (Figures 13–13 and 13–14).

Pseudocysts

Pseudocysts are focal collections of pancreatic fluid that usually evolve from acute fluid collections and inflammatory exudates. Their size is variable, but larger cysts often measure 5 cm to 10 cm in diameter. Pseudocysts have a dense peripheral fibrous capsule, which usually requires several weeks to mature. Pancreatic pseudocysts can persist for a relatively long time and may result in pain, secondary infection, hemorrhage, or biliary-duct obstruction. Helical CT is excellent for demonstrating the pseudocyst capsule, which can show significant enhancement following bolus-contrast administration. The degree of enhancement may relate to the ''maturity'' of the capsule and be a reliable indication for percutaneous drainage (21). Most often, though, the decision to drain pseudocysts is dependent equally on the patient's clinical condition. Complications of pseudocysts

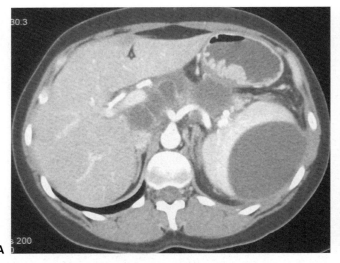

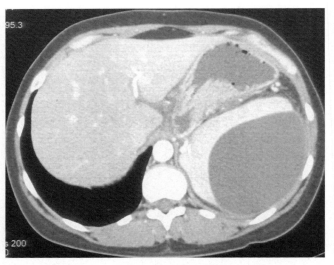

FIG. 13–13. Pancreatitis with pseudocyst tracking beneath the splenic capsule. **A,B:** Multidetector CT demonstrates inflammation of the pancreatic gland with pseudocysts noted. Fluid also tracts beneath the splenic capsule, resulting in a splenic pseudocyst. Intrasplenic pseudocysts make the spleen more prone to rupture, even with minor trauma.

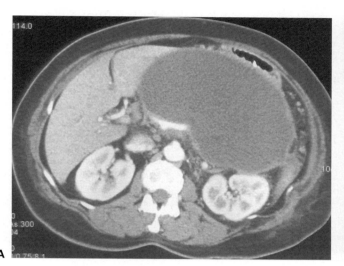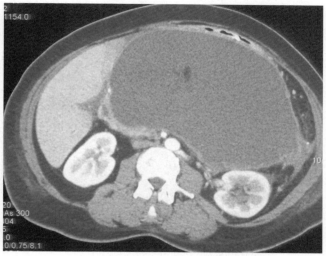

FIG. 13–14. Twenty-centimeter pseudocyst compressing the stomach. **A,B:** Multidetector CT demonstrates the large pseudocyst that compresses the stomach and subsequently was drained with a cystogastrostomy at surgery. Initial catheter drainage was unsuccessful.

also include compression and occlusion of the splenic vein, which can result in extensive formation of venous collaterals around the spleen and stomach. In time, this may become a source of GI bleeding (Figures 13–15 and 13–16).

Computed tomography with multiplanar reconstruction (MPR) is valuable in helping to determine the optimal pathway for pseudocyst drainage. Procedures such as cystgastrostomy can be planned with the use of sagittal and 3D volume mapping. Computed tomography also can document successful drainage of these collections (Figure 13-17).

Pancreatic Necrosis

Pancreatic necrosis represents a severe complication of acute pancreatitis (22). Necrosis tends to occur early in the course of the disease. The diagnosis of necrosis is based on demonstrating a focal or diffuse well-marginated area of parenchymal nonenhancement. The region should be at least 3 cm or larger in diameter or involve more than one-third of the gland. Excellent correlation between the lack of pancreatic enhancement on CT and necrosis has been docu-

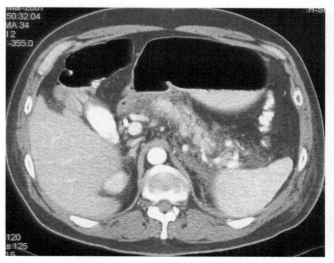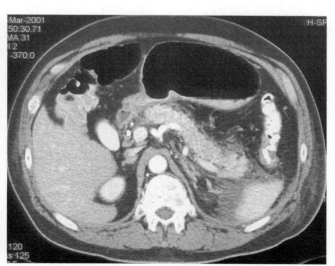

FIG. 13–15. Acute pancreatitis with perisplenic inflammation. **A,B:** Inflamed and edematous pancreatic gland with peripancreatic inflammation. Fluid tracks into left anterior pararenal space and surrounds the splenic capsule

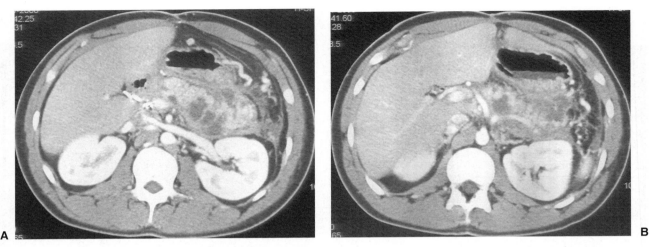

FIG. 13–16. Acute pancreatitis with splenic-vein occlusion. **A,B:** Dilated gastroepiploic vessels are seen anterior to stomach due to splenic-vein occlusion secondary to repeated episodes of pancreatitis. Computed-tomography also demonstrates inflammation especially of the body and tail of the pancreas with multiple pseudocysts noted.

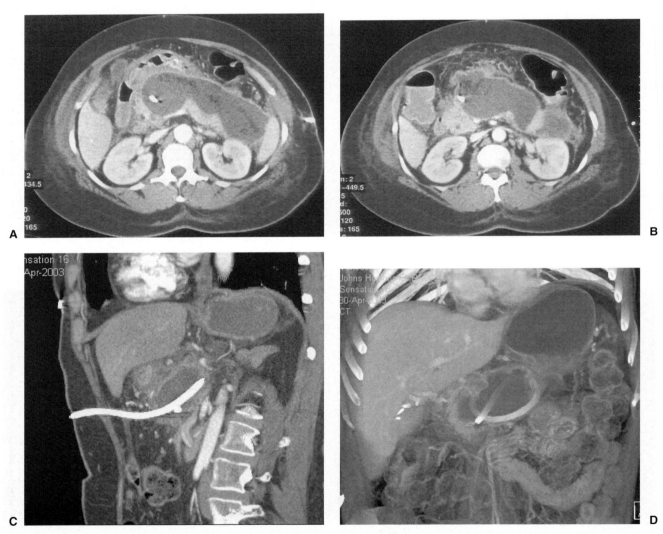

FIG. 13–17. Pancreatic pseudocyst with drain in place. **A,B:** Computed tomography can be used to direct placement of drains into pseudocysts, as well as monitor positioning of tube and success of drainage. **C,D:** Three-dimensional mapping may be useful for better definition of drain positioning and optimization of drain placement.

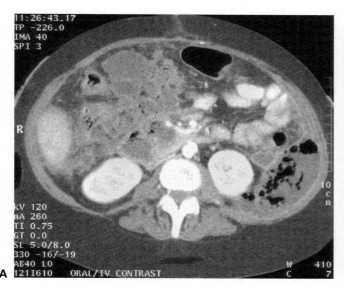
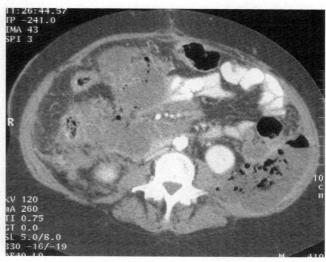

FIG. 13–18. Necrotizing pancreatitis with pancreatic abscess. **A,B:** Computed tomography demonstrates extensive inflammation of the pancreatic gland with fluid tracking into mesentery and perirenal spaces. Multiple air bubbles in pancreatic bed, mesentery, and in posterior left pararenal space are consistent with abscess formation. Patient was treated with aggressive surgical management.

mented. Edematous forms of acute pancreatitis with diminished glandular enhancement must not be confused with the nonenhancement of necrosis. Infected pancreatic necrosis is recognized on helical CT as bubbles of gas within areas of the pancreas, or as a collection of gas and tissue within the retroperitoneum. Massive infected necrosis ("emphysematous pancreatitis") carries a grave prognosis (Figures 13–18 and 13–19).

Several authors have discussed the importance of parameters such as contrast-injection rate and contrast volumes, as well as timing of data acquisition relative to contrast bolus, in determining the absolute values of pancreatic enhancement in the normal gland (23–25). Kim et al. found that higher dose (2 mL per kilogram versus 1.5 mL per kilogram) and faster injection rates (5 mL per second versus 3 mL per second) increased the maximum pancreatic enhancement value by 13 HU to 24 HU (23). Others, including Bonaldi et al., found that, although peak enhancement increased, overall image quality was similar (24). Tublin et al. noted that, by varying injection rates between 2.5 mL per second and 5.0 mL per second, peak pancreatic enhancement. as well time to peak enhancement, varied. At 2.5 mL

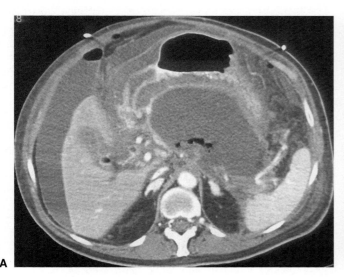
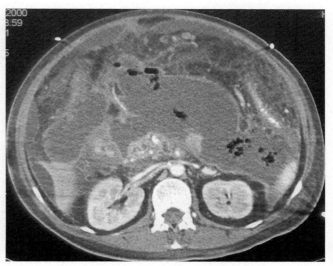

FIG. 13–19. Pancreatic necrosis with pancreatic abscess. **A,B:** Diffuse inflammation of pancreas and peripancreatic tissues with multiple air bubbles within pseudocysts, and peripancreatic tissue most compatible with pancreatic necrosis and abscess formation.

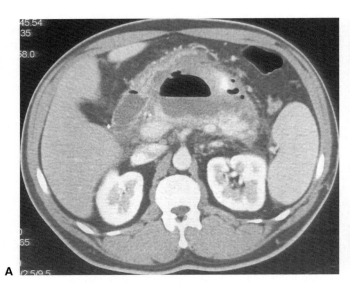
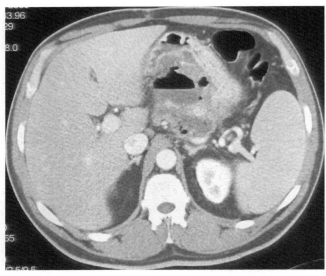

FIG. 13–20. Pancreatic abscess with infected pseudocyst. **A,B:** Computed tomography demonstrates air–fluid level within pseudocyst, as well as tiny air bubbles in and around the pancreatic gland. This subsequently was drained surgically.

per second, the pancreas reached a peak enhancement of 65 HU at 69 seconds, while at 5.0 mL per second, the peak enhancement was 84 HU at 43 seconds.

Pancreatic Abscess

Pancreatic abscesses represent focal areas of infection in or around the pancreatic gland. Abscesses usually present 4 or more weeks after the onset of acute pancreatitis, and probably result from secondary infection of pancreatic-fluid collections or from areas of focal necrosis. The helical-CT diagnosis is suggested with the demonstration of a focal fluid collection containing gas bubbles. The nearby pancreas remains visible and enhances following contrast administration. Clinical correlation or percutaneous aspiration often is required to make the diagnosis. Even in the absence of air, the possible presence of abscess always should be considered in any febrile patient with a persistent fluid collection. One CT finding that may be helpful in suggesting infection is a mottled appearance within the area of inflammation (Figures 13–20 and 13–21).

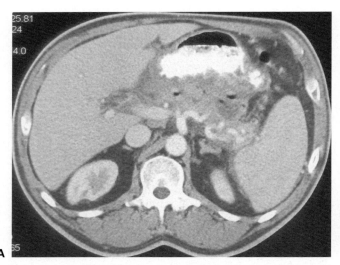
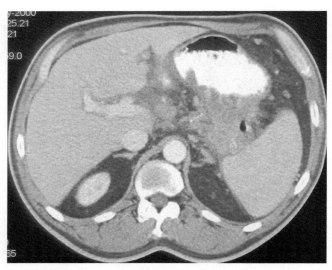

FIG. 13–21. Pancreatic abscess. **A,B:** Multidetector CT defines inflamed pancreatic gland with air bubbles in the tail of the pancreas, consistent with early abscess formation. This was treated without surgical intervention. Air bubbles usually are pathnomonic of infection or abscess, but occasionally can be due to fistulaezation.

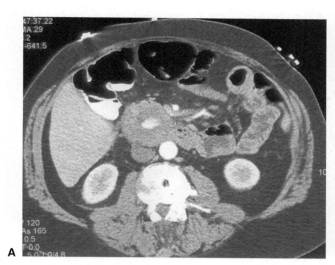 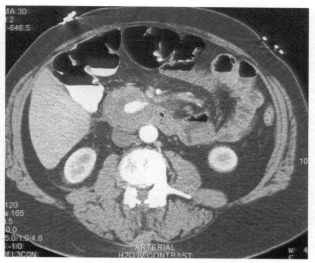

FIG. 13–22. Pseudoaneurysm as a complication of prior pancreatitis. **A,B:** Enlarged pancreatic head with hypervascular lesion in pancreatic head consistent with a pseudoaneurysm. Patient developed a retroperitoneal hematoma. The pseudoaneurysm was defined best on arterial-phase imaging.

Vascular Complications and Hemorrhage

Pseudocysts and chronic pancreatitis can result in vascular occlusion of the splenic vein, superior mesenteric vein, and/or portal vein. Splenic-vein thrombosis is most common, and results in complications such as gastric varices. Helical CT can depict accurately sites of vascular thrombosis and demonstrate collateral vascular pathways. Hemorrhage, in cases of pancreatitis, results from enzymatic autodigestion of arterial walls. This may lead to a confined perivascular blood leak or subsequent pseudoaneurysm formation. Injuries commonly involve the splenic artery or the pancreatic-

duodenal or the gastroduodenal arteries, which are related intimately to the pancreas. An arterial pseudoaneurysm may result and often is the underlying etiology in cases of massive hemorrhage. Computed tomography with arterial-phase MDCT can detect routinely the presence and location of pseudoaneurysms. Three-dimensional CT angiography (CTA) may be helpful in defining the specific site of the pseudoaneurysm. In these cases, the importance of rapid contrast bolus (3 cc per second minimum) and arterial-phase imaging cannot be overemphasized (26–28) (Figures 13–22 and 13–23).

Bleeding also can occur into a preexisting pseudocyst.

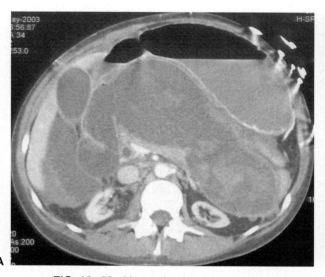 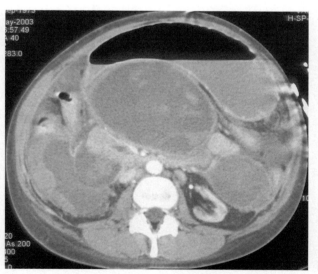

FIG. 13–23. Hemorrhagic pancreatitis with bleed into multiple pseudocysts in a patient with lupus. **A,B:** Sequence of images demonstrates severe fluid collection with areas of high CT attenuation compatible with hemorrhage. The patient was treated surgically with drainage of the pseudocysts.

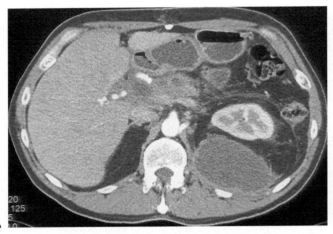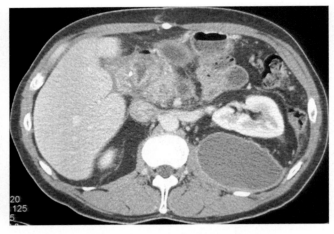

FIG. 13–24. Acute pancreatitis with fluid collection in left posterior pararenal space. **A,B:** Fluid collection is defined in left posterior pararenal space with secondary displacement of the kidney anteriorly. Inflamed pancreatic gland is demonstrated as well.

Helical CT often is very helpful in identifying the source of hemorrhage. Acute hemorrhage secondary to a bleeding pseudocyst or pseudoaneurysm has an associated mortality rate of 12% to 37% (26–28).

Involvement of Adjacent Organs

Classically, pancreatitis is a disease process where spread is not limited by adjacent organs, mesenteries, or the omentum. While pancreatitis most commonly involves the pararenal spaces and lesser sac, it can extend to and involve adjacent organs. Renal involvement typically results in inflammatory extension into the anterior and posterior pararenal space. The left pararenal space most commonly is involved, except when the cause of pancreatitis is postprocedural, such as post-ERCP pancreatitis, where right-sided in-

volvement is more common. On occasion, a pseudocyst can tract into the perirenal space and even beneath the renal capsule. At times, this pseudocyst can even simulate a renal cyst on select images. When pancreatic fluid tracts beneath the capsule, it can result in a Page kidney, due to compressive forces on the renal parenchyma. Percutaneous drainage may be needed to drain the subcapsular fluid. Other unusual complications include renal vascular abnormalities such as narrowing of the renal vein, renal-vein thrombosis, perirenal varices, and asymmetric renal enhancement due to extrinsic pressure on one of the renal arteries. In one series of acute pancreatitis, 7% of cases had renal and perirenal complications (29) (Figure 13-24).

Splenic involvement by pancreatitis is not uncommon, especially when one considers the intimate relationship of the tail of the pancreas and the splenic hilum (30,31) (Figure

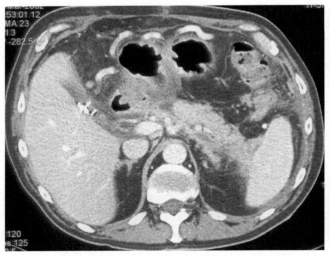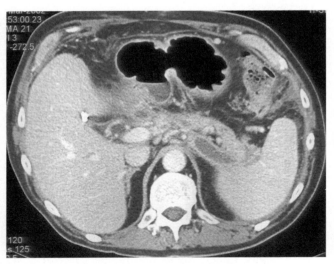

FIG. 13–25. Splenic-vein thrombosis due to repeated episodes of pancreatitis. **A,B:** Multidetector CT demonstrates pancreatic inflammation with evidence of thrombosis splenic vein.

13-25). In addition to vascular complications ranging from splenic-artery pseudoaneurysm to splenic-vein occlusion, pseudocysts may tract deep into the spleen. This can result in complications such as intrasplenic pseudocysts, splenic infarction, and intrasplenic hemorrhage. Intrasplenic pseudocysts may distend the splenic capsule so that even minor trauma may result in splenic rupture. Splenic abscess may develop as a rare complication of pancreatitis. Although splenic involvement by pancreatitis occurs in only 1% to 5% of patients, it can be life threatening, and CT can be used as a guide to monitor these patients and determine when aggressive intervention is necessary to avoid catastrophic clinical outcomes. Portal-vein thrombosis is another complication of acute pancreatitis (Figure 13-26).

Interventional Guidance in Pancreatitis: Role of CT

Although the detailed role of CT in the guidance of interventional procedures in pancreatitis is beyond the scope of this chapter, a few brief comments are in order. Although there often has been discussion as to the role of interventional percutaneous drainage of pancreatic abscess, pancreatic necrosis, or pseudocyst in regard to timing of surgical intervention, it generally is accepted that percutaneous drainage is a safe and effective technique even in patients with infected acute necrotizing pancreatitis. As noted by Freeny, sepsis was controlled in 74% of patients, permitting elective surgery for treatment of pancreatic fistulae, and 47% were cured without the need for surgery (32). Computed tomography is used routinely for guidance in catheter placement, as well as to monitor response. In these cases, 3D display of the relationship of the catheter to the fluid collection may prove useful (32).

Chronic Pancreatitis

Repeated episodes of pancreatitis lead to a series of changes, which can result in glandular atrophy and subsequent glandular scarring and fibrosis. Pancreatic calcifications involving part or the entire gland may occur as an isolated event or part of the process of glandular atrophy. Calcifications are associated most commonly with chronic alcoholic pancreatitis. In this process, the ducts become occluded with proteinaceous plugs that eventually accumulate calcium carbonate. Duct obstruction results in changes of duct ectasia and glandular fibrosis. In most cases, the calcifications are 1 mm to 5 mm, although larger calcifications do occur. Occasionally, these calcifications become located strategically and may obstruct the distal common bile duct. Lesniak et al. noted that calcifications also may develop in pancreatitis secondary to hyperparathyroidism, tropical pancreatitis, and idiopathic pancreatitis, while other causes of pancreatitis including gallstones, drugs, trauma, and viruses do not cause pancreatic calcifications (33) (Figures 13–27, 13–28, 13–29, and 13–30).

One of the classic diagnostic dilemmas with CT in the past has been the differential diagnosis of acute pancreatitis on a background of chronic pancreatitis simulating a pancreatic neoplasm. This is especially common in the pancreatic head, where areas of the gland may appear masslike, especially relative to areas of glandular atrophy. With MDCT and rapid-contrast bolus, this is less of a problem, but occasionally it remains a diagnostic challenge, especially in the patient with changing clinical symptoms and weight loss. Two strategies can be employed depending on the clinical scenario. One is to perform a fine-needle biopsy, which is diagnostic when positive. Another acceptable strategy is to perform a repeat CT scan in 4 weeks to 8 weeks. In most

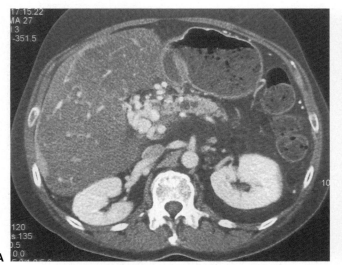
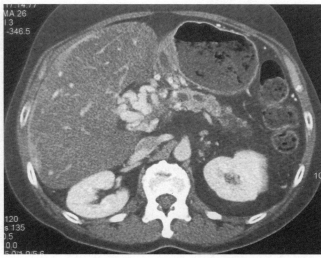

A   B

FIG. 13–26. Cavernous transformation of the portal vein in a patient with repeated episodes of pancreatitis. **A,B:** Inflammation of the pancreas is demonstrated with multiple tubular vessels in porta hepatis, compatible with cavernous transformation of the portal vein.

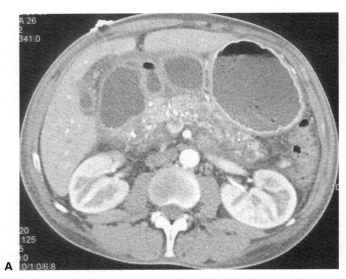
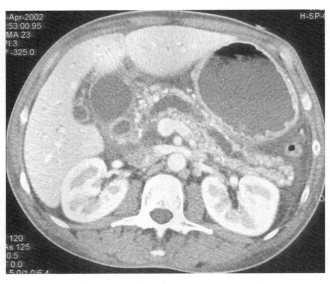

FIG. 13–27. Acute and chronic pancreatitis with dilated pancreatic duct. **A,B:** Study demonstrates dilated pancreatic duct with extensive calcifications, compatible with chronic pancreatitis. There also is diffuse inflammation of the gland and peripancreatic tissues compatible with acute pancreatitis as well.

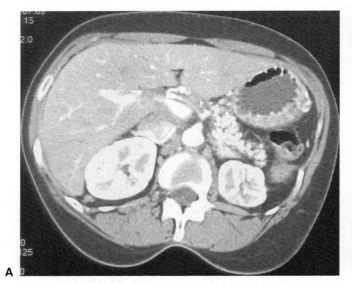
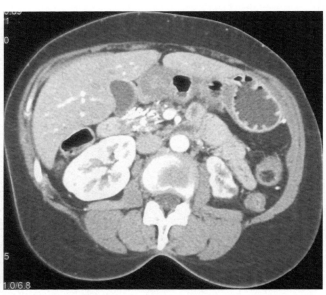

FIG. 13–28. Chronic pancreatitis in a patient with a history of repeated episodes of pancreatitis. **A,B:** Extensive calcifications are seen throughout the pancreatic gland, compatible with the diagnosis of chronic pancreatitis.

CHAPTER 14

MDCT Evaluation of the Spleen

Satomi Kawamoto, Elliot K. Fishman

INTRODUCTION

Until the advent of cross-sectional imaging, splenic pathology was exceedingly difficult to diagnose. This perception changed with the advent of computed tomography (CT), which quickly became recognized as the standard for splenic imaging (1–3). Computed tomography can easily and rapidly image the spleen, and it is valuable in the diagnosis of a variety of congenital, inflammatory, traumatic, and neoplastic lesions of the spleen, in addition to identifying certain normal variants that may present problems. Spiral CT is used widely for evaluation of the abdomen, especially the liver and pancreas (4–6), because of its ability to scan during a single breath hold during peak contrast enhancement. This produces a volumetric scan, which essentially eliminates data misregistration and minimizes motion artifacts. More recently, multidetector CT (MDCT) has become accepted as the state-of-the-art modality for evaluation of the upper abdomen (7–10). The unique advantages of MDCT over single-detector spiral CT include improved temporal resolution, improved spatial resolution in the z-axis, increased concentration of intravascular-contrast material, decreased image noise, efficient X ray tube use, and longer anatomic coverage (11). These factors improve evaluation of abdominal visceral imaging, including the spleen, particularly in the detection of subtle parenchymal disease and vascular pathology. This chapter will discuss the many advantages that MDCT offers in evaluating the spleen.

TECHNIQUE

In most cases, evaluation of the spleen is done in conjunction with the liver and pancreas. In only a few instances is direct evaluation of the spleen requested or required. The spleen usually is imaged using the same parameters as for the liver. Typically, 100 mL to 120 mL of nonionic contrast is administered at a rate of 2 mL to 3 mL per second. Rates higher than this are used occasionally when the exam is targeted for vascular mapping, but in the routine patient such rapid injection rates are not necessary. Scanning begins at or near the termination of injection, usually 50 seconds to 70 seconds. Optimizing injection timing for splenic evaluation is not as important as for other organs such as the liver and pancreas. However, slower injection rates and delayed scanning can result in an inability to detect subtle splenic abnormalities.

Individual scanning parameters vary depending on the CT scanner. Ideally, thin-detector collimation (2.5 mm) is preferred for evaluation of the upper abdomen (12). Pitch can be increased to approximately 6 to 8 without significant image compromise. Reconstructed images are reformatted routinely using 3-mm to 5-mm increments. Reconstructions every 1 mm or 2 mm are helpful to improve quality of three-dimensional (3D) images, which can be obtained using a variety of postprocessing software packages. In select cases where directed evaluation of a known splenic lesion is desired, image quality can be improved by decreasing the collimation, pitch, and reconstruction interval. Delayed scans, obtained several minutes after injection, may be useful in cases of confusing splenic pathology, or to help differentiate an heterogeneously enhancing normal spleen from an abnormal spleen.

Volume acquisition of MDCT datasets in conjunction with improvement in 3D software markedly improved 3D and multiplanar imaging capabilities as compared to single-detector CT (13). Three-dimensional and multiplanar reconstructions are very helpful in the demonstration of splenic and perisplenic processes (Figures 14–1 and 14–2). Coronal and sagittal views often help clarify confusing cases where the origin of a particular mass or lesion is uncertain (Figure 14-3). At times, certain processes, such as splenic infarcts and lacerations, are demonstrated better with additional views. Software packages on most MDCT scanners allow for convenient multiplanar reconstruction of an acquired volumetric dataset within minutes. The reconstructed images can be reviewed in real time using an interactive-display format.

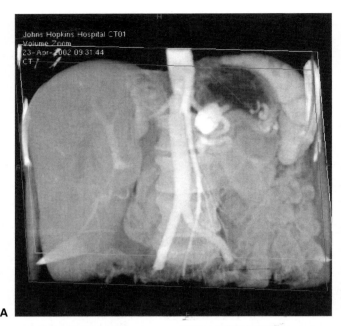

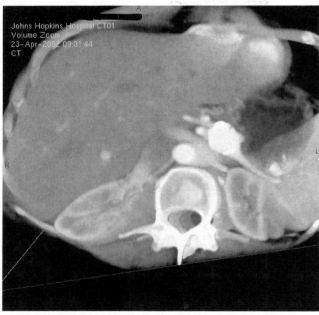

FIG. 14–1. Splenic-artery aneurysm in 58-year-old female. There is a 2.2-cm aneurysm in the proximal portion of the splenic artery with peripheral calcification. **A:** Anterior coronal and **(B)** superior axial-3D images nicely demonstrate the aneurysm with peripheral calcification.

THE NORMAL SPLEEN

The spleen is an intraperitoneal organ and lies deep in the left upper quadrant of the abdomen, closely abutting the left hemidiaphragm. The lateral border along the abdominal wall has a smooth convex surface margin. The medial visceral surface faces the posterior wall of the stomach anteriorly and the upper part of the left kidney posteriorly. The

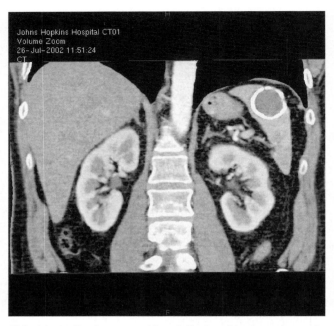

FIG. 14–2. Benign cyst with calcified wall in the spleen of a 46-year-old male. Coronal reconstruction image of the spleen demonstrates cyst with dense rim calcification within the spleen. Calcified cysts often result from prior trauma with hemorrhage.

hilum of the spleen receives the reflections of its supporting mesenteries, the gastrosplenic and splenorenal ligaments.

Anatomically, the spleen is divided into two compartments: white pulp and red pulp, separated by an ill-defined interphase known as the marginal zone. The white pulp is made up of lymphatic follicles and reticuloendothelial cells and is the site of the spleen's immunological and cytopoietic functions. The red pulp consists of a complex network of sinusoids and splenic cords, which contain macrophages and function as a filter and blood-flow regulator. The red pulp is responsible for erythrocyte storage, as well as macrophage proliferation and differentiation (14).

On noncontrast CT, CT-attenuation values of the normal spleen are in the range of 40 Hounsfield units (HU) to 65 HU, slightly lower (5 HU to 10 HU) than those for the normal liver (1,15). The spleen is evaluated optimally with intravenous (IV) contrast enhancement. Following bolus-intravenous-contrast administration, the normal spleen enhances heterogeneously, unlike the liver. This heterogeneity is assumed to result from the variable rates of blood flow through the cords of the red pulp (16). Some of the flow is through the "open circulation," reaching the splenic veins after traversing the splenic cords, resulting in relatively slow flow. The remaining flow is through the "closed circulation," or more rapid course, directly reaching the splenic veins without intervening flow through the splenic cords. Contrast material flowing through the rapid pathway will enhance particular portions of the spleen before others. In combination, these variable pathways contribute to overall

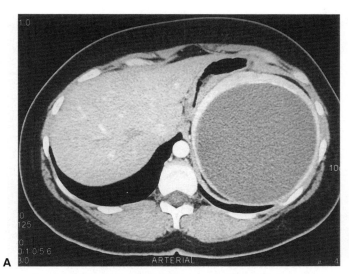

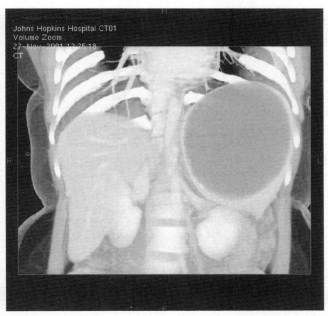

FIG. 14–3. Splenic cyst in a 38-year-old female. **A:** Axial MDCT shows a 12-cm cyst in the spleen with focal-wall calcifications. The spleen is enlarged and the splenic parenchyma is stretched peripherally. This cyst is thought to be a posttraumatic pseudocyst. **B:** The coronal reconstruction and **(C)** anterior coronal view of volume-rendering 3D images nicely demonstrate the extent of the cyst in an additional plane.

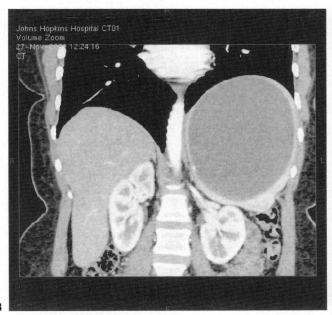

heterogeneous enhancement of normal spleen following bolus-contrast administration. This effect is transient and can be appreciated only for a very brief time following a rapid injection. At least 50% of normal spleens demonstrate heterogeneous enhancement on dynamic CT (17). This particularly is pronounced on MDCT due to high levels of bolus-contrast opacification. It also is more pronounced with faster injection rates, and when scanning begins soon after initiation of contrast administration (arterial phase) (18).

The pattern of normal splenic enhancement can vary greatly among patients. Several patterns have been encountered in clinical practice among normal subjects. A serpentine cordlike arciform distribution of enhancement seen homogeneously throughout the splenic tissue is the most common pattern (6,18). This has been termed an arciform

or ''Moiré'' pattern (Figure 14-4). Peripheral opacification of the spleen with relative delayed enhancement of the central splenic tissue is another form of normal enhancement, often seen in patients with portal hypertension. Occasionally, the spleen enhances irregularly and cannot be characterized readily (Figure 14-5). However, if the pattern is distributed homogeneously, it is likely a variation of normal enhancement. The key finding to suggest a normal variant of enhancement is usually the lack of a focal abnormality. Delayed images of the spleen are very helpful when uncertainty persists. Diffuse forms of normal splenic heterogeneity are transient and typically disappear on delayed imaging (Figure 14-5).

Normal heterogeneous splenic enhancement can be marked in patients with decreased cardiac output or heart

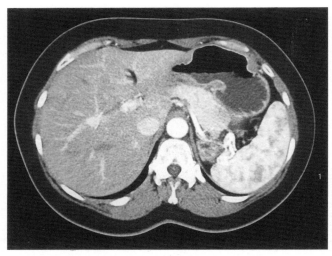

FIG. 14–4. Normal spleen in a 48-year-old female. Normal heterogeneous splenic enhancement results from differential flow through the red pulp. Serpentine enhancement, as in this case, is the most common pattern.

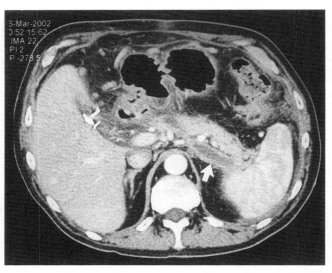

FIG. 14–6. Acute pancreatitis with splenic-vein thrombosis in a 62-year-old male. Pronounced heterogeneous contrast enhancement of the spleen. The splenic vein is occluded completely (*arrow*) due to pancreatitis.

failure. Secondary delayed transit can result from splenic-vein occlusion (Figure 14-6), portal hypertension (Figure 14-7), or portal-vein thrombosis (16). When encountering a patient with exaggerated heterogeneous enhancement, the above factors should be considered, with careful attention to the region of the splenic vein and pancreas to exclude a vascular thrombosis or occlusion from an adjacent pancreatic tumor (Figure 14-5).

Focal regions of heterogeneous splenic enhancement are invariably abnormal and represent true splenic pathology. Often, foci of involvement as small as 1 mm to 2 mm

in diameter can be detected with MDCT scanning. Punctate foci are always abnormal and commonly result from an inflammatory or infectious insult. Regional or geographic areas of decreased-contrast enhancement on MDCT following bolus-contrast administration are other patterns of abnormal enhancement. Etiologies of these regional or geographic perfusion abnormalities include infections, neoplasms, and infarction. In some of these patients, delayed scans may appear normal; however, the focal or punctate nature of the

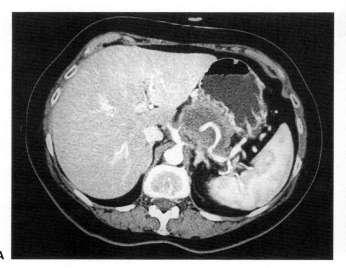

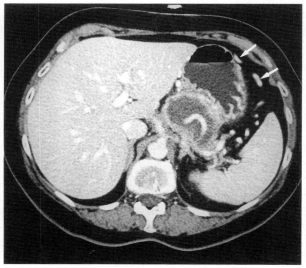

FIG. 14–5. Pancreatic cancer in a 71-year-old male. **A:** Arterial-phase image shows encasement of the splenic artery and occlusion of the splenic vein. Note heterogeneous contrast enhancement of the spleen. **B:** Venous-phase image demonstrates increased collateral veins around the stomach (*arrows*). The spleen is enhanced homogeneously on venous-phase image.

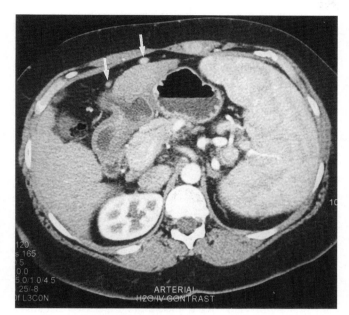

FIG. 14–7. Splenomegaly in a 52-year-old female with cirrhosis and portal hypertension. The spleen demonstrates heterogeneous contrast enhancement. Note recanalized umbilical vein (*arrows*).

initial splenic-enhancement heterogeneity is the key differential point in diagnosing the pattern as abnormal.

SPLENOMEGALY

Splenic size can vary at different ages, in different individuals, and under different conditions. In the adult, the spleen typically weighs approximately 150 grams and measures approximately 12 cm in length, 7 cm in breadth, and 4 cm in thickness (14). Various indices have been described for calculating splenic size. In practice, however, most observers assess splenic volume by subjective evaluation of the CT based on experience (19).

A variety of disease processes can result in splenomegaly. Computed tomography can determine whether the spleen is enlarged, and the degree of splenomegaly. However, the MDCT appearance often is nonspecific. Clinical correlation is essential for accurate diagnosis in these cases.

Altered splenic blood flow in liver cirrhosis with portal hypertension and/or splenic, hepatic or portal vein thrombosis is one of the most common causes of splenic enlargement. The diagnosis is made easily with MDCT when characteristic alterations in the size and shape of the liver are observed, along with ascites and collateral venous channels (Figure 14-7). Multidetector CT can demonstrate collateral-venous pathways of portal hypertension and provide an accurate demonstration of venous patency and flow dynamics. Multidetector CT also can suggest an underlying cause in cases of splenomegaly from isolated splenic vein thrombosis or occlusion, as seen in patients with pancreatitis or pancreatic carcinoma.

Infiltrating conditions from malignant diseases such as lymphoma and leukemia also can cause splenomegaly. They may result in microscopic changes reflected in an overall increase in the size of the spleen. With MDCT, subtle abnormalities of enhancement now can be appreciated in cases of splenic enlargement that were previously undetectable on conventional CT. Presence of abdominal lymph-node enlargement may suggest lymphoma or leukemia. Chronic lymphocytic leukemia can result in massive splenomegaly (Figure 14-8).

Many infectious processes can result in splenic enlargement. These include bacterial endocarditis and viral infections such as mononucleosis (Figure 14-9). Granulomatous infection, such as tuberculosis or histoplasmosis, may cause splenomegaly in the acute phase, but more typically presents as a normal-sized spleen with scattered granulomata. Patients with acquired immunodeficiency syndrome (AIDS) frequently demonstrate splenomegaly, which often is the result of superimposed infection (20). Because splenomegaly in AIDS patients also may result from diffuse lymphomatous involvement, differentiating infectious from malignant splenomegaly in these patients can be extremely difficult.

Systemic processes such as sarcoidosis and Gaucher's disease can present as splenomegaly with focal masses simulating malignant tumors. The CT appearance may mimic lymphoma. In one review of the CT findings in 59 patients with sarcoidosis, variable degrees of splenomegaly were seen in 33% of patients, including 6% with marked splenomegaly. Multiple low-attenuation splenic nodules were seen in 15% of patients (Figures 14–10 and 14–11) (21). Ancillary findings of parenchymal lung disease and adenopathy strongly suggest the diagnosis of sarcoidosis. In Gaucher's disease, splenomegaly with discrete areas of low attenuation correspond to local deposits of glucocerebroside within the reticuloendothelial cells in the spleen (Figure 14-12).

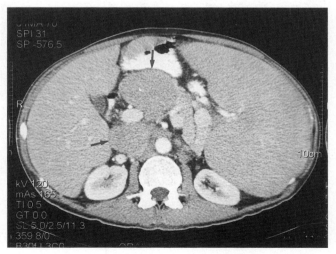

FIG. 14–8. Chronic lymphocytic leukemia in a 64-year-old male. The spleen is markedly enlarged. A large confluent nodal mass is visible in the porta portocaval, and hepatis regions (*arrows*).

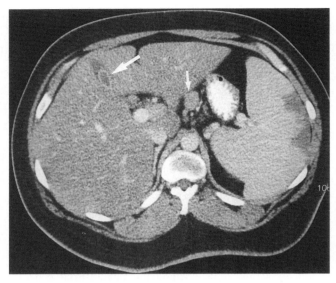

FIG. 14–9. A 43-year-old male with acute mononucleosis with Epstein–Barr virus. The spleen is moderately enlarged. There are multiple peripheral wedge-shaped low-attenuation lesions indicating infarcts. Adenopathy in the gastrohepatic ligament also is seen (*small arrow*). The gallbladder wall is diffusely thickened (*large arrow*).

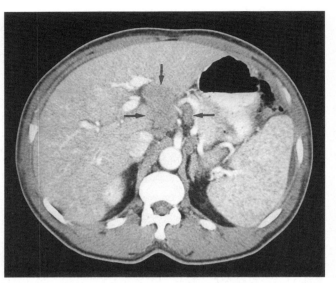

FIG. 14–11. Sarcoidosis in a 58-year-old male. Numerous tiny granulomas are visible throughout the spleen. The liver also is heterogeneous in attenuation. Enlarged lymph node is present in the porta hepatis and along the celiac axis (*arrows*). Trace ascites are seen around the spleen.

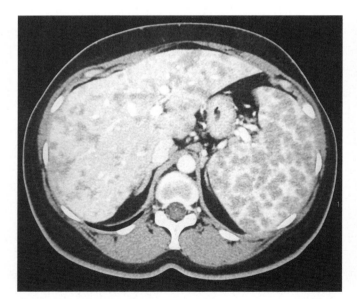

FIG. 14–10. Sarcoidosis in a 47-year-old female. The spleen is moderately enlarged. The liver and spleen show innumerable small low-attenuation lesions. The liver biopsy showed numerous granulomas consistent with sarcoidosis.

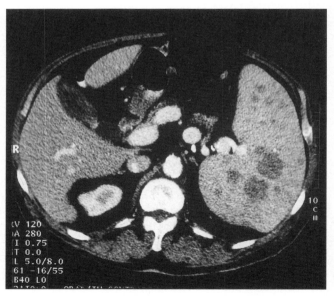

FIG. 14–12. Gaucher disease in 71-year-old male. Spleno-megaly with discrete areas of low attenuation correspond to local deposits of glucocerebroside within the reticuloendothe-lial cells in the spleen. This appearance also can be seen with lymphoma or metastases.

NORMAL VARIANT AND CONGENITAL ANOMALIES

Accessory Spleen

Accessory spleens are found in 10% to 20% of cases at autopsy examination (22). Size varies from a few millimeters to several centimeters in diameter. They are located near the spleen, especially within the gastrosplenic ligament and greater omentum (14). In most patients, it has no clinical significance, but occasionally it is confused with tumor when the location is atypical (23). In patients with previous splenectomy, accessory spleens can enlarge significantly. Ectopic splenic tissue also may be caused by autotransplantation of splenic cells within the peritoneal cavity due to traumatic disruption of the splenic capsule. In this condition, called splenosis, the nodules that develop after splenectomy are more numerous and widespread than accessory spleens (Figure 14–13) (22). When confusion exists, comparison of attenuation of the normal spleen and accessory spleen before and after intravenous-contrast enhancement is useful. The accessory spleen tends to exhibit the same pattern of contrast enhancement as the spleen (17). In problematic cases, nuclear scintigraphy with technetium-99m sulfur colloid is useful (24).

Wandering Spleen

In this rare condition, the spleen does not have fixed ligamentous attachment, which allows the spleen to move about in the abdomen. Clinically it may present as an unexplained abdominal mass with or without intermittent abdominal pain. Torsion of the wandering spleen is an unusual cause of acute abdomen secondary to compromised vascular supply, and can lead to splenic ischemia or infarction. Computed tomography can confirm the absence of the spleen in its expected location and the presence of wandering spleen in the abdomen or pelvis, seen as a soft tissue mass. In splenic torsion, CT demonstrates minimal or nonenhancement. A whorled appearance of twisted splenic pedicle and adjacent fat vessels also may be observed (25,26). If there is uncertainty as to whether the mass truly represents an ectopically located spleen, technetium-99m sulfur-colloid scan may help provide accurate diagnosis (19).

Polysplenia and Asplenia

Polysplenia is a rare congenital anomaly and consists of situs ambiguous with features of bilateral left sidedness. It is more common in females, and in most cases multiple spleens are present in either the right or left upper quadrant. The spleens are always on the same side as the stomach, typically along the greater curvature (27). Other abdominal anomalies include anomalous positions of abdominal viscera, short pancreas, and abnormal rotation of the bowel (28). In an autopsy series of 146 patients with polysplenia, heterotaxy of abdominal viscera was seen in 56% and cardiac anomalies in over 50%, including bilateral superior vena cava, interruption of the inferior vena cava with azygos continuation, ventricular septal defect, and ostium primum defect (29). However, many patients with polysplenia have mild congential heart disease or none at all (27), and the associated abnormalities may be discovered as an incidental finding on CT during adulthood (30).

Asplenia is characterized by an absent spleen, situs ambiguous, and multiple anomalies, including cardiovascular anomalies, intestinal malrotation, and genitourinary-tract anomalies. Asplenia occurs more frequently in males. The cardiovascular anomalies typically are more complex than those seen with polysplenia, accounting for much of the high mortality. Death occurs in the first year of life in up to 80% of these patients (31). Children with asplenia syndrome have a significantly greater incidence of sepsis, which also contributes to high mortality rate (32).

NEOPLASM

Lymphoma

Lymphoma is the most common malignancy involving the spleen. Although primary splenic lymphoma (Figure 14–14) is rare and constitutes approximately 1% to 2% of all lymphomas (33,34), staging laparotomy reveals clinically unsuspected involvement of the spleen in approximately one third of patients with previously untreated disease (35–37).

Splenomegaly is the most common CT finding; how-

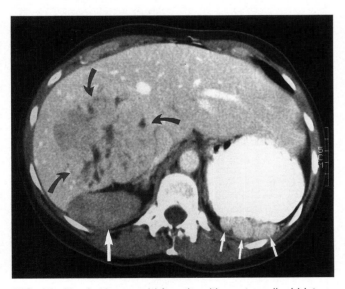

FIG. 14–13. A 48-year-old female with past medical history of splenectomy after ruptured spleen due to motor-vehicle accident. Computed tomography was performed for evaluation of liver mass. A large mass in the right lobe of the liver was found to be fibrolamellar-hepatocellular carcinoma (*black curved arrows*). A 6 cm × 3 cm focus of splenic tissue posterior to the right lobe of the liver was identified at the time of right hepatectomy (*large white arrow*). Also note splenosis posterior to the stomach (*small white arrows*).

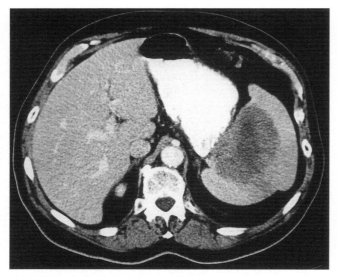

FIG. 14–14. A 74-year-old man with diffuse large-cell lymphoma of the spleen. The spleen is enlarged and there is a large area of low attenuation in the center of the spleen.

ever, the size of the spleen is normal in up to one third of patients with lymphomatous involvement (36,37). Moreover, in up to 30% of patients with lymphoma, splenic enlargement is not due to lymphoma unless the spleen is markedly enlarged (greater than 400 g) (36). Other CT manifestations of lymphoma involving the spleen may include miliary nodules, multifocal lesions (1 cm to 10 cm) (Figure 14-15), and/or a solitary mass (Figure 14-14) (33). Focal lymphomatous lesions are lower in attenuation than the normal spleen on CT. By eliminating data misregistration with a single breath-hold acquisition and improving contrast dynamics, MDCT likely increases detection of small miliary nodular lesions, which were difficult to detect on conven-

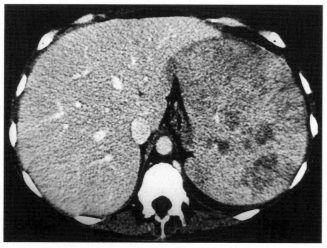

FIG. 14–15. Hodgkin's disease in a 35-year-old female. The spleen is markedly enlarged and there are multiple focal-nodular lesions.

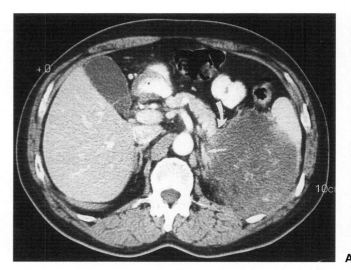

A

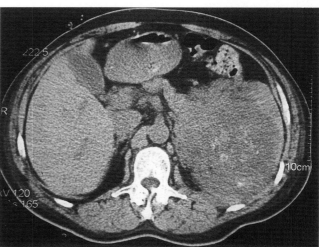

B

FIG. 14–16. Diffuse large-cell lymphoma in a 56-year-old male. **A:** Large splenic tumor extends beyond the splenic capsule, invading the pancreatic tail (*large curved arrow*). The left adrenal gland (*small arrow*) also is surrounded by the tumor. **B:** Seven weeks after (**A**), the patient developed acute chest pain and shortness of breath. The spleen had enlarged and developed spontaneous hemorrhage.

tional CT (38). Necrosis of large lesions can mimic cystic masses (39). Splenic lymphoma usually is confined to the splenic capsule, but local extension with invasion into adjacent structures has been reported (Figure 14-16) (39,40). Ancillary findings of adenopathy in the chest or abdomen also may help to diagnose lymphoma. In patients with non-Hodgkin lymphoma, splenic involvement is associated with paraaortic adenopathy in approximately 70% (41).

Leukemia

The spleen often demonstrates marked enlargement in patients with leukemia. The spleen usually maintains a homogeneous enhancement pattern. Focal leukemic infiltration (chloroma) is very rare (42). It is not possible with CT to differentiate among the various forms of leukemia. There may be lymphadenopathy in the chest or abdomen.

Patients with splenomegaly from leukemia infiltration are more prone to spontaneous infarction and rupture. Splenic rupture is an uncommon but life-threatening complication of leukemia and lymphoma (Figure 14-16), and its incidence has been reported in 0.72% of adults (43) and 0.18% of children with leukemia (44). Systemic fungal infection is a serious complication in patients with leukemia who have neutropenia after chemotherapy. The spleen is the second most common solid organ, after the liver, involved with systemic fungal infection. Computed tomography is the modality of choice to evaluate possible splenic microabscess and may show multiple low-attenuation lesions in the spleen.

PRIMARY TUMORS

Primary malignant tumors of the spleen are a rare entity, and angiosarcoma is the most common malignant primary nonlymphoid tumor of the spleen (45). Angiosarcoma has been caused by thorotrast exposure (46), in which the characteristic opacification of the liver, spleen, and lymph nodes is associated. Angiosarcoma has a poor prognosis and may present with acute abdominal symptoms secondary to spontaneous splenic rupture (45). On CT, the tumors demonstrate an aggressive growth pattern and can be single or multiple. Cystic and necrotic areas may be seen within the tumor (19). Spiral CT may show immediate focal intense enhancement with progressive centripetal enhancement of the lesion, which can help distinguish angiosarcoma from a benign tumor (47).

Benign tumors of the spleen include cysts, hemangiomas, lymphangiomas, and hamartomas. Splenic cysts can be congenital-epithelial (true cysts) cysts, posttraumatic pseudocysts (false cysts), and/or parasitic cysts due to Echinococcal infection. Parasitic cysts are most common worldwide, but are distinctly unusual in most Western countries (48,49). True epithelial-lined cysts are relatively uncommon, constituting fewer than 20% of splenic cysts (19). Congenital-epithelial cysts are well-defined low-density lesions. The borders are defined sharply, and there is no appreciable contrast enhancement following bolus-contrast administration. Computed tomography may show cyst-wall trabeculation or peripheral septation. Rarely, wall calcification is observed (50). Nonepithelial (false) cysts are thought to result from previous trauma, and a calcified wall is identified in 25% to 30% of patients (Figures 14-2 and 14-3) (48,50). It often is impossible to distinguish a true cyst from a false splenic cyst, but this usually is of little practical significance. The real diagnostic dilemma stems from differentiating a cyst from a splenic abscess or tumor; in this regard, MDCT is helpful.

Pancreatic pseudocysts may present as a splenic or perisplenic-cystic lesion (Figure 14-17). Pseudocysts can become quite large, completely surrounding and engulfing the spleen. Associated findings of acute or chronic pancreatitis

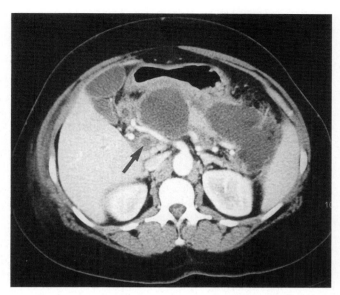

FIG. 14–17. A 58-year-old male with acute pancreatitis. Pancreatic pseudocysts involve the entire pancreas and extend to the spleen. Note thrombosed portal vein (*arrow*).

usually are present and help establish the diagnosis. Pancreatitis often occludes the splenic vein and may result in areas of splenic infarction (51). These patients also are prone to spontaneous splenic rupture even with mild trauma.

Splenic hemangioma is the most common primary splenic tumor (48). It often is the cavernous variety, and lesions can vary in size from a few millimeters to several centimeters. Hemangiomas often are multiple in cases (Figure 14-18) of Klippel–Trenauney–Weber syndrome (52,53). Central punctate calcifications can be seen in the solid portions, and curvilinear calcifications may be seen in the pe-

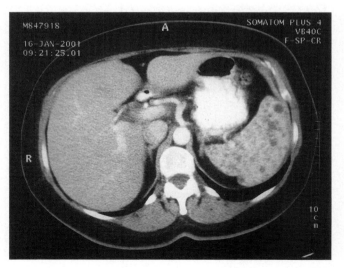

FIG. 14–18. Multiple hemangiomas in a 55-year-old-female. Multiple low-attenuation lesions up to 1 cm scattered throughout the spleen.

riphery of the cystic areas (54,55). Multidetector CT can demonstrate low-density lesions with peripheral enhancement, reflecting the vascular nature of these lesions. The splenic hemangioma, however, may not necessarily demonstrate the typical ''filling-in'' seen with hepatic hemangiomas (52).

Lymphangioma can be single or multiple, and filled with proteinaceous material (49). In cystic lymphangioma, CT demonstrates thin-walled well-marginated cysts, often in a subcapsular location. No contrast enhancement is noted after intravenous-contrast administration (55). Computed-tomography-attenuation measurements vary from 15 HU to 35 HU (56).

METASTASES

Metastatic lesions to the spleen are uncommon, with an autopsy incidence varying from 2% to 8%, despite the fact that the spleen has a rich blood supply (49,57). However, they are far more common than primary splenic tumors. Although cases of isolated metastasis have been reported, they usually are seen in patients with widespread metastases. Autopsy studies reveal that the primary sites for splenic metastasis include malignant melanoma, breast, ovary, lung, colon, and rectum (57,58).

On CT, splenic metastases usually appear as multiple nodules of decreased attenuation (Figure 14-19). Cystic metastasis may occur with metastasis from ovary, breast, endometrium, and melanoma (19). Peritoneal implants in patients with ovarian, gastrointestinal-tract, and/or pancreatic cancer may cause scalloping of the capsular surface of the spleen. Direct invasion into the splenic hilum also can occur with pancreatic or gastric malignancies. Differentiation of cystic-splenic metastasis from a benign cyst often is difficult. Mul-

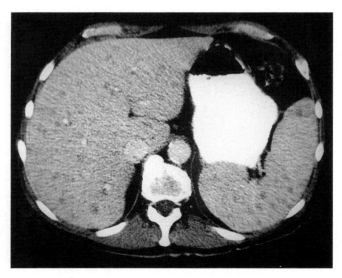

FIG. 14–19. An 81-year-old male with malignant melanoma. Multiple small low-attenuation lesions in the liver and spleen represent metastases.

tidetector CT is helpful in evaluating enhancing components of the lesion that favor a diagnosis of malignancy.

INFECTION

Splenic abscess is a rare yet potentially lethal disease process. The high morbidity is due in part to vague clinical symptoms, which often lead to a delay in diagnosis. Prior to the advent of cross-sectional imaging, a high percentage of abscesses went undetected until the time of surgery or autopsy. The most common organisms are staphylococci, streptococci, anaerobes, and aerobic gram-negative rods, including Salmonella. In neutropenic hosts, fungi, predominantly *Candida* species, may cause splenic abscesses (59). Patients predisposed to splenic-abscess formation include those with diabetes, alcoholism, or IV drug abuse. Endocarditis, splenic trauma, splenic infarction, or infection in adjacent organs also can result in splenic abscess. Computed tomography has proven accurate for the early diagnosis of abscesses, especially in the immunocompromised host. Early detection with CT often can alter and direct appropriate clinical management (60).

Splenic abcesses typically are focal, hypodense, and slightly lobulated in shape. A thick enhancing capsule may be seen following bolus-contrast administration (Figure 14-20). The presence of gas within the abscess is seen occasionally (Figure 14-21), and CT is the most reliable method of identifying small amounts of gas (55). Multidetector CT virtually can eliminate partial volume averaging, which aids in the detection of small gas bubbles. Computed tomography also can demonstrate an air–fluid or fluid–fluid level (60). The CT appearance often is similar to that of splenic infarction, chronic intrasplenic hemorrhage, cyst, or even cystic tumor.

Fungal infection in the immunocompromised host can have a specific appearance. Multiple 2-mm to 5-mm low-density lesions suggest the diagnosis of fungal microabscesses, usually due to candidiasis (61,62). Individuals with AIDS can develop similar hypodense lesions, usually the result of *Pneumocystis carinii* infection, disseminated tuberculosis (Figure 14-22), or mycobacterium-avium-intracellulare (MAI) infection (63). Liver involvement often is apparent as well. Multidetector CT enhances the detection of these smaller lesions with dynamic-contrast enhancement and continuous data acquisition. At times, infectious deposits can coalesce into larger areas of splenic involvement. Low-density adenopathy with peripheral rim enhancement is a supportive finding for tuberculosis (Figure 14-22) (64,65). Diffuse punctate calcifications may appear in the spleen, as well as liver and lymph nodes, following therapy for *P. carinii* infection (66–68).

Certain viral illnesses, such as mononucleosis, can result in splenomegaly without frank abscess formation (Figure 14-9). In such cases, MDCT usually reveals nonspecific splenic enlargement. Spontaneous splenic rupture is an ex-

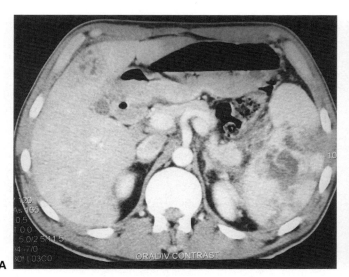 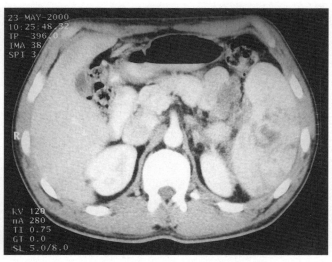

A   B

FIG. 14–20. Occupationally acquired glanders disease. *Burkholderia mallei* is a gram-negative bacillus, and glanders disease is *Burkholderia mallei* (formerly *Pseudomonas mallei*) infection. **A:** The liver and spleen are both enlarged, with several confluent low-attenuation septated abscesses within the liver and spleen. Multiple infarcts also are present in the periphery of the spleen. **B:** Eight days after **(A)**, abscesses in the liver and spleen are decreased in size and splenic infarcts have become indistinct.

tremely rare but life-threatening complication of mononucle-osis, which requires immediate splenectomy (69).

INFARCT

Multidetector CT is suited ideally for evaluation of vascular pathology. Patients may present with pain in the left upper quadrant, although many cases are clinically silent. Splenic infarcts are relatively common, and usually result from embolic occlusion of the splenic artery (e.g., bacterial endocarditis, mitral-valve disease) (Figures 14–23 and 14–24). Other causes include local thromboses, especially in hematological disorders (e.g., sickle-cell anemia, myelofibrosis, leukemia, and lymphoma), vasculitis, pancreatic dis-

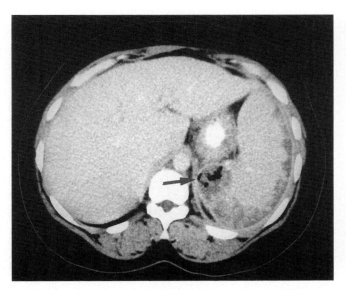

FIG. 14–21. Splenic infarcts and abscess in a 39-year-old female. Low-attenuation lesions in the periphery of the spleen represent infarcts. There is gas density within the medial portion of the spleen (*arrow*), compatible with splenic abscess developed in the area of infarction.

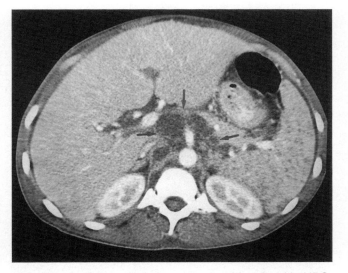

FIG. 14–22. Tuberculosis in a 32-year-old male with AIDS. The spleen is minimally enlarged and there are multiple small (less than 5 mm) low-attenuation lesions. Note low-attenuation adenopathy along the celiac axis and paraaortic and aortocaval regions (*arrows*). A small amount of ascites is present around the spleen.

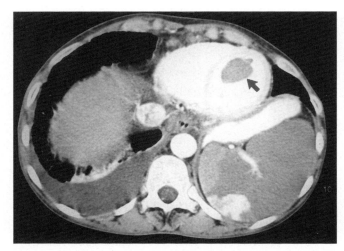

FIG. 14–23. Splenic infarct in a 40-year-old female with HIV infection. The spleen is enlarged and almost completely infarcted. Note filling defect within the left ventricle indicating thrombus (*arrow*).

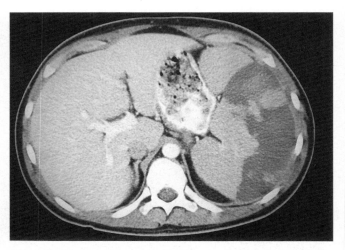

FIG. 14–25. Splenomegaly of unknown etiology in a 27-year-old male. The patient is status postrenal transplant and developed left upper-quadrant discomfort without history of trauma. There is global infarct of the enlarged spleen.

ease, and splenic artery aneurysm (1). Splenic infarct also may occur as a complication or result of transcatheter embolization of the hepatic artery (70). Splenomegaly itself may result in infarction due to relative ischemia (Figure 14-25). Patients with splenomegaly and portal hypertension also have increased risk of splenic infarct. Areas of splenic infarcts are known to predispose to splenic rupture and superimposed infection (Figure 14-21) (1).

Patients with sickle-cell disease often have repeated episodes of splenic infarct. In homozygous sickle-cell disease, areas of calcification frequently are seen within the spleen (Figure 14-26). These eventually result in a shrunken spleen containing diffuse microscopic deposits of calcium and iron, a small and densely calcified spleen on CT.

Focal splenic infarcts typically appear with MDCT as

wedge-shaped zones of decreased attenuation that extend to the surface of the spleen (Figure 14-24). However, infarcts also may appear as heterogeneous, poorly marginated, low-attenuation lesions that are indistinguishable from other splenic lesions such as abscesses or tumors (71). The appearance of infarcts can vary depending on age, usually becoming less dense and increasingly well defined with time (71). Infarcts may disappear, or heal with fibrosis and form multiple scars, which appear on CT as notching of the splenic contour.

Global infarction can result in diffuse hypodensity and can mimic splenic abscess or tumor. Multidetector CT during peak contrast enhancement allows reliable demonstra-

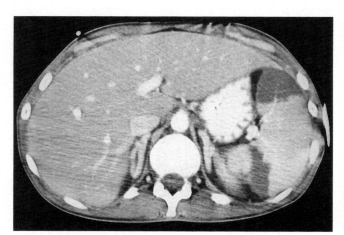

FIG. 14–24. Multiple large infarcts in the spleen of a 39-year-old female. The patient has bacterial endocarditis and also had infarcts of the kidneys bilaterally.

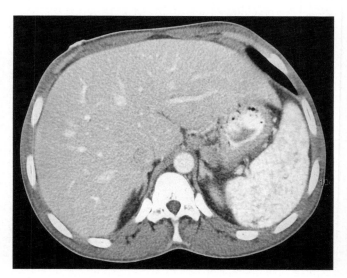

FIG. 14–26. An 18-year-old male with homozygous sickle-cell disease. The spleen is diffusely dense, representing calcium deposition.

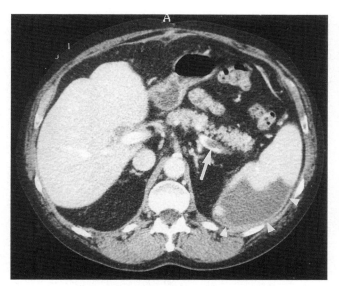

FIG. 14–27. Splenic infarct in a 63-year-old male. Peripheral low attenuation in the spleen indicates infarct. Note capsular enhancement indicating "rim sign," due to perfusion from capsular vessels (*arrowheads*). Thrombosis is seen in the splenic vein (*arrow*).

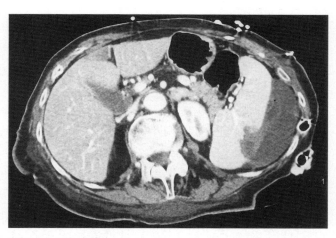

FIG. 14–28. Splenic laceration and subcapsular hematoma in an 82-year-old female. There is a peripheral geographic area of decreased attenuation within the splenic parenchyma, representing lacerations. Crescent area of decreased attenuation along the lateral aspect of the spleen indicates subcapsular hematoma.

tion of the splenic artery and vein, which may be helpful in differentiating extensive abscess or tumor from global infarction. Some cases of global infarction maintain enhancement of the splenic periphery, the so-called "rim sign," due to perfusion from capsular vessels (Figure 14-27).

The most common cause of splenic-vascular occlusion is pancreatic disease, usually due to pancreatitis or pancreatic carcinoma. Multidetector CT is useful for patients with suspected pancreatic neoplasms. It especially is useful in the preoperative staging of pancreatic cancer. Because of the data continuity provided by MDCT, improved multiplanar reconstruction is obtainable and can demonstrate vascular encasement or occlusion (9,10). It also is very useful in detecting splenic- or hepatic-artery pseudoaneurysms, a relatively common complication of pancreatitis (72). Peak contrast enhancement allows for detection of pseudoaneurysms as small as 1 cm in diameter. Severe cases of pancreatitis can develop large pseudocysts that can track into the splenic hilum, resulting in vascular occlusion and infarction (51).

TRAUMA

The spleen is the most frequently injured organ in blunt abdominal trauma. Computed tomography is extremely sensitive in the detection of splenic injury (73–75). Computed tomography can detect the presence or absence of splenic injury in nearly 100% of patients (73,75). Multidetector CT can provide a whole-body "screen" in a matter of minutes. With the increasing availability of CT in the trauma setting (many centers now have CT scanners on site in the emergency room), CT has become the modality of choice for imaging the trauma patient because it can rapidly image multiple organs simultaneously.

Blunt splenic injury may cause a splenic laceration or hematoma. Lacerations appear as linear or geographic low-attenuation defects (Figure 14-28). If the laceration traverses two capsular surfaces, it is called a fracture (Figure 14-29) (3). Even if a splenic laceration is not seen, the presence of focal hyperdense perisplenic clotted blood suggests the diagnosis of splenic trauma. It often is referred to as the "sentinel-clot" sign, and mean CT attenuation of clotted

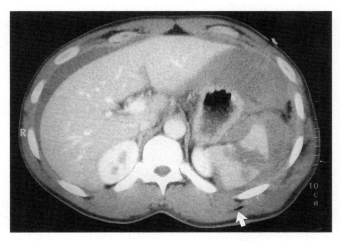

FIG. 14–29. Splenic fracture in a 38-year-old male who had a stab wound to the back. There is an extensive hemorrhage surrounding the spleen and hemoperitoneum. A large splenic laceration traverses two capsular surfaces. Note small subcutaneous air in the posterior left back indicating stab-wound site (*arrow*).

blood is greater than 60 HU (76). A subcapsular hematoma appears as a crescentic collection along the margin of the spleen, which flattens the normally convex margin (Figure 14-28). The hematoma may have a layered onion-skin appearance due to alternating layers of clotted and unclotted blood, if there are repeated episodes of bleeding. Extension of the hematoma into the spleen results in a splenic hematoma, which has a more irregular shape. Over several days to weeks, splenic hematomas become less dense and still may be visible years later in the form of a nonepithelial cyst, often with a calcified wall.

Intravenous-contrast enhancement is essential for detection of splenic hematomas because they can be equal in attenuation to the normal spleen immediately after injury (3). As the normal spleen enhances brightly against the injured tissue, lacerations and hematomas are more apparent with bolus-contrast enhancement, and viable splenic tissue can be differentiated easily from surrounding clot. Furthermore, single breath-hold acquisition using MDCT markedly diminishes data misregistration, which is problematic with conventional CT, due to variable diaphragmatic excursions in the upper abdomen. Multidetector CT ensures continuous coverage of the entire spleen free from breathing artifact, enhancing detection of small splenic lacerations. In some patients, splenic-vascular lesions or active vascular-contrast extravasation may be seen. In these cases, CT can play a valuable role in selecting patients who may be treated with transcatheter endovascular therapy (77).

The normal mottled appearance of the enhanced spleen should not be mistaken for splenic trauma. From past experience, dynamic enhancement with spiral scanning does not create diagnostic difficulty (78). Furthermore, in the setting of the acutely ill or injured patient, the benefits of spiral scanning far outweigh this potential pitfall (6). If uncertainty about splenic enhancement persists, delayed scans of the spleen always can be performed. A normal spleen usually will demonstrate a homogeneous appearance on delayed scans. In the vast majority of patients, however, delayed scans are not necessary.

Delayed splenic rupture is a well-defined clinical entity, often occurring more than 48 hours after trauma. The reported prevalence of delayed rupture is 0.3% to 20% of patients (79). Many of these cases likely represent small splenic lacerations without subcapsular hemorrhage, undetected at the initial time of trauma. Multidetector CT is very useful in detecting subtle splenic lacerations, and from previous experience has been helpful in identifying those patients with subtle injuries who are at increased risk for delayed rupture. In these patients, careful hemodynamic monitoring is warranted.

REFERENCES

1. Rabushka LS, Kawashima A, Fishman EK. Imaging of the spleen: CT with supplemental MR examination. *Radiographics* 1994; 14:307–332.
2. Piekarski J, Federle MP, Moss AA, et al. Computed tomography of the spleen. *Radiology* 1980;135:683–689.
3. Freeman JL, Jafri SZ, Roberts JL, et al. CT of congenital and acquired abnormalities of the spleen. *Radiographics* 1993;13:597–610.
4. Zeman RK, Zeiberg AS, Davros WJ, et al. Routine helical CT of the abdomen: image quality considerations. *Radiology* 1993; 189:395–400.
5. Zeman RK, Fox SH, Silverman PM, et al. Helical (spiral) CT of the abdomen. *AJR Am J Roentgenol* 1993;160:719–725.
6. Urban BA, Fishman EK. Helical CT of the spleen. *AJR Am J Roentgenol* 1998;170:997–1003.
7. Ji H, McTavish JD, Mortele KJ, et al. Hepatic imaging with multidetector CT. *Radiographics* 2001;21 Spec No:S71–S80.
8. Foley WD, Mallisee TA, Hohenwalter MD, et al. Multiphase hepatic CT with a multirow detector CT scanner. *AJR Am J Roentgenol* 2000; 175:679–685.
9. Horton KM, Fishman EK. Multidetector CT angiography of pancreatic carcinoma: part 2, evaluation of venous involvement. *AJR Am J Roentgenol* 2002;178:833–836.
10. Horton KM, Fishman EK. Multidetector CT angiography of pancreatic carcinoma: part I, evaluation of arterial involvement. *AJR Am J Roentgenol* 2002;178:827–831.
11. Rydberg J, Buckwalter KA, Caldemeyer KS, et al. Multisection CT: scanning techniques and clinical applications. *Radiographics* 2000; 20:1787–1806.
12. Foley WD. Special focus session: Multidetector CT: Abdominal visceral imaging. *Radiographics* 2002;22:701–719.
13. Ros PR, Ji H. Special focus session: Multisection (multidetector) CT: Applications in the abdomen. *Radiographics* 2002;22:697–700.
14. Williams PL, Warwick R, Dyson M, Bannister LH, eds. *Gray's anatomy*, 37th ed. New York: Churchill Livingstone, 1989.
15. Nelson RC, Chezmar JL, Peterson JE, et al. Contrast-enhanced CT of the liver and spleen: comparison of ionic and nonionic contrast agents. *AJR Am J Roentgenol* 1989;153:973–976.
16. Miles KA, McPherson SJ, Hayball MP. Transient splenic inhomogeneity with contrast-enhanced CT: mechanism and effect of liver disease. *Radiology* 1995;194:91–95.
17. Glazer GM, Axel L, Goldberg HI, et al. Dynamic CT of the normal spleen. *AJR Am J Roentgenol* 1981;137:343–346.
18. Donnelly LF, Foss JN, Frush DP, et al. Heterogeneous splenic enhancement patterns on spiral CT images in children: minimizing misinterpretation. *Radiology* 1999;210:493–497.
19. Warshauer DM, Koehler RE. Spleen. In: Lee JKT, Sagel SS, Stanley RJ, Heiken JP, eds. *Computed body tomography with MRI correlation*, 3rd ed. New York: Lippincott-Raven, 1998; 845–872.
20. Jeffrey RB Jr, Nyberg DA, Bottles K, et al. Abdominal CT in acquired immunodeficiency syndrome. *AJR Am J Roentgenol* 1986;146:7–13.
21. Warshauer DM, Dumbleton SA, Molina PL, et al. Abdominal CT findings in sarcoidosis: radiologic and clinical correlation. *Radiology* 1994; 192:93–98.
22. Wadham BM, Adams PB, Johnson MA. Incidence and location of accessory spleens. *N Engl J Med* 1981;304:1111.
23. Azar GB, Awwad JT, Mufarrij IK. Accessory spleen presenting as adnexal mass. *Acta Obstet Gynecol Scand* 1993;72:587–588.
24. Beahrs JR, Stephens DH. Enlarged accessory spleens: CT appearance in postsplenectomy patients. *AJR Am J Roentgenol* 1980;135:483–486.
25. Raissaki M, Prassopoulos P, Daskalogiannaki M, et al. Acute abdomen due to torsion of wandering spleen: CT diagnosis. *Eur Radiol* 1998; 8:1409–1412.
26. Emery KH. Splenic emergencies. *Radiol Clin North Am* 1997; 35:831–843.
27. Applegate KE, Goske MJ, Pierce G, et al. Situs revisited: imaging of the heterotaxy syndrome. *Radiographics* 1999;19:837–852; discussion 853–834.
28. Gayer G, Apter S, Jonas T, et al. Polysplenia syndrome detected in adulthood: report of eight cases and review of the literature. *Abdom Imaging* 1999;24:178–184.
29. Peoples WM, Moller JH, Edwards JE. Polysplenia: a review of 146 cases. *Pediatr Cardiol* 1983;4:129–137.
30. Winer-Muram HT, Tonkin IL, Gold RE. Polysplenia syndrome in the asymptomatic adult: computed tomography evaluation. *J Thorac Imaging* 1991;6:69–71.
31. Rose V, Izukawa T, Moes CA. Syndromes of asplenia and polysplenia. A review of cardiac and non-cardiac malformations in 60 cases with

special reference to diagnosis and prognosis. *Br Heart J* 1975; 37:840–852.

32. Waldman JD, Rosenthal A, Smith AL, et al. Sepsis and congenital asplenia. *J Pediatr* 1977;90:555–559.

33. Ahmann DL, Kiely JM, Harrison EG Jr, et al. Malignant lymphoma of the spleen. A review of 49 cases in which the diagnosis was made at splenectomy. *Cancer* 1966;19:461–469.

34. Spier CM, Kjeldsberg CR, Eyre HJ, et al. Malignant lymphoma with primary presentation in the spleen. A study of 20 patients. *Arch Pathol Lab Med* 1985;109:1076–1080.

35. Castellino RA, Hoppe RT, Blank N, et al. Computed tomography, lymphography, and staging laparotomy: correlations in initial staging of Hodgkin disease. *AJR Am J Roentgenol* 1984;143:37–41.

36. Kadin ME, Glatstein E, Dorfman RF. Clinicopathologic studies of 117 untreated patients subjected to laparotomy for the staging of Hodgkin's disease. *Cancer* 1971;27:1277–1294.

37. Kim H, Dorfman RF. Morphological studies of 84 untreated patients subjected to laparotomy for the staging of non-Hodgkin's lymphomas. *Cancer* 1974;33:657–674.

38. Castellino RA. Hodgkin disease: practical concepts for the diagnostic radiologist. *Radiology* 1986;159:305–310.

39. Harris NL, Aisenberg AC, Meyer JE, et al. Diffuse large cell (histiocytic) lymphoma of the spleen. Clinical and pathologic characteristics of ten cases. *Cancer* 1984;54:2460–2467.

40. Karpeh MS Jr, Hicks DG, Torosian MH. Colon invasion by primary splenic lymphoma: a case report and review of the literature. *Surgery* 1992;111:224–227.

41. Veronesi U, Musumeci R, Pizzetti F, et al. Proceedings: The value of staging laparotomy in non-Hodgkin's lymphomas (with emphasis on the histiocytic type). *Cancer* 1974;33:446–459.

42. Hahn PF. Biliary system, pancreas, spleen, and alimentary tract. In: Stark DD, Bradley WG, eds. *Magnetic resonance imaging*, 3rd ed. Missouri: Mosby, 1999: 471–501.

43. Canady MR, Welling RE, Strobel SL. Splenic rupture in leukemia. *J Surg Oncol* 1989;41:194–197.

44. Athale UH, Kaste SC, Bodner SM, et al. Splenic rupture in children with hematologic malignancies. *Cancer* 2000;88:480–490.

45. Smith VC, Eisenberg BL, McDonald EC. Primary splenic angiosarcoma. Case report and literature review. *Cancer* 1985;55:1625–1627.

46. Levy DW, Rindsberg S, Friedman AC, et al. Thorotrast-induced hepatosplenic neoplasia: CT identification. *AJR Am J Roentgenol* 1986; 146:997–1004.

47. Reddy SC. Hemangiosarcoma of the spleen: helical computed tomography features. *South Med J* 2000;93:825–827.

48. Garvin DF, King FM. Cysts and nonlymphomatous tumors of the spleen. *Pathol Annu* 1981;16:61–80.

49. Morgenstern L, Rosenberg J, Geller SA. Tumors of the spleen. *World J Surg* 1985;9:468–476.

50. Dachman AH, Ros PR, Murari PJ, et al. Nonparasitic splenic cysts: a report of 52 cases with radiologic–pathologic correlation. *AJR Am J Roentgenol* 1986;147:537–542.

51. Fishman EK, Soyer P, Bliss DF, et al. Splenic involvement in pancreatitis: spectrum of CT findings. *AJR Am J Roentgenol* 1995;164:631–635.

52. Pakter RL, Fishman EK, Nussbaum A, et al. CT findings in splenic hemangiomas in the Klippel–Trenaunay–Weber syndrome. *J Comput Assist Tomogr* 1987;11:88–91.

53. Moss CN, Van Dyke JA, Koehler RE, et al. Multiple cavernous hemangiomas of the spleen: CT findings. *J Comput Assist Tomogr* 1986; 10:338–340.

54. Ros PR, Moser RP Jr, Dachman AH, et al. Hemangioma of the spleen: radiologic–pathologic correlation in ten cases. *Radiology* 1987; 162:73–77.

55. Urrutia M, Mergo PJ, Ros LH, et al. Cystic masses of the spleen: radiologic–pathologic correlation. *Radiographics* 1996;16:107–129.

56. Pistoia F, Markowitz SK. Splenic lymphangiomatosis: CT diagnosis. *AJR Am J Roentgenol* 1988;150:121–122.

57. Berge T. Splenic metastases. Frequencies and patterns. *Acta Pathol Microbiol Scand [A]* 1974;82:499–506.

58. Marymont JH GS. Patterns of metastatic cancer in the spleen. *Am J Clin Pathol* 1963;40:58–66.

59. Haynes BF. Enlargement of lymph nodes and spleen. In: Wilson JD, Braunwald E, Isselbacher KJ, Petersdorf RG, Root RK, eds. *Harrison's principles of internal medicine*, 12th ed. New York: McGraw–Hill, 1991: 356–359.

60. van der Laan RT, Verbeeten B Jr, Smits NJ, et al. Computed tomography in the diagnosis and treatment of solitary splenic abscesses. *J Comput Assist Tomogr* 1989;13:71–74.

61. Shirkhoda A. CT findings in hepatosplenic and renal candidiasis. *J Comput Assist Tomogr* 1987;11:795–798.

62. Pastakia B, Shawker TH, Thaler M, et al. Hepatosplenic candidiasis: wheels within wheels. *Radiology* 1988;166:417–421.

63. Radin R. HIV infection: analysis in 259 consecutive patients with abnormal abdominal CT findings. *Radiology* 1995;197:712–722.

64. Epstein BM, Mann JH. CT of abdominal tuberculosis. *AJR Am J Roentgenol* 1982;139:861–866.

65. Im JG, Song KS, Kang HS, et al. Mediastinal tuberculous lymphadenitis: CT manifestations. *Radiology* 1987;164:115–119.

66. Lubat E, Megibow AJ, Balthazar EJ, et al. Extrapulmonary *Pneumocystis carinii* infection in AIDS: CT findings. *Radiology* 1990; 174:157–160.

67. Fishman EK, Magid D, Kuhlman JE. *Pneumocystis carinii* involvement of the liver and spleen: CT demonstration. *J Comput Assist Tomogr* 1990;14:146–148.

68. Radin DR, Baker EL, Klatt EC, et al. Visceral and nodal calcification in patients with AIDS-related *Pneumocystis carinii* infection. *AJR Am J Roentgenol* 1990;154:27–31.

69. Aldrete JS. Spontaneous rupture of the spleen in patients with infectious mononucleosis. *Mayo Clin Proc* 1992;67:910–912.

70. Takayasu K, Moriyama N, Muramatsu Y, et al. Splenic infarction, a complication of transcatheter hepatic arterial embolization for liver malignancies. *Radiology* 1984;151:371–375.

71. Balcar I, Seltzer SE, Davis S, et al. CT patterns of splenic infarction: a clinical and experimental study. *Radiology* 1984;151:723–729.

72. Nino-Murcia M, Jeffrey RB Jr, Beaulieu CF, et al. Multidetector CT of the pancreas and bile duct system: value of curved planar reformations. *AJR Am J Roentgenol* 2001;176:689–693.

73. Federle MP, Griffiths B, Minagi H, et al. Splenic trauma: evaluation with CT. *Radiology* 1987;162:69–71.

74. Jeffrey RB, Laing FC, Federle MP, et al. Computed tomography of splenic trauma. *Radiology* 1981;141:729–732.

75. Wing VW, Federle MP, Morris JA Jr, et al. The clinical impact of CT for blunt abdominal trauma. *AJR Am J Roentgenol* 1985; 145:1191–1194.

76. Orwig D, Federle MP. Localized clotted blood as evidence of visceral trauma on CT: the sentinel clot sign. *AJR Am J Roentgenol* 1989; 153:747–749.

77. Shanmuganathan K, Mirvis SE, Boyd-Kranis R, et al. Nonsurgical management of blunt splenic injury: use of CT criteria to select patients for splenic arteriography and potential endovascular therapy. *Radiology* 2000;217:75–82.

78. Fishman EK. Spiral CT: applications in the emergency patient. *Radiographics* 1996;16:943–948.

79. Leppaniemi A, Haapiainen R, Standertskjold-Nordenstam CG, et al. Delayed presentation of blunt splenic injury. *Am J Surg* 1988; 155:745–749.

CHAPTER 15

SDCT/MDCT of the Esophagus

Karen M. Horton, Elliot K. Fishman

INTRODUCTION

Computed tomography (CT) is useful in the evaluation of benign and malignant diseases of the esophagus. Although endoscopy and barium studies often are considered the diagnostic modalities of choice, they image only the mucosa, providing little information about intramural or extraluminal spread of disease. Therefore, CT has come to play an important role in evaluation of esophageal pathology owing to its unique ability to visualize accurately and rapidly the lumen, wall, adjacent structures, and lymphadenopathy, as well as distant metastases. Although the accuracy of CT has been debated in the past, spiral and multidetector CT (MDCT) have specific advantages that can overcome many of the prior limitations. This chapter will discuss the current role of CT in evaluation of the esophagus with particular emphasis on esophageal carcinoma.

TECHNIQUE

Accurate imaging of the esophagus requires the administration of both oral and intravenous contrast, with careful attention to technique.

For esophageal imaging, 500 cc of a 3% oral Hypaque (Hypaque; Amersham Health, Princeton, NJ) solution is administered routinely approximately 30 minutes prior to the scan in order to distend fully the stomach and proximal small-bowel loops. An additional 250 cc of oral contrast is given immediately prior to scanning to ensure maximal distention of the stomach and gastric cardia. Once the patient is positioned on the scanning table, an esophageal paste is administered immediately prior to the start of the intravenous injection (1). The paste (Esoph-O-CAT, E-Z-M Co., Westbury, NY) allows good opacification of the esophagus without creating streak artifacts. An alternative new barium-paste mixture also is available, consisting of carboxy-methyl-cellulose sodium paste containing barium sulfate (2). This esophageal contrast reportedly improves opacification rates of the esophageal lumen compared with studies using Esoph-O-CAT (2). Although these barium pastes do not necessarily distend the esophagus, they do coat it well. If esophageal distention is desired, effervescent granules, similar to those used for double-contrast upper-gastrointestinal series, may be administered. This especially is helpful when better visualization of the gastroesophageal junction is needed.

The administration of intravenous contrast is essential for complete evaluation of esophageal disease, especially if extraluminal extension of disease is to be evaluated accurately. One-hundred-and-twenty cubic centimeters of Omnipaque 350 (Amersham Health, Princeton, NJ) routinely was administered intravenously, at a rate of 2 cc to 3 cc per second. Scanning begins approximately 50 seconds after the initiation of the injection. This corresponds to the portal-venous phase of liver enhancement and will maximize the detection of metastases to the liver in patients with esophageal cancer. Using a single-detector row scanner, 5-mm collimation with a table speed of 8 mm per second and a reconstruction interval of 5 mm usually is adequate for most indications. If necessary, 3-mm slices can be obtained in selected cases. With new MDCT scanners, the 4-mm × 2.5-mm collimator setting typically would be used to create 5-mm slices; however, if necessary, 3-mm slices also can be created from the original acquisition. Newer 16 slice MDCT scanner allows 0.75 mm collimation. The thinner collimation especially is useful in patients with esophageal cancer and local spread of tumor. Images should be obtained from above the thoracic inlet through the liver, as malignant tumors of the esophagus often spread to the liver and to the lymph nodes in the gastrohepatic ligament and around the celiac axis.

Imaging at deep inspiration with a single breath hold results in better distention of the posterior wall of the trachea. This may be helpful when assessing tracheal invasion by the tumor (3). The use of multidetector scanners allows a more rapid acquisition and therefore requires a shorter breath hold, which helps reduce respiratory and motion artifacts and misregistration.

3D IMAGING

Three-dimensional (3D) reconstruction of CT data has been possible for almost 20 years. However, early systems were crude and offered only simplistic renderings of the surfaces of structures such as bone. They offered little application for imaging of the gastrointestinal tract. Fortunately, major advancements in both CT-scanner technology and computer hardware and software have now made powerful and affordable 3D imaging systems available. Current systems offer real-time volume-rendering software, which is easy to use and simple to incorporate into existing practices. The Siemens 3D-Virtuoso or Leonardo (Siemens Medical Solutions, Iselin, NJ) currently is used. It has been found that 3D volume rendering can be a valuable adjunct to axial imaging in patients with complicated esophageal pathology, such as esophageal perforation, tracheoesophageal fistula, and in patients with local extension of esophageal malignancies (4).

NORMAL ESOPHAGUS

The esophagus is a muscular tube that transports food and liquid from the pharynx to the stomach and prevents the reflux of stomach contents. The esophageal wall is comprised of five distinct layers: mucosa, muscularis mucosa, submucosa, and the inner and outer muscularis propria. There is no serosal layer. Thus, malignant disease can spread easily to adjacent mediastinal structures. These distinct esophageal-wall layers typically cannot be distinguished on CT scans, even when thin-collimation MDCT is performed.

On CT, the esophagus routinely is well visualized because of natural contrast provided by the surrounding lung and mediastinal fat planes. In normal patients, the esophagus typically is collapsed, although it may contain a small amount of air on several individual slices, especially in anxious patients (5).

The normal esophageal wall is very thin, usually less than 3 mm when the esophagus is distended (6). Wall thickness greater than 5 mm definitely is abnormal (7). As the esophagus traverses the diaphragmatic hiatus to join the cardia of the stomach, the wall normally may appear thickened due to the presence of the lower esophageal sphincter. This should not be confused with pathology at the gastroesophageal junction. If there is question of pathology at the gastroesophageal junction, better distension of the segment can be obtained by the use of effervescent granules.

ESOPHAGEAL CANCER

Esophageal carcinoma comprises approximately 1% of all cancers and 7% of the gastrointestinal-tract malignancies diagnosed in the United States each year (8). The estimated number of new cases in the United Staes each year is approximately 12,000 (8).

Males have a four times greater risk of developing esophageal cancer compared to females, and the risk increases with age. In the past, over 90% of esophageal malignancies were squamous-cell carcinomas, with adenocarcinomas comprising only a small minority of tumors. However, in the last two decades, the incidence of adenocarcinomas has increased, and now the ratio is approximately 60% squamous cell and 40% adenocarcinoma (8–11).

The two most common risk factors for the development of squamous-cell carcinoma of the esophagus are tobacco and alcohol consumption (8,9). There also are many conditions that predispose to the development of squamous-cell carcinoma of the esophagus, including caustic stricture, achalasia, celiac disease, radiation, Plummer–Vinson syndrome, history of oral or pharyngeal cancer, and tylosis palmaris and plantaris (12).

Adenocarcinoma historically had comprised only a minority of esophageal cancers. However, in the last 20 years, a changing epidemiology has been observed in the United States, where the incidence of adenocarcinoma has risen significantly (8,9,13). The reason for this trend is not understood fully. Adenocarcinoma usually arises in Barrett's mucosa, a sequela of long-term gastroesophageal reflux.

Surgery continues to be the most important treatment for patients with either histology who have localized disease. Although advances in surgical techniques have lowered operative mortality and shortened hospital stay, the surgery remains challenging, with a reported operative mortality of approximately 30% (13). Neoadjuvant-chemoradiation therapy combined with surgery may help improve survival (14). Recent trends include using chemotherapy and radiation therapy to downstage patients before performing surgery. Initial results with this protocol have been positive, almost doubling the 5-year survival rate, compared with surgery alone (14). However, the 5-year survival rate for patients with esophageal cancer continues to be poor, as most patients still present with metastatic or locally advanced-stage disease (15). In some countries, including China, where the incidence of esophageal cancer is greater, screening programs have led to earlier diagnosis and improved survival rates (8).

STAGING AND TREATMENT

Adequate preoperative staging of esophageal cancer is essential to determine whether therapy should be directed toward cure or palliation. The Tumor Nodes and Metastases (TNM) system is used widely for the staging of esophageal cancer, and is based on information obtained from a variety of sources: endoscopy, biopsy, endoscopic ultrasonography, barium studies, CT, bone scintigraphy, etc. (Table 15.1).

In patients with limited disease, esophagectomy is the treatment of choice, with or without pre- or postoperative chemoradiation therapy. Extraesophageal extension of disease typically precludes curative surgery, although in some patients preoperative chemotherapy and radiation may reduce the local disease enough so that surgical resection is

TABLE 15–1. *TNM staging of esophageal carcinoma*

Tis—Carcinoma in situ
T1—invasion of lamina propria or submucosa
T2—invasion of muscularis propria
T3—invasion of adventitia
T4—invasion of adjacent structure

N0—no regional nodes involved
N1—regional nodes involved

M0—no distant metastasis
M1—distant metastasis (including nodes outside mediastinum)

Stage 0—Tis, N0, M0
Stage I—T1, N0, M0
Stage IIA—T2/T3, N0, M0
Stage IIB—T1/T2, N1, M0
Stage III—T3, N1, M0 or T4, N0/1, M0
Stage IV—T1–4, N0/1, M1

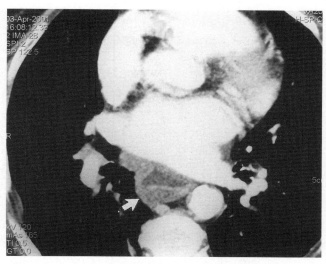

FIG. 15–1. Contrast-enhanced MDCT scan in a patient with esophageal cancer demonstrates eccentric wall thickening of the mid-esophagus (*arrow*). The esophagus also is minimally dilated.

possible. Palliative procedures include surgery, radiotherapy, chemotherapy, esophageal stents, and laser therapy.

CT IMAGING

Although the initial diagnosis of esophageal cancer typically is made with endoscopy or contrast esophagography, CT plays a valuable role in treatment planning, as well as an important role in preoperative staging. A preoperative CT can demonstrate tumor size, local extension, and invasion of adjacent organs, as well as the presence of significant adenopathy and distant metastases (11). Early studies found that CT was more accurate than magnetic resonance (MR) for staging patients with esophageal cancer (16,17). However, a recent study has found that MR and CT are comparable in predicting tumor resectability (9).

Primary Tumor

Very little has been reported about CT evaluation of early stage esophageal tumors. A limitation of CT staging of esophageal tumors is its inability to determine the exact depth of tumor infiltration of the esophageal wall, which is important for staging early carcinoma. Endoscopic ultrasound offers a distinct advantage over CT in patients with tumors confined to the esophageal wall, restaging of tumor depth after chemoradiation therapy, and in detection of anastomotic recurrence (18). Although it is true that early or superficial esophageal tumors may not be visible on CT scans, most malignant esophageal tumors are at an advanced stage at the time of diagnosis (TNM Stage III), and therefore the primary tumor typically is visible on CT in untreated patients. In a recent study of 39 patients with esophageal cancer, CT was able to identify the esophageal neoplasms in all patients (19).

The primary tumor can appear as a focal area of wall thickening (greater than 5 mm), circumferential thickening,

or a discrete soft-tissue mass (Figures 15–1 and 15–2). Computed tomography is accurate at judging tumor size, and there is a reported association between lesions greater than 3.0 cm in width on CT and the presence of periesophageal spread (19,20). Computed-tomography estimates of tumor length may not be as accurate, especially if only axial images are reviewed. However, the use of multiplanar reconstruction or 3D imaging may improve evaluation of tumor length and extension into the gastric cardia. In addition, the ability to visualize the tumor in 3D may help define better tumors at the gastroesophageal junction. The extent of tumors in this location traditionally is difficult to appreciate using axial images alone. Complications resulting from the primary tumor, such as obstruction (Figure 15-2) or perforation, also can be detected with CT.

Positron-emission tomography (PET) also has been investigated as a tool to detect and stage esophageal cancer (Figures 15–3 and 15–4). In a recent study of 32 patients with esophageal cancer, PET detected the primary tumor in 25 of 32 patients (78.1%) (21).

Local Extension

Advanced tumors are characterized by mediastinal extension of tumor with or without local adenopathy (Figure 15-5). Mediastinal invasion can involve the periesophageal fat, tracheobronchial tree, aorta, pericardium, or diaphragm. Although CT cannot always determine the intramural tumor depth, CT often can detect transmural spread of tumor into the periesophageal fat. The periesophageal fat normally demonstrates low (fat) attenuation on CT. In patients with esophageal cancer, early periesophageal invasion may appear as increased attentuation of the fat surrounding the

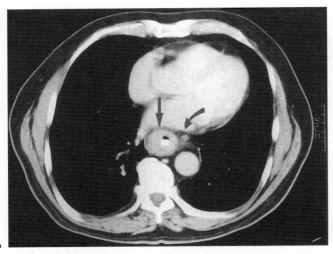
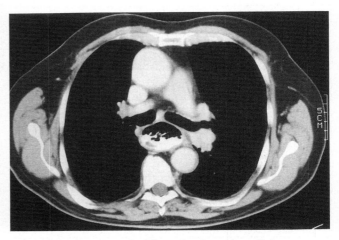

FIG. 15–2. Contrast-enhanced CT in a patient with esophageal cancer. **A:** There is circumferential thickening of the lower esophagus (*arrow*). There also is a small adjacent lymph node (*curved arrow*). **B:** Computed tomography scan at a level superior to **(A)** demonstrates a distended esophagus with residual contrast compatible with partial obstruction.

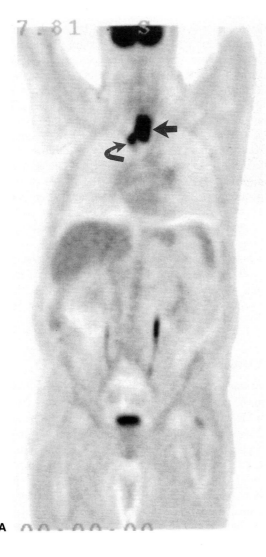

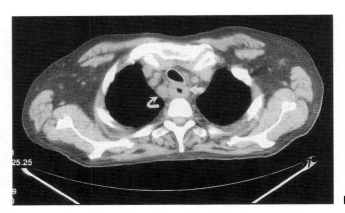

FIG. 15–3. **A:** Positron emission tomography scan in patient with esophageal cancer demonstrates the primary mass (*arrow*), as well as metastatic right paratracheal lymph node (*curved arrow*). **B:** Contrast-enhanced CT in the same patient demonstrates the esophageal thickening (*arrow*) and node (*curved arrow*).

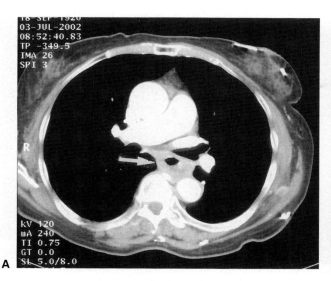
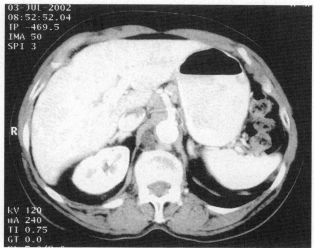

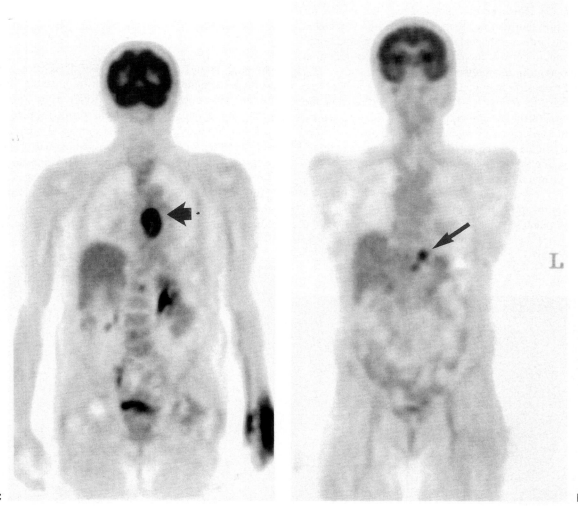

FIG. 15–4. **A:** Contrast-enhanced CT in patient with esophageal cancer demonstrates the esophageal mass (*arrow*). **B:** Axial scan at a more inferior level shows enlarged nodes in the gastrohepatic region and near the superior mesenteric artery. **C:** Positron-emission-tomography scan in the same patient shows increased activity in the chest corresponding to the primary esophageal mass (*arrow*). **D:** Positron-emission-tomography scan in the same patient shows the increased activity in the nodes (*arrow*).

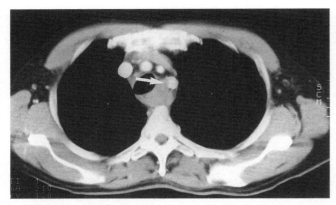

FIG. 15–5. Contrast-enhanced CT scan in a patient with esophageal cancer demonstrates mediastinal extension of the tumor, which is causing mass effect on the trachea and is encasing the left subclavian artery (*arrow*).

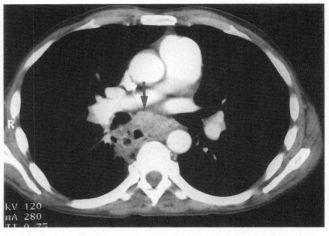

FIG. 15–7. Contrast-enhanced CT scan of a patient with esophageal cancer shows mediastinal extension of the tumor (*arrow*). The tumor has invaded the mediastinum and is invading the main-stem bronchus and medial portion of the right lower lobe.

esophagus (22). However, this appearance is not specific for tumor invasion and can occur in patients with esophagitis or in patients with esophageal cancer after chemoradiation. It is important to know if there is a prior history of radiation or chemotherapy in this patient population.

Local extension may involve the tracheobronchial tree (Figures 15–6, 15–7, and 15–8). This is suspected when the posterior wall of the airway is displaced or compressed by the adjacent tumor mass or when a discrete fistula is visualized. These fistulae may be small (less than 2 mm) and therefore 3D imaging especially is helpful for this indication (Figure 15-8). Virtual bronchoscopy also can be helpful in select cases.

Invasion of the aorta is more difficult to assess accurately. A fat plane separates the normal esophagus from the

aorta. Picus has reported that if 90 degrees or more of the aorta is in contact with the tumor (no discrete fat plane between), invasion is suggested strongly (23). An interesting study, by Wayman et al. (24), performed supine and prone CT imaging in 39 patients with esophageal carcinoma. It was felt that the combination of the supine and prone imaging improved accuracy for determining the presence of aortic invasion when compared with the supine images alone (24). Similarly, tumor invasion of the pericardium is suspected if the normal surrounding fat plane is obliterated. Computed tomography does not appear to be able to detect accurately

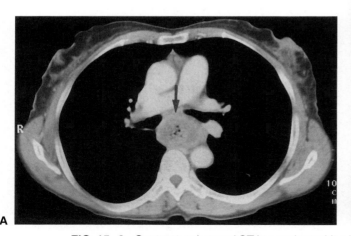

A

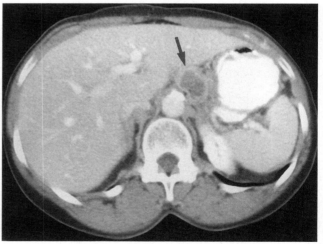

B

FIG. 15–6. Contrast-enhanced CT in a patient with a large esophageal cancer. **A:** Computed tomgraphy at the level of the pulmonary-artery bifurcation demonstrates a large subcranial mass abutting both main-stem bronchi (*arrow*). **B:** Axial contrast-enhanced CT scan at a level inferior to **(A)** demonstrates cystic nodes in the upper abdomen (*arrow*). At surgery, metastatic nodes were detected and the mass was found to have invaded the carina.

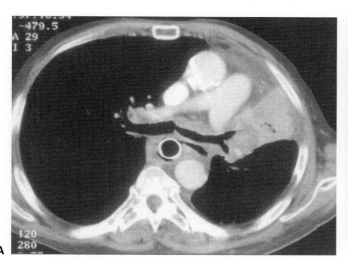
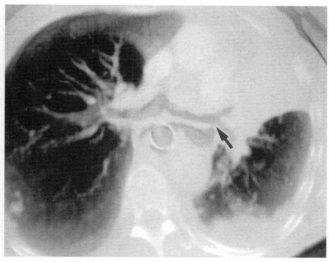

FIG. 15–8. **A:** Contrast-enhanced axial CT in a patient with locally invasive esophageal cancer and a stent. The tumor involved the airway and caused obstruction of the left upper lobe. **B:** Three-dimensional volume-rendered CT in the same patient demonstrates the fistula (*arrow*) from the tumor to the left main-stem bronchus.

diaphragmatic invasion (25), although this typically does not preclude attempt at surgical resection.

Although fat-plane obliteration is a reliable sign of tumor involvement of adjacent structure, the absence of distinct fat planes can occur as a normal variant in cachectic patients, or in patients who have received radiation therapy or surgery (26). In these situations, the fat planes may be absent throughout the mediastinum (6). However, invasion is likely if the fat plane is obliterated at the site of suspected invasion, but intact at other nearby levels. Overall, the reported sensitivity of CT for detecting mediastinal invasion in patients with esophageal carcinoma ranges from 88% to 100%, with a specificity ranging between 85% to 100% (22,23,26,27). In a study performed by Takashima et al. of 35 patients with esophageal cancer, MR and CT demonstrated similar accuracy in predicting resectability, with an accuracy of 87% and 84%, respectively (16). Three-dimensional imaging may improve visualization of the prior tumor and local extension (4). Positron-emission-tomography CT also may prove useful in this clinical application.

Adenopathy

The sensitivity of CT for detection of mediastinal lymphadenopathy is lower, as metastatic involvement of periesophageal nodes may not result in significant enlargement (25). In a study by Picus, almost all of the periesophageal nodes containing tumor measured less than 7 mm, indistinguishable on CT from uninvolved nodes (23). Although some studies suggest a decreased postoperative survival rate in patients with localized nodal spread, at this time metastases to small periesophageal nodes is not considered a contraindication to surgical resection (28).

The accuracy of CT for predicting abdominal-lymph-

node involvement ranges between 83% and 87% (3,19). Computed tomography is accurate, especially in the detection of enlarged nodes in the celiac and left gastric region, a common site of nodal disease (Figures 15–2, 15–6, and 15–9). However, CT is limited by this size criterion. Small nodes can contain malignant tumor. This point was stressed in a recent article by Romagnuolo et al., which compared CT and endoscopic ultrasound in the detection of metastases to the celiac-axis nodes in a group of patients with esophageal cancer. The sensitivity and specificity of spiral CT for diagnosing metastatic nodes in the celiac-axis region was 53% and 86%, respectively (18).

Recently, PET has been used for the staging of esophageal cancer (Figures 15–3 and 15–4). A recent study by Kim et al. compared the accuracy of PET versus CT in evaluating lymph-node metastases in patients with squamous carcinoma of the esophagus. In 53 patients, PET detected 56 metastatic-node groups (52% sensitivity, 94% specificity) compared with CT, which detected 16 metastatic-node groups (15% sensitivity, 96.7% specificity) (29). In another study by Kato et al., fluorodeoxyglucose (FDG)-PET showed a 78% sensitivity and 93% specificity for detecting lymph-node metastases, which was better than CT (61% sensitivity, 71% specificity). Positron-emission tomography used in conjunction with CT may improve preoperative staging of esophageal carcinoma (21).

Distant Metastases

Spiral CT is well suited for the detection of metastases to the solid abdominal organs. Computed tomography has an established role in the detection of liver metastases in patients with a variety of primary tumors (Figure 15-10).

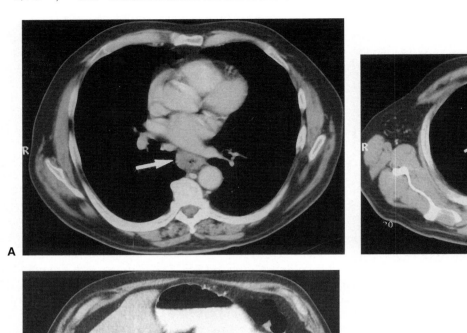

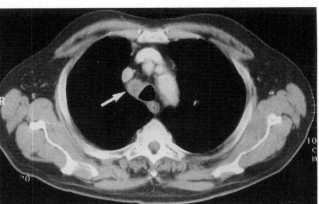

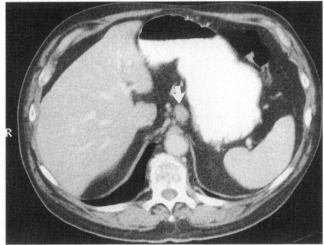

FIG. 15–9. Contrast-enhanced CT in a patient with esophageal cancer metastatic to mediastinal and gastrohepatic-ligament nodes. **A:** There is circumferential thickening of the mid-esophagus (*arrow*) compatible with known esophageal cancer. **B:** Axial scan through the chest demonstrates an enlarged right paratracheal lymph node (*arrow*). **C:** Axial scan through the upper abdomen demonstrates an enlarged lymph node in the gastrohepatic ligament (*arrow*).

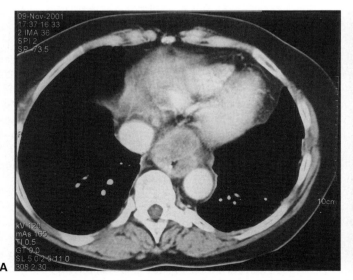

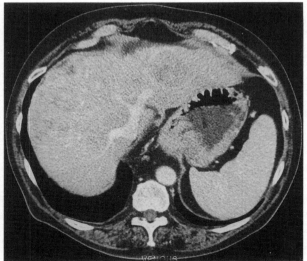

FIG. 15–10. **A:** Contrast-enhanced MDCT demonstrates a bulky esophageal tumor. **B:** Axial scan through the upper abdomen demonstrates liver metastases.

The detection of liver masses with standard incremental CT varies from series to series, but usually ranges between 60% and 75% (30–32). However, the sensitivity of spiral CT for the detection of masses 1 cm or greater in size is approximately 90% (33). The accuracy of MR and CT for evaluation of liver metastases is equivalent, but these data were for standard dynamic-CT scanning (34). In that series of 478 patients with colorectal cancer, the specificity for both CT (97%) and magnetic-resonance imaging (MRI) (94%) for the detection of liver metastases was similar to most published series. The sensitivities of the two techniques in this study were 62% and 70%, respectively (34). Although MRI can detect smaller lesions than CT, these tiny lesions cannot be characterized definitively as benign or malignant, and usually require continued follow up to assess for growth in size or number. Currently, spiral CT or MDCT is the preferred method for liver evaluation.

Multidetector CT scanning with rapid intravenous (IV) contrast injection is considered the preferred technique for liver imaging. With MDCT, the entire liver can be imaged in one breath-hold sequence lasting 10 seconds. Faster scanning eliminates respiratory misregistration and allows imaging during the optimal window for lesion contrast enhancement. A study of the detection of hepatic masses using spiral CT demonstrated a better than 90% sensitivity for detecting liver lesions greater than 1 cm in size, and a 56% sensitivity for detecting lesions less than 1 cm (33). This represents an improvement compared with traditional incremental-CT scanning. The sensitivity of CT for the detection of liver metastases is likely to increase as MDCT scanners become more widely available and allow thinner collimation and increased resolution.

On CT, liver metastases usually appear as hypodense lesions. Most metastases are visualized best during the portal-venous phase of liver enhancement, and therefore careful coordination of contrast injection and the timing of data acquisition is crucial for maximum sensitivity. Metastases usually are multiple and vary in size. If only one lesion is detected, CT or ultrasound-guided biopsy can be performed to obtain pathologic confirmation.

Positron-emission tomography also has been used for the detection of distant metastases in patients with esophageal carcinoma. In a study by Lightdale et al., PET had a sensitivity of 91% and a specificity of 93% in the detection of distant metastases (11). This corresponded to an accuracy of 91%. However, although the use of PET in this clinical setting is promising, it still is limited in its availability.

Postoperative Esophagus

The most common surgical procedure performed today for the treatment of malignant disease of the esophagus is the partial esophagogastrectomy. This consists of a transhiatal esophagectomy followed by either a gastric pull up or co-lonic interposition (Figure 15-11). The surgical procedure is complex and can result in a number of postsurgical complications, including anastomotic leak (Figure 15-12) or stricture, mediastinal abscess, chylothorax, or lymphocele (35). Complications can occur in up to 50% of patients (36).

Anastomotic stricture or recurrence can be difficult to appreciate on CT scans, unless it results in a significant obstruction. The exact location of the esophago-stomach anastomosis is not always obvious on CT and is appreciated better on video-swallowing examinations or endoscopy. Postsurgical leaks at the anastomosis can be recognized by extraluminal air or extravasation of oral contrast.

Mediastinal abscess is an important potential complication of esophagectomy, which usually results from a contained leak. The abscess usually will begin at the anastomosis, although it may extend locally. It can be suspected by the development of fever, leukocytosis, and chest pain. On CT, a mediastinal abscess appears as a loculated fluid collection in the mediastinum, which typically demonstrates an enhancing wall and may contain gas or an air–fluid level.

Chylothorax also is a well-recognized complication of transhiatal esophagectomy, occurring in between 0.8% and 3% of patients (37). Chylothorax results from injury to the thoracic duct (37,38). During esophagectomy, the thoracic duct may be injured, usually between the diaphragmatic hiatus and the carina, where the duct is a prevertebral structure coursing behind the esophagus before crossing to the left of the spine at the T4–5 level. On CT, a persistent or increasing pleural effusion is demonstrated. Computed tomography sometimes can distinguish a chylous effusion from nonchylous effusion by noting a fat–fluid level in the chylous effusion. However, in most cases, correlation with thoracentesis and laboratory analysis is necessary for specific diagnosis.

A lymphocele is another complication resulting from injury to the thoracic duct during surgery. It represents a more localized fluid collection on CT, compared to a layering and free-flowing chylothorax. After esophagectomy, a lymphocele may occur in the thorax or upper abdomen (38).

It is important for the radiologist to be familiar with the normal postoperative appearance and to be aware of the potential complications in order to evaluate optimally these patients in the postoperative period.

Recurrence

Even after curative resection, a large number of patients with esophageal carcinoma experience recurrence. In a study by Morita of 187 cases of after-curative esophagectomy for squamous-cell carcinoma, over 50% of the patients died of recurrence (39). The most common recurrence patterns included lymphatic (48%), hematogenous (24%), mixed lymphatic and hematogenous (23%), and intramural recurrence (4%). The most common organs involved with recurrence are lung, liver, and bone (40). Thus, although endoscopy and endoscopic ultrasound are effective in diagnosis of anastomotic tumor recurrence, as well as regional lymph-node

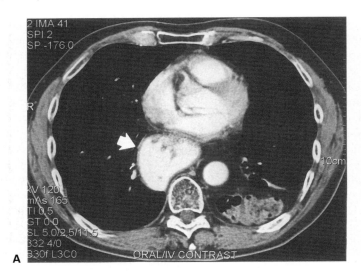

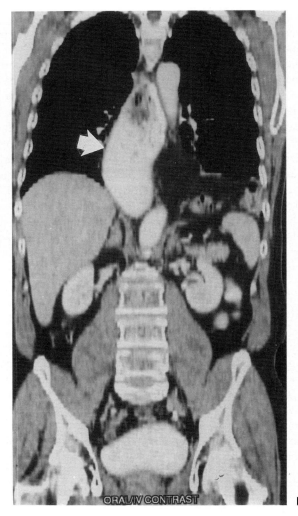

FIG. 15–11. Contrast-enhanced CT in a patient after esophagectomy with gastric pull up. **A:** Axial scan demonstrates the gastric pull up in the chest (*arrow*). **B:** Coronal multiplanar reconstruction again demonstrates the normal CT appearance of a gastric pull up (*arrow*).

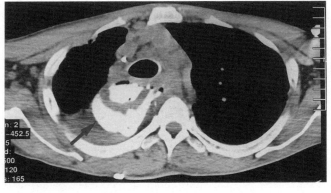

FIG. 15–12. Computed tomography scan with oral contrast only in a patient with esophageal cancer after esophagectomy with gastric pull up. There is extravasation of contrast at the esophagogastric anastomosis (*arrow*).

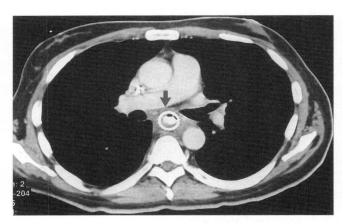

FIG. 15–13. Contrast-enhanced CT in a patient with recurrent esophageal cancer. An esophageal stent (*arrow*) has been placed for palliation.

involvement, CT is important for follow up in order to detect distant metastases. The prognosis following recurrence is extremely poor. However, recent advancements with neoadjuvant-chemoradiation therapy combined with surgery may help improve survival by decreasing recurrence rates (14). Treatment of recurrence can include additional chemotherapy or palliative stents (Figures 15–8 and 15–13).

BENIGN DISEASES

Benign Esophageal Tumors

Benign esophageal tumors such as leiomyoma, lipoma, fibroma, neurofibroma, hamartoma, or hemangioma may be incidental findings on CT. These tumors typically are intramural and smooth in contour. Only large tumors (greater than 1 cm to 2 cm) will be detected on CT. In some cases, CT may allow definitive diagnosis or be employed as a problem-solving tool. For instance, the diagnosis of lipoma can be made confidently on CT, which will demonstrate characteristic fat attenuation. Similarly, esophageal cysts, such as congenital-duplication cysts or acquired-retention cysts, may demonstrate water attentuation on CT depending on the contents of the cyst. Esophageal leiomyomas typically appear as homogeneous low-density or isodense masses with smooth or lobulated margins (41).

Esophageal Varices

In patients with portal hypertension, increased resistance to portal-venous flow in the liver results in the development of portosystemic collaterals. The most common and clinically relevant collaterals involve the paraesophageal-venous plexus. Owing to the high-resistance flow in the liver, blood flows from the portal system retrograde through the left coronary vein or short gastric veins to the esophageal-venous plexus and eventually empties into the azygous system.

Spiral CT with intravenous contrast is an excellent modality for the detection and evaluation of portosystemic shunts in patients with portal hypertension (42) (Figures 15–14 and 15–15). The sensitivity of CT for the detection of varices is superior to a barium esophagram. In addition, CT allows for better evaluation of the extent and size of varices, as well as the ability to detect other portosystemic collaterals (43).

The CT appearance of esophageal varices varies depending on the size and extent of involvement. Usually, on unenhanced scans, esophageal varices appear as thickening or nodularity of the esophageal wall. With IV contrast, esophageal varices will appear as enhancing vascular structures within the esophageal wall (44). On noncontrast scans, large varices can simulate adenopathy in the posterior mediastinum, which is a potential pitfall.

Computed-tomography angiography with volume rendering also can be used to evaluate better portosystemic col-

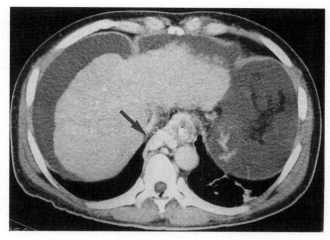

FIG. 15–14. Contrast-enhanced CT in a patient with portal hypertension demonstrates esophageal varices (*arrow*). In addition, ascites are present.

laterals (Figure 15-15). In particular, the CT appearance of esophageal varices is distinctive. Furthermore, the use of 3D reconstruction with volume rendering clearly demonstrates esophageal-venous collaterals and their relationship to the portal- and systemic-venous systems (45).

Esophagitis

There are many causes of esophagitis, including gastro-esophageal reflux, radiation therapy, corrosive ingestions,

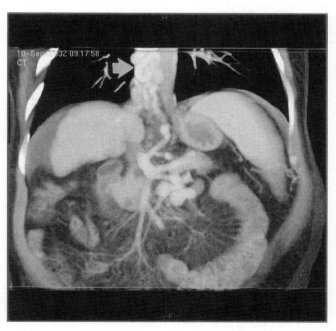

FIG. 15–15. Three-dimensional volume-rendered CT angiography in coronal projection demonstrates esophageal varices (*arrow*).

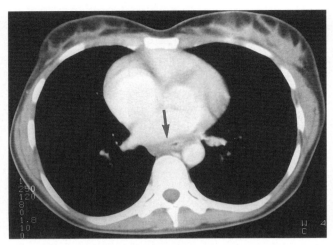

FIG. 15–16. Contrast-enhanced CT in a patient with esophagitis demonstrates circumferential wall thickening of the esophagus (*arrow*). The wall has a low-density appearance compatible with edema.

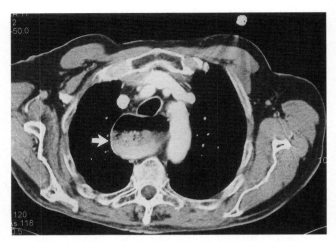

FIG. 15–18. Contrast-enhanced CT in a patient with achalasia demonstrates marked dilation of the esophagus (*arrow*). There is retained contrast and debris within the esophagus. Also note that the esophageal wall is not thickened.

Crohn's disease, and a variety of infections. Immunosuppressed patients particularly are prone to certain esophageal infections, such as Candida, herpes simplex, cytomegalovirus, and tuberculosis. Candidiasis is the most common cause of infection esophagitis and is caused by spread of the fungus from the oropharynx to the esophagus.

Regardless of the etiology, the CT findings of esophagitis usually consist of nonspecific diffuse esophageal wall thickening (Figures 15–16 and 15–17). Occasionally, deep esophageal ulceration is identified. If ulceration, intramural dissection, and fistula formation are identified, tuberculosis should be considered as the possible etiologic agent (46).

Achalasia

Achalasia is a motor disorder of the esophagus characterized by inadequate relaxation of the lower esophageal

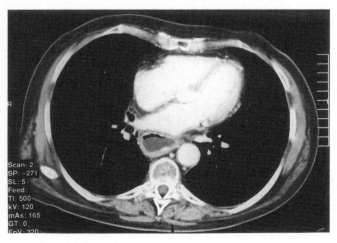

FIG. 15–17. Contrast-enhanced CT in a patient with esophagitis demonstrates circumferential wall thickening. There also is fluid distention of the esophagus.

sphincter and failure of organized peristalsis in the lower esophagus. Although the condition usually is evaluated with barium studies and endoscopy, CT plays a role.

Computed tomography in patients with achalasia demonstrates moderate-to-marked dilatation of the esophagus, with a mean esophageal diameter of 4.5 cm at the level of the carina (47) (Figure 15-18). There often is an abrupt transition from the dilated esophagus to normal at the gastroesophageal junction. Air, fluid, or food particles often are present in the lumen. The esophageal wall usually is of normal thickness.

Since achalasia is associated with the development of esophageal carcinoma, CT can detect and demonstrate the extent of esophageal neoplasms occurring in these patients.

Esophageal Perforation

Perforation of the esophagus is a life-threatening condition that must be recognized early in order to decrease morbidity and mortality. It may occur spontaneously, or because of chest trauma, foreign-body aspiration, esophageal neoplasms, or endoscopic procedures. Although contrast radiography is considered to be the radiographic standard for the evaluation of patients with suspected esophageal perforation, up to 10% of patients with esophageal perforation may have false-negative findings on contrast esophagram (48). In addition, if the clinical symptoms are atypical, CT may be performed early in the clinical course and may be the first to suggest the diagnosis (49). Therefore, recognition of the CT findings in esophageal perforation is important. In addition, CT can detect extraluminal complications of perforation such as pneumomediastinum, mediastinal abscess, and empyema.

Computed tomography is useful in the diagnosis of esophageal perforation and may help direct surgical manage-

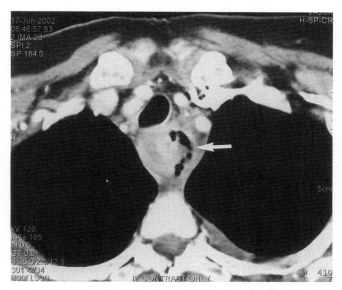

FIG. 15–19. Contrast-enhanced CT in a patient after upper endoscopy demonstrates periesophageal inflammation, as well as extraluminal air (*arrow*). This is compatible with esophageal perforation.

ment. Extraluminal air is the most useful CT finding, occurring in over 90% of cases (49) (Figure 15-19). Although mediastinal air is a sensitive indicator of esophageal perforation, it is not specific. Patients with pneumothorax or pneumoperitoneum may have extension of air into the mediastinum without esophageal injury. Other CT findings include the presence of mediastinal fluid, pleural fluid, or esophageal-wall thickening. Extravasated oral contrast may be demonstrated when the perforation is transmural. In cases of contained intramural perforation, CT will demonstrate intramural air and/or contrast.

In patients with esophageal carcinoma as the cause of the perforation, CT can evaluate the location of the mass and assess for local extension and distant metastases. In patients with suspected esophageal injury and/or perforation after ingestion of a caustic substance, CT can be performed, as there is a risk of perforation of the acutely inflamed esophagus during endoscopy.

CONCLUSION

With the introduction of MDCT, along with significant improvements in 3D-imaging software and hardware, CT has come to play a vital role in imaging both benign and malignant diseases of the esophagus. It can be used to detect and stage malignancies of the esophagus, as well as to identify and classify a variety of nonneoplastic conditions.

REFERENCES

1. NIH Consensus. *Helicobacter pylori* in peptic ulcer disease. *JAMA* 1994; 272:65–69.
2. Noda Y, Ogawa Y, Nishioka A, et al. New barium paste mixture for helical (slip-ring) CT evaluation of the esophagus. *Comput Assist Tomogr* 1996;20:773–776.
3. Wolfman NT, Scharling ES, Chen MY. Esophageal squamous carcinoma. *Radiol Clin North Am* 1994;32:1183–1201.
4. Griffith JF, Kew J, Chan ACW, et al. 3D CT of esophageal cancer. *Eur J Radiol* 1999;32:216–220.
5. Goldwin RL, Heitzman ER, Proto AV. Computed tomography of the mediastinum. Normal anatomy and indications for the use of CT. *Radiology* 1977;124:235–241.
6. Noh HM, Fishman EK, Forastiere AA, et al. CT of the esophagus: spectrum of disease with emphasis on esophageal carcinoma. *Radiographics* 1995;15:1113–1134.
7. Desai RK, Tagliabue JR, Wegryn SA, et al. CT evaluation of wall thickening in the alimentary tract. *Radiographics* 1991;11:771–783.
8. Levine MS, Halvorsen RA. Carcinoma of the esophagus. In: Gore RM Levine MS, eds. *Textbook of gastrointestinal radiology*. Philadelphia: WB Saunders, 2000:403–433.
9. Levine MS. Esophageal cancer: radiologic diagnosis. *Radiol Clin North Am* 1997; 35:265–279.
10. Daly JM, Fry WA, Little AG, et al. Esophageal cancer: results of an American College of Surgeons patient care evaluation study. *Am Coll Surg* 2000;190:562–573.
11. Lightdale CJ. Positron emission tomography: another useful test for staging esophageal cancer. *J Clin Oncol* 2000;18:3199–3201.
12. Kumbasar B. Carcinoma of esophagus: radiologic diagnosis and staging. *Eur J Radiol* 2002;42:170–180.
13. Heitmiller RF, Jones B. Transient diminished airway protection after transhiatal esophagectomy. *Am J Surg* 1991;162:442–446.
14. Forasriere AA, Orringer MB, Perez-Tamayo C, et al. Preoperative chemoradiation followed by transhiatal esophagectomy for carcinoma of the esophagus: final report. *J Clin Oncol* 1993;11:1118–1123.
15. Lowe VJ, Stack BC Jr. Esophageal cancer and head and neck cancer. *Semin Roentgenol* 2002;37:140–150.
16. Takashima S, Takeuchi N, Shiozaki H, et al. carcinoma of the esophagus: CT versus MR imaging in determining resectability. *AJR Am J Roentgenol* 1991;156:297–302.
17. Quint LA, Glazer GM, Orringer MB, et al. Esophageal carcinoma: CT findings. *Radiology* 1985;155:171–175.
18. Romagnuolo J, Scott J, Hawes RH, et al. Helical CT versus EUS with fine needle aspiration for celiac nodal assessment in patients with esophageal cancer. *Gastrointest Endosc* 2002;55:648–654.
19. Drudi FM, Trippa F, Cascone F, et al. Esophagram and CT vs endoscopic and surgical specimens in the diagnosis of esophageal carcinoma. *Radiol Med (Torino)* 2002;103:344–352.
20. Lefor AT, Merino M, Steinberg SM, et al. Computerized tomographic prediction of extraluminal spread and prognostic implications of lesion width in esophageal cancer. *Cancer* 1988;62:1287–1292.
21. Kato H, Kuwano H, Nakajima M, et al. Comparison between positron emission tomography and computed tomography in the use of the assessment of esophageal carcinoma. *Cancer* 2002;15:921–928.
22. Coulomb M, Lebas JF, Sarrazin R, et al. Oesophageal cancer extension. Diagnostic contribution and effects of therapy of computed tomography (French). *J Radiol* 1981;62:475–487.
23. Picus D, Balfe DM, Koehler RE, et al. Computed tomography in the staging of esophageal carcinoma. *Radiology* 1983;146:433–438.
24. Wayman J, Chakraverty S, Griffin SM, et al. Evaluation of local invasion by esophageal carcinoma—a prospective study of prone computed tomography scanning. *Postgrad Med J* 2001;77:181–184.
25. van Overhagen H, Lameris JS, Berger MY, et al. CT assessment of resectability prior to transhiatal esophagectomy for esophageal/gastroesophageal junction carcinoma. *J Comput Assist Tomogr* 1993; 17:367–373.
26. Daffner RH, Halber MD, Postlethwait RW, et al. CT of the esophagus. II. Carcinoma. *AJR Am J Roentgenol* 1979;133:1051–1055.
27. Halvorsen RA Jr, Thompson WM. Computed tomographic staging of gastrointestinal malignancies. Part I. Esophagus and stomach. *Invest Radiol* 1987;22:2–16.
28. Rosenberg JC, Franklin R, Steiger Z. Squamous cell carcinoma of the thoracic esophagus: an interdisciplinary approach. *Curr Probl Cancer* 1981;5:1–52.
29. Kim K, Park SJ, Kim BT, et al. Evaluation of lymph node metastases in squamous cell carcinoma of the esophagus with positron emission tomography. *Ann Thorac Surg* 2001;71:290–294.

30. Wernecke K, Rummeny E, Bongartz G, et al. Detection of hepatic masses in patients with carcinoma: comparative sensitivities of sonography, CT and MR imaging. *AJR Am J Roentgenol* 1991;157:731–739.

31. Miller WJ, Baron RL, Dodd GD 3rd, et al. Malignancies in patients with cirrhosis: CT sensitivity and specificity in 200 consecutive transplant patients. *Radiology* 1994;193:645–650.

32. Matsui O, Tacashima T, Kadoya M, et al. liver metastases from colorectal cancer; detection with CT during arterial portography. *Radiology* 1987;165:65–69.

33. Kuszyk BS, Bluemke DA, Urban BA, et al. Portal-phase contrast enhanced helical CT for the detection of malignant hepatic tumors: sensitivity based on comparison with intraoperative and pathologic findings. *AJR Am J Roentgenol* 1996;166:91–95.

34. Zerhouni EA, Rutter C, Hamilton SR, et al. CT and MR imaging in the staging of colorectal carcinoma: report of Radiology Diagnostic Oncology Group II. *Radiology* 1996;200:443–451.

35. Tunaci A. postoperative imaging of gastrointestinal tract cancers. *Eur J Radiol* 2002;42:224–230.

36. Kararia K, Harvey JC, Pina E, et al. Complications of transhiatal esophagectomy. *J Surg Oncol* 1994;57:157–163.

37. Orringer MB, Bluett M, Deeb GM. Aggressive treatment of chylothorax complicating transhiatal esophagectomy without thoracotomy. *Sugery* 1988;104:720–726.

38. Reichle RL, Fishman EK, Nixon MS, et al. Evaluation of the postsurgical esophagus after partial esophagogastrectomy for esophageal cancer. Normal postoperative appearance and complications. *Invest Radiol* 1993;28:247–257.

39. Morita M, Kuwano H, Ohno S, et al. Characteristic and sequence of recurrence patterns after curative esophagectomy for squamous cell carcinoma. *Surgery* 1994;116:1–7.

40. Isono K, Onoda S, Okuyama K, et al. Recurrence of intrathoracic esophageal cancer. *Jpn J Clin Oncol* 1985;15:49–60.

41. Yang PS, Lee KS, Lee SJ, et al. Esophageal leiomyoma: radiologic findings in 12 patients. *Korean J Radiol* 2001;2:132–137.

42. Cho KC, Patel YD, Wachsberg RH, et al. Varices in portal hypertension: evaluation with CT. *Radiographics* 1995;15:609–622.

43. Balthazar EJ, Naidich DP, Megibow AJ, et al. CT evaluation of esophageal varices. *AJR Am J Roentgenol* 1987;148:131–135.

44. Clark KE, Foley WD, Lawson TL, et al. CT evaluation of esophageal and upper abdominal varices. *J Comput Assist Tomogr* 1980;4:510–515.

45. Henseler KP, Pozniak MA, Lee FT Jr, et al. Three-dimensional CT angiography of spontaneous portosystemic shunts. *Radiographics* 2001;21:691–704.

46. deSilva R, Stoopack PM, Raufman JP. Esophageal fistulas associated with mycobacterial infection in patients at risk for AIDS. *Radiology* 1990;175:449–453.

47. Rabushka LS, Fishman EK, Kuhlman JE. CT evaluation of achalasia. *J Comput Assist Tomogr* 1991;15:434–439.

48. Bladergroen MR, Lowe JE, Postlethwait RW. Diagnosis and recommended management of esophageal perforation and rupture. *Ann Thorac Surg* 1986;42:235–239.

49. White CS, Templeton PA, Attar S. Esophageal perforation: CT findings. *AJR Am J Roentgenol* 1993;160:767–770.

CHAPTER 16

SDCT/MDCT of the Stomach

Karen M. Horton, Elliot K. Fishman

INTRODUCTION

Although barium studies and endoscopy classically have been considered the diagnostic modalities of choice for the evaluation of gastric pathology, computed tomography (CT) is used increasingly as the first-line imaging study in patients with a variety of symptoms. It is imperative, therefore, that the radiologist be familiar with the CT appearance of the normal stomach, as well as the appearance of a variety of gastric conditions. In addition, CT also plays an important role in the staging and follow up of gastric malignancies once the diagnosis has been established.

The recent technical advancement in CT, along with current interest in the use of water- and air-contrast techniques, suggests that the usefulness of CT in the evaluation of gastric pathology may increase.

TECHNIQUE

For adequate CT examination of the stomach, careful technique is essential. The key to CT imaging of the stomach is gastric distention, as wall thickening can be simulated by underdistention or masked by pathology. Gastric distention can be accomplished by positive-contrast solutions such as Hypaque (Amersham Health, Princeton, NJ), by neutral agents such as water, or by negative contrast agents such as air.

Positive Contrast

In abdominal imaging, positive-contrast agents such as Hypaque (Amersham Health, Princeton, NJ) have traditionally been used. A 3% oral Hypaque solution (500 cc–750 cc) is administered routinely 30 minutes to 60 minutes before the scan in order to fill the stomach and small-bowel loops. An additional 250 cc of oral contrast is given immediately prior to scanning to ensure maximal distention of the stomach.

Although widely used, there are some concerns that positive-contrast agents may obscure pathology when the gastrointestinal wall is enhanced simultaneously with intravenous (IV) agents (1,2). In addition, there are reports of inadequate mixing of these agents with gastrointestinal contents, sometimes resulting in "pseudotumors" (3,4). Finally, the use of positive-oral-contrast agents interferes with manipulation of the dataset in CT angiography. Therefore, investigators have explored the use of alternative oral-contrast agents for use with abdominal CT.

Water Contrast

Several investigators have advocated the use of water as a low-density contrast agent for imaging of the stomach and upper gastrointestinal tract (1,5–8). Water is safe, well tolerated, and inexpensive. Water may allow better visualization of the enhanced wall of the stomach and small bowel and will not interfere with CT angiography, as has been described with positive-contrast agents (1,2) (Figure 16-1). Limitations of the use of water include suboptimal evaluation of the distal small bowel and colon, and potential confusion between water-filled bowel loops and abnormal abdominal-fluid collections (abscess). These theoretical concerns usually are not a problem when IV contrast is administered, because even nondistended bowel loops have a characteristic wall enhancement and fold pattern that allows identification. However, water would limit the ability to diagnose extravasation of contrast from gastrointestinal perforation and therefore, for this clinical indication, positive-contrast agents are preferred (5). Some authors have advocated giving positive contrast initially, followed by water (9). The positive contrast will opacify the distal small-bowel loops, whereas the water will distend the stomach and proximal small bowel.

The use of water in patients with suspected gastric pathology is preferred. If water contrast is desired, 750 cc of water is given 20 minutes to 30 minutes prior to

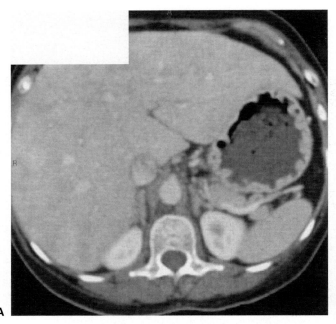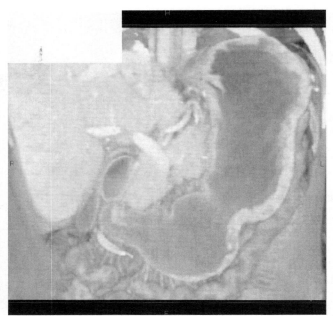

FIG. 16–1. Contrast-enhanced axial MDCT scan in a normal patient demonstrates distention of the stomach with water. **A:** Axial scan shows the normal gastric wall and folds. **B:** Coronal 3D volume-rendered image nicely demonstrates the gastric anatomy and normal fold pattern.

the exam. An additional 250 cc of water is given to the patient immediately before scanning begins.

Air Contrast

If air contrast is desired, effervescent citrocarbonate granules (4 g to 6 g) can be given with 30 cc of water. Gaseous distention alone, while good for evaluation of stomach pathology, does not provide adequate contrast for the remainder of the bowel. Gas granules also can be administered after the patient has consumed the Hypaque or water for additional air distention of the stomach. Air, like water, is a low density contrast agent and therefore allows better visualization of bowel-wall enhancement and will not interfere with CT angiography.

Oil-based agents also have been investigated as potential CT oral-contrast agents, (10) and do allow adequate depiction of the gastric wall, but they are not well tolerated by patients and typically will cause steatorrhea.

IV Contrast

Regardless of the oral-contrast agent used, the administration of IV contrast is essential for complete evaluation of the stomach. Spiral CT and multidetector CT (MDCT) combine rapid scanning and rapid infusion of contrast, resulting in better visualization of bowel loops and gastric wall. Subtle changes often are well visualized. Typically, 120 cc of Omnipaque 350 (Amersham Health, Princeton, NJ) is injected intravenously, at a rate of 2 cc to 3 cc per

second. Scanning begins approximately 45 seconds after the initiation of the contrast injection.

Scan Protocol

With a single-detector row spiral scanner, 5-mm collimation is adequate. A 3-mm reconstruction interval is helpful if three-dimensional (3D) imaging is to be performed. However, when imaging gastric pathology, the preference is to use a multidetector row scanner. It is faster, allows thinner collimation, and has better resolution compared to traditional single-detector row scanners. A Siemens Somatom Volume Zoom (Siemens Medical Solutions, Iselin, NJ) is currently used, which can be eight times faster than traditional 1-second single-detector row spiral scanners. Depending on the collimator setting, the Volume Zoom can acquire up to 4 slices per 0.5-second rotation, nearly eliminating motion artifacts. In addition, these scanners allow thinner slices than single-detector spiral scanners; 1.00-mm to 1.25-mm slices are easily obtainable. Even thinner slices (0.75 mm) can be obtained with the new 16 slice MDCT scanners. The thinner collimation definitely improves the quality of the 3D dataset in terms of gastric imaging, as well as CT angiography.

When imaging a patient with gastric pathology, the 4-mm × 1.0-mm collimator setting is used; 1.25-mm slices then are generated. Using this setting, the abdomen (diaphragm-to-iliac crest) can be scanned in 20 seconds. Depending on the indication, dual-phase imaging may be performed. Arterial-phase images are acquired 25 seconds after the start of the injection; venous-phase images are acquired 50 seconds after the start of the injection. This allows optimal visualization of both the gastric arteries and veins, as well as optimal detection of liver metastases.

3D Imaging

Three-dimensional imaging of the gastrointestinal tract, the colon in particular, has gained much attention since it first was proposed in 1993. At that time, 3D imaging was limited by computer speed and performance. Early reports of 3D CT imaging of the stomach (CT gastroscopy) were limited to surface-rendering techniques, that is, shaded surface. However, with improvements in computer technology and speed, most manufacturers now also offer volume rendering (VR). Volume rendering is superior to shaded surface for imaging the stomach and gastric vessels. The Siemens 3D Virtuoso Imaging package currently is used. This software includes real-time volume rendering, as well as fly-through capabilities.

At John Hopkins Medical Institutions, after the data are acquired (1.25-mm slices reconstructed at 1-mm intervals), they are transferred over an Ethernet to an Infinite Reality or Onyx workstation with Reality Engine graphics (Silicon Graphics, Mt. View, CA) or an O2 workstation for interac-

tive volume rendering. Simple two-dimensional (2D) multiplanar reconstructions (MPR) of the CT data allow quick visualization of the stomach in the axial, sagittal, and coronal planes (Figure 16-2). Most radiologists are familiar and comfortable with 2D MPR. It is quick and available on all workstations. An abnormality detected in one plane can be visualized immediately in the other two planes. It often is helpful to start with the MPR and then proceed with the 3D.

The 3D volume set can be manipulated using different orientations or cut planes in order to demonstrate best the stomach and pathology (Figure 16-3). This flexibility is a distinct advantage over traditional axial images. In addition to the use of cut planes, the radiologist has the ability to change the opacity, brightness, window width, and level. This allows the radiologist to accentuate certain structures.

In addition, the CT data of the stomach also can be manipulated to simulate images as seen by the endoscopist for "virtual gastroscopy" (4,11,12) (Figure 16-4). Early studies of this technique were limited, mostly due to computer limitations. In a study by Springer et al. of both cadavers and patients, the endoluminal views using shaded-surface display (SSD) correlated well with endoscopy except for artificial smoothing of surface structures and density limitations created by the shaded-surface technique (SST) (4). The quality of virtual gastroscopy is improved with the use of

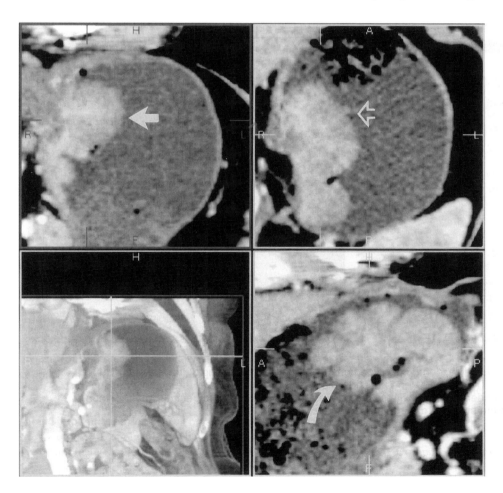

FIG. 16-2. Multiplanar reconstruction in a patient with gastric cancer. The mass can be visualized simultaneously in the coronal (*solid arrow*), axial (*open arrow*), and sagittal (*curved arrow*) planes.

geons recommend laparotomy in all cases of gastric cancer for either curative resection or palliation, obviating the need for a CT scan. Conversely, many surgeons rely on CT findings to help stage the malignancy, plan patient therapy, and plan the surgical approach. The reported accuracy of CT in gastric-cancer staging has varied widely in the literature, partially owing to differences in scanning techniques over the past two decades. With the advent of spiral CT, and more recently MDCT, combining narrow collimation and close interspace scanning, it is likely that the accuracy of CT will improve. In a study by Hori et al. using single-detector CT (SDCT) of patients with advanced gastric cancers, water was used as an oral-contrast agent. Computed tomography detected 95% of the advanced cacinomas and 93% of the early carcinomas (8). In a different study of gastric-cancer staging at CT by Baert et al., CT was able to detect 22 of 24 cancers (91%)(7). Computed tomography has some limitation when staging gastric cancers, as it cannot always determine the level of invasion within the gastric wall (19). Endoscopic ultrasound is more sensitive for visualizing the individual gastric-wall layers.

In addition to the use of water as oral contrast, there may be some benefit to performing dual-phase imaging of the abdomen when staging patients with gastric carcinoma, as supported in studies by Hundt et al. and Mani et al. (20,21). Hundt et al. performed dual-phase imaging of the abdomen during the arterial and venous phases of enhancement and were able to detect 97.5% (39 of 40) of cancers (20). The CT staging correlated with the surgical and pathological staging in 79% of the patients. The major limitation to staging in that study was difficulty in detecting tumor invasion in normal-sized lymph nodes.

Mani et al. also performed dual-phase imaging, but at 45 seconds and 3 minutes after IV-contrast injection (21). They found that the 45-second scan was helpful for determination of the depth of the tumor and invasion through the gastric wall and correctly determined the depth of tumor invasion in 17 of 20 patients (21). The 3-minute delay was not found to be helpful. It is not clear why they chose such a long scan delay and decided not to image during the arterial phase, which would be beneficial for displaying the arterial anatomy. The optimal protocol for imaging patients with gastric malignancies has yet to be determined. However, it is clear that a portal-venous-phase scan is necessary in order to detect potential liver metastases. The addition of arterial-phase imaging also may be helpful in select cases.

In addition, 3D imaging may help improve the staging accuracy of CT. In a study by Lee et al. of patients with advanced gastric cancer, the combination of 3D imaging with axial images allowed more accurate staging than with axial images alone (16).

CT IMAGING

Primary Tumor

Common CT appearances of primary gastric carcinoma include discrete soft-tissue mass with or without ulceration

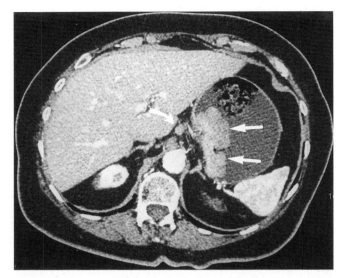

FIG. 16–6. Contrast-enhanced axial MDCT demonstrates a large enhancing mass along the medial wall of the stomach (*arrows*); this was an adenocarcinoma of the stomach. A small lymph node is noted in the gastrohepatic ligament (*curved arrow*).

or wall thickening, which may be focal or diffuse (*linitis plastica*)(14) (Figures 16–6, 16–7, and 16–8). The average wall thickness in gastric carcinoma is 2 cm, ranging from 6 mm to 4 cm. Owing to limited spatial resolution, CT often is not able to distinguish the layers within the gastric wall, and therefore is not able to determine depth of tumor invasion. However, CT is able to demonstrate accurately wall thickening, which has been shown to correlate directly with probability of transmural extension. Patients with diffuse infiltration of the stomach can present with *linitis plastica*. In these cases, the stomach wall thickens and often will allow only limited gastric distention.

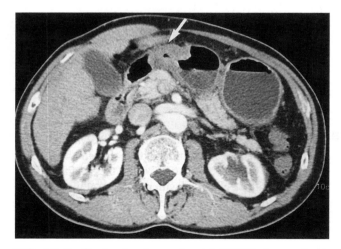

FIG. 16–7. Contrast-enhanced axial MDCT demonstrates focal circumferential narrowing at the gastric atrum (*arrow*). This was an adenocarcinoma.

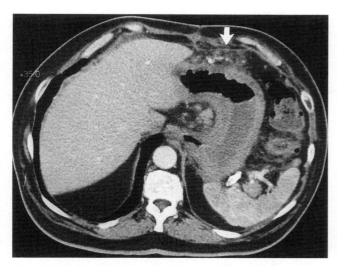

FIG. 16–8. Contrast-enhanced axial MDCT demonstrates diffuse circumferential thickening of the stomach. There is limited gastric distention. This is an example of linitis plastica. There also is minimal stranding in the fat anterior to the stomach (*arrow*), compatible with carcinomatosis.

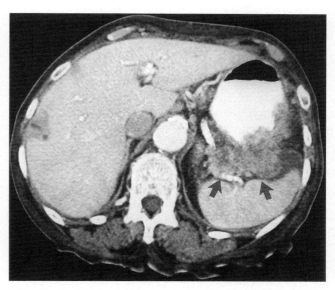

FIG. 16–9. Contrast-enhanced MDCT in a patient with gastric cancer demonstrates extraluminal extension of the tumor posterior to the stomach (*arrows*). There also is liver metastasis.

In a study by Cho et al. using water contrast, dynamic scanning, rapid IV-contrast injection, and dual-phase-image acquisition, 88% of the primary gastric cancers were detected. This detection rate potentially could improve if spiral scanning were use (22). Three-dimensional imaging of the stomach may improve the rate of tumor detection. In a study by Lee et al. of 31 patients with early gastric cancer, the investigators were able to detect 93.5% of the tumors when using 3D CT. Only 64.5% of the tumors were detected on axial images alone (15).

Local Extension

Stage-III tumors are characterized by extragastric extension of tumor with or without regional adenopathy (Figure 16-9). Early perigastric invasion may appear as increased attenuation of the fat surrounding the stomach, or obliteration of fat planes separating the stomach from adjacent organs (i.e., pancreas). Although fat-plane obliteration is a reliable sign of extragastric tumor invasion, the absence of distinct fat planes can occur as a normal variant in cachectic patients, or in patients with inflammatory conditions such as pancreatitis. The most problematic area for CT in staging gastric neoplasms is in determining pancreatic invasion (23,24). The inability of CT to distinguish between inflammation and tumor when fat planes are obliterated has limited the usefulness of CT in staging the primary tumor in earlier studies. Three-dimensional imaging, which allows real-time manipulation of the dataset, may help visualize better local extension of tumor and invasion of adjacent organs.

Adenopathy

The detection of adenopathy is important in the evaluation of gastric carcinomas, as perigastric lymph-node in-

volvement decreases the median survival rate by 65% (25). Nodal spread of disease may extend into or around the gastrohepatic ligament (Figures 16–6 and 16–10). Nodes in this region are considered suspicious for harboring malignancy if they are greater than 8 mm in diameter (26). Although the best indication of lymph-node involvement is enlargement, it has been shown that normal-sized nodes may contain tumor, whereas some enlarged nodes do not. Multiple enlarged nodes are more likely to be malignant than a solitary en-

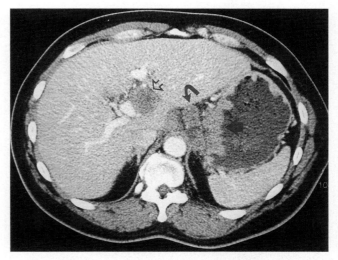

FIG. 16–10. Contrast-enhanced MDCT demonstrates a gastric tumor on the medial wall of the stomach involving the cardia. Nodes are present in the gastrohepatic ligament (*curved arrow*). In addition, there is liver metastasis (*open arrow*).

larged node (27). Another factor that may help distinguish metastatic from normal nodes is lack of enhancement.

The reported sensitivity of CT for detection of adenopathy in patients with adenocarcinoma of the stomach ranges between 47% and 97% (23,28,29). Although the use of spiral CT may help improve results, the major limitation with CT continues to be the inability to detect microscopic involvement of normal-sized nodes.

Distant Metastases

Spiral CT is excellent for the detection of distant metastases in patients with gastric cancer, as it combines rapid imaging and intravenous-contrast injection with 3D-imaging-display capabilities. Common sites for gastric metastatic disease include the liver, adrenal glands, and bone (Figure 16-9 and 16–10); in addition, gastric cancer can involve the ovaries (Krukenberg tumor). Gastric cancer also may be associated with carcinomatosis (Figure 16-11).

Spiral scanning with rapid IV-contrast injection is considered the preferred technique for liver imaging. A study of the detection of hepatic masses using SDCT demonstrated better than 90% sensitivity for detecting lesions over 1 cm in size, and 56% sensitivity for detecting lesions less than 1 cm (30). This is an improvement compared with traditional CT scanning, and it is likely that these numbers will improve with MDCT.

Postoperative Stomach and Recurrence

In patients with limited disease, partial gastrectomy is the treatment of choice. The median survival for patients after subtotal gastrectomy is 18 months and after total gastrectomy only 12 months. The success of gastrectomy depends on the extent of gastric-wall invasion and lymphatic spread. Chemoradiation protocols are being tested in an attempt to improve survival after gastrectomy. After treatment, these patients are followed regularly with endoscopy and CT in order to identify recurrence.

In a study by Ha et al. of 36 patients with tumor recurrence after gastrectomy, 69% of recurrences involved nodal spread along the celiac axis or hepatic pedicle, 28% of recurrences involved the anastomotic site or gastric stump, 22% involved the pancreas, and 11% occurred in the anterior abdominal wall (31). A similar study by Mullin of 38 patients with recurrent tumor after gastrectomy for carcinoma also demonstrated that the majority of recurrence involved regional lymph nodes or metastases to organs such as the liver, lung, adrenals, or bone (32). Occasionally, the recurrence can be extensive, involving peritoneal implants and carcinomatosis.

Endoscopic ultrasound, upper endoscopy, and barium studies often are capable of detecting recurrence at the anastomosis or in the gastric stump, but they are unable to image tumor spread to the abdominal wall or distant organs. In addition, CT is a useful guide for percutaneous biopsy of suspicious lesions.

LYMPHOMA

Gastric lymphoma comprises approximately 1% to 5% of all gastric malignancies and represents the most common extranodal site of non-Hodgkin's lymphoma (33). The majority of cases are non-Hodgkin's lymphomas, predominately of the diffuse histiocytic subtype. The CT appearance of gastric lymphoma is variable. Gastric lymphoma may appear as diffuse or segmental wall thickening, with an average wall thickness of 4 cm to 5 cm (33,34). Alternately, gastric lymphoma may present as a localized polypoid mass, with or without ulceration (14). Most patients with gastric lym-

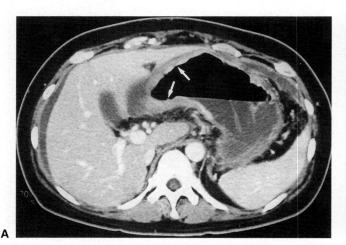 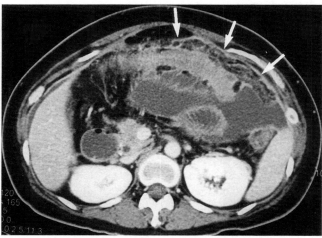

FIG. 16–11. A: Contrast-enhanced MDCT demonstrates circumferential thickening and narrowing of the gastric atrum (*arrows*). There also is minimal fluid surrounding the liver and in the left upper quadrant. **B:** Axial-enhanced scan at a more inferior level than **(A)** demonstrates loculated fluid in the mesentery, as well as mesenteric, stranding compatible with carcinomatosis (*arrows*). The colon also is thickened.

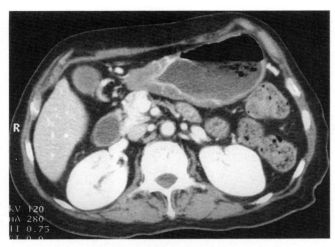

FIG. 16–12. Contrast-enhanced CT demonstrates circumferential narrowing and thickening of the gastric antrum. This was a lymphoma.

phoma have associated adenopathy, which often is bulky and may extend below the left renal hilum.

The CT appearance of gastric lymphoma may mimic adenocarcinoma of the stomach (Figures 16–12 and 16–13). Several key findings have been identified that may help distinguish the two malignancies. First, the gastric wall in lymphoma tends to be thicker (4 cm to 5 cm) and more lobular than in adenocarcinoma (1 cm to 3 cm). In addition, although lymphadenopathy may occur in both gastric lymphoma and adenocarcinoma, adenopathy in gastric lymphoma tends to be bulkier and often extends below the level of the renal hilum. Finally, although gastric lymphomas may appear as large bulky tumors, they often are pliable and rarely result in gastric-outlet obstruction (13).

Spiral CT is valuable both for patients with primary gastric lymphoma and for detection of secondary gastric invasion by lymphoma in patients with more extensive disease. Accurate staging of disease is enhanced with narrower scan collimation and interscan gaps. Water as oral contrast also may be helpful in identifying more subtle cases. In addition, it is necessary to optimize organ enhancement and disease detection in the liver, spleen, and kidneys. Solid-organ involvement is being detected more commonly, especially in patients whose lymphoma is a result of immunosuppression, such as acquired-immunodeficiency syndrome (AIDS) or following organ transplantation. With the increased use of CT, cases of incidental gastric lymphoma are being seen. These cases are uncommon but identifiable, especially if careful attention is paid to scan protocols.

Mucosa-associated-lymphoid-tissue (MALT) lymphoma is a low-grade lymphoma that is being recognized with increased frequency. It is thought to be associated with *H. pylori*. This tumor differs from the typically high-grade non-Hodgkin's gastric lymphoma. In a series of 40 patients with gastric MALT lymphoma by Kessar et al., the most frequent finding was gastric-wall thickening (35). The wall thickening usually is minimal and may not be detected on CT, especially if the stomach is not maximally distended (Figure 16–14). Associated adenopathy or extragastric distention is not common (35).

Treatment consists of surgery with postoperative-chemoradiation therapy. Radiotherapy alone may be effective in patients with Stage-I and -II disease. Chemotherapy is indicated in patients with disseminated disease.

Gastrointestinal Stromal Tumors

Gastrointestinal stromal tumors (GIST) are gastrointestinal neoplasms that arise from mesenchymal cells in the

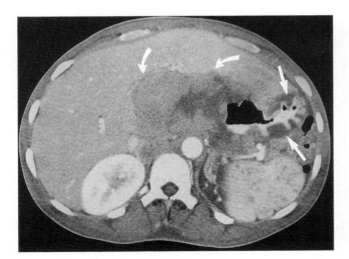

FIG. 16–13. Contrast-enhanced MDCT demonstrates low-density circumferential thickening of the stomach (*arrows*). Bulky adenopathy is noted around the stomach and the gastrohepatic ligament (*curved arrows*). This was a lymphoma.

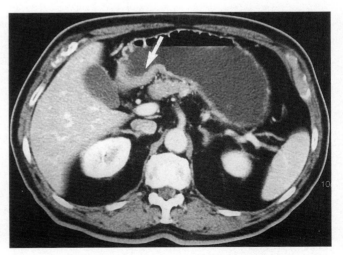

FIG. 16–14. Contrast-enhanced MDCT with water as oral contrast demonstrates subtle thickening of the gastric antrum (*arrow*). This was MALT lymphoma. There was no associated adenopathy.

bowel wall. These tumors, which formerly were referred to as smooth-muscle tumors such as leiomyomas or leiomyosarcomas, have undergone pathological reclassification. They encompass several different histological varieties that demonstrate variability in differentiation and are categorized based on immunohistochemical and ultrastructural studies (36). Stromal tumors can be classified histologically as myogenic (arising from smooth muscle), neurogenic (arising from neural elements), or less-differentiated tumors, referred to as GIST. Stromal tumors with smooth-muscle differentiation formerly were called leiomyoma or leiomyosarcoma. They account for only 1% of gastric tumors, and usually occur in adults (37).

On CT, these tumors vary in appearance and size. Ninety percent of gastric leiomyosarcomas occur in the fundus or body of the stomach (38). Small tumors will appear as masses arising from the smooth-muscle layers of the bowel wall (Figures 16-15 and 16-16). As the tumors grow, they stretch the overlying mucosa and can ulcerate. When large (greater than 5 cm), the tumors often grow exophytically and may contain areas of central necrosis or calcification (39). When the tumors are large and exophytic, it may be difficult to appreciate their gastric origin on axial scans (Figure 16-17). Multiplanar reconstructions and 3D imaging can be helpful to characterize better the mass and its relationship to the stomach. Adenopathy is uncommon, unlike patients with gastric adenocarcinoma or lymphoma.

Computed tomography usually cannot differentiate between malignant and benign gastric-stromal tumor unless obvious local invasion or metastatic disease is detected (37). However, small tumors (less than 4 cm to 5 cm) usually are benign. Malignant stromal tumors can invade adjacent

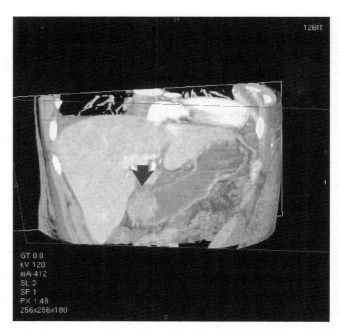

FIG. 16–16. Coronal 3D volume-rendered image in a patient with abdominal pain demonstrates a 2.5-cm smooth mass in the gastric antrum (*arrow*). At surgery, this was a GIST with smooth-muscle differentiation.

organs and can metastasize hematogenously, usually to the lung, liver, or peritoneal surfaces (39). Metastatic lesions also may appear cystic owing to central necrosis. It is important to investigate carefully all cystic lesions in the liver in patients with GIST, as the cystic metastases can mimic benign liver cysts.

METASTASES

Metastases to the stomach occur in approximately 2% of patients who die of cancer each year. Metastases that involve the stomach by hematogenous spread include melanoma, breast, lung, and ovary (Figures 16-18 and 16–19). Cancers of the esophagus and colon can spread to the stomach by lymphatic invasion. The stomach also may be involved by direct extension of local malignancies originating in the colon, pancreas, or liver (40,41). Patients can present with a variety of symptoms, including gastrointestinal bleeding, anemia, epigastric pain, and gastric-outlet obstruction.

The CT appearance of metastatic disease of the stomach is variable. It can appear as a solitary mass, multiple masses (melanoma), or rigid wall thickening, as in *linitis plastica* (breast). The appearance of metastatic disease can be indistinguishable from primary gastric malignancies, stressing the importance of clinical information (27). Tumor implants on the stomach are especially common in processes such as ovarian cancer.

GASTRIC VARICES

Gastric varices are tortuous distended collateral vessels fed mainly from the coronary vein, which may develop in

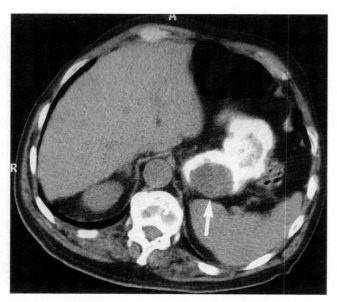

FIG. 16–15. Unenhanced CT with oral contrast demonstrates 3.5-cm smooth mass within the gastric lumen (*arrow*). This was a benign GIST.

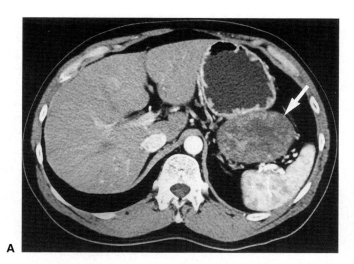

A

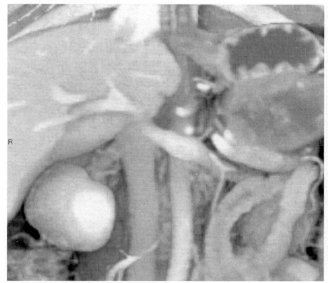

B

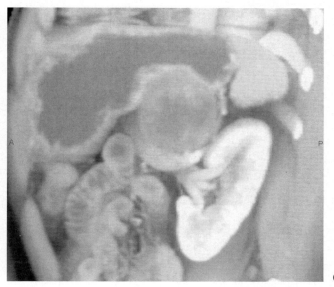

C

FIG. 16–17. A: Contrast-enhanced MDCT with water as oral contrast demonstrates a large soft-tissue mass in the left upper quadrant (*arrow*), abutting the stomach. It is an exophytic GIST. **B, C:** Coronal **(B)** and sagittal **(C)** 3D volume-rendered images demonstrate the relationship of the mass to the stomach.

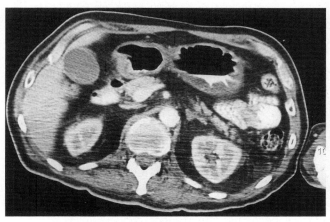

FIG. 16–18. Contrast-enhanced CT demonstrates circumferential thickening of the stomach. There was limited gastric distention. At endoscopy, metastatic melanoma was discovered infiltrating the stomach.

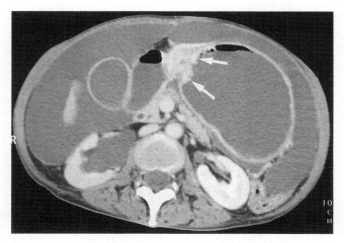

FIG. 16–19. Contrast-enhanced CT demonstrates gastric distention. There is a focal mass in the gastric atrum (*arrows*). The patient had a history of breast cancer. At endoscopy, metastatic breast cancer was diagnosed. There also is extensive ascites and hydronephrosis of the right kidney.

association with esophageal varices in patients with cirrhosis and portal hypertension. While intra- or extrahepatic obstruction leads to esophageal and gastric varices, isolated splenic-vein occlusion leads to the development of gastric varices without accompanying esophageal collaterals. Gastric varices may occur in any region of the stomach, but are located most commonly in the fundus. Although gastric varices do not bleed as frequently as esophageal varices, hemorrhage from gastric collaterals can be more severe.

The ability of endoscopic and conventional esophagram to diagnose gastric varices is limited, especially if not accompanied by esophageal varices. In the past, angiography was considered the most reliable method for diagnosis of gastric varices. With the advent of CT, contrast-enhanced

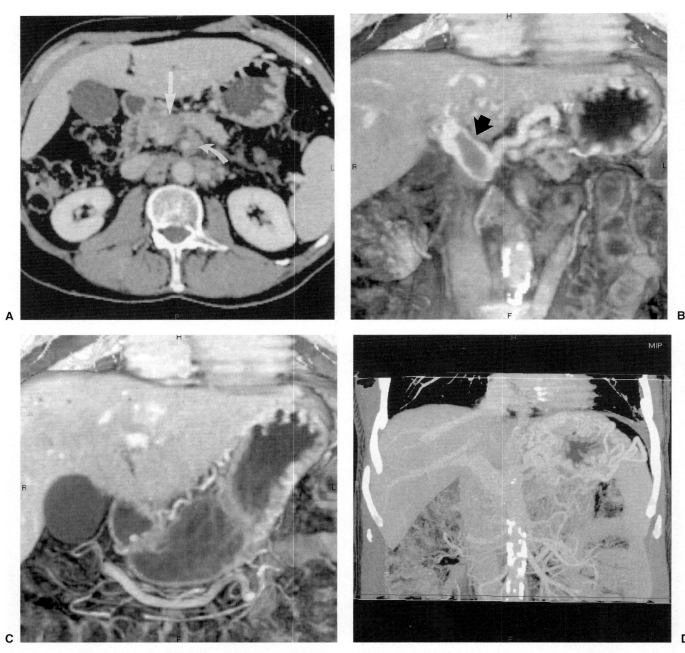

FIG. 16–20. A: Contrast-enhanced MDCT demonstrates a mass in the neck of the pancreas (*straight arrow*) that has occluded the splenic vein and encased the superior mesenteric artery (*curved arrow*). **B:** Coronal 3D volume-rendered image demonstrates thrombus in the portal vein (*arrow*), and occlusion of the splenic vein. **C:** Coronal 3D volume-rendered image demonstrates gastric collaterals resulting from the splenic-vein occlusion. **D:** Maximum-intensity projection nicely shows the extensive gastric varices.

CT quickly proved to be a sensitive method for the detection of gastric varices (42). In recent years, spiral CT with IV contrast has been shown to be an accurate modality for the detection and evaluation of portosystemic shunts in patients with portal hypertension (43).

The CT appearance of gastric varices varies depending on the size and extent of involvement. Usually, on unenhanced scans, gastric varices appear as a scalloped lobulated gastric border. With IV contrast, gastric varices will appear as enhancing tubular and rounded structures within the gastric wall. On noncontrast scans, large varices can simulate adenopathy in the posterior mediastinum, which is a potential pitfall (13,14).

Computed-tomography angiography with volume rendering and 3D-image display also can be used to evaluate better gastric varices and their relationship to the portal- and systemic-venous systems (44) (Figure 16-20).

GASTRITIS

There are many causes of gastritis, including infections (*H. pylori*, Cryptosporidia, CMV), inflammatory conditions (Crohn's disease, eosinophilic gastroenteritis, Zollinger–Ellison syndrome), radiation, and ingestion of alcohol, corrosive agents, or drugs.

On CT, gastritis usually appears as a gastric fold and wall thickening, regardless of etiology. The thickened wall typically has soft-tissue density, although, if there is significant edema, the wall may have a low density (14) (Figure 16-21). In some patients, owing to significant edema and hyperemia, a layered appearance can be seen in the gastric wall after intravenous contrast. This will be most apparent on early phase imaging and helps to confirm the diagnosis, as neoplasms of the stomach will not respect the bowel-wall layers and typically will not result in this layered appearance. Gastritis does not have to involve the stomach diffusely, and thus can appear as focal or segmental thickening (Figure 16-

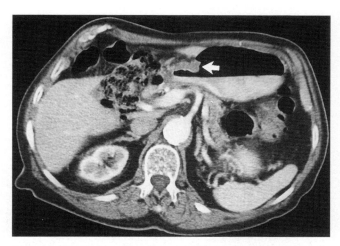

FIG. 16–22. Contrast-enhanced CT demonstrates focal circumferential thickening of the gastric antrum (*arrow*). At CT, this was suspicious for neoplasm; however, at endoscopy, focal gastritis with ulceration was discovered.

22). *H. pylori* gastritis in particular can simulate a gastric neoplasm, as it often results in circumferential antral-wall thickening or focal thickening along the greater curvature (45).

Adequate gastric distention is necessary in order to avoid confusing wall thickening from gastritis with underdistention. The CT appearance of gastritis and gastric cancer often overlap, requiring biopsy for the definitive diagnosis.

CONCLUSION

Although CT is not the primary imaging modality for gastric disease, it plays a significant role in the evaluation and staging of gastric carcinoma and in the imaging of a variety of benign diseases. With the increased use of water as an oral-contrast agent, along with the introduction of MDCT and continued advancements in 3D volume rendering, the role of CT in the evaluation of gastric diseases continues to evolve.

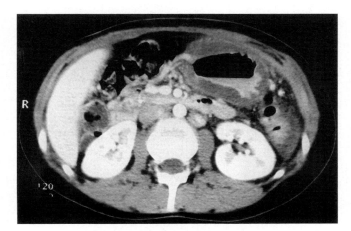

FIG. 16–21. Contrast-enhanced MDCT demonstrates diffuse circumferential thickening of the stomach. This appears low in density. At endoscopy, diffuse gastritis was diagnosed.

REFERENCES

1. Horton KM, Fishman EK. Helical CT of the stomach: evaluation with water as an oral contrast agent. *AJR Am J Roentgenol* 1998; 171:1373–1376.
2. Horton KM, Eng J, Fishman EK. Normal enhancement of the small bowel: evaluation with spiral CT. *J Comput Assist Tomogr* 2000; 24:67–71.
3. Raptopoulos V, Davis MA, Davidoff A, et al. Fat density oral contrast agent for abdominal CT. *Radiology* 1987;164:653–656.
4. Springer P, Dessl A, Giacomuzzi SM. Virtual computed tomography gastroscopy; a new technique. *Endoscopy* 1997;29:632–634.
5. Winter TC, Ager JD, Nghiem HV, et al. Upper gastrointestinal tract and abdomen: water as an orally administered contrast agent for helical CT. *Radiology* 1996;201:365–370.
6. Gossios KJ, Tsianos EV, Demou LL, et al. Use of water or air as oral contrast media for computed tomographic study of the gastric wall:

comparison of the two techniques. *Gastrointest Radiol* 1991; 16:293–297.

7. Baert AL, Roex L, Marchal G, et al. Computed tomography of the stomach with water as an oral contrast agent: technique and preliminary results. *J Comput Assist Tomogr* 1989;13:633–636.

8. Hori S, Tsuda K, Murayama S, et al. CT of gastric carcinoma; preliminary results with a new scanning technique. *Radiographics* 1992; 12:257–268.

9. Matsuoka Y, Masumoto T, Koga H, et al. Positive and negative oral contrast agents for combined abdominal and pelvic helical CT: first iodinated agent and second water. *Radiat Med* 2000;18:213–216.

10. Ramsay DW, Markham DH, Morgan B, et al. The use of dilute Cologen as a fat density oral contrast medium in upper abdominal computed tomography, compared with the use of water and positive oral contrast media. *Clin Radiol* 2001;56:670–673.

11. Lee DH. Two-dimensional and three-dimensional imaging of gastric tumors using spiral CT. *Abdom Imaging* 2000;25:1–6.

12. Wood BJ, O'Malley ME, Hahn PF, et al. Virtual endoscopy of the gastrointestinal system outside the colon. *AJR Am J Roentgenol* 1998; 171:1367–1372.

13. Savader BL, Fishman EK. CT evaluation of the stomach. *Contemp Diagnost Radiol* 1992;15:1–5.

14. Fishman EK, Urban BA, Hruban RH. CT of the stomach: spectrum of disease. *Radiographics* 1996;16:1035–1054.

15. Lee DH, Ko YT. The role of 3D spiral CT in early gastric carcinoma. *J Comput Assist Tomogr* 1998;22:709–713.

16. Lee DH, Ko YT. Advanced gastric carcinoma: the role of three-dimensional and axial imaging by spiral CT. *Abdom Imaging* 1999; 24:111–116.

17. Eisenberg RL. Gastric ulcers. In: Eisenberg RL, ed. *Gastrointestinal radiology: A pattern approach*. Philadelphia, PA: Lippincott-Raven, 1996;196–197.

18. Consensus NIH. *Helicobacter pylori* in peptic ulcer disease. *JAMA* 1994;272:65–69.

19. Rossi M, Broglia L, Maccioni F, et al. Hydro-CT in patients with gastric cancer: preoperative radiologic staging. *Eur Radiol* 1997;7:659–664.

20. Hundt W, Braunschweig R, Reiser M. Assessment of gastric cancer: value of breathhold technique and two phase spiral CT. *Eur Radiol* 1999;9:68–72.

21. Mani NB, Suri S, Gupta S, et al. Two-phase dynamic contrast-enhanced computed tomography with water-filling method for staging gastric cancer. *Clin Imaging* 2001;25:38–43.

22. Cho JS, Kim JK, Rho SM, et al. Preoperative assessment of gastric cancer: value of two-phase dynamic CT with mechanical IV injection of contrast material. *AJR Am J Roentgenol* 1994;163:69–75.

23. Sussman SK, Halvorsen RA, Illescas FF, et al. Gastric adenocarcinoma: CT versus surgical staging. *Radiology* 1988;167:335–340.

24. McFee AS, Aust JB. Gastric carcinoma and the CAT scan. *Gastroenterology* 1981;80:196–198.

25. Bedikian AY, Chen TT, Khankhanian N, et al. The natural history of gastric cancer and prognostic factors influencing survival. *J Clin Oncol* 1984;2:302–310.

26. Balfe DM, Mauro MA, Koehler RE, et al. Gastrohepatic ligament: normal and pathologic CT anatomy. *Radiology* 1984;150:485–490.

27. Komaki S. Gastric carcinoma. In: Meyers MA, ed. *Computed tomography of the gastrointestinal tract*. New York: Springer, 1986;23–54.

28. Dehn TC, Reznek RH, Nockler IB, et al. The preoperative assessment of advanced gastric cancer by computed tomography. *Br J Surg* 1984; 71:413–417.

29. Cook AO, Levine BA, Sirinek KR, et al. Evaluation of gastric adenocarcinoma; abdominal computed tomography does not replace celiotomy. *Arch Surg* 1986;121:603–606.

30. Kuszyk BS, Bluemke DA, Urban BA, et al. Portal-phase contrast enhanced helical CT for the detection of malignant hepatic tumors: sensitivity based on comparison with intraoperative and pathologic findings. *AJR Am J Roentgenol* 1996;166:91–95.

31. Ha HK, Kim HH, Lee MH, et al. Local recurrence after surgery for gastric carcinoma. *AJR Am J Roentgenol* 1993;161:975–977.

32. Mullin D, Shirkhoda A. Computed tomography after gastrectomy in primary gastric carcinoma. *J Comput Assist Tomogr* 1985;90:30–33.

33. Megibow AJ, Balthazar EJ, Nadich DP, et al. Computed tomography of gastrointestinal lymphoma. *AJR Am J Roentgenol* 1983;141:541–547.

34. Buy JN, Moss AA. Computed tomography of gastric lymphoma. *AJR Am J Roentgenol* 1982;138:859–865.

35. Kessar P, Norton A, Rohatiner AZ, et al. CT appearances of mucosa-associated lymphoid tissue (MALT) lymphoma. *Eur Radiol* 1999; 9:693–696.

36. Occhionorelli S, Mitaritonno M, Penella A, et al. Gastrointestinal stromal tumor (GIST): case report. *G Chir* 2001;22:65–69.

37. McLeod AJ, Zornoza J, Shirkoda A. Leiomyosarcoma: computed tomographic findings. *Radiology* 1984;152:133–136.

38. Gore RM, Levine MS, Laufer I. Textbook of gastrointestinal radiology. Philadelphia: WB Saunders, 1994;703–708.

39. Pannu HK, Hruban RH, Fishman EK. CT of gastric leiomyosarcoma: patterns of involvement. *AJR Am J Roentgenol* 1999;173:369–373.

40. Menuck L, Amberg J. Metastatic disease involving the stomach. *J Comput Assist Tomogr* 1975;11:283–287.

41. Radin DR, Halls JM. Cavitary metastases of the stomach and duodenum. *J Comput Assist Tomogr* 1987;11:283–287.

42. Balthazar EJ, Naidich DP, Megibow AJ, et al. CT evaluation of esophageal varices. *AJR Am J Roentgenol* 1987;148:131–135.

43. Cho KC, Patel YD, Wachsberg RH, et al. Varices in portal hypertension: evaluation with CT. *Radiographics* 1995;15:609–622.

44. Matsumoto A, Kitamoto M, Imamura M, et al. Three-dimensional portography using mulitslice helical CT is clinically useful for management of gastric fundic varices. *AJR Am J Reontgenol* 2001; 176:899–905.

45. Urban BA, Fishman EK, Hruban RH. *Helicobacter pylori* gastritis mimicking gastric carcinoma at CT evaluation. *Radiology* 1991; 179:689–691.

CHAPTER 17

SDCT/MDCT of the Small Intestine

Karen M. Horton, Elliot K. Fishman

INTRODUCTION

Radiologists always have played an important role in the diagnosis of small-bowel pathology, as the mesenteric small bowel is the least accessible portion of the gastrointestinal tract to the gastroenterologist. Owing to the length of the small intestine, endoscopes are not able to maneuver the entire course of the small bowel; therefore, radiological studies are necessary for complete evaluation. Barium small-bowel follow through still is performed routinely as the first radiological imaging study in patients with suspected small-bowel disease, and it is able to display the mucosa of the duodenum, jejunum, and ileum in exquisite detail. However, due to the superimposition of small-bowel loops and nonuniform distention, segments of the small bowel may not be visualized adequately. In a detailed analysis of small-bowel series by Goldberg et al., inadequate evaluation of the proximal ileum was noted in 35% of patients, of the distal ileum in 32% of patients, and of the jejunum in 24% of patients (1). In another study of small-bowel series by Garvey et al., the proximal ileum was not evaluated optimally in 28% of patients (2). Enteroclysis can overcome many of the limitations of the small-bowel follow through by maximally distending the entire small bowel, and it certainly is more sensitive for the diagnosis of small-bowel neoplasms and low-grade obstructions (3–5). However, both techniques are limited in their ability to detect intramural and extramural disease, which often is important for the accurate diagnosis of many small-bowel conditions.

Computed tomography (CT) overcomes many of the shortcomings of traditional barium studies by allowing visualization of the entire small bowel, intramural disease, as well as extraluminal disease. In addition, owing to continued technical advancements in CT technology and three-dimensional (3D) imaging software, CT now allows unparalleled evaluation of the small intestine and mesenteric vessels. Computed tomography quickly has become a valuable part of the work up of patients with suspected small-bowel disease. This chapter will review the current role of CT for the evaluation of small-bowel pathology, with an emphasis on the use of multidetector CT (MDCT).

TECHNIQUE

The optimal CT technique to image patients with small-bowel disease has changed over the years, reflecting the rapid changes in CT-scanner technology and the development of 3D-imaging software. In the early days of CT, scan times per slice were slow (5 seconds to 15 seconds) and allowed only relatively thick collimation (e.g., 8 mm to 10 mm). This resulted in partial volume averaging and problems related to motion artifacts. However, despite these limitations, the value of CT for diagnosing small-bowel disease was recognized. As scanner technology improved with the introduction of spiral CT and, more recently MDCT, the role of CT in imaging the small intestine has evolved, as has the optimal technique.

Oral Contrast

Positive oral-contrast agents such as diluted iodinated or barium solutions have been used traditionally for abdominal CT imaging. These agents are safe, fairly well tolerated, and adequately opacify the small intestine. They appear white on CT, which allows easy identification of the small bowel and colon, and allows reliable detection of extravasation of contrast from the bowel. Although these agents have been well accepted over the years, they may no longer be optimal, given the improvement in CT technology. For example, these agents can mix unevenly with gastric and intestinal fluid, resulting in pseudotumors (6,7). In addition, since these agents are high in density, they may obscure the enhancing bowel wall when intravenous (IV) contrast is administered rapidly and subsecond scanning is performed. For example, after rapid IV-contrast injection and fast scanning, the normal small-bowel wall enhances to approximately 110 Hounsfield units (HU) (8). Furthermore, if 3D imaging of

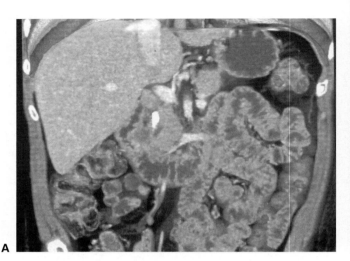

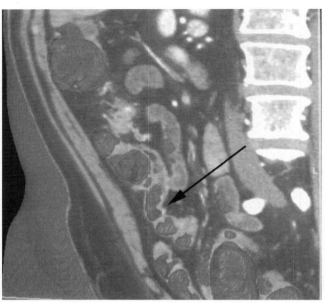

A

B

FIG. 17–1. Normal CT appearance of the small bowel using water as oral contrast. **A:** Coronal 3D volume-rendered MDCT demonstrates the normal appearance of the small intestine when water is given as oral contrast and when there is a good IV-contrast bolus. The individual small loops and folds can be identified readily. **B:** Volume-rendered 3D MDCT in a coronal plane demonstrates the normal appearance of the terminal ileum (*arrow*).

the small bowel or mesenteric vessels is planned, the use of high-density oral agents will necessitate extensive editing. Therefore, radiologists are starting to realize the value of using low-density agents as oral contrast for CT. These agents allow excellent visualization of the enhancing wall and do not interfere with 3D imaging. The benefits of using water as an oral CT contrast agent for gastric imaging have been well documented in the literature (9–11). More recently, the value of using water for CT imaging of the small bowel and colon has been investigated. Currently, the John Hopkins Medical Institutions use water as oral contrast when detailed CT imaging of the small bowel or mesenteric vessels is required. Water is safe, well tolerated, and allows exquisite visualization of the enhancing bowel wall and abdominal vessels (Figures 17–1 and 17–2). One relative disadvantage of water is that, since it is emptied rapidly from the stomach and moves quickly through the small intestine, it sometimes results in suboptimal distension of the distal small bowel (8). However, when IV-contrast bolus is administered, the normal bowel wall and fold pattern can be visualized (Figure 17-1) and abnormalities still can be detected when loops are not distended completely. Alternatively, oral metoclopromide can be administered to improve ileal distension (12). Another potential disadvantage of using a low-density agent such as water is the difficulty in identifying extravasation of bowel contents. If this is a concern, positive contrast agents can be used for this clinical indication; however, it is felt that water is a useful CT oral-contrast agent for many small-bowel conditions.

IV Contrast

Intravenous contrast is essential for a comprehensive CT examination of the small bowel and mesentery. There are a few indications, such as small-bowel hemorrhage, when noncontrast scans can be helpful. However, for most conditions, IV contrast is preferred. At this facility, nonionic iodinated contrast agents (Omnipaque 350, Amersham Health, Princeton, NJ) administered via a power injector are used exclusively. For many clinical indications, an injection rate of 2 cc to 3 cc per second is adequate; however, faster injection rates may be helpful (3 cc to 5 cc per second) if detailed vascular mapping is required.

Scanning Protocol

For routine abdominal CT scans for indications such as abdominal pain, positive oral-contrast agents and IV contrast are administered, and scans are performed using 5-mm slice thickness. However, if specific small-bowel pathology is suspected, customized protocols are used. For a detailed CT examination of the small bowel, water as oral contrast is administered, typically 750 cc 20 minutes prior to the exam, followed by an additional 250 cc immediately before the scan. This ensures opacification of the small bowel, as well as the stomach. Intravenous contrast is administered at a rate of 3 cc to 5 cc per second through a peripheral angiocatheter. Depending on the indication, arterial- and/or portal-venous imaging is performed using 25-second and 50-second scan delays, respectively. A MDCT scanner is used so that thinner collimation can be obtained. For instance, this facility uses the Siemens Plus 4 Volume Zoom multidetector scanner. For small-bowel imaging, the 4-mm × 2.5-mm collimator setting can be used to obtain high-resolution 3-mm slices. Alternatively, the 4-mm × 1-mm setting allows 1.0-mm to 1.25-mm slices to be acquired, which allows detailed imaging of the mesenteric vasculature. We also have a new 16 slice scanner (Siemens Sensation 16) that allows 0.75 mm slices.

3D Imaging

Although 3D CT imaging has been possible for almost 20 years, the quality, affordability, and speed have improved enough only recently that it is beginning to be incorporated into clinical practice. Among the different rendering algorithms available, volume rendering is superior for small-bowel imaging and vascular imaging. Maximum-intensity projection (MIP) also can be helpful when evaluating the mesenteric vessels.

At this institution, the data are transferred over an Ethernet to an Infinite Reality or Onyx workstation with Reality Engine graphics (Silicon Graphics, Mt. View, CA), or an O2 workstation for interactive volume rendering. Simple two-dimensional (2D) multiplanar reconstructions (MPR) of the CT data allow quick visualization of the abdomen in the axial, sagittal, and coronal planes. An abnormality detected in one plane can be visualized immediately in the other two planes. It often is helpful to start with the MPR and then proceed with the 3D reconstructions.

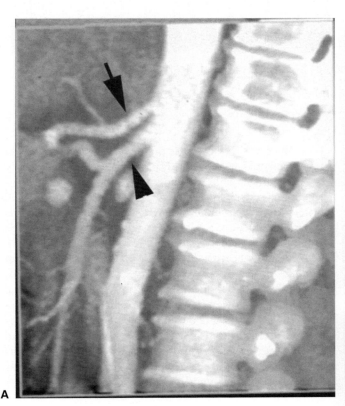

A

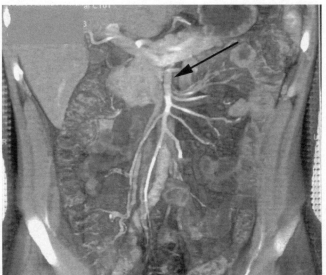

B

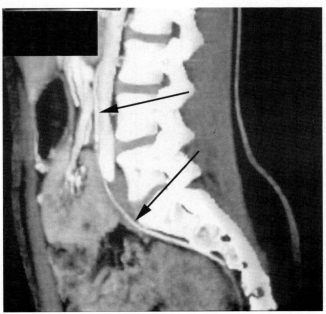

C

FIG. 17–2. A: Sagittal 3D volume-rendered MDCT demonstrates the normal anatomy of the celiac axis (*arrow*) and superior mesenteric artery (*arrowhead*). **B:** Coronal 3D volume-rendered MDCT demonstrates the normal anatomy of the superior mesenteric artery (*arrow*). Even the small branches can be identified. **C:** Sagittal 3D volume-rendered MDCT demonstrates the normal anatomy of the inferior mesenteric artery (*arrows*). *(continued)*

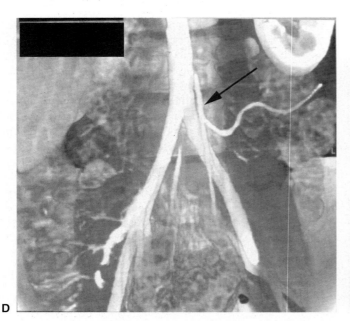
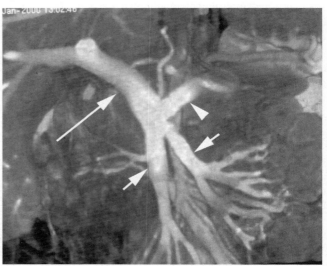

FIG. 17–2. *Continued.* **D:** Coronal 3D volume-rendered MDCT again demonstrates the normal anatomy of the inferior mesenteric artery (*arrow*). **E:** Volume-rendered 3D MDCT in the venous phase demonstrates the normal venous anatomy. Portal vein, *long arrow*; splenic vein, *arrowhead*; superior mesenteric vein, *short arrows*.

The 3D volume set can be manipulated using different orientations or cut planes in order to demonstrate best the small bowel and pathology. This flexibility is a distinct advantage over traditional axial images and barium studies, as it allows optimal visualization of every small-bowel loop. The radiologist is able to adjust the window level, center, brightness, and opacity in order to accentuate certain structures, such as the small-bowel wall or vasculature.

In addition, the CT data of the small intestine can be manipulated to simulate images as seen by the endoscopist for "virtual enteroscopy" (Figure 17-3). This virtual fly through of the small intestine has been described, but it is not performed routinely owing to the redundancy of the small bowel. Often it is not necessary to fly through the intestine because the radiologist simply can use the clip planes and different orientation planes to visualize the entire bowel.

NORMAL SMALL BOWEL AND MESENTERY

The small bowel consists of three distinct segments: the duodenum, jejunum, and ileum. Each is imaged well with CT. The small intestine usually measures less than 2.5 cm in diameter on CT, although the jejunum can measure as much as 3.5 cm in some people. Typically, the jejunum will be more distended (3 cm) than the ileum (2.5 cm). The terminal ileum usually measures 2 cm or less (13). When loops are distended well, the wall thickness should be less than 3 mm (14,15). Underdistension of the small bowel will result in the appearance of wall thickening, which can simulate or, in some cases, mask pathology.

When water is given as oral contrast, the small-bowel loops and fold pattern are displayed optimally, especially with multiplanar or 3D imaging (Figure 17-1). Three-dimensional imaging allows the same CT dataset to be displayed differently. For example, the information can be displayed using traditional CT parameters or the settings can be manipulated to simulate a small-bowel series (Figure 17-4).

In addition to examining the small intestine, CT can evaluate the mesenteric vessels (16). When dual-phase scanning has been performed, detailed maps of the mesenteric arteries and veins can be generated easily using 3D volume-rendering software (Figure 17-2). Even small distal branches of the vessels can be visualized if thin collimation is obtained (17). These vascular maps especially are useful for evaluating patients with suspected ischemia and for identifying vascular invasion in patients with neoplasms.

SMALL-BOWEL PATHOLOGY

Small-bowel Neoplasms

Early diagnosis of small-bowel tumors continues to pose a significant challenge to both clinicians and radiologists. Small-bowel neoplasms are relatively uncommon; they represent fewer than 25% of all gastrointestinal neoplasms and fewer than 2% of all malignant tumors (18). The annual incidence of small-bowel tumors is only 0.5 to 1.0 per 100,000 people in the Western hemisphere (19). Owing to their rarity, the diagnosis of small-bowel neoplasms sometimes is overlooked clinically (20). In addition, patients often present with very nonspecific symptoms such as abdominal

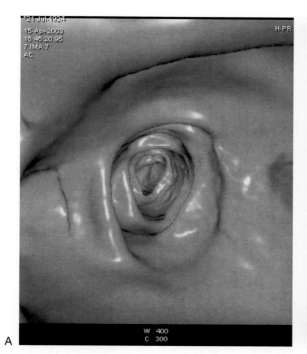 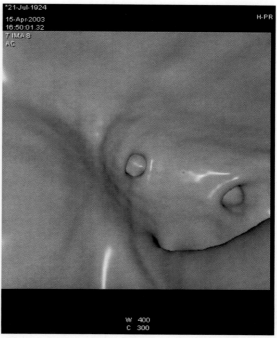

A

B

COLOR FIG. 2–19. Virtual colonoscopy with color mapping. **A,B:** Use of color allows realistic imaging in endoscopic projection. **A:** Normal haustral folds of the ascending colon are shown; (**B**) shows diverticula in sigmoid colon.

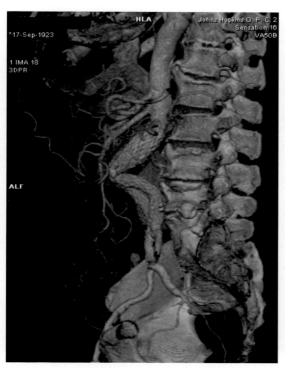 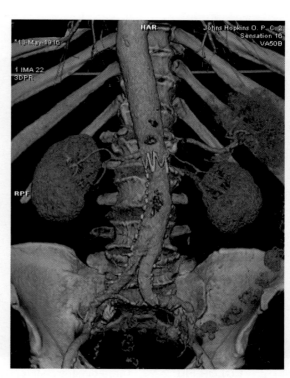

B

COLOR FIG. 2–20. Failing endovascular stent for repair of abdominal aorta. **A,B:** Stress-related failure of endovascular stent is defined in gray scale (**A**) and color (**B**). The color image gives a more realistic 3D effect.

COLOR FIG. 2–21. Endovascular stent in color display. **A,B:** Imaging of endovascular stent in gray scale (**A**) and color (**B**) shows the advantage of color in defining the stent, whereas gray-scale image optimally shows the native aorta with aneurysm.

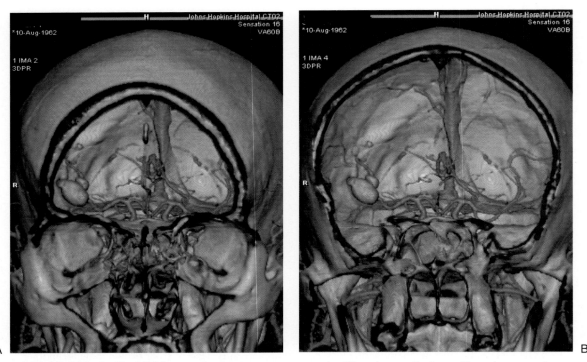

COLOR FIG. 2–22. Middle cerebral artery aneurysm in 3D volume display with color mapping. **A,B:** Detailed 3D mapping defines middle cerebral artery aneurysm. Color imaging in this case adds to the realism of images and provides increased 3D feel to the images.

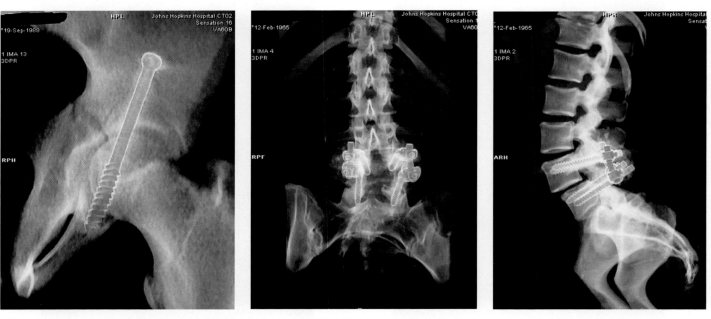

COLOR FIG. 2–23. Three-dimensional rendering of orthopedic hardware using color mapping to optimize image display. **A:** Screw in place for repair of acetabular fracture. Note detail of the ridges of the screw. **B,C:** Postoperative study following fusion of lower lumbar spine. Note detail of 3D volume-rendered images despite significant artifact on axial images (not shown).

COLOR FIG. 3–3. Conceptual basis of virtual endoscopy (colonoscopy). Spiral CT data were obtained at 3-m collimation, pitch 2, and reconstructed at 1-mm intervals at a 36-cm DFOV. The patient had undergone colonic cleansing for fiberoptic colonoscopy and had air insufflated into the colon with a Foley catheter. **B:** PVR view of the carcinoma with 60-degree FOV. Note the nodularity of the inner colonic surface. *Arrow*, residual lumen through the lesion. Rendering a series of images obtained at viewpoints coursing through the lumen, one can create an animation simulating fiberoptic colonoscopy. In this patient, the virtual camera captured the proximal aspect of the lesion and permitted endoscopic views of the cecum; the fiberoptic scope could not be passed through the constricted lumen.

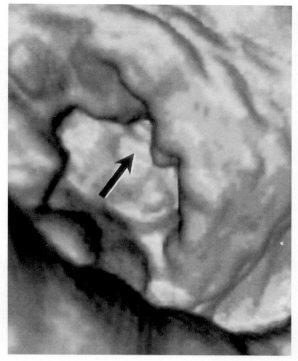

B

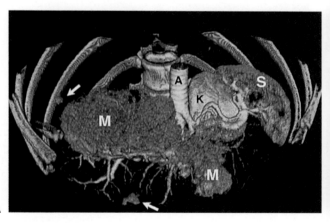

A

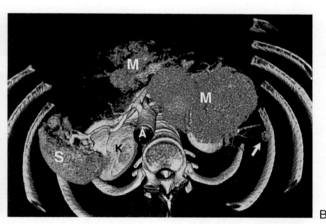

B

COLOR FIG. 3–4. Fly around of focal hepatic masses: focal nodular hyperplasia (FNH). **A** and **B:** Two different PVRs of hyperenhancing hepatic lesions imaged with 5-mm collimation, pitch 1.5, in the arterial phase of bolus IV contrast enhancement. Images were created with Voxel View 2.5 with a 60-degree FOV and the opacity table adjusted to emphasize contrast enhancement and osseous structures. Normal liver parenchyma is transparent. The relationship of the multiple masses (*M*) to the portal venous system can be visualized on static images or when a series of images is viewed as an animation. *Arrows*, small foci of FNH; *A*, abdominal aorta; *K*, left kidney; *S*, Spleen. **C:** Volume-rendered view of a slab of data 50 mm thick from the same patient. In this view, normal liver parenchyma is semitransparent and the relationship of the FNH foci to the portal venous system (*arrows*) is illustrated. Note that the hepatic masses (*M*) are assigned the same color as the spleen, owing to similar attenuation values achieved with contrast enhancement.

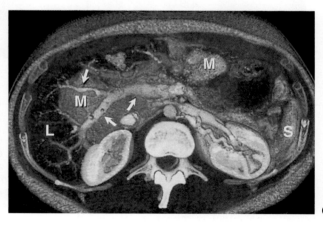

C

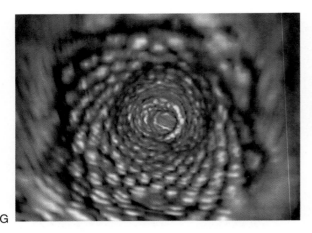

COLOR FIG. 3–5. Perspective rendering of the airways. Spiral CT volumes were acquired with 1-mm collimation, pitch 2, and reconstructed at 0.5-mm -1.0-mm intervals, unless indicated otherwise, and rendered with a 60-degree FOV. **G:** Tracheal stent. Follow-up PVR view (80-degree FOV) of spiral CT in a patient with tracheal stenosis shows wide patency of the trachea after placement of expandable metallic stents. The stent could be assigned a different color than the tracheal wall because of the higher attenuation values in the metal, which aids in visualization.

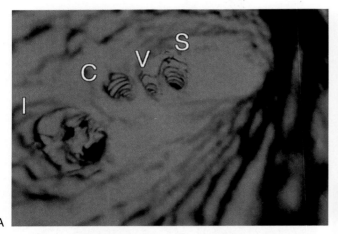

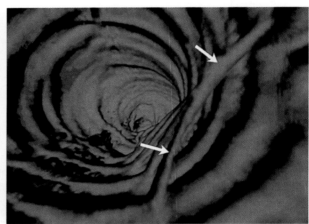

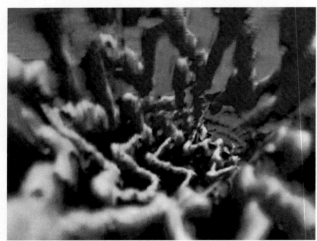

COLOR FIG. 3–7. Endoscopic imaging of the thoracic aorta. Images were acquired with 3-mm collimation, pitch 1.5–2.0, during bolus IV injection of iodinated contrast at 4–5 cc/sec and rendered with PVR. **A:** PVR view showing the innominate (*I*), left common carotid (*C*), left vertebral (*V*), and left subclavian (*S*) arteries arising from the aortic arch as viewed from the ascending aorta. **B:** Type B aortic dissection. Infero-superior view from the descending thoracic aorta shows a dissection flap (*arrows*) demarcating the true and false lumina. Prominent corrugations in the aortic wall predominantly reflect pulsatility of the thoracic aorta during the CT acquisition. **C:** Aortic stent graft. Metallic struts of a covered thoracic aortic stent graft can be depicted along the aortic wall to visualize adequacy of stent deployment and the configuration of the aortic lumen.

COLOR FIG. 3–9. Fly around of the abdominal aorta. By assuming a viewpoint inside the volume, a unique perspective can be obtained allowing the viewer to move around and between structures to optimize visualization of the anatomy of interest. **A:** Oblique supero-inferior view (60 degree) of the left renal artery (*arrows*) in a patient with an infrarenal abdominal aortic aneurysm. Calcific plaque at the ostium is evident. The splenic (*SP*) and superior mesenteric (*SM*) arteries also are visible. *A*, aorta **B:** Antero-posterior view of the left renal artery (80-degree FOV) in a patient with moderate renal artery stenosis (*arrows*). In this case, early enhancement of the left renal vein obscured visualization of the renal artery, so the viewpoint was positioned *between* the renal artery and the vein, obviating the need to perform spatial editing of the data.

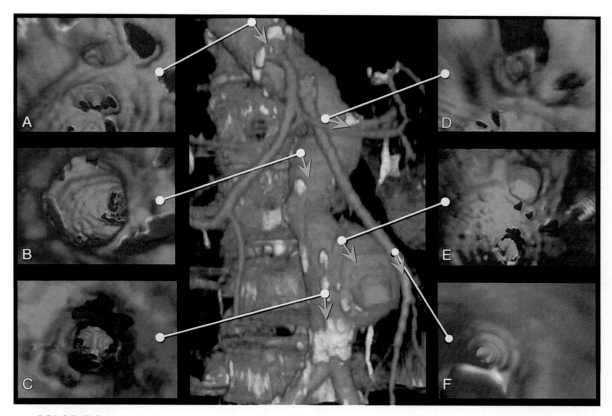

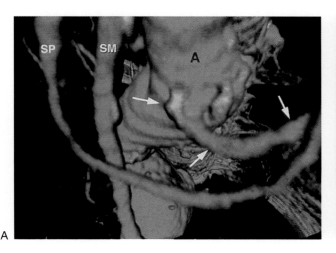
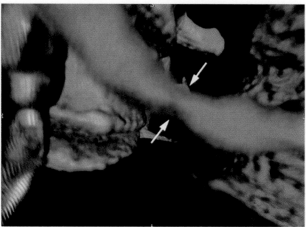

COLOR FIG. 3–8. Endoscopic imaging of the abdominal aorta. Multiple frames were captured from an endoscopic fly through of a patient with an infrarenal abdominal aortic aneurysm performed with PVR on spiral CT data obtained with 3-mm collimation, pitch 2, during injection of IV iodinated contrast at 5 cc/sec. Center image depicts the general morphology of the abdominal aorta. Calcific plaque has been assigned a white color and can be depicted as distinct from contrast column due to attenuation higher than the aortic lumen. Lines with arrows show viewpoint and viewing directions for multiple endoluminal views shown in (**A-F**). **A:** Celiac and superior mesenteric artery (SMA) origins. Note foci of atherosclerotic plaque at the ostium of the SMA. **B:** Mid-aortic view showing plaque and proximal neck of aneurysm. **C:** Caudal aorta showing aortic bifurcation and heavy calcific plaque. **D:** Left renal artery origin with ostial plaque, but no significant stenosis. **E:** Endoluminal view of focal ulcer in the anterior/left aspect of the aneurysm. The aortic bifurcation is visible in the lower portion of image, but better shown in (**C**). **F:** SMA fly through. Second- through fourth-order branch vessels can be viewed routinely from an endoscopic perspective provided there is adequate vascular enhancement. Focal calcific plaque in the distal SMA is seen in the lower portion of the image and branching is seen in the distance. Renderings performed by Yasayuki Kobayashi, MD.

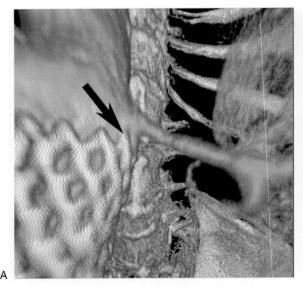

A

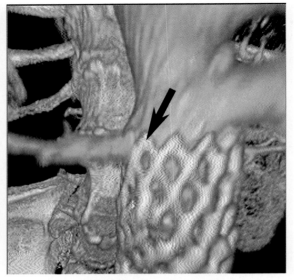

B

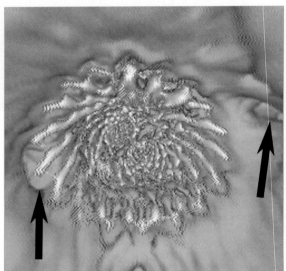

C

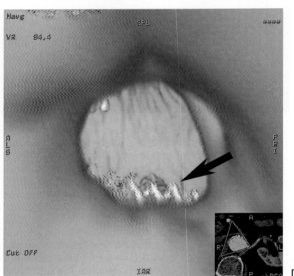

D

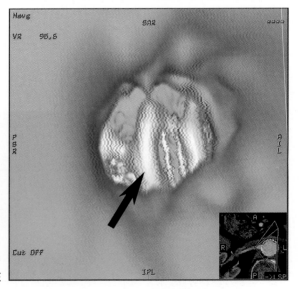

E

COLOR FIG. 3–11. Renal arteries. Multidetector CT reconstructed with 1.25-mm section thickness. **A,B:** Left and right renal arteries, respectively, with an aortic stent graft (*arrow*) that originated close to both renal ostea. The exact relationship between the stent graft and the renal artery ostea is difficult to ascertain. **C:** Perspective volume rendering within the suprarenal aorta, looking inferiorly. The *arrows* identify the renal artery ostea. From this perspective, the relationship of the renal artery ostea and the stent graft remains difficult to assess. **D,E:** Perspective volume rendering from within the left and right renal arteries, respectively, looking in to the aorta. The left renal artery origin is encroached upon minimally, but the right renal artery origin is obstructed nearly completely by the stent graft.

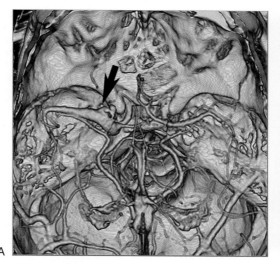

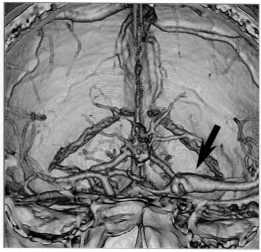

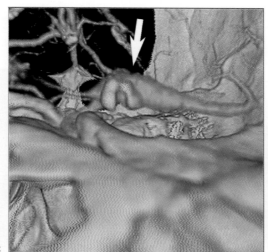

COLOR FIG. 3–12. Intracranial arteries. Multi-detector CT reconstructed with 0.625-mm section thickness. **A:** Volume rendering viewed from above after the superior aspect of the skull has been removed. There is a fusiform aneurysm of the left-middle cerebral artery (*arrow*). **B:** Frontal view of the aneurysm shows the aneurysm (*arrow*) with the A1 segment originating medially. **C:** Perspective volume-rendered view seen from the floor of the anterior cranial fossa demonstrates the aneurysm (*arrow*) rendered from within the craium.

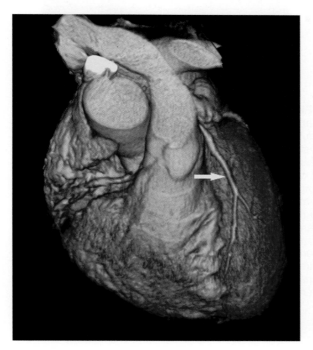

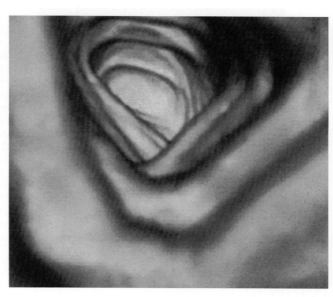

COLOR FIG. 4–1. Cardiac MDCT. Note normal left coronary artery on volume-rendered image (*arrow*).

COLOR FIG. 4–3. Virtual endoscopic image of normal colon with MDCT colonography.

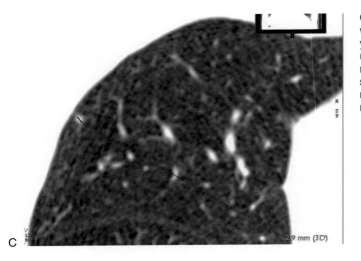

COLOR FIG. 5–4. Prevalence screen in a 57-year-old man with a 2-pack-year history of cigarette smoking who quit 7 years ago. There are three noncalcified solid pulmonary nodules. Nodules have been stable on CT scans obtained 3 months later and again at 6 months. Continued followup CT scans will be performed at 12 months, 18 months, and 24 months from the initial CT. (**C**) 2.9-mm right middlelobe nodule.

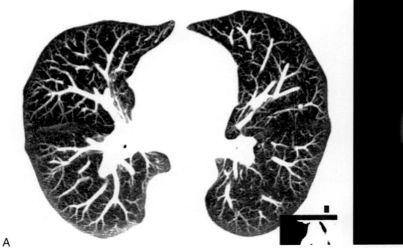

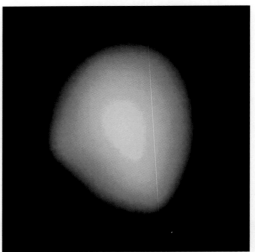

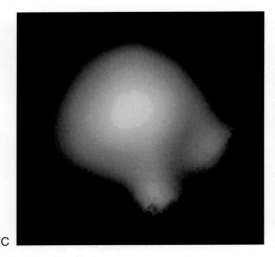

COLOR FIG. 5–5. Alternate imaging viewing methods. **A:** Sliding-slab maximum-intensity projection (MIP) image of the same nodule illustrated in Fig. 4(**B**), in which the 1.25-mm images are stacked together to yield an image that shows the relationship of vessels to the nodule. These usually are viewed in cine-mode or scrolling-mode on a computer workstation, and may enhance the conspicuity of small nodules. **B,C:** Volumetric CT of the same nodule volume in the (**B**) anterior and (**C**) inferior projections: The Advance Lung Analysis software package displays nodule dimensions as 7.1 × 5.6 × 6.6 mm, and calculates nodule volume as 67 mm³. Serial measurements of nodule volume can be used to calculate tumor doubling time. By viewing the nodule in three dimensions, variations in shape may be appreciated that are not shown on two-dimensional images alone.

COLOR FIG. 9–2. Volume rendering, normal trachea. **B**: Internal volume-rendered display (virtual bronchoscopy). Same data set as in (**A**). View from above looking towards carina.

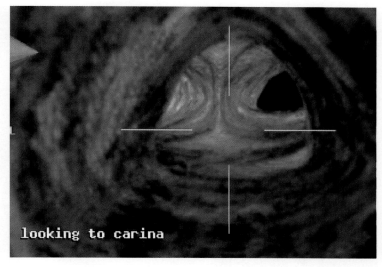

B

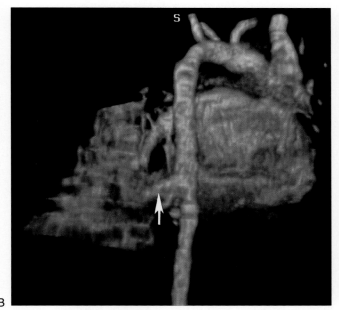

B

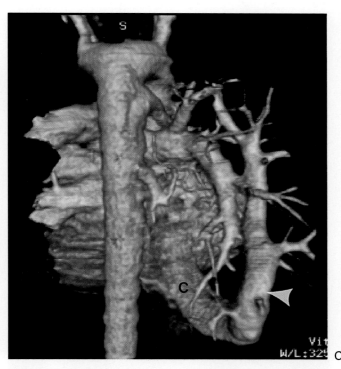

C

COLOR FIG. 9–11. Lung mass, intralobar pulmonary sequestration. **B**: 3D volume rendering viewed from behind shows the feeding artery (*arrow*) arising from the aorta and extending to the lower lobe sequestration. Drainage was via a pulmonary vein, which entered the left atrium. The course of the artery and vein and their relationship to adjacent structures are seen better when the vascular structures, heart, and lung are viewed simultaneously.

COLOR FIG. 9–12. Scimitar syndrome with partial anomalous venous return. **C**: Volume-rendered 3D display. With this technique, it is possible to depict the entire course of the vessel on one image. *C*, inferior vena cava; *arrowhead*, anomalous vein.

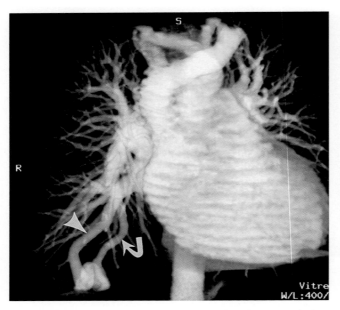

COLOR FIG. 9–13. Pulmonary AVM. 3D volume rendering in a young adult. The feeding artery (*arrow*) originates from the anterior segment artery of the right lower lobe. The draining vein (*arrowhead*) drains into the right inferior pulmonary vein.

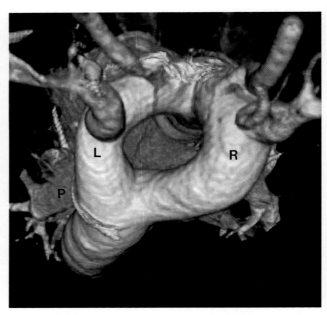

COLOR FIG. 9–14. Double aortic arch. B: Volume-rendered image (posterior view) in the same patient shows that the two arches unite just above the level of the pulmonary artery (*P*): *R*, right arch; *L*, left arch; *PA*, main pulmonary artery.

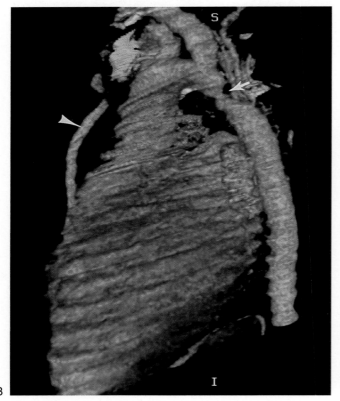

COLOR FIG. 9–16. Aortic coarctation. B: Post-ductal coarctation (*arrow*) in a young adult. Note the large mammary artery collateral vessel (*arrowhead*).

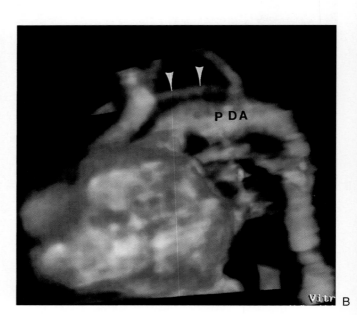

COLOR FIG. 9–17. Interrupted aortic arch. B: Volume-rendered reconstruction shows a markedly hypoplastic transverse arch (*arrowhead*) and a large patent ductus arteriosus (PDA) that supplies the distal aorta. The volume-rendered reconstruction facilitates display of this complex anatomy.

COLOR FIG. 9–27. Chest-wall deformity secondary to prior pneumonectomy. A preoperative CT scan was done to assess the volume of the right hemithorax prior to insertion of a chest prosthesis. Coronal volume-rendered image shows a small right hemithorax and dextroscoliosis of the thoracic spine (*S*).

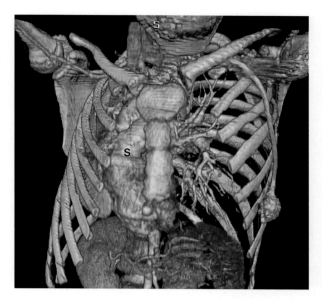

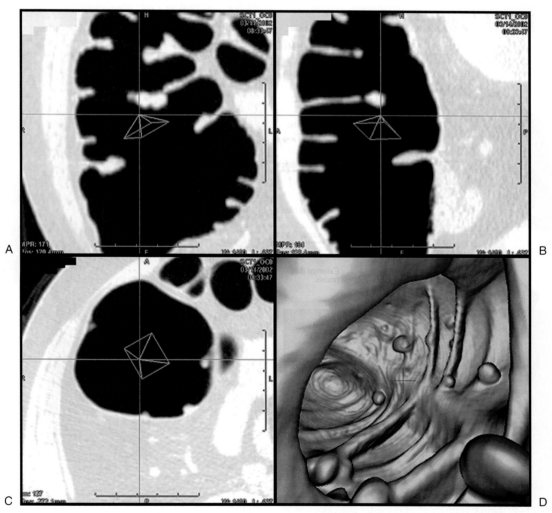

COLOR FIG. 19–1. Computed-tomography colonography with MDCT. Coronal (**A**), sagittal (**B**), and axial (**C**) viewing of CT data obtained at 1.25-mm sections, reconstructed at 1.25-mm intervals. Air-distended lumen demonstrates the colonic surface to good advantage. Pyramidal shape within the lumen demonstrates camera viewing direction for virtual endoscopy. Virtual endoscopic image (**D**) demonstrates multiple polyps in the cecum, ranging in size from 3 mm to 7 mm in diameter.

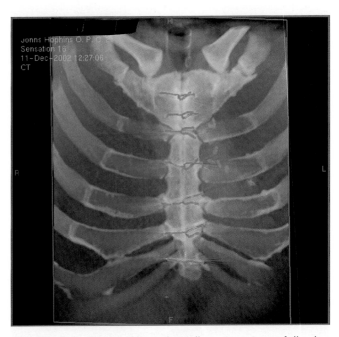

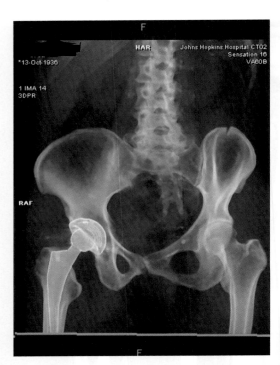

COLOR FIG. 25–25. Normal median sternotomy following coronary-artery bypass surgery. Three-dimensional mapping was done in a patient with persistent chest pain. A successful median sternotomy without evidence of complication is seen on this examination.

COLOR FIG. 25–26. Total hip replacement. Patient had experienced pain, and the study was done to rule out a loose prosthesis. Three-dimensional mapping using color coding demonstrates the prosthesis to be in satisfactory position with no evidence of loosening.

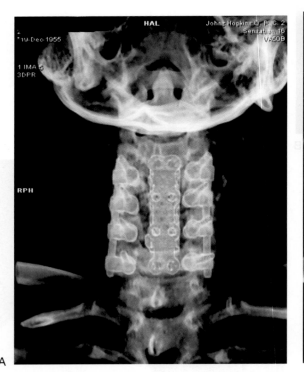

A

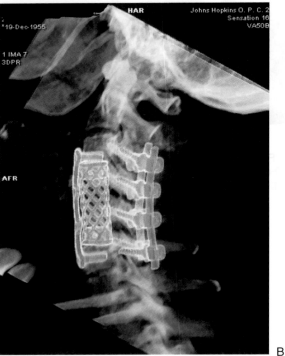

B

COLOR FIG. 25-27. Post C4-C5 corpectomy and removal of epidural abscess with spinal fusion. **A,B:** Extensive hardware is in place involving multiple vertebral bodies and posterior elements and shows a good postoperative result. Note how the metal artifact is minimized by the use of 3D mapping with volume rendering.

COLOR FIG. 28–1. Coronary-calcification scoring study **B:** Computer-assisted highlighting program is used to help define the full extent of calcification on a semiautomated system approach.

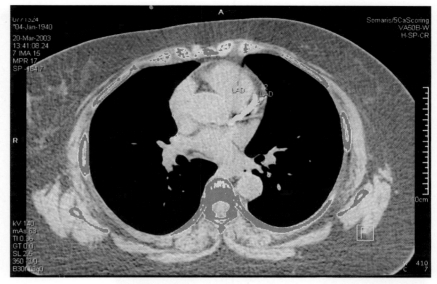

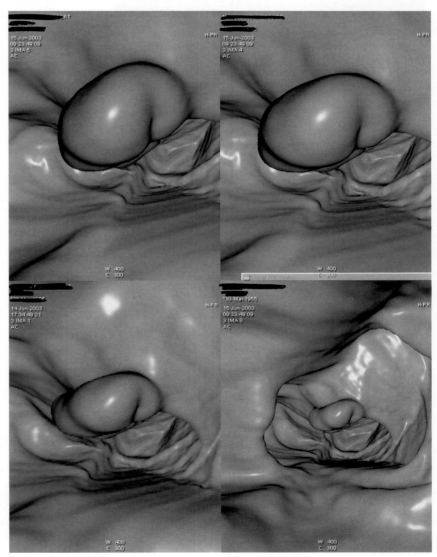

COLOR FIG. 28–4. Virtual colonoscopy. **A,B:** Computed tomography detects colonic polyp on this screening exam. The keys to a successful exam include adequate colonic distension, good patient prep, and good flythru software.

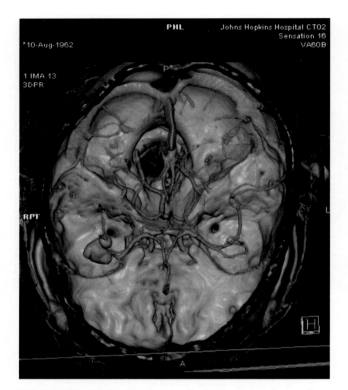

COLOR FIG. 29–2. Middle cerebral artery aneurysm. Composite image demonstrates a middle cerebral-artery aneurysm by using a display combining multiplanar and 3D imaging. The extent of the aneurysm is defined best on the 3D map done interactively with volume rendering.

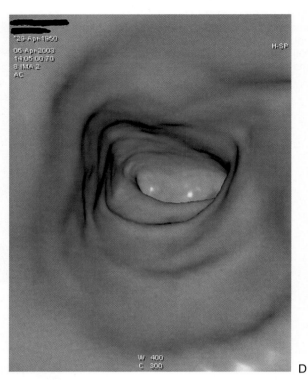

COLOR FIG. 29–7. Computed tomography small bowel enteroclysis. The spectrum of imaging now possible with volume visualization is shown clearly in this case. Image (**D**) is an endoluminal view of the small bowel.

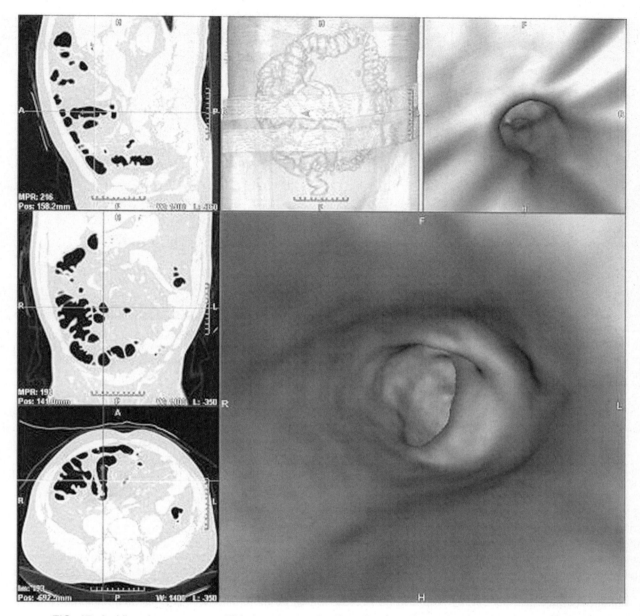

FIG. 17–3. Virtual enteroscopy. This is an example of available software using TeraRecon. Individual air-filled small-bowel loops can be visualized.

pain or bleeding (20). Small-bowel tumors tend to be small initially, and they may be difficult to diagnose by conventional radiological studies (21).

Today, the small-bowel series and enteroclysis still are used for evaluation of suspected small-bowel tumors. Enteroclysis is considered more sensitive in patients in whom there is a high suspicion of tumors (3–5,20,22). In addition to the contrast-fluoroscopy studies, CT now is recognized as an important tool for evaluation of these patients. Computed tomography has the advantage of visualizing both the entire GI tract and extraluminal structures such as lymph nodes.

When performing CT in patients with suspected small-bowel disease, adequate opacification of the small intestine is essential. In the past, high volumes of positive oral-contrast agents would be administered to opacify completely the small bowel. However, as discussed earlier in the chapter, the use of water as oral contrast may have some benefits for this indication, as it allows exquisite visualization of the enhancing bowel wall. Regardless of the type of oral contrast administered, intravenous contrast is essential for this clinical indication. Usually, scans obtained during the portal-venous phase are adequate, and 5-mm slice thickness is adequate; however, if 3D reconstruction is anticipated, thinner collimation (3 mm) can be helpful.

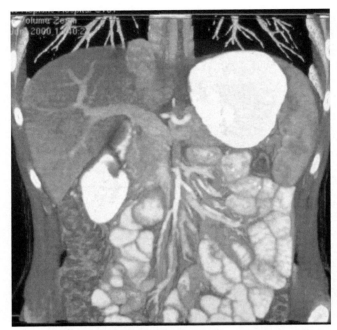

FIG. 17–4. Coronal volume-rendered MDCT in a normal patient using water as oral contrast. The parameters have been adjusted so that the intraluminal water appears white to simulate a standard small-bowel series.

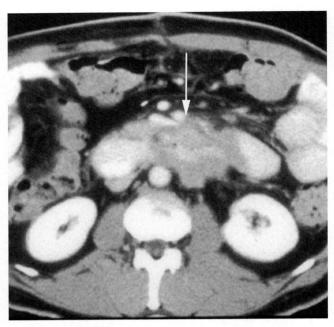

FIG. 17–5. Axial contrast-enhanced CT demonstrates a circumferential mass in the third portion of the duodenum (*arrow*). This was an adenocarcinoma.

Adenocarcinoma

Adenocarcioma is the most common primary malignancy of the small intestine, and the duodenum is the site most frequently involved (23). On CT, adenocarcinoma of the small bowel can have variable appearances. It typically will appear as a focal area of wall thickening causing luminal narrowing (24,25) (Figures 17–5 and 17–6). However, polypoid masses or infiltrative lesions also have been reported. These tumors often are rigid and fibrotic and therefore can result in early obstruction. Occasionally, the tumors will have the classic barium appearance of an applecore lesion. Ulceration of tumors also has been reported in up to 40% of cases (26); however, it may not be visualized readily on CT scans (27).

In addition to detecting primary adenocarcinoma of the small bowel, CT can aid in staging by detecting local extension, adenopathy, or distant metastasis (28). Local extension can be seen in patients in whom the tumor shows extension beyond the bowel wall into the adjacent fat or adjacent structures. Computed tomography can detect enlargement of the enteric lymph nodes, which may be involved with tumor (24). However, as in other malignancies, CT is not always sensitive in detecting malignant nodes, as CT basically uses size criteria, and even small nodes can harbor tumors. Computed tomography is excellent for the detection of distant metastases, of which the liver is the most common site (29). Typically, small-bowel adenocarcinoma metastatic to the liver will appear as low-density masses, which are visualized best during the portal-venous phase of enhancement.

Survival of patients with adenocarcinoma depends on the stage at diagnosis. Treatment consists of early resection, if possible. However, the majority of patients are at an advanced stage at the time diagnosis; consequently, they have a poor outcome (18). Chemotherapy sometimes can be beneficial; radiation therapy usually is not indicated.

Carcinoid

Carcinoid is the next most common small-bowel malignancy, representing approximately 25% of all primary small-bowel tumors (18). Unlike adenocarcinoma, carcinoid tumors are more common in the ileum than in the jejunum or duodenum. These are slow-growing tumors, first appearing as submucosal nodules. In the past, at this stage, the small-bowel series or enteroclysis would be much more sensitive for detection (22). However, given improvements in CT scanning and technique, the submucosal carcinoid tumor occasionally can be identified with CT (Figure 17-7), appearing as an intramural mass demonstrating increased enhancement. Since approximately 30% of carcinoid tumors are multicentric, multiple nodules can be identified (24). As the tumor grows, it usually extends into the adjacent mesentery. As this point, the CT appearance is fairly characteristic, usually appearing as an ill-defined low-density mesenteric mass. Calcification can be seen in up to 70% of cases (30) (Figure 17-8). The mesenteric mass often has a spiculated appearance owing to the desmoplastic reaction. This reaction can encase mesenteric vessels and occasionally will cause ischemia in the affected bowel loops (Figure 17-9). Although

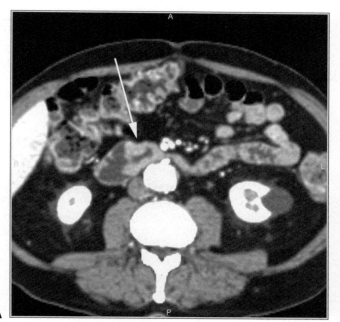 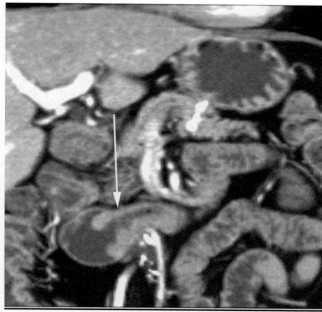

A   B

FIG. 17–6. A: Axial contrast-enhanced MDCT demonstrates a focal mass at the junction of the second and third portions of the duodenum (*arrow*). **B:** Coronal volume-rendered 3D image again demonstrates the mass (*arrow*). This was an adenocarcinoma.

the mesenteric mass typically is a soft-tissue density, cystic carcinoid tumors have been described. These mesenteric masses also are active hormonally.

Metastasis from carcinoid tumors typically involves the liver. These are best demonstrated on arterial-phase imaging, where they will enhance brightly owing to their increased vascularity (Figure 17-10). On portal-venous-phase imaging or delayed imaging through the liver, these lesions may become isodense. If metastatic carcinoid tumor is suspected,

dual-phase imaging of the liver should be performed in order to detect subtle liver metastasis.

The 5-year survival rate for patients with carcinoid of the small bowel is approximately 54% (31). When complete resection of the tumor is possible, the survival rate increases

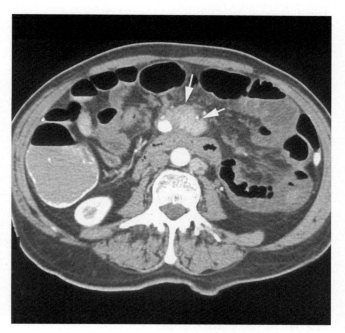

FIG. 17–7. Coronal volume-rendered 3D MDCT with intravenous contrast demonstrates a 2-cm submucosal mass in the proximal jejunum (*arrow*). This was a carcinoid tumor.

FIG. 17–8. Axial contrast-enhanced MDCT demonstrates a mesenteric mass (*arrows*) with calcification in a patient with carcinoid tumor.

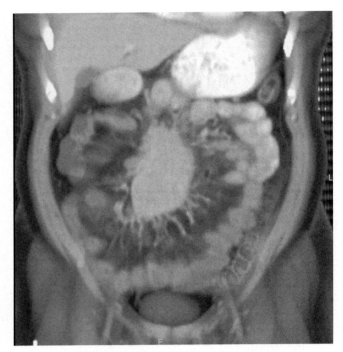

FIG. 17–9. Coronal contrast-enhanced MDCT demonstrates a large mesenteric mass compatible with carcinoid tumor. The adjacent small-bowel loops are thickened, compatible with ischemia resulting from the desmoplastic reaction.

to 75% (31). If there is distant metastasis, the 5-year survival rate is less than 20% (31). In addition to surgery, chemoembolization of the liver metastases occasionally is performed to relieve pain and may prolong survival. Radiation usually is not helpful.

Lymphoma

The third most common small-bowel malignancy is non-Hodgkin's lymphoma. This can involve portions of the gastrointestinal (GI) tract, but is more common in the stomach (32). Primary small-bowel lymphomas have a better prognosis than carcinomas. Four major patterns of small-bowel lymphoma have been identified on radiographic studies (24). First, lymphoma can appear as multiple nodules within the small bowel. It can originate at multiple sites along the small intestine, which can differentiate it from adenocarcinoma and carcinoid tumor. Second, it can appear as a single mass lesion, which varies in size and can lead to intussusception. Third, it can be infiltrating and appear as wall thickening with destruction of the normal small-bowel folds. Unlike adenocarcinoma, these tumors typically are soft and are unlikely to result in obstruction. In addition, because the tumor infiltrates the muscular layer of the wall, it can inhibit peristalsis and result in aneurysmal dilatation of the affected bowel loops (18,26,27) (Figure 17-11). This has been described in up to 50% of cases (26). The fourth pattern is that of exophytic mass, which can ulcerate.

In addition to primary small-bowel lymphomas, non-Hodgkin's lymphoma can develop within the small-bowel

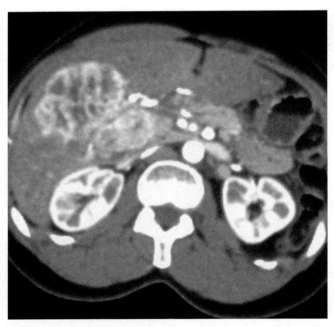

FIG. 17–10. Contrast-enhanced MDCT in a patient with carcinoid tumor demonstrates hypervascular liver metastasis.

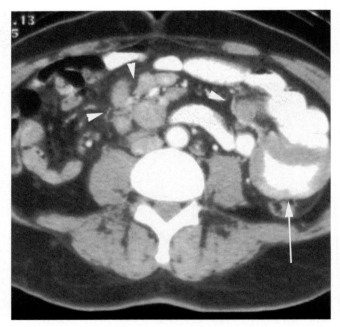

FIG. 17–11. Contrast-enhanced MDCT in a patient with small-bowel lymphoma demonstrates multiple mesenteric nodes (*arrowheads*) and aneurysmal dilatation of a small bowel loop in the left abdomen (*arrow*).

mesentery and infiltrate the adjacent small-bowel loops as it enlarges. Treatment usually consists of chemotherapy, and surgery may be performed.

Gastrointestinal Stromal Tumors (GIST)

The fourth most common small-bowel malignancy is gastrointestinal stromal tumors (GISTs), which arise from smooth-muscle cells within the wall of the small intestine and most commonly occur in the jejunum or ileum (33). Gastointestinal stromal tumors are least common in the duodenum. These tumors formally were referred to as leiomyomas or leiomyosarcoma. They are more common in males than females and are more common in the 5th and 6th decades (34). They represent 9% of all small-bowel malignant tumors (18,33). It often is difficult to distinguish benign from malignant GIST based on the radiographic appearance unless obvious metastases are present. These tumors can be characterized as benign, borderline, low malignant potential, or malignant based on the pathologic appearance. Therefore, they need to be removed for accurate evaluation.

Gastrointestinal stromal tumors typically appear exophytic and can be bulky (33,35) (Figures 17–12 and 17–13). Central necrosis or ulceration also is common. They can be so large that the site of origin is difficult to identify. The communication of the tumor with the intestinal lumen also may be difficult to appreciate. However, 3D imaging can help to clarify the findings on the axial images.

Tumor spread usually is through direct extension into adjacent organs or hematogeneously to the liver. Liver me-

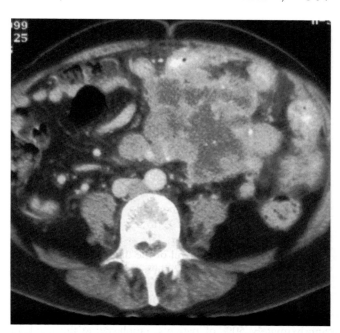

FIG. 17–13. Contrast-enhanced CT image demonstrates a large necrotic mass in the mesentery. At surgery, a large GIST was diagnosed. These often are large and exophytic.

tastasis can appear low density or cystic, and peritoneal metastasis also may be seen. Treatment usually consists of surgical resection. Tumor survival is increased for smaller tumors (less than 5 cm) (18).

SMALL-BOWEL INFLAMMATORY DISEASE

Crohn's Disease

Although contrast studies still are the cornerstone in radiological evaluation of patients with Crohn's disease, CT is beginning to play a more dominant role. Barium studies, such as small-bowel series and enteroclysis, are able to demonstrate exquisite mucosal detail but give very little information about extramural disease, which often is crucial for evaluating these patients. Therefore, CT always has been a valuable adjunct to barium studies owing to its ability to image extraluminal extension of disease. Computed tomography can affect significantly patient management by demonstrating extraluminal abscesses, fistulae, or involvement of other adjacent organs (36). With improvements in 3D-imaging technology, CT also can be used to demonstrate mural disease. The early mucosal changes of Crohn's disease are not always visualized reliably with CT, and these may be demonstrated better with barium studies. However, with thinner collimation and IV contrast, ulcers within the wall can be visualized on CT.

As Crohn's disease can affect any portion of the GI tract, good opacification of the entire tract is necessary. Traditionally, a patient with Crohn's disease was evaluated

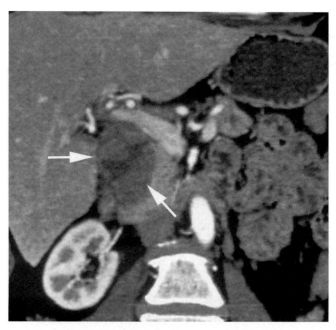

FIG. 17–12. Coronal volume-rendered 3D MDCT demonstrates a low-density mass with central necrosis in the region of the second portion of the duodenum (*arrows*). This was a benign GIST.

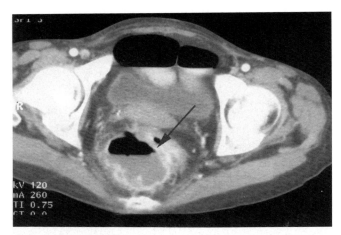

FIG. 17–20. Contrast-enhanced MDCT in a patient with Crohn's disease demonstrates a large abscess in the perirectal region (*arrow*).

not contain contrast material or air. Three-dimensional imaging can be helpful to visualize better these small fistulae.

In addition to the standard CT examination, CT enteroclysis also is performed at some institutions (45). This technique involves infusing a large volume of water-soluble contrast or methylcellulose solution, optimally distending the entire small bowel. This may be a more sensitive technique to detect low-grade obstructions or subtle mucosal disease.

SMALL-BOWEL OBSTRUCTION

Small-bowel obstruction is a common clinical entity that usually is suspected based on clinical signs and symp-

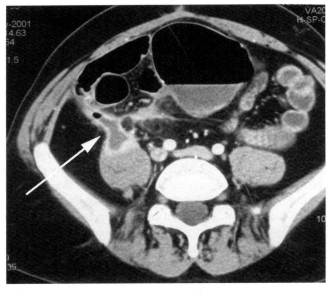

FIG. 17–21. Contrast-enhanced MDCT in a patient with Crohn's disease demonstrates an abscess involving the right psoas muscle (*arrow*).

toms and confirmed with radiological studies. Although the barium small-bowel series traditionally has been the radiological study ordered in these patients, CT is now often the first examination ordered, as it offers distinct advantages. First, CT is fast; with the newer MDCT scanners, the entire abdomen and pelvis can be imaged in 10 seconds to 15 seconds with spectacular resolution. In urgent cases, CT can be performed immediately. Even without administration of oral-contrast agents, CT can detect obstruction, as obstructed loops are distended with enteric fluid. Second, CT is not only able to diagnose the presence of obstruction, but also often can identify the cause. Computed tomography has proven to be more sensitive and specific than barium studies, and it is much better than plain films and barium studies in its ability to determine the level and cause of the obstruction and to detect complications, especially in cases of longstanding or high-grade obstruction (46,47). Many studies have confirmed the value of CT for this clinical indication and have demonstrated a sensitivity of 94% to 100% and an accuracy of 90% to 95% (5,47). Studies have demonstrated that CT is able to identify correctly the cause of obstruction in 73% to 95% of cases (46,48–51) and can distinguish reliably obstruction from ileus (52,53).

The CT diagnosis of small-bowel obstruction is based on the presence of a transition between dilated and nondilated bowel loops. Collapsed small-bowel loops always will be present distal to the site of the small-bowel obstruction unless the obstruction occurs at the ileocecal valve, in which case the colon will be decompressed. The greater the difference in caliber between proximal and distal loops, the more reliable the CT diagnosis and the more severe the degree of obstruction. However, there are no exact CT criteria to gauge accurately the degree of obstruction. If oral contrast successfully traverses the site of transition, a partial obstruction is likely. If oral contrast does not traverse the transition, it does not necessarily indicate a complete obstruction.

The ability to view the CT data in more than one plane can be useful in the evaluation of patients with small-bowel obstruction, as the exact site of transition may be difficult to detect on axial images. Multiplanar reconstruction now is available widely and it is easy to use. The use of MPR for this clinical indication has been shown to increase diagnostic confidence (54). The usefulness of 3D imaging in the setting of small-bowel obstruction has yet to be determined. However, 3D imaging is more flexible than simple MPR, as the data can be viewed from any imaging plane or angle. Similarly, the value of MDCT for this clinical indication has not yet been explored completely, but it is likely that the thinner collimation and higher resolution obtainable with these systems will improve CT diagnosis of small-bowel obstruction (55).

The major causes of small-bowel obstruction can be classified into three distinct categories: extrinsic causes, intrinsic causes, and intraluminal causes (56).

Extrinsic causes include adhesions, hernias, and extrinsic masses. Adhesions are the most common cause of small-

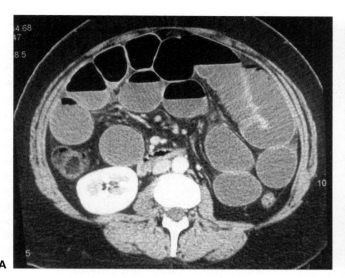

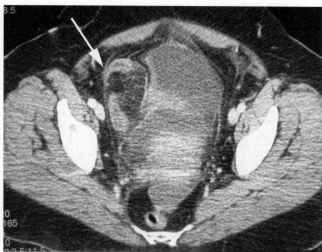

FIG. 17–22. A: Contrast-enhanced MDCT in a patient with abdominal pain demonstrates moderate dilatation of the proximal small bowel. **B:** The distal small-bowel loops are collapsed (*arrow*), compatible with obstructions. This was due to adhesions.

bowel obstruction, and usually form after surgery, although severe peritoneal inflammation also can result in adhesion formation. The CT diagnosis of adhesions usually is made when all other possible causes have been ruled out (Figure 17-22). Typically, although the level of transition is identified, the fibrous bands are not visible. Hernias also are a common cause of obstruction and occur when there is prolapse of the bowel loop through a defect in the abdominal or pelvic wall (Figure 17-23). These external hernias are

most common in the inguinal and femoral canals, periumbilical regions, and at sites of previous surgery (57). Other sites of external hernias include spegalian, obturator, and ventral hernias. Hernias can be diagnosed by identifying bowel loops through the defects. If there is a transition in caliber of the loops proximal and distal to the hernia site, it is obstructed. If the hernia cannot be reduced, it is incarcerated. The presence of wall thickening and inflammatory stranding within a hernia suggests associated ischemia and requires urgent surgical attention (Figure 17-24). Internal hernias also can occur through peritoneal defects and are most common in the paraduodenal and transmesenteric regions. Masses ex-

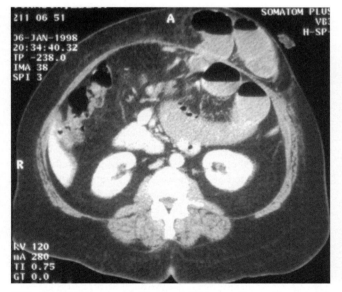

FIG. 17–23. Contrast-enhanced CT in a patient with abdominal pain demonstrates an abdominal-wall hernia with dilated small-bowel loops. The distal small bowel and colon are decompressed. This is compatible with a small-bowel obstruction due to an incisional hernia.

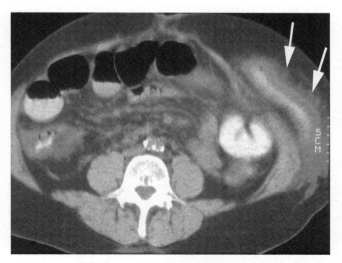

FIG. 17–24. Contrast-enhanced CT in a patient with severe abdominal pain demonstrates an incisional hernia in the left abdomen (*arrows*). The herniated small-bowel loop is thickened moderately with stranding compatible with ischemia.

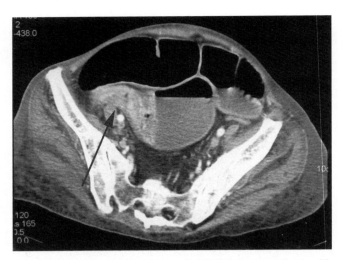

FIG. 17–25. Contrast-enhanced MDCT in a patient with Crohn's disease demonstrates moderate dilatation of the small bowel. In the right lower quadrant (*arrow*) there is an inflamed small-bowel loop. The small-bowel obstruction was caused by active inflammation due to the patient's Crohn's disease.

trinsic to the bowel also can result in small-bowel obstructions. These tumors include carcinoid, lymphoma, and peritoneal carcinomatosis (56). In these instances, a mass will be identified as the cause of the obstruction.

Intrinsic causes of small-bowel obstruction include small-bowel neoplasms, such as adenocarcinoma, and inflammatory or infectious entities. For example, Crohn's disease may result in small-bowel obstruction, either due to acute inflammation with small-bowel thickening or focal strictures (Figure 17-25). Other intrinsic causes include intramural hemorrhage (anticoagulation or ischemia) and can lead to small-bowel obstruction.

Intraluminal entities are the least common cause of obstruction and can be caused by ingested foreign matter, bezoars, gallstones, meconium, or ascaris (58). Enteroenteric intussusception is an intraluminal obstruction that can result from various extrinsic, intrinsic, or intraluminal causes. In most cases, a lead point will cause a loop of bowel and its associated mesentery to invaginate into the lumen of a distal small-bowel loop, resulting in a characteristic CT appearance (59).

Mesenteric Ischemia

Acute Ischemia

Mesenteric ischemia is a fairly common but complex disorder that results from insufficient blood flow to the intestines. It can be classified into two main categories: acute ischemia and chronic ischemia.

The most common cause of acute mesenteric ischemia is an embolism to the superior mesenteric artery (60), the emboli typically arising from the heart. In addition to emboli,

acute thrombosis can occur in the superior mesenteric artery or superior mesenteric vein, thereby resulting in acute mesenteric ischemia (60). Acute mesenteric ischemia also can be caused by low-flow states (61). In this instance, the mesenteric arteries and veins are patent, but the blood flow through them is slowed and is not adequate to deliver necessary oxygenated blood to the intestine. The usual cause is decreased cardiac output resulting from primary cardiac disease, infarction, arrhythmia, or hypovolemia. Acute small-bowel ischemia also can occur as a result of small-bowel obstruction. A strangulated or incarcerated small-bowel loop can comprise the mesenteric vessels and result in ischemia of the infected loops (62). In these cases, there will be an associated small-bowel obstruction and the strangulated loops will appear thickened with mesenteric stranding and congestion. This is a surgical emergency requiring immediate attention.

Computed tomography can be used to evaluate patients with suspected acute mesenteric ischemia. For this clinical indication, a special protocol is necessary. Typically, thin collimation is used for adequate visualization of the mesenteric arteries and veins; dual-phase imaging also is required. A 4-mm × 1-mm collimator setting was used to create 1.25-mm slices. These are reconstructed at 1-mm intervals, producing high-resolution 3D images of the mesenteric vasculature. A rapid IV-contrast bolus is necessary for adequate opacification of the vessels. Nonionic contrast is injected at a flow rate of 3 cc to 5 cc per second. Arterial-phase images are obtained 25 seconds after injection; portal-phase images are obtained 50 seconds after injection. Three-dimensional imaging is essential for this clinical indication, as the mesenteric arteries and veins are very small and not visualized well in the axial plane. Three-dimensional imaging with volume rendering allows complete evaluation of mesenteric arteries and veins to identify potential causes of ischemia (16). Thrombosis can be identified easily within the superior mesenteric artery and vein (Figures 17–26 and 17–27). In addition, other causes of ischemia, such as encasement of the mesenteric vessels by tumors, can be detected. Nonocclusive ischemia can be difficult to diagnose on CT angiography, as the mesenteric vessels will appear patent, although they may be small or constricted as a result of the hypotension.

In addition to abnormalities in the mesenteric vasculature, CT can detect enhancement changes in the bowel wall. This is appreciated best when water is given as oral contrast and IV-contrast injection is administered. In cases of acute mesenteric ischemia, the affected small-bowel loops often are thickened, which is nonspecific (Figure 17-28). Decreased, delayed, or absence of enhancement has been reported in affected bowel loops, but is less common. There may be low density within the bowel wall resulting from edema (63,64). Intramural hemorrhage also is an associated finding with ischemia (65). The presence of intramural gas (pneumatosis) (Figure 17-29) is a late finding. This is a more specific but less common sign of ischemic bowel disease and usually indicates irreversible infarction. Pneumatosis

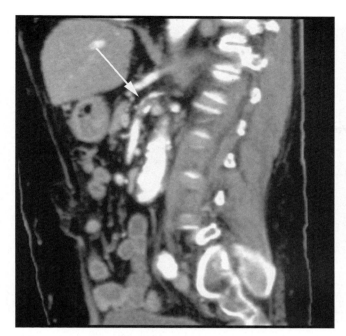

FIG. 17–26. Sagittal volume-rendered 3D MDCT demonstrates acute thrombosis in the proximal portion of the superior mesenteric artery (*arrow*).

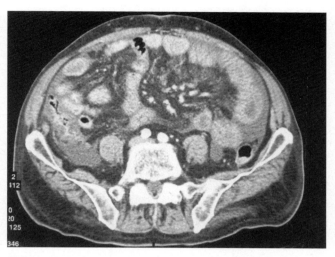

FIG. 17–28. Contrast-enhanced CT in a patient with severe abdominal pain demonstrates diffused thickening of the small bowel and right colon. No thrombosis was identified. Based on the clinical information, this was thought to be due to ischemia resulting from hypotension.

can have associated gas within the mesenteric vessels and/or portal vein.

Shock bowel is a subtype of nonocclusive ischemia that typically occurs in the trauma setting when a patient becomes acutely hypovolemic. Although contrast is delivered to the gut, there is a slow washout. On CT, this will result in persistent increased enhancement of the bowel wall (66–68) (Fig-

ure 17-30). There may be associated findings including a flattened inferior vena cava, which also signifies a hypovolemic state. Usually, the CT findings of shock bowel resolve with the correction of the hypovolemia.

In addition to changes in the bowel wall, the affected loops may be dilated owing to an interruption in peristalsis (69). There may be associated inflammatory changes in the mesentery, as well as free fluid (70). These findings are visualized well when thin collimation is used and 3D imaging is available (16). Computed-tomography evaluation for acute mesenteric ischemia is improved with MDCT, which provides thinner collimation, faster scanning, and increased

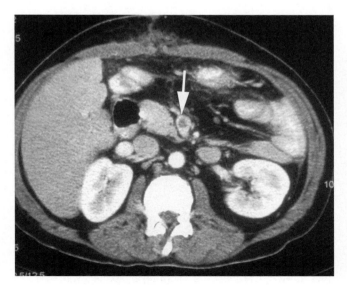

FIG. 17–27. Contrast-enhanced CT in a patient with severe abdominal pain demonstrates thickening of the small-bowel loops. A thrombosis is demonstrated in the superior mesenteric vein (*arrow*).

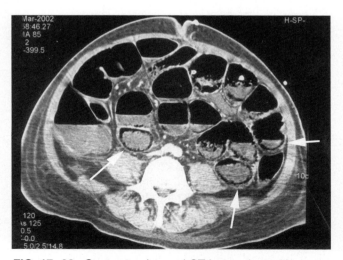

FIG. 17–29. Contrast-enhanced CT in a patient with severe abdominal pain demonstrates pneumatosis involving multiple small-bowel loops (*arrows*).

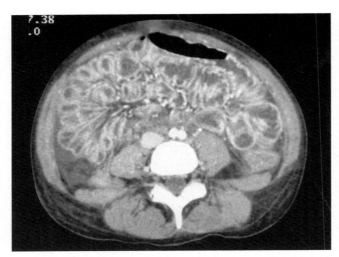

FIG. 17–30. Contrast-enhanced CT in a patient after trauma demonstrates persistent enhancement of the small bowel. This is an example of shock bowel.

resolution, resulting in a more comprehensive visualization of the small bowel and mesenteric vessels.

Chronic Ischemia

Chronic mesenteric ischemia is relatively uncommon and often diagnosed late, given the nonspecific symptoms (71). Patients often suffer from vague abdominal pain and weight loss, which is not recognized clinically. Chronic mesenteric ischemia typically occurs in older patients and is due to long-standing atherosclerotic disease, which has resulted in arterial insufficiency (72). Patients present with nonspecific abdominal pain, often associated with meals. The patient frequently will complain of periumbilical or epigastric pain within 15 minutes after meals (72). This may increase in severity and persist for up to 3 hours. This often is the clinical clue that significant ischemia is present.

Atherosclerotic disease of the mesenteric arteries is common in older patients even without mesenteric ischemia (72–75). In order to develop symptoms, usually two of the three major vessels supplying the bowel must be infected. In the past, when chronic mesenteric ischemia was suspected clinically, an angiogram would be performed in order to evaluate the celiac axis, superior mesenteric artery, and inferior mesenteric artery. This was considered to be the gold standard for diagnosis of the entity. The angiogram usually will demonstrate a minimum 70% narrowing of at least two of the major arterial vessels. Although angiography still is used for this indication, CT now plays a valuable role, given the recent technical improvements (76). Computed-tomography angiography (CTA) now can be performed easily to evaluate all of the mesenteric arteries and vessels including distal branches, and identify areas of stenosis, areas of calcified atherosclerotic plaque, and luminal narrowing (Figure 17-31). Another common finding on angiography and

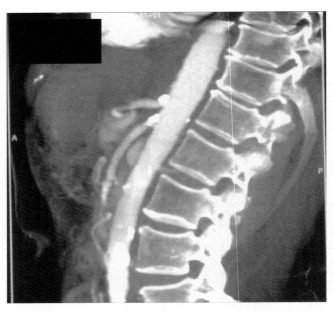

FIG. 17–31. Lateral CT angiography demonstrates a focal calcification at the origin of the celiac axis and SMA in a patient with chronic mesenteric ischemia.

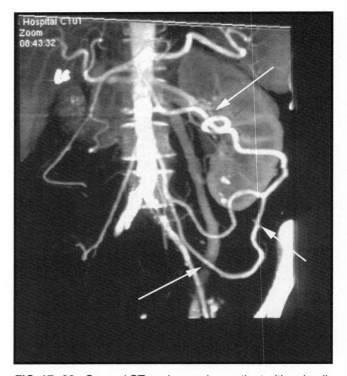

FIG. 17–32. Coronal CT angiogram in a patient with episodic abdominal pain demonstrates collateral filling of the superior mesenteric artery. The superior mesenteric artery is filled in a retrograde manner. The collaterals are visualized well (*arrows*).

computed tomography with chronic mesenteric ischemia is the presence of associated collateral vessels, which have appeared over time in an attempt to maintain adequate blood supply to the gut (Figure 17-32). These include collaterals connecting the celiac axis to the superior mesenteric artery, which usually involve pancreaticoduodenal arteries running between the gastric duodenal artery and proximal superior mesenteric artery (76). The other main route of collateral vessels connects the superior mesenteric artery to the inferior mesenteric artery and includes the paracolic arcade and the marginal artery of Drummond (76). These collaterals are identified easily on CTA.

Treatment for chronic mesenteric ischemia usually involves surgery with bypass grafting. However, more recently, transluminal angioplasty and percutaneous stents have been used successfully to treat this condition less invasively (77).

CONCLUSION

With continued advancements in technology, the value of CT evaluation of small-bowel pathology continues to expand. Computed tomography reliably can detect a variety of small-bowel conditions and acts as an important adjunct to endoscopy and barium studies for optimal patient management. As scanners provide thinner collimation, greater imaging speed, and increased resolution, the role of CT in the diagnosis of gastrointestinal disease will continue to evolve.

REFERENCES

1. Goldberg HI, Caruthers SB Jr, Nelson JA, et al. Radiographic findings of the National Cooperative Crohn's Disease Study. *Gastroenterology* 1979;77:925–937.
2. Garvey DJ, de Lacey G, Wilkins RA. Preliminary colon cleansing for small-bowel examinations: results and implications of a prospective survey. *Clin Radiol* 1985;36:503–506.
3. Maglinte DDT, Kelvin FM, O'Connor K, et al. Current status of small bowel radiography. *Abdom Imaging* 1996;21:247–257.
4. Maglinte DDT, Hall R, Miller RE, et al. Detection of surgical lesions of the small bowel by enteroclysis. *Am J Surg* 1984;147:225–229.
5. Maglinte DDT, Burney BT, Miller RE. Lesions missed on small-bowel follow-through: analysis and recommendations. *Radiology* 1982;144:737–739.
6. Springer P, Dessl A, Giacomuzzi SM. Virtual computed tomography gastroscopy; a new technique. *Endoscopy* 1997;29:632–634.
7. Raptopoulos V, Davis MA, Davidoff A, et al. Fat density oral contrast agent for abdominal CT. *Radiology* 1987;164:653–656.
8. Horton KM, Eng J, Fishman EK. Normal enhancement of the small bowel: Evaluation with spiral CT. *J Comput Assist Tomogr* 2000;24:67–71.
9. Winter TC, Ager JD, Nghiem HV, et al. Upper gastrointestinal tract and abdomen: water as an orally administered contrast agent for helical CT. *Radiology* 1996;201:365–370.
10. Gossios KJ, Tsianos EV, Demou LL, et al. Use of water or air as oral contrast media for computed tomographic study of the gastric wall: comparison of the two techniques. *Gastrointest Radiol* 1991;16:293–297.
11. Baert AL, Roex L, Marchal G, et al. Computed tomography of the stomach with water as an oral contrast agent: technique and preliminary results. *J Comput Assist Tomogr* 1989;13:633–636.
12. Theoni RF, Filson RG. Abdominal and pelvic CT: use of oral metoclopromide to enhance bowel opacification. *Radiology* 1988;169:391–393.
13. Birnbaum BA. Computed tomography of the small bowel: Technique and principles of interpretation. In: Herlinger H, Birnbaum BA, eds. *Clinical imaging of the small intestine. Vol. I.* New York: Springer–Verlag, 1999;153–166.
14. Gore RM, Balthazar EJ, Gharemani GC, et al. CT features of ulcerative colitis and Crohn's disease. *AJR Am J Roentgenol* 1996;167:3–15.
15. Megibow AJ. Techniques of gastrointestinal CT. In: Gore RM LM, Laufer I, eds. *Textbook of gastrointestinal radiology.* Philadelphia, PA: WB Saunders, 1993;103–112.
16. Horton KM, Fishman EK. Multidetector CT in the evaluation of mesenteric ischemia: Can it be done? *Radiographics* 2001;21:1463–1473.
17. Horton KM, Fishman EK. Volume-rendering 3D CT of the mesenteric vasculature: normal anatomy, anatomic variants and pathologic correlation. *Radiographics* 2002;22:161–172.
18. Maglinte DDT, Herlinger H. Small bowel neoplasms. In: Herlinger HMD, Birnbaum BA, eds. *Clinical imaging of the small intestine.* New York: Springer–Verlag, 1999;377–438.
19. Chow JS, Chen CS, Ahsan H, et al. A population-based study of the incidence of malignant small bowel tumors: SEER, 1973–1990. *Int J Epidemiol* 1996;25:722–728.
20. Maglinte DDT, O'Connor K, Bessette J, et al.. The role of the physician in the late diagnosis of primary malignant tumors of the small intestine. *Am J Gastroenterol* 1991;86:304–308.
21. Zollinger RM Jr. Primary neoplasms of the small intestine. *Am J Surg* 1986;151:654–658.
22. Bessette JR, Maglinte DDT, Kelvin FM, et al. Primary malignant tumors in the small bowel: a comparison of the small-bowel enema and conventional follow-through examination. *AJR Am J Roentgenol* 1989;153:741–744.
23. Brookes VS, Waterhouse JAH, Powel DJ. Malignant lesions of the small intestine. *Br J Surg* 1968;55:405–410.
24. Buckley JA, Jones B, Fishman EK. Small bowel cancer: imaging features and staging. *Radiol Clin North Am* 1997;35:381–402.
25. Ekberg O, Ekholm S. Radiology in primary small bowel adenocarcinoma. *Gastrointest Radiol* 1980;5:49–53.
26. Dudiak KM, Johnson CD, Stephens DH. Primary tumors of the small intestine: CT evaluation. *AJR Am J Roentgenol* 1989;152:995–998.
27. Laurent F, Raynaud M, Biset JM, et al. Diagnosis and categorization of small bowel neoplasms: role of computed tomography. *Gatroinest Radiol* 1991;16:115–119.
28. Merine D, Fishman EK, Jones B. CT of the small bowel and mesentery. *Radiol Clin North Am* 1989;27:707–715.
29. Kuszyk BS, Bluemke DA, Urban BA, et al. Portal-phase contrast-enhanced helical CT for the detection of malignant hepatic tumours: sensitivity based on comparison with intraoperative and pathologic findings. *AJR Am J Roentgenol* 1996;166:91–95.
30. Pantingrag-Brown L, Buetow PC, Carl NJ, et al. AFIP Calcification and fibrosis in mesenteric carcinoid tumor: CT findings and pathologic correlation. Society of Gastrointestinal Radiologists, 24th Annual Meeting, Tucson, AZ 1995;71(abst).
31. Gore RM. Small bowel cancer. Clinical and pathologic features. *Radiol Clin North Am* 1997;35:351–360.
32. Brady LW, Asbell SO. Malignant lymphoma of the gastrointestinal tract. *Radiology* 1980;137:291–298.
33. Bruenton J. Imaging of gastrointestinal tract tumors. Adenocarcinoma of the small intestine. In: Bruenton JN, ed. *Imaging of gastrointestinal tract tumors.* Berlin, Heidelberg, Germany: Springer–Verlag, 1990;130–137.
34. Shiu MH, Farr GH, Egeli RA, et al. Myosarcomas of the small and large intestine: a clinicopathological study. *J Surg Oncol* 1983;24:67–72.
35. Megibow AJ, Balthazar EJ, Hulnick DH, et al. CT evaluation of gastrointestinal tract leiomyomas and leiomyosarcomas. *AJR Am J Roentgenol* 1985;144:727–731.
36. Fishman E, Wolf E, Jones B, et al. CT evaluation of Crohn's disease: effect on patient management. *AJR Am J Roentgenol* 1987;148:537–540.
37. Caroline D, Friedman A. The radiology of inflammatory bowel disease. *Med Clin North Am* 1994;78:1353–1385.
38. Farmer RG, Whelan G, Fazio VW. Long term follow-up of patients with Crohn's disease. Relationship between clinical pattern and prognosis. *Gastroenterology* 1985;88:1818–1825.
39. Gore RM, Marn CS, Kirby DF, et al. CT findings in ulcerative, granulomatous and indeterminate colitis. *AJR Am J Roentgenol* 1984;2:279–284.

abdomen or extension of the sigmoid colon out of the pelvis into the lower abdomen. Chiladiti's syndrome occurs when there is interposition of the right colon between the liver and diaphragm.

COLONIC PATHOLOGY

Colitis

Inflammation of the colon may occur from a variety of causes, including infection, ischemia, or inflammatory conditions. The inflammatory disorders to be discussed include pseudomembranous colitis, ischemic colitis, Crohn's colitis, and ulcerative colitis.

Pseudomembranous Colitis

Pseudomembranous colitis (PMC) results from toxins produced by an overgrowth of the organism *Clostridium difficile*, and results in a profuse watery diarrhea with abdominal pain and fever (6). Although first reported as a complication of antibiotic therapy, PMC also has been reported with hypotensive episodes, chemotherapeutic agents, and following abdominal surgery. The diagnosis typically is made with stool assay for the *C. difficile* toxin, but the clinical presentation often is nonspecific and the radiologist may be the first to suggest the diagnosis.

The most common, but nonspecific, CT finding in patients with PMC is thickening of the colonic wall, which may be circumferential or eccentric (Figure 18-1). In a series of 64 patients with PMC studied by Boland et al., 85% showed some colonic abnormality, usually nonspecific

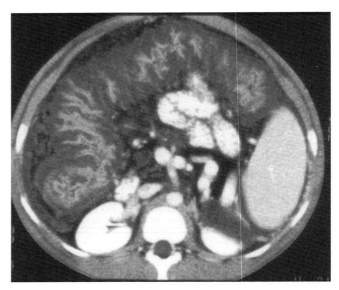

FIG. 18–2. Contrast-enhanced CT in a patient with PMC demonstrates dramatic mucosal enhancement. The submucosa is low density, compatible with edema. There is only minimal pericolonic stranding and minimal ascites.

thickening (7). In a different series, the colonic-wall thickness ranged between 3 mm and 32 mm (average 14.7) (8). In another series by Philpotts, the average colonic-wall thickness in patients with PMC was 10.7 mm (9). In general, the amount of bowel-wall thickening in PMC is greater than in other inflammatory/infectious diseases of the colon, with the exception of Crohn's disease, and is a helpful differentiation point (8,10). In patients with PMC, the bowel wall may be low in attenuation due to edema, or the mucosa may enhance significantly after IV contrast secondary to hyperemia, but this is not specific for the condition (Figure 18-2).

In addition to wall thickening, the colon often is dilated due to the transmural inflammation affecting peristalsis. Mild pericolonic stranding also may be present. Although pericolonic stranding is a nonspecific finding occurring in many other inflammatory and infectious colonic diseases, the pericolonic stranding in PMC often is disproportionately mild compared to the marked colonic-wall thickening, as the condition predominantly affects the mucosa and submucosa (11) (Figure 18-1). The "target sign" originally reported in ulcerative colitis and Crohn's disease also has been reported in PMC (Figure 18-3). When haustral folds are thickened significantly, they can appear as broad transverse bands that may trap oral contrast. This is known as the "accordion sign" (8). The accordion sign is very suggestive of PMC, but typically occurs only in severe cases and therefore is not sensitive.

Pseudomembranous colitis is classically a pancolitis, but it can involve any segment of the colon (12) (Figure 18-4). In some patients, it may begin in the rectum and progress retrograde to involve the left colon. Alternatively, PMC can be limited to the right side of the colon with sparing of

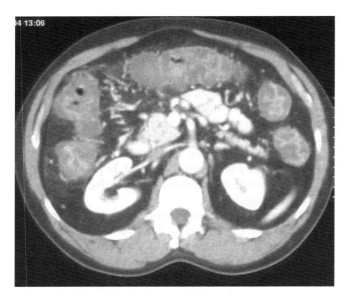

FIG. 18–1. Contrast-enhanced CT in a patient with severe abdominal pain and fever demonstrates marked circumferential thickening of the entire colon. There is increased mucosal enhancement. Minimal pericolonic stranding is noted. Toxin assay was positive for pseudomembranous colitis.

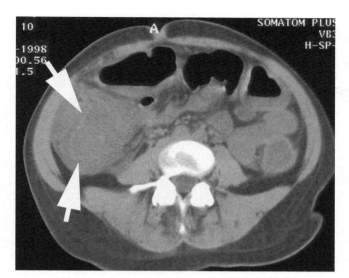

FIG. 18–3. Unenhanced CT scan of a patient with PMC demonstrates circumferential thickening of the colon. The right colon is more involved than the left colon. Individual layers can be identified within the right colon (*arrows*) due to submucosal edema.

the left colon in 30% to 40% of the cases (13). Isolated involvement of segments of the colon and rectum also has been reported (8,13). Ascites has been reported to occur in up to 35% of patients with PMC, but is neither sensitive nor specific for the diagnosis (8,11,14).

A recent retrospective study by Kirkpatrick et al. reported the accuracy of CT in diagnosing PMC (12). Over a 4-year period, 54 patients with positive stool assays and CT scans were identified and matched with 56 control patients.

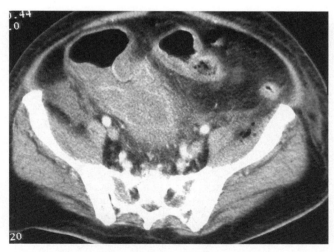

FIG. 18–4. Contrast-enhanced MDCT in a patient with PMC demonstrates marked circumferential thickening of the sigmoid colon. There is minimal involvement of the descending colon. However, the right colon and transverse were not involved. This is an example of segmental involvement of the colon by PMS.

When a diagnostic criterion of colonic-wall thickness greater than 4 mm was combined with pericolonic stranding, wall nodularity, accordion signs, or unexplained ascites, the sensitivity for PMC was 70%, with a specificity of 93% (12).

Treatment for PMC usually consists of metronidozole. If not treated aggressively, severe sepsis and bowel perforation can occur. Pseudomembranous colitis can result in significant patient morbidity and mortality (15,16). A small number of patients with a fulminant form of PMC may not respond to medical therapy, and therefore require surgical intervention, such as colectomy (17). Although CT is valuable in diagnosing PMC and determining the extent of involvement and the presence of complications, it cannot determine reliably which patients will require surgery (11).

Ischemic Colitis

Ischemic colitis results from insufficient blood flow to the colon. It is the most common vascular disorder of the intestine in elderly patients and usually is due to hypoperfusion or hypotension rather than vascular occlusion (18). Although an underlying etiologic factor may be present, most cases are considered unexplainable or idiopathic.

In a recent study of 54 patients with confirmed ischemic colitis, a precipitating cause was discovered in only 43% of cases, whereas in 57% of cases no etiology was determined (19). Given the prevalence of vascular disease in patients over the age of 70, it is assumed that the cause is related to atherosclerosis (19,20). The episode is likely to occur when there is an increased demand for flow in a patient with only marginal baseline colonic blood flow. Patients typically present with vague abdominal pain accompanied by bloody diarrhea. The damage of the ischemic attack depends on the acuteness and duration of the process, as well as the presence of adequate collaterals. In mild cases, only the mucosa is involved, as it is most vulnerable to ischemic insult (21). In more severe cases, the damage may involve the mucosa and submucosa, resulting in transmural ischemia or even infarction.

Most of the CT literature regarding the effectiveness of CT in the diagnosis of ischemic colitis was written before the availability of spiral CT, and therefore describes late findings in ischemia, such as pneumatosis or bowel infarction (22–26). With the current widespread use of spiral scanners and MDCT, it is likely that CT will enable diagnosis at an earlier stage.

The most common CT finding in ischemic colitis is bowel-wall thickening. In a recent series by Balthazar et al. of 54 patients with proven ischemic colitis, the average wall thickness was 8 mm, with a range of 2 mm to 20 mm (19). The entire colon can be affected, although patchy or segmental areas are more common (27) (Figures 18–5 and 18–6). In the series by Balthazar et al., 89% of cases demonstrated segmental involvement with a mean length of 19 cm (19). Any segment of the colon can be involved, depending on the etiology. As most cases are a result of nonocclusive is-

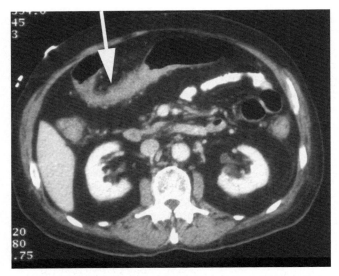

FIG. 18–5. Contrast-enhanced CT scan in a patient with ischemia colitis demonstrates segmental involvement of the transverse colon (*arrow*).

chemia, the watershed regions are the most commonly affected, usually at the splenic flexure, left colon, or rectosigmoid junction. Right-sided ischemic colitis and necrosis have been reported as a complication of hemorrhagic shock after blunt or penetrating trauma (28). Right-sided ischemic colitis also can be associated with small-bowel ischemia when thrombosis of the superior mesenteric artery or vein is present (25) (Figure 18-7). In addition, ischemic colitis has been described proximal to an obstructing colon cancer, which can be misinterpreted as tumor extension if it is adjacent to the primary tumor (29). In patients with colon cancer, ischemic segments have been reported at sites distant from the obstructing mass (29).

Colonic thickening usually is circumferential, but may appear homogeneous or heterogeneous, depending on the extent of submucosal edema, inflammation, or hemorrhage. A halo also may be present. As with mesenteric ischemia, if transmural ischemia or infarction has occurred, pneumatosis may be present (Figure 18-7) (30). Pneumatosis with or without air in the mesenteric vessels or portal vein is an ominous finding in patients with colonic ischemia, suggesting necrosis (26,31) (Figures 18–8 and 18–9). In addition to wall thickening, free fluid or mesenteric stranding also may be present, but these are not specific signs of ischemia.

Unlike mesenteric ischemia, which usually is more severe and more likely to be related to arterial thrombosis, colonic ischemia typically resolves with conservative management, such as bowel rest, IV fluids, and occasionally antibiotics. The injury resolves spontaneously in over 50% of cases in 1 week to 2 weeks (32). The bowel may return to normal or, if transmural ischemia was present, a focal or segment stricture may result. If the episode is severe or related to occlusive disease, surgical intervention may be necessary.

Inflammatory Bowel Disease

Both Crohn's disease and ulcerative colitis may involve the colon. Although the findings can overlap, there often are distinguishing features present. Computed tomography can aid in differentiating Crohn's disease and ulcerative colitis when barium studies are equivocal. Crohn's disease most

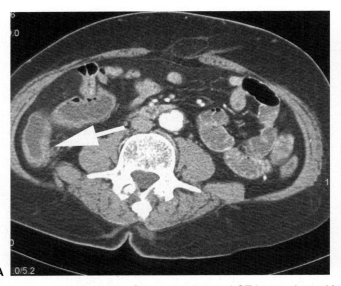
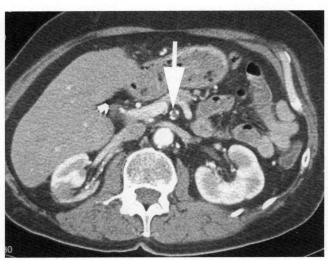

A / **B**

FIG. 18–6. Contrast-enhanced CT in a patient with severe abdominal pain and elevated lactic acid. **A:** Minimal thickening of the right colon is noted (*arrow*). **B:** Calcified atherosclerotic plaque is noted in the superior mesenteric artery; in addition, thrombosis is noted (*arrow*). This is an example of ischemic colitis caused by an embolism to the superior mesenteric artery.

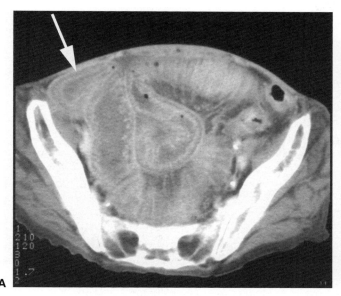

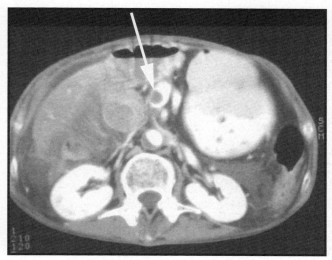

FIG. 18–7. A: Contrast-enhanced CT in a patient with extensive ischemia demonstrates thickening and submucosal edema of both the small bowel and right colon (*arrow*). Minimal ascites also is noted. **B:** Nonocclusive thrombus is noted in the superior mesenteric vein (*arrow*).

often will involve the right colon and distal ileum (Figure 18-10), although the disease may affect any portion of the gastrointestinal tract from the mouth to the anus. Ulcerative colitis typically appears predominantly left sided or is diffuse. Isolated involvement of the right colon is rare (Figures 18–11 and 18–12). The combination of both colonic and small-bowel involvement highly favors the diagnosis of Crohn's disease. Ulcerative colitis never involves the small bowel, with the exception of limited involvement of the terminal ileum due to backwash ileitis. In these cases, the terminal ileum may be thickened and usually is dilated in contrast to patients with Crohn's disease, where the terminal ileum will be thickened and narrowed.

Both conditions will produce colon wall thickening. However, the mean wall thickness in Crohn's colitis (11 mm–13 mm) usually is greater than in ulcerative colitis (7.8 mm)(9) (Figure 18-13). In advanced cases of Crohn's dis-

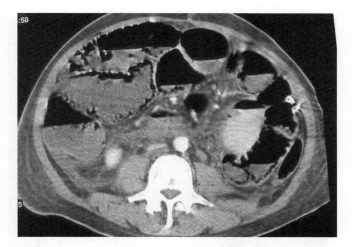

FIG. 18–9. Contrast-enhanced CT in a patient with severe ischemia demonstrates pneumatosis involving multiple loops of both small bowel and colon. This is compatible with infarction. Minimal ascites and subcutaneous edema also are noted.

FIG. 18–8. Coronal multiplanar reconstruction in a patient with ischemia demonstrates pneumatosis involving the right colon (*arrows*).

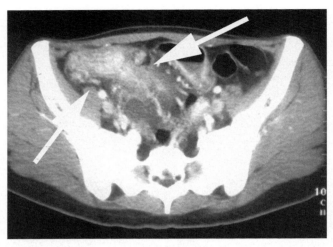

FIG. 18–10. Contrast-enhanced CT in a patient with Crohn's disease demonstrates extensive inflammation involving the terminal ileum and right colon (*arrows*). There is mucosal enhancement, as well as submucosal edema, noted.

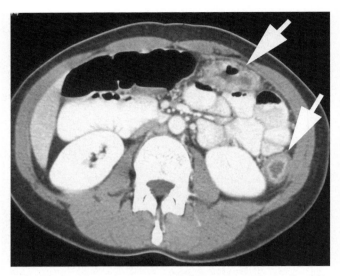

FIG. 18–12. Contrast-enhanced CT in a patient with Crohn's disease demonstrates circumferential thickening of the descending colon (*arrows*). The right colon was not involved.

ease, the wall often measures more than 1 cm in thickness (33). Wall thickening in ulcerative colitis may be diffuse and symmetric, whereas wall thickening in Crohn's most often is eccentric (33). The asymmetry of the disease involvement in Crohn's disease can result in the formation of pseudodiverticula, which appears as outpouchings of the colon formed opposite eccentric regions of scarring and fibrosis. This discontinuous appearance ("skip areas") is an important feature distinguishing Crohn's disease from ulcerative colitis, which usually appears confluent, continuous, and circumferential. In both ulcerative colitis and Crohn's disease, the inflamed wall may appear either homogeneous or heterogeneous. Submucosal inflammation produces a

low-density mural layer in both conditions. Similarly, fat can be deposited in the colonic submucosa, producing a "halo" (34). This is more common in ulcerative colitis, especially when the rectum is involved (Figure 18-14).

Proliferation of mesenteric fat is seen almost exclusively in Crohn's disease, while the proliferation of perirectal fat is nonspecific and can be present in Crohn's disease, ulcerative colitis, pseudomembranous colitis, and/or radiation colitis (35).

The presence of mesenteric lymphadenopathy suggests Crohn's disease rather than ulcerative colitis, although it is not specific for inflammatory bowel disease. In patients with

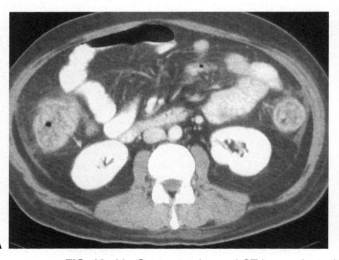

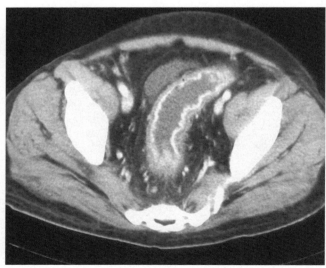

A   B

FIG. 18–11. Contrast-enhanced CT in a patient with Crohn's disease. **A:** Diffuse colonic thickening is noted. There is minimal pericolonic stranding in this patient with Crohn's disease. **B:** Computed-tomography scan through the sigmoid colon also demonstrates thickening, as well as mucosal enhancement.

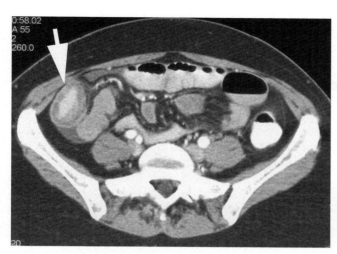

FIG. 18–13. Contrast-enhanced CT in a patient with Crohn's disease demonstrates circumferential thickening of the right colon only (*arrow*). There is minimal free fluid near the right colon.

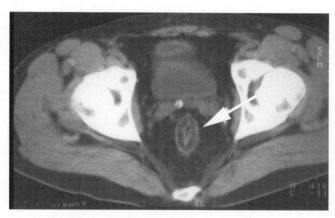

FIG. 18–14. Contrast-enhanced CT in a patient with ulcerative colitis demonstrates submucosal fat deposition in the rectum (*arrow*). There also is an increased amount of perirectal fat.

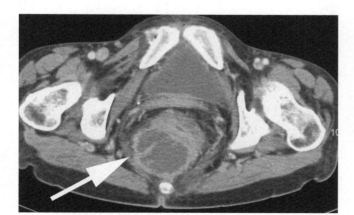

FIG. 18–15. Contrast-enhanced CT in a patient with Crohn's disease demonstrates a perirectal abscess (*arrow*).

Crohn's disease, the mesenteric nodes should measure 1 cm or less. Larger nodes should raise the possibility of bowel malignancy, since patients with Crohn's disease are at increased risk for the development of adenocarcinoma of both the colon and small bowel (36).

Crohn's patients can experience significant complications such as abscess, obstruction, and/or fistulae (37) (Figures 18–15, 18–16, and 18–17). These are much more common in Crohn's disease than in ulcerative colitis. In a study

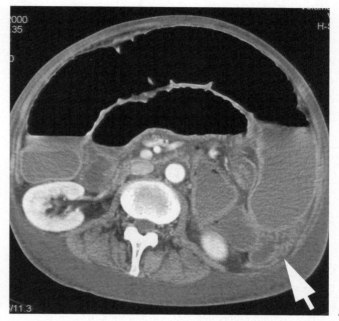

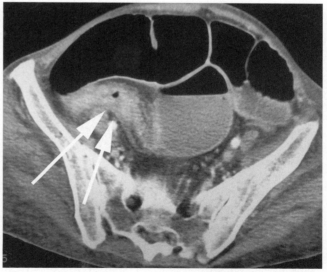

FIG. 18–16. Contrast-enhanced CT in a patient with Crohn's disease demonstrates significant small-bowel dilation. **A:** The colon (*arrow*) is not distended. **B:** Computed-tomography scan at a slightly inferior level than **(A)** demonstrates significant circumferential thickening of the terminal ileum (*arrows*). This is an example of Crohn's disease causing a small-bowel obstruction.

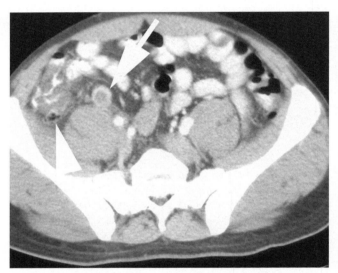

FIG. 18–17. Contrast-enhanced CT in a patient with Crohn's disease and fever demonstrates a fistula from the small bowel to the psoas muscle (*arrow*). There also is fluid within the fistula compatible with abscess.

of 80 patients with symptomatic Crohn's disease, 28% of patients had CT scans that revealed previously unexpected findings and subsequently led to a change in medical or surgical management (10). These findings included fistulae, abscess, avascular necrosis of the femoral head, osteomyelitis, and venous thrombosis.

Although patients with ulcerative colitis tend to have fewer complications than patients Crohn's disease, they can present with severe colonic inflammation and toxic megacolon, which is life threatening. They also are at significant risk for the development of colon cancer and may undergo prophylactic colectomy.

APPENDICITIS

Appendicitis is a common cause of acute abdominal pain and typically results in emergency surgery (38,39). Patients usually present with acute right-lower-quadrant pain, nausea, vomiting, and elevated white blood cell count.

Computed tomography has been shown to have a high sensitivity and specificity for the diagnosis of acute appendicitis in adults and has been shown to be slightly more accurate than ultrasonography (40). The widespread use of CT for appendicitis has resulted in a drop in the negative appendectomy rate, from 20% to 7% (41). Even early studies with conventional CT demonstrated a high accuracy (42,43). However, there continues to be controversy about the optimal CT technique and protocol. Most studies agree that the use of thin collimation (5 mm or less) is helpful for reliable identification of the appendix (44). Some researchers advocate performing a focused examination of the right lower quadrant (45–47), whereas others prefer to scan the entire

abdomen and pelvis (48), which allows for potential diagnosis of alternative pathology if appendicitis is not present. In addition, there is controversy about whether IV contrast is essential. Some researchers advocate noncontrast CT for appendicitis, whereas others feel that IV contrast can be helpful to diagnose appendicitis, as well as extraappendiceal pathology (49,50). Similarly, while most radiologists agree that enteric contrast is essential, some advocate the use of rectal contrast with or without oral contrast (45,49,51). Overall, considering the various protocols, the accuracy of CT for the diagnosis of appendicitis ranges between 94% and 98% (45,47–50,52). Much of the success depends on the experience of the radiologist interpreting the study.

A dilated (more than 6 mm) fluid-filled appendix that

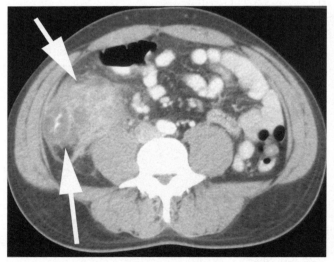

FIG. 18–18. A: Contrast-enhanced CT in a patient with right lower-quadrant pain demonstrates dilation of the appendix with wall thickening (*arrow*). The right colon (*arrowhead*) also is thickened. **B:** Computed-tomography scan at a slightly more inferior level than (**A**) demonstrates phlegmon and abscess due to perforation of the appendix.

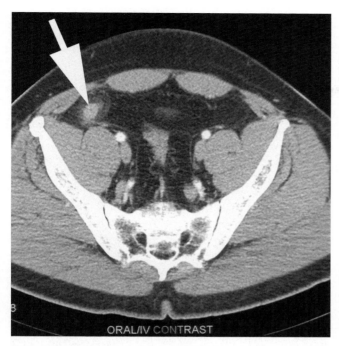

FIG. 18–19. Contrast-enhanced CT in a patient with right lower-quadrant pain demonstrates circumferential thickening of the appendix (*arrow*) with periappendiceal stranding. The CT appearance is compatible with acute appendicitis.

does not fill with enteric contrast is the most specific helical-CT finding in patients with acute appendicitis (Figure 18-18). Associated fat stranding is a sensitive finding, but only 80% specific (53) (Figure 18-19). The combination of an enlarged appendix and periappendiceal stranding occurs in 93% of cases (53). Other findings include focal cecal-apical thickening, adenopathy, paracolic gutter fluid, and thickening of the colon or small bowel. The presence of an appendicolith is not common, but is specific for the diagnosis (54) (Figure 18-20). In addition to being able to diagnose acute

appendicitis, CT also is valuable for detection of complications such as periappendiceal abscess, phlegmon, perforation, or small-bowel obstruction (Figure 18-18).

Although CT has a high sensitivity and specificity for the diagnosis of acute appendicitis, other disorders may mimic both the clinical presentation and CT findings (54). For example, a dilated appendix can be seen in other diseases of the appendix, including mucocele and carcinoid or mucin-secreting tumors of the appendix. Other inflammatory conditions such as Crohn's disease, ovarian pathology, Meckel's diverticulitis, and epiploic appendagitis can cause right lower-quadrant pain and inflammation.

DIVERTICULITIS

Colonic diverticular disease is very common. Diverticulosis is present in almost 80% of the population by age 85 (55), and it is estimated that 10% to 35% of patients with diverticulosis will develop diverticulitis (56). The diagnosis of diverticulitis can be made with contrast enema, CT, or colonoscopy. Computed tomography largely has replaced the water-soluble contrast enema at most centers for the diagnosis of diverticulitis. In a recent series by Ambrosetti et al. of 420 patients with diverticulitis, all patients underwent both contrast enema and CT (57). The performance of CT was significantly better than contrast enema. The sensitivity of CT and contrast enema was 98% versus 92%, respectively (57). In addition, CT was able to detect an abscess in 69 patients, whereas enema identified abscess only in 29 patients (57). In another large series by Kircher et al. of 312 patients, CT was found to have a 99% accuracy for the diagnosis of diverticulitis (58). Computed tomography also has the advantage of establishing alternative diagnoses if diverticulitis is not present in patients with acute left-lower-quadrant pain. In one study, CT suggested an alternative diagnosis in 78% of cases in whom diverticulitis was not present (59).

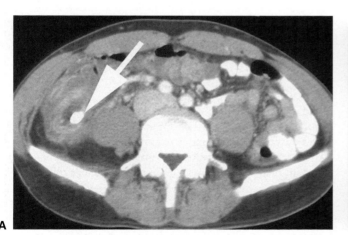
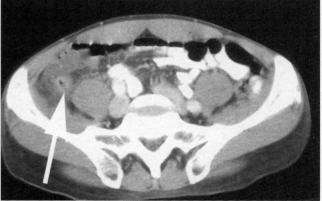

FIG. 18–20. A: Contrast-enhanced CT in a patient with severe right-lower-quadrant pain demonstrates an appendicolith (*arrow*). There also is circumferential thickening of the right colon. **B:** Computed-tomography scan at a slightly inferior level than **(A)** demonstrates thickening and dilation of the appendix (*arrow*) along with periappendiceal inflammation.

A tailored CT examination in patients with suspected diverticulitis should include thin collimation (5 mm or less) through the lower abdomen and pelvis. Most centers scan the entire abdomen and pelvis at 5 mm, since diverticulitis can affect any segment of the colon and because other conditions such as small-bowel obstruction, acute cholecystitis, ileitis, ureteral-stone disease, or ovarian pathology may mimic the clinical presentation (41). The colon can be opacified with either oral or rectal contrast, which improves visualization of the colon and bowel wall. Although spiral CT with rectal contrast and without IV contrast has been shown to be highly accurate for diagnosis (59), the administration of IV contrast is helpful in the detection and characterization of colonic inflammation, improves visualization of the bowel wall, and helps define pericolonic abscess (60). In patients with clinically suspected diverticulitis, the preference is to perform CT of the entire abdomen and pelvis with oral and IV contrast. In urgent or equivocal cases, rectal contrast is administered. Since colonic opacification and distention is achieved best with rectal contrast (59), this is a common practice at many institutions.

Computed tomography findings in patients with acute diverticulitis usually consist of bowel wall thickening, stranding in the pericolonic fat, and the presence of diverticula (Figure 18-21). In a series of 114 patients with diverticulitis who underwent CT scanning, bowel wall thickening was found in 108 patients (95%) and pericolonic fat stranding in 104 patients (91%). Discrete diverticula could be identified in 57 patients (50%) (58). Other findings include fascial thickening, free fluid, and free air. Complications of diverticulitis that can be detected on CT include abscess (Figure 18-22), phlegmon, and rarely frank perforation with pneumoperitoneum. If necessary, CT also can be used in percutaneous drainage of pericolonic abscesses.

Computed tomography findings in patients with diverticulitis can mimic CT findings in patients with colon cancer,

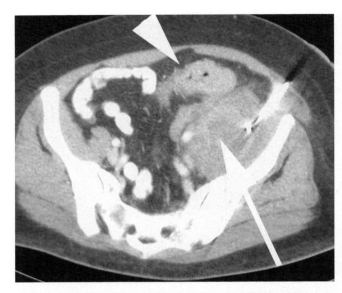
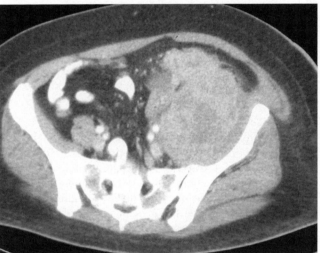

FIG. 18–22. A: Contrast-enhanced CT in a patient with acute diverticulitis demonstrates thickening of the sigmoid colon (*arrowhead*). There also is inflammation and abscess involving the psoas muscle (*arrow*) on the left. A percutaneous drain was placed. **B:** Computed-tomography scan at a slightly more inferior level than **(A)** demonstrates the abscess involving the left iliacus muscle.

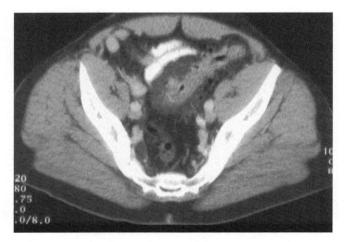

FIG. 18–21. Contrast-enhanced CT in a patient with acute diverticulitis demonstrates diverticula, stranding, and thickening of the sigmoid colon.

and it can be difficult to distinguish between the two conditions (Figure 18-23). The presence of fluid in the mesentery and vascular engorgement tends to favor the diagnosis of diverticulitis (61), whereas the presence of pericolonic adenopathy tends to favor the diagnosis of cancer (62).

COLORECTAL CANCER

Colorectal cancer is a common malignancy, resulting in significant morbidity and mortality. Approximately 130,000 new cases were diagnosed in the United States in 2000, and approximately 56,000 deaths were attributed to the disease

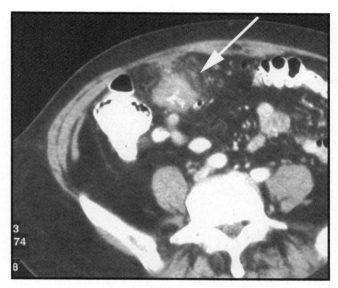

FIG. 18–23. Contrast-enhanced CT scan in a patient with acute abdominal pain demonstrates a focal area of thickening involving the transverse colon (*arrow*). Minimal pericolonic stranding is noted. The CT appearance was suspicious for carcinoma; however, at endoscopy, focal diverticulitis was diagnosed.

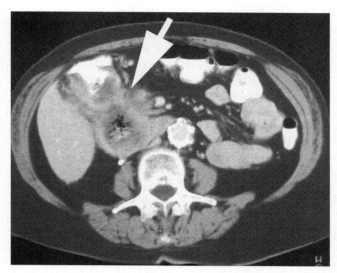

FIG. 18–24. Contrast-enhanced CT scan in a patient with colon cancer demonstrates a large mass involving the right colon (*arrow*). Central necrosis is noted within the mass. This happens when the mass outgrows its blood supply.

during the same year. Although initial diagnosis often is made with fiberoptic colonoscopy, CT is beginning to play a more active role in primary detection of colon cancer, as well as in detection of precancerous polyps. This is discussed in detail in Chapter 19. In addition to its role in colon-cancer screening, CT continues to play a significant role in the staging of adenocarcinoma of the colon and rectum once the diagnosis has been established. Preoperative CT scanning typically is performed if there is suspicion for: i) hematogeneous or distal nodal (e.g., paraaortic) metastases, ii) invasion into adjacent organs or abscess formation, iii) unexplained or atypical symptomatology, and iv) unusual histology (e.g., lymphoma). The major goal of CT is to determine if there is direct invasion of adjacent organs, enlargement of local nodes, or evidence of distant metastases. Computed tomogrtaphy also is performed commonly for follow up of patients to determine response to treatment and to evaluate for recurrent disease.

Primary Tumor

The sensitivity of CT for the detection of primary colorectal cancer is reported to range between 75% and 85% (63). However, most of these studies were performed on dynamic or early spiral scanners, and CT technology has improved significantly over the past few years. Computed tomography previously had been limited in its detection of small tumors (<2 cm). Recent advancements in spiral CT and MDCT, as well as the use of 3D CT (virtual colonoscopy) with interactive multiplanar views, have improved the

sensitivity of CT for the detection of both colon cancer and precancerous polyps. Computed tomography in patients with colorectal cancer typically demonstrates a discrete soft-tissue density mass with irregular borders. Larger masses may have a low-density necrotic center or occasionally may contain gas, resembling an abscess (Figure 18-24). However, a significant percentage of colorectal cancers will not present as a discrete mass, but as a focal or circumferential area of wall thickening. In particular, rectal cancers may appear as symmetric wall thickening that narrows the lumen (Figure 18-25). Thus, sometimes it is difficult to distinguish prospectively carcinoma from other processes that result in bowel-

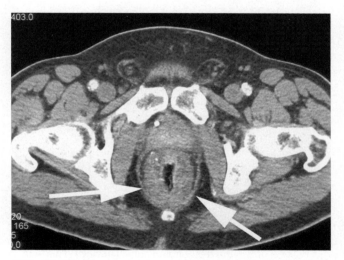

FIG. 18–25. Contrast-enhanced CT scan in a patient with rectal carcinoma demonstrates circumferential thickening of the rectum (*arrows*).

wall thickening, such as diverticulitis. In a study by Padidar et al. of 69 patients with sigmoid diverticulitis and 29 patients with sigmoid colon cancer, the presence of fluid in the root of the sigmoid mesentery and engorgement of adjacent sigmoid mesenteric vasculature favored the diagnosis of diverticulitis, whereas the presence of local adenopathy favored diverticulitis (61,62).

Complications of primary colonic malignancies, such as obstruction, perforation, abscess, and fistula can be visualized readily on CT (Figure 18-26). Occasionally CT is the first indication of the diagnosis of colon cancer when a patient presents emergently with acute abdominal pain resulting from such complications.

Owing to its ability to visualize the colon and surrounding structures, CT also can detect pericolonic extension of disease (Figure 18-27). Computed tomography is more accurate than magnetic resonance (MR) in staging the local extent of tumor, particularly for rectal cancers and detection of penetration of the lamina propria (64). Local extension of tumor on CT can appear as extracolonic tumor mass or simply thickening and infiltration of pericolonic fat. Extracolonic spread of tumor also is suggested by loss of fat planes between the colon and adjacent organs (Figure 18-26), although this is not specific, as fat planes can be lost in patients with cachexia, or after radiation or chemotherapy. In a study by Freeney et al., the sensitivity and specificity of CT for the detection of local tumor extension was 61% and 81%, respectively (63). A study by Acunas et al. demonstrated a sensitivity and specificity of 60% and 67%, respectively (65). In general, the lower sensitivity results reflect the ina-

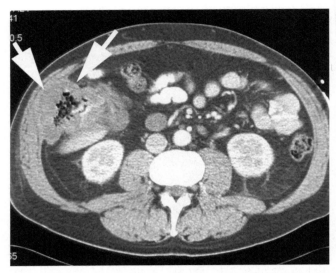

FIG. 18–27. Contrast-enhanced CT scan in a patient with colon cancer demonstrates a large right-sided colonic mass invading the abdominal-wall muscles (*arrows*).

bility of CT to detect microscopic extramural tumor extension.

Nodal Disease

Computed tomography can detect lymphadenopathy within the abdomen with a high sensitivity, but equal accuracy compared with MR (64). The presence of lymph nodes

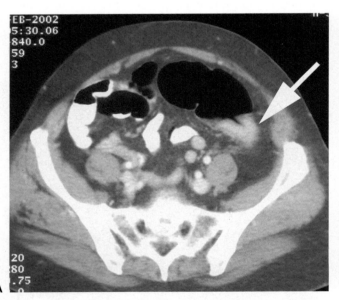
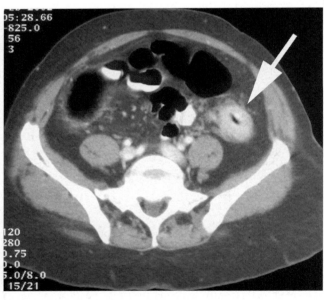

FIG. 18–26. A: Contrast-enhanced CT scan demonstrates dilation of the colon. There is a focal narrowing in the descending colon (*arrows*). This was a colon cancer causing partial obstruction. **B:** Computed-tomography scan at a slightly more inferior level than **(A)** demonstrates circumferential thickening of the descending colon in the region of the carcinoma. Minimal pericolonic stranding is suspicious for tumor extension.

measuring more than 1 cm to 1.5 cm is considered pathologic. However, enlarged nodes do not necessarily contain tumor and simply may be reactive. Conversely, microscopic tumor may involve normal-sized nodes. Therefore, although CT has a high specificity (96%) for the detection of metastatic lymph nodes, the sensitivity is only 26% (63). In most cases, however, the inability of CT to detect lymph nodes involved with tumor does not present a clinical problem, as regional lymph-node dissection is performed routinely at surgery. FDG–positron-emission tomography (FDG–PET) may be useful in this clinical setting to detect the presence of metastatic nodes.

The nodal pathways for the spread of colon cancer have been well described and tend to follow the blood supply (66–70). Adenocarcinoma of the right colon typically involves the lymphatics located near the cecum and ascending colon first, then involves ileocolic nodes and nodes in the root of the mesentery. Tumors located in the proximal transverse-colon spread along the mesocolon and drain into the lymphatics located along the right- or middle-colic vessels to reach the root of the mesocolon, anterior to the head of the pancreas. Tumors located in the distal transverse colon or splenic flexure spread via nodes near the left middle-colic vasculature to the region of the inferior mesenteric vein, below the body and tail of the pancreas. Tumors involving the descending and sigmoid colon spread to the lymphatics located along the left-ascending colic artery and sigmoidal artery, and subsequently drain to nodes near the root of the inferior mesenteric artery.

Distant Metastases

The liver is the most common site for metastatic disease in patients with colorectal cancer. Computed tomography is considered the primary imaging modality for the detection of liver metastasis. The accuracy of dynamically enhanced CT and unenhanced magnetic resonance imaging (MRI) in the detection of metastatic liver disease appears to be equivalent at 85%. In a series of 478 patients with colorectal cancer, the specificity of both CT (97%) and MRI (94%) for the detection of liver metastases was similar to prior published series (64). The sensitivities of the two techniques in this study were 62% and 70%, respectively (64). Although MRI can detect smaller lesions, it often is impossible to characterize them definitively as benign or malignant. Serial scanning often is required when small lesions are detected with either modality.

Most liver metastases due to colorectal cancer will appear hypodense on contrast-enhanced CT of the liver (Figure 18-28). For optimal detection, the liver should be opacified well and imaging should be performed during the portal-venous phase of enhancement (50 seconds to 60 seconds after IV injection).

In addition to liver metastases, colorectal cancer also can result in metastases to bones, lung, adrenal gland, or peritoneum (Figure 18-28). Mucinous colorectal tumors also can spread to the surface of intraabdominal organs and produce pseudomyxoma peritonei.

Recurrent Disease

In addition to the routine use of CT in staging colorectal cancer, CT is used frequently for follow up of patients during and after treatment. Computed tomography is an effective tool to monitor treatment response, as well as to detect recurrent disease. Recurrent disease can occur at the surgical site or in distant organs such as the liver, lungs, or lymph nodes.

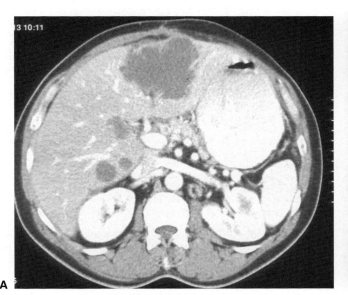
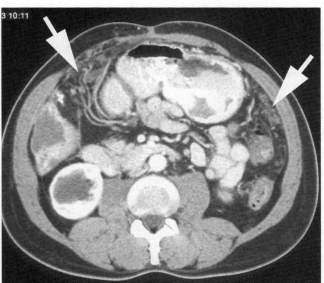

A   B

FIG. 18–28. A: Contrast-enhanced CT scan in a patient with colon cancer demonstrates multiple liver metastases. **B:** Axial CT scan at a slightly more inferior than **(A)** demonstrates nodularity of the omentum compatible with carcinomatosis (*arrows*).

CONCLUSIONS

Improvements in CT and computer technology have led to increased applications for CT imaging of the gastrointestinal tract, including the colon. Computed tomography now is used commonly for the evaluation of patients with inflammatory and neoplastic diseases of the colon, and in many instances can obviate the need for other radiological studies, such as the barium enema. Further developments in CT technology with 16-slice scanners and advanced postprocessing and display techniques likely will increase the role of CT for the evaluation of colonic pathology.

REFERENCES

1. Amin Z, Boulos PB, Lees WR. Technical report: spiral CT pneumocolon for suspected colonic neoplasms. *Clin Radiol* 1996;51:56–61.
2. Solomon A, Michowitz M, Papo J, et al. Computed tomographic air enema technique to demonstrate colonic neoplasms. *Gastrointest Radiol* 1986;11:194–196.
3. Gossios KJ, Tsianos EV, Kontogiannis DS, et al. Water as contrast medium for computed tomography study of colonic wall lesions. *Gastrointest Radiol* 1992;17:125–128.
4. Angelelli G, Macarini L, Lupo L, et al. Rectal carcinoma: CT staging with water as contrast medium. *Radiology* 1990;177:511–514.
5. Fisher JK. Abnormal colonic wall thickening on computed tomography. *J Comput Assist Tomogr* 1983;7:90–97.
6. Kelly CP, Pothoulakis C, LaMont JT. *Clostridium difficile* colitis. *N Engl J Med* 1994;330:257–262.
7. Boland GW, Lee MJ, Cats AM, et al. Antiobiotic-induced diarrhea: specificity of abdominal CT for the diagnosis of *Clostridium difficile* disease. *Radiology* 1994;191:103–106.
8. Fishman EK, Kavuru M, Jones B, et al. Pseudomembranous colitis: CT evaluation of 26 cases. *Radiology* 1991;180:57–60.
9. Philpotts LE, Heiken JP, Westcott MA, et al. Colitis: use of CT findings in differential diagnosis. *Radiology* 1994;190:445–449.
10. Fishman EK, Wolf EJ, Jones B, et al. CT evaluation of Crohn's disease, effect on patient management. *AJR Am J Roentgenol* 1987;148:537–540.
11. Kawamoto S, Horton KM, Fishman EK. Pseudomembranous colitis: can CT predict which patients will need surgical intervention? *J Comput Assist Tomogr* 1999;23:79–85.
12. Kirkpatrick IDC, Greenberg HM. Evaluating the CT diagnosis of *Clostrium difficile* colitis. *AJR Am J Roentgenol* 2001;176:635–639.
13. Ros PR, Buetow PC, Pantograg-Brown L, et al. Pseudomembranous colitis. *Radiology* 1996;198:1–9.
14. Jafri SF, Marshall LB. Ascites associated with antibiotic associated pseudomembranous colitis. *South Med J* 1996;89:1014–1017.
15. Jobe BA, Grasley A, Deveney KE, et al. *Clostridium difficile* colitis: an increasing hospital-acquired illness. *Am J Surg* 1995;169:480–483.
16. Morris JB, Zollinger RM Jr, Stellato TA. Role of surgery in antibiotic-induced pseudomembranous enterocolitis. *Am J Surg* 1990;160:535–539.
17. Bradley SJ, Weaver DW, Maxwell NP, et al. Surgical management of pseudomembranous colitis. *Am Surg* 1988;127:329–332.
18. Reinus JF, Brand L, Boley SJ. Ischemic disease of the bowel. *Gastroenterol Clin North Am* 1990;19:319–343.
19. Balthazar EJ, Yen BC, Gordon RB. Ischemic colitis: CT evaluation of 54 cases. *Radiology* 1999;211:381–388.
20. Bower TC. Ischemic colitis. *Surg Clin North Am* 1993;73:1037–1053.
21. Chou CK. CT manifestations of bowel ischemia. *AJR Am J Roentgenol* 2002;178:87–91.
22. McKinsey JF, Gewertz BL. Acute mesenteric ischemia. *Surg Clin North Am* 1997;77:307–318.
23. Smerud MJ, Johnson CD, Stephens DH. Diagnosis of bowel infarction: a comparison of plain films and CT scans in 23 cases. *AJR Am J Roentgenol* 1990;154:99–103.
24. Clark RA. Computed tomography of bowel infarction. *J Comput Assist Tomogr* 1987;11:757–762.
25. Federle MP, Chun G, RBJ, et al. Computed tomographic findings in bowel infarction. *AJR Am J Roentgenol* 1984;142:91–95.
26. Jones B, Fishman EK, Siegelman SS. Ischemic colitis demonstrated by computed tomography. *J Comput Assist Tomogr* 1982;6:1120–1123.
27. Brandt LJ, Boley SJ. Ischemic and vascular lesions of the bowel. In: Sleisenger MHFJ, ed. *Gastrointestinal disease: pathophysiology, diagnosis, management*. Philadelphia: WB Saunders, 1993:1940–1945.
28. Ludwig KA, Quebbeman EJ, Bergstein JM, et al. Shock-associated right colon ischemia and necrosis. *J Trauma* 1995;39:1171–1174.
29. Ko GY, Ha HK, Lee HJ, et al. Usefulness of CT in patients with ischemic colitis proximal to colonic cancer. *AJR Am J Roentgenol* 1997;168:951–956.
30. Alpern MB, Glazer GM, Francis IR. Ischemic or infarcted bowel: CT findings. *Radiology* 1988;166:149–152.
31. Connor K, Jones B, Fishman EK. Pneumatosis intestinalis: role of computed tomography in diagnosis and management. *J Comput Assist Tomogr* 1984;8:269–275.
32. Bakal CW, Sprayregen S, Wolf EL. Radiology in intestinal ischemia. *Surg Clin North Am* 1992;72:125–141.
33. Gore RM, Marn CS, Kirby DF, et al. CT findings in ulcerative, granulomatous, and indeterminate colitis. *AJR Am J Roentgenol* 1984;143:279–284.
34. Jones B, Fishman EK, Hamilton SR, et al. Submucosal accumulation of fat in inflammatory bowel disease: CT/pathologic correlation. *J Comput Assist Tomogr* 1986;10:759–763.
35. Krestin GP, Beyer D, Steinbrich W. Computed tomography in the differential diagnosis of the enlarged retrorectal space. *Gastrointest Radiol* 1986;11:364–369.
36. Kerber GW, Frank PH. Carcinoma of the small intestine and colon as a complication of Crohn disease: radiologic manifestations. *Radiology* 1984;150:639–645.
37. Kerber GW, Greenberg M, Rubin JM. Computed tomography evaluation of local and extraintestinal complications of Crohn's disease. *Gastrointest Radiol* 1984;9:143–148.
38. Addiss DG, Shaffer N, Fowler BS, et al. The epidemiology of appendicitis and appendectomy in the United States. *Am J Epidemiol* 1990;132:910–925.
39. Garcia-Pena BM, Mandl KD, Kraus SJ, et al. Ultrasonography and limited computed tomography in the diagnosis and management of appendicitis in children. *JAMA* 1999;282:1041–1046.
40. Wise SW, Labruski MR, Kasales CJ, et al. Comparative assessment of CT and sonographic techniques for appendiceal imaging. *AJR Am J Roentgenol* 2001;176:933–941.
41. Rao PM. CT of diverticulitis and alternative conditions. *Semin Ultrasound CT MR* 1999;20:86–93.
42. Balthazar EJ, Megibow AJ, Siegel SE, et al. Appendicitis: prospective evaluation with high resolution CT. *Radiology* 1991;180:21–24.
43. Malone AJ, Wolf CR, Malmed AS. Diagnosis of acute appendicitis: value of unenhanced CT. *AJR Am J Roentgenol* 1993;160:763–766.
44. Weltman DI, Yu J, Krumenacker J Jr, Huang SPM. Diagnosis of acute appendicitis: comparison of 5 and 10 mm CT sections in the same patient. *Radiology* 2000;216:172–177.
45. Mullins ME, Kircher MF, Ryan DP, et al. Evaluation for suspected appendicitis in children using limited helical CT and colonic contrast material. *AJR Am J Roentgenol* 2001;176:37–41.
46. Rhea JT, Rao PM, Noveliine RA, et al. A focused appendiceal CT technique to reduce the cost of caring for patients with clinically suspected appendicitis. *AJR Am J Roentgenol* 1997;169:113–118.
47. Rao PM, Rhea JT, Novelline RA. Helical CT technique for the diagnosis of appendicitis: prospective evaluation of a focused appendix CT examination. *Radiology* 1997;202:139–144.
48. Raman SS, Lu DS, Kadell BM, et al. Accuracy of nonfocused helical CT for the diagnosis of acute appendicitis. *AJR Am J Roentgenol* 2002;178:1319–1325.
49. Rao PM, Rhea JT, Novelline RA, et al. Helical CT combined with contrast material administered only through the colon for imaging of suspected appendicitis. *AJR Am J Roentgenol* 1997;169:1275–1280.
50. Jacobs JE, Birnbaum BA, Macari M, et al. Acute appendicitis: comparison of helical CT diagnosis focused appendiceal technique with oral contrast material versus nonfocused technique with oral and intravenous contrast material. *Radiology* 2001;220:683–690.
51. Funaki B, Grosskreutz SW, Funaki CN. Using unenhanced helical CT with enteric contrast material for suspected appendicitis in patients

treated at a community hospital. *AJR Am J Roentgenol* 1998; 171:997–1001.

52. Lane MJ, Katz DS, Ross BA, et al. Unenhanced helical CT for suspected acute appendicitis. *AJR Am J Roentgenol* 1997;168:405–409.

53. Rao PM, Rhea JT, Novelline RA. Sensitivity and specificity of the individual CT signs of appendicitis: experience with 200 helical appendiceal CT examinations. *J Comput Assist Tomogr* 1997; 21:686–692.

54. Curtin KR, Fitzgerald SW, Nemcek AA, et al. CT diagnosis of acute appendicitis: imaging findings. *AJR Am J Roentgenol* 1995; 164:905–909.

55. Almy TP, Howell DA. Diverticular disease of the colon. *N Engl J Med* 1980;320:324–331.

56. Ferzoco LB, Raptopoulos VWS. Acute diverticulitis. *N Engl J Med* 1998;338:1521–1526.

57. Ambrosetti P, Jenny A, Becker C, et al. Acute left colonic diverticulitis—compared performance of computed tomography and water-soluble contrast enema: prospective evaluation of 420 patients. *Dis Colon Rectum* 2000;43:1363–1367.

58. Kircher MF, Rhea JT, Kihiczak D, et al. Frequency, sensitivity and specificity of individual signs of diverticulitis on thin-section helical CT with colonic contrast material in 312 cases. *AJR Am J Roentgenol* 2002;178:1313–1318.

59. Rao PM, Rhea JT, Novelline RA, et al. Helical CT with only colonic material for diagnosing diverticulitis: prospective evaluation of 150 patients. *AJR Am J Roentgenol* 1998;170:1445–1449.

60. Urban BA, Fishman EK. Tailored helical CT evaluation of acute abdomen. *Radiographics* 2000;20:725–749.

61. Padidar AM, Jeffrey RB Jr, Mindelzun RE, et al. Differentiating sig-moid diverticulitis from carcinoma on CT scans: mesenteric inflammation suggests diverticulitis. *AJR Am J Roentgenol* 1994;163:81–83.

62. Chintapali KN, Chopra S, Ghiatas AA, et al. Diverticulitis versus colon cancer: differentiation with helical CT findings. *Radiology* 1999; 210:429–435.

63. Freeny PC, Marks WM, Ryan JA, Bolen JW. Colorectal carcinoma evaluation with CT: preoperative staging and detection of postoperative recurrence. *Radiology* 1986;158:347–353.

64. Zerhouni EA, Rutter C, Hamilton SR, et al. CT and MR imaging in the staging of colorectal carcinoma: report of Radiology Diagnostic Oncology Group II. *Radiology* 1996;200:443–451.

65. Acunas B, Rozanes I, Acunas G, et al. Preoperative CT staging of colon carcinoma (excluding the recto-sigmoid region). *Eur J Radiol* 1990;11:150–153.

66. Iyer RB, Silverman PM, DuBrow RA, et al. Imaging in the diagnosis, staging and follow-up of colorectal cancer. *AJR Am J Roentgenol* 2002; 179:3–13.

67. Gore RM. Colorectal cancer: clinical and pathologic features. *Radiol Clin North Am* 1997;35:404–429.

68. Charnsangavej C. Pathways of lymph node metastases in cancer of the gastrointestinal and hepatobiliary tracts. In: Meyers MA, ed. *Dynamic radiology of the abdomen*. New York, NY; Springer–Verlag, 2000; 287–308.

69. McDanial KP, Charnsangavej C, DuBrow RA, et al. Pathways of nodal metastasis in carcinomas of the cecum, ascending colon, and transverse colon: CT demonstration. *AJR Am J Roentgenol* 1993;161:61–64.

70. Balfe D, Semin M. Colorectal cancer. In: Husband JES, Reznek RH, eds. *Imaging in oncology*. Oxford, UK; Isis Medical Media, 1998; 129–150.

CHAPTER 19

Multidetector CT of the Large Intestine: Virtual Colonoscopy

John Paul Schreiber II, R. Brooke Jeffrey, Jr., Marta Davila, Christopher F. Beaulieu

INTRODUCTION

Colorectal cancer is the second leading cause of cancer-related death in the United States, and the third most common cancer overall (1). It is believed widely that almost all cases of colorectal cancer begin with the development of benign colonic polyps. Early detection and removal of adenomatous polyps has proven to reduce mortality from colorectal cancer (2). The American Cancer Society now recommends annual fecal occult blood testing/physical examination and screening sigmoidoscopy every 5 years for all adults over the age of 50 (3). Further recommendations include either a double-contrast barium enema or fiberoptic colonoscopy every 5 years to 10 years. The latter recommendations are based on the fact that nearly half of all colon cancers occur proximal to the sigmoid flexure.

Computed-tomography (CT) imaging of the colon for polyp detection initially was described in 1983 (4); however, it was not until the advent of spiral CT in 1994 that virtual colonoscopy or CT colonography (CTC) was introduced by Vining and Gelfand. This technique facilitated display of three-dimensional (3D) endoluminal images of the colon (5). This examination involves thin-section CT of the cleansed colon after distention with either room air or CO_2 gas. The dataset then is reviewed, using both two-dimensional (2D) and 3D images of the colorectal mucosal surface (Figure 19-1). During the past 8 years there has been intense research and development in this field, greatly aided by technological advances such as the advent of multidetector CT (MDCT) and improved computer-processing ability/software (6). Advantages of CTC compared to conventional colonoscopy include safety and the ability to demonstrate the entire colon in both antegrade and retrograde directions with subsequent visualization of both sides of the haustral folds. Lesions can be localized accurately relative to extracolonic landmarks.

This technique has proven efficacy in the evaluation of the proximal large bowel in patients with both incomplete conventional colonoscopy and obstructing distal lesions, as well as in frail debilitated patients (7,8). Ultimately, the goal is for this examination to be a viable option for population screening.

DATA ACQUISITION AND INTERPRETATION

Owing to the rapid evolution of imaging and computer technology, there currently is not a consensus on optimal techniques for performance and interpretation of CTC (9,10). A substantial body of literature has developed on the topic, however, with current techniques having been reviewed by several authors (6,11,12). Most recently, acquisition techniques have begun to take advantage of faster imaging and thinner sections available with MDCT technology (13,14). These concepts are developed further in the following paragraphs.

Bowel Preparation

Our current bowel-cleansing technique consists of oral phosphosoda in two 30-cc doses, one taken the evening prior to the exam and the other on the morning of the exam. This approach appears to result in less residual fluid than polyethylene-glycol (PEG) preparations (15), but is not appropriate for patients with renal insufficiency who may not tolerate the phosphate load or fluid shifts. Many investigators have used PEG solutions as the standard bowel preparation prior to performing fiberoptic colonoscopy. Specialized commercial-preparation kits also are available now, based on magnesium citrate and derived from the dry prep designed for barium-enema examinations (EZ–EM, Westbury, CT). Thorough cleansing of the bowel of residual fecal material

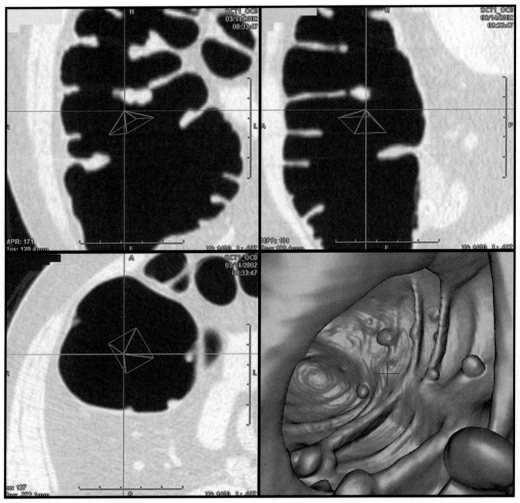

FIG. 19–1. Computed-tomography colonography with MDCT. Coronal **(A)**, sagittal **(B)**, and axial **(C)** viewing of CT data obtained at 1.25-mm sections, reconstructed at 1.25-mm intervals. Air-distended lumen demonstrates the colonic surface to good advantage. Pyramidal shape within the lumen demonstrates camera viewing direction for virtual endoscopy. Virtual endoscopic image **(D)** demonstrates multiple polyps in the cecum, ranging in size from 3 mm to 7 mm in diameter. (See Color Fig. 19–1D)

and fluid is critical to the success of the examination. Unfortunately, the preparation also is the least-tolerated portion of the examination. Research currently is underway on various forms of tagging of fluid and residual fecal material with barium- or iodine-containing agents (16,17). In some institutions, the resulting high-density material is removed electronically in what has been termed digital-subtraction bowel cleansing (18,19).

Bowel Insufflation and Data Acquisition

The patient arrives in the CT suite approximately 2 hours to 3 hours after the final dose of the bowel-cleansing agent. At this time, evacuation of as much residual liquid and solid fecal material as possible typically has been achieved. A Foley catheter is inserted into the rectum and air or continuous CO_2 is insufflated into the rectum while

the patient is rolled in multiple positions to facilitate colonic distension. Carbon dioxide has been proposed for colonic distension because it is absorbed more rapidly by the colon and therefore may be tolerated better (20); however, CO_2 requires continuous insufflation with a specialized pump, adding expense and logistical complications. After insufflation, a scout radiograph is used to assess colonic distention. Some investigators also have used spasmolytic agents such as glucagon to reduce bowel peristalsis and resulting motion artifact; however, the largest study to date addressing this subject showed no added benefit to the use of spasmolytics, and their use remains controversial at this time (21).

The abdomen and pelvis are scanned in both supine and prone position using MDCT. With 4-slice imaging, a 4-mm $\times$ 2.5-mm detector configuration is used, and images are reconstructed with 2.5-mm nominal widths at 1.25-mm intervals. With this configuration at a table feed of 7.5 mm per gantry-rotation period, the abdomen and pelvis are imaged within 40 seconds. A relatively low radiation dose is obtained with the use of 120 kVp and 48 mAs (60 mA at a 0.8 second gantry-rotation period) (22). Imaging at 15-mm table feed per gantry rotation results in a 20-second acquisition, suitable for older patients who may have difficulty holding their breath for 40 seconds. In this case, we use 120 kVp and 96 mAs (120 mA at a 0.8 second gantry-rotation period) is used. While some investigators continue to perform CTC with 5-mm sections, there has been a trend towards thinner sections as scanners have advanced, with some now routinely using 1.0-mm to 1.25-mm sections. Imaging parameters can be adjusted to the technical parameters of the CT scanner, and protocols used by numerous institutions, including very low-dose parameters, have been published (22). Consensus has been reached that both supine and prone imaging are required to evaluate fully the colon (9,23). This allows retained fluid and fecal material to move to dependent portions of the colon and also provides for optimal distension of most segments (21).

Image Processing and Interpretation

While bowel preparation is critical and data acquisition is important, a crucial element in CT-colonography performance relates to the data interpretation by the radiologist. This has been the subject of considerable research and debate, but as yet there is no clear consensus on the best means of data visualization and interpretation. Early work focused on the use of 3D viewing of endoscopic images for polyp detection. However, this view is unfamiliar to radiologists and the attenuation information inherent in axial 2D sections is important for diagnosis. One straightforward approach that has gained popularity is to review axial 2D sections in a stack or cine format, followed by selective 3D viewing of areas of possible polyps (24). There are a number of potential interpretive pitfalls with both 2D and 3D viewing (25,26). Examples of polyps, as well as potential pitfalls or mimics, are shown in Figures 19–2 through 19–6. Experimental studies have suggested an incremental benefit of 3D for detecting surface abnormalities (27,28), but 3D imaging in itself is not sufficient for accurate interpretation. Various forms of advanced 3D-image displays also have been developed (Figure 19-7) with the goal of providing a more thorough and efficient means than virtual endoscopic displays for viewing the colon (29–32). Images need to be reviewed at lung window settings with correlation of supine and prone images to allow for discrimination between retained mobile feces and stationary polyps.

A significant limitation of CTC is the extensive time required for interpretation of the large datasets. Average interpretation times for experienced readers are approximately 15 minutes per exam, with reported ranges of 10 minutes (33) to well over 30 minutes (24,34). This factor, and the tedium of reviewing large numbers of images, has provided motivation for advanced viewing modes (Figure 19-7), and

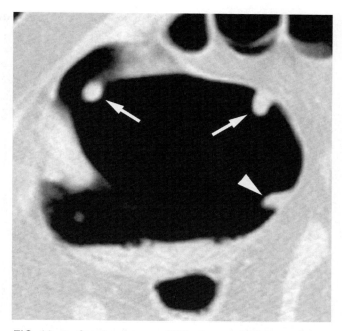

FIG. 19–2. Small polyps on CTC. *Arrows* depict a pedunculated and a sessile polyp on the anterior aspect of the colonic wall, each 5 mm in diameter. *Arrowhead* demonstrates a portion of a haustral fold. Note difficulty in distinguishing polyps from haustral folds on a single 2D section.

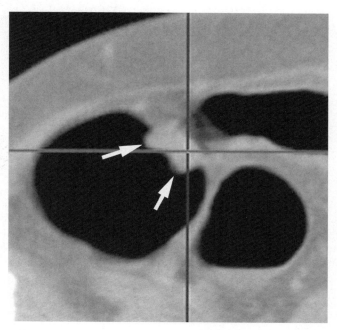

FIG. 19–3. Polyp in the cecum measuring 13 mm across, but with a relatively flat bilobed profile (*arrows*). Lesions such as this may be clinically significant but difficult to detect.

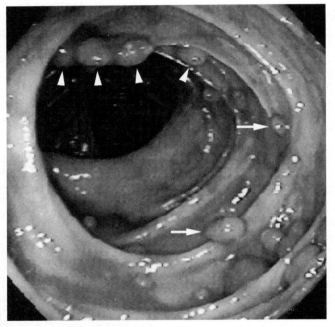

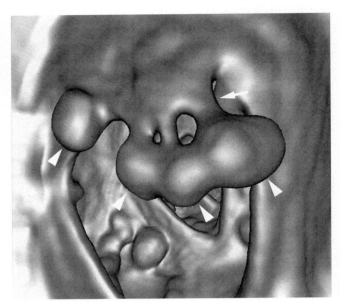

FIG. 19–4. A: Pedunculated polyps in the ascending colon. Four separate polyp heads are identified (*arrowheads*). These hang dependently from the anterior aspect of the colon along a haustral fold. Polyp stalk of one lesion is indicated by an *arrow*. **B:** Endoluminal volume-rendered image of same pedunculated polyps. **C:** Fiberoptic colonoscopic view demonstrating the polyps along the anterior colonic wall (*arrowheads*), as well as multiple other small relatively sessile lesions (*arrows*).

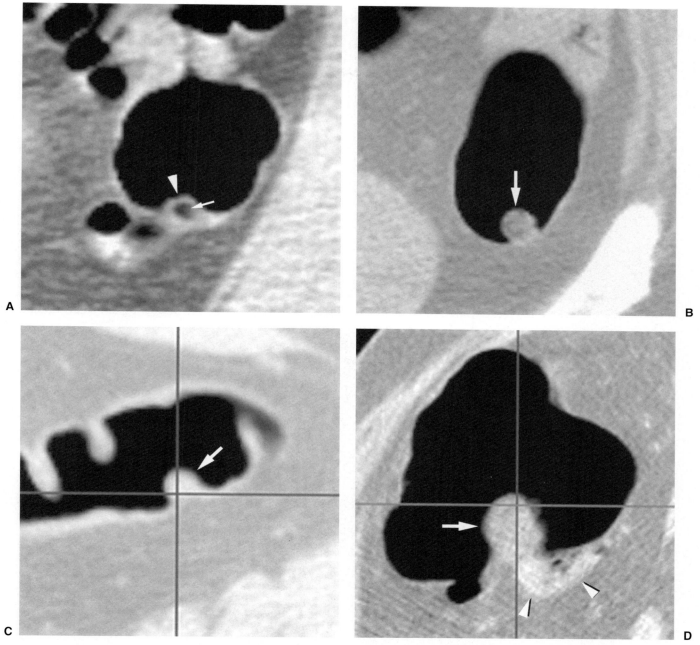

FIG. 19–5. Polyp mimics. **A:** Retained fecal material (*arrowhead*) with a polypoid morphology. Presence of low-attenuation gas within center of lesion (*arrow*) is diagnostic of retained feces, and not present in true polyps. **B:** Retained fecal material (*arrow*) demonstrating heterogeneous attenuation with some areas approaching fat density. Adenomatous polyps have uniform soft-tissue attenuation. Computed-tomography data courtesy of Dr. Judy Yee, UCSF/San Francisco VAMC. **C:** Thickened fold in sigmoid colon mimicking a polyp (*arrow*). **D:** Ileocecal valve. Typical morphology of terminal ileum (*arrowheads*) inserting in the cecum confirms this structure as the ileocecal valve (*arrow*).

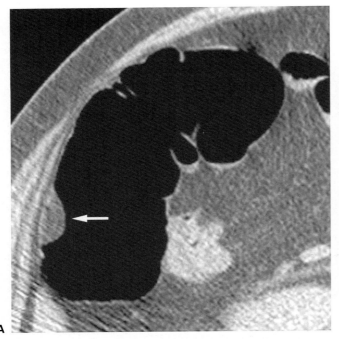

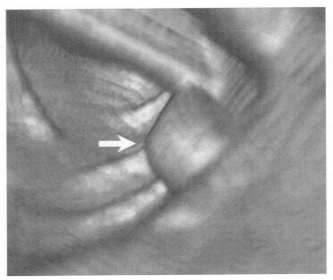

FIG. 19-6. A: Polypoid lesion in hepatic flexure with fat attenuation, representing a 2-cm lipoma. **B:** Endoluminal volume rendering demonstrating polypoid mass, highlighting the importance of evaluating morphology and attenuation within a lesion. (See Color Fig. 19-6B)

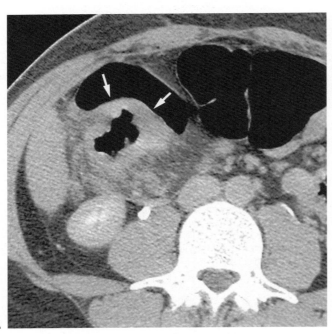

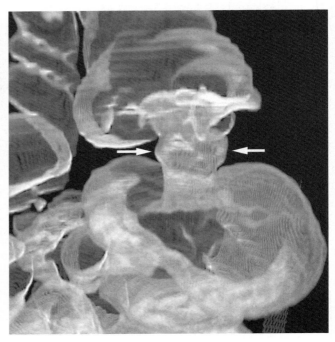

FIG. 19-7. A: Axial CT section demonstrating a constricting annular mass in the hepatic flexure (*arrows*). Infiltration of surrounding fat is visible, consistent with extracolonic extension. **B:** External 3D volume rendering, "tissue-transition projection" demonstrating familiar applecore-type morphology of adenocarcinoma of the colon.

for the development of computer-aided detection methods for polyps discussed later in this chapter.

Finally, the interpreter also must detect and characterize incidental extracolonic findings. It is not surprising that benign lesions such as gallstones and hepatic and renal cysts, as well as more-threatening lesions such as solid renal masses and abdominal aortic aneurysms, are encountered in the population undergoing CTC (35).

CLINICAL RESULTS

A discussion of the efficacy of CTC must compare the sensitivity and specificity of this technique with the accepted gold standard of conventional colonoscopy. There has long been debate about what constitutes a clinically significant size of a polyp. Many endoscopists advocate removal of all polyps discovered at colonoscopy, regardless of size. The practical necessity of this approach has been questioned by Glick and others (36,37), who pointed out that only about 1% of adenomas less than 1 cm in diameter harbor invasive cancer. By comparison, polyps 1 cm to 2 cm generally are neoplastic, and about 10% are malignant (38,39); however, most malignancies occur beyond the 15-mm threshold (40). It may be argued that polyps greater than 15 mm in diameter should be the primary goal for detection and removal. A more conservative threshold would be detection of polyps 1 cm or greater, but as yet there has been no clear consensus regarding the critical size for detection.

The sensitivity and specificity of CTC are dependent directly on polyp size, with the lowest sensitivity being for polyps less than 6 mm. Many observers feel that the lower size for lesion detection should be 1 cm, and the available data will be described with regard to this threshold (Table 19.1). In an early publication, Hara et al. studied 70 consecutive patients who underwent both conventional and CTC (41). This study had a sensitivity and specificity of 75% and 90%, respectively, for identifying patients with adenomas greater than 1 cm. The authors pointed out that false-negative results were due to a combination of perceptive errors and suboptimal patient preparation. They ascribed their false-positive observations to respiration artifact and perceptive errors such as misidentification of stool. A major benefit of MDCT has been the elimination of respiratory artifacts seen with slower scanners (13,14).

The efficacy of CTC in polyp detection has been studied in larger trials independently by Yee et al. and Fenlon et al. (33,42). In a study involving 300 patients that compared CTC and traditional colonoscopy with histologic findings, Yee et al. reported a sensitivity of 90% (74 of 82) for the detection of polyps 10 mm or larger. In a study of 100 patients, Fenlon et al. reported a sensitivity of 91% for polyps greater than 10 mm in size. They also reported a positive and negative predictive value of 96% each for polyps greater than 9 mm in diameter. More recently, similarly encouraging results have been reported with thin-section low-dose MDCT (43).

There is growing evidence that CTC also is effective in evaluating larger colorectal masses in symptomatic patients

TABLE 19–1. *CT colonography performance data*

Author (ref.)	Total no. of patients	No. of polyps > 1 cm	Sensitivity (%)*		Specificity (%)*	Inclusion criteria **
			By polyp	By patient	By patient	
Hara (67)	10	5	100	NR	NR	Patients with known polyps
Hara (38)	70	15	Obs. A: 73	Obs. A: 75	Obs. A: 91	35 patients with known polps
			Obs. B: 67	Obs. B: 75	Obs. B: 90	35 patients with high probability
Royster (53)	20	22	100	100	NA	All 20 patients had known masses
Dachman (21)	44	6†	Obs. A: 83	Obs. A: NR	Obs. A: 93	High probability
			Obs. B: 83	Obs. B: NR	Obs. B: 86	
Rex (57)	46	14††	50	80	89	Screening
Morrin (5)	40	21	95	NR	89	High probability
Macari (54)	37	3	100	100	100	Screening
Fenlon (30)	100	22	91	96	96	High probability
Hara (11)	160‡	10	80	78	93	High probability
Yee (39)	300	82	90	100	NR	High probability
Laghi (44)	165	12	92	92	97	High probability
Belloni (46)	100	12	92	NR	NR	High probability
Macari (40)	105	14	93	NR	98	High probability

Note: Conventional colonoscopy was the standard of reference for all detected polyps. NR = not reported.
* Reported data are for detection of polyps ≥ 1 cm, unless specified.
** High probability is indicated by family or personal history of colorectal cancer, personal history of adenomatous polyps, positive fecal occult blood test, rectal bleeding, iron-deficiency anemia, weight loss, recent sigmoidoscopy demonstrating one or more polyps, or altered bowel habit.
† Polyps 8 mm or larger.
†† Including 3 flat adenomas.
‡ Includes patients studied with multidetector row CT only.

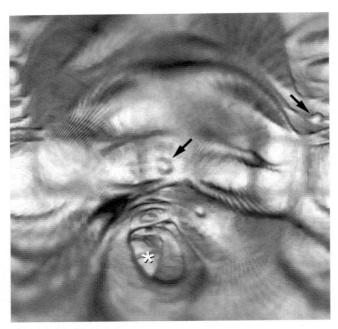

FIG. 19–8. Advanced viewing modes—Mercator projection. Sixteen virtual endoscopic-camera views were used to composite a single image demonstrating the circumference of the colonic segment across the center of the image, where a 7-mm polyp is illustrated (*arrow*). Upper and lower portions of the image demonstrate colon in antegrade or retrograde directions. *Asterisk* demonstrates a portion of the more proximal colonic lumen. Other small polyps also are visible. (See Color Fig. 19–8)

(Figure 19-8). Lees and Gillams submitted a cohort of 1250 symptomatic patients who had CTC, over 1150 of whom had corroboration with colonoscopy, laparotomy, or a minimum of 6-months clinical follow up (44). This study included the use of intravenous (IV) contrast material, which is not in general use at this time but has been studied as an improvement to CTC for polyp detection and characterization (45). They concluded that CTC is reliable for the detection of cancer in symptomatic patients with a sensitivity of 98.7% and a specificity of 98.2%. They detected 232 of 235 cancers in the cohort. One cancer was missed secondary to inadequate patient bowel preparation and subsequently was found on a follow-up CT. The other two were Duke's A 'flat' cancers. These cancers, which arise in so-called "flat adenomas," are important to consider. This pathologic sequence through a flat adenoma has an unclear contribution to the natural history of colon cancer but may be responsible for 15% to 20% of cases (46).

A recent publication by Laghi et al. studied 165 patients with suspected colorectal lesions referred for conventional colonoscopy who underwent preliminary CTC (47). Thirty colorectal carcinomas and 37 polyps were found at conventional colonoscopy. Computed-tomography colonography correctly identified all carcinomas and had a 92% sensitivity for polyps greater than 10 mm. The per-patient sensitivity and specificity were 92% and 97%, respectively.

Lastly, long-awaited results were submitted at the Radiological Society of North America (RSNA) (2002) from the American College of Radiology Imaging Network (ACRIN) Study that constructed a multicenter performance evaluation of CTC. In a sample of 94 cases with 50% disease prevalence, CTC demonstrated high accuracy for the detection of polyps greater than 1 cm. Accuracy was measured by the average area under the receiver operator characteristic (ROC) curve, which was 0.89 (48).

While these recent results are encouraging, they are difficult to extrapolate to a screening population given the high disease prevalence in the study groups. Further studies still are required to assess the performance of this study in large screening populations with low disease prevalence. To date, CTC has proven efficacious in symptomatic patients, as well as patients with obstructing distal lesions. Belloni et al. have demonstrated the potential efficacy of this procedure for following patients after polypectomy by conventional colonoscopy, showing a sensitivity of 92.6% for polyps when directly comparing CT and conventional colonoscopy (49).

CT COLONOGRAPHY IN THE SCREENING POPULATION

The United States government has endorsed these screening methods by establishing coverage for all Medicare beneficiaries. It has been proposed that all individuals over 50 years of age should undergo comprehensive evaluation of the entire large bowel, which currently is accomplished best by conventional colonoscopy (1). This argument is supported strongly by large studies performed independently by Imperiale et al. and Lieberman et al., who reported similar findings (3,50). These studies included large cohorts of asymptomatic patients who underwent colonoscopic screening. More than 50% of patients in both studies had large polyps or carcinomas seen only in the proximal colon, and would not have been detected with flexible sigmoidoscopy. The results of the National Polyp Study also were striking, demonstrating convincingly that colonoscopic polypectomy resulted in a lower-than-expected incidence of colorectal cancer (2). These findings support the well-established view that colorectal adenomas progress to adenocarcinomas, as well as the practice of finding and eliminating polyps to prevent colorectal cancer.

It is clear that comprehensive evaluation of the large bowel will be central to colorectal cancer screening in the near future. Computed-tomography colonography has demonstrated efficacy in the detection of polyps greater than 1 cm in patients with high disease prevalence, but its utility can be extrapolated only in a screening population with low disease prevalence. The current gold standard for complete evaluation of the large bowel is fiberoptic colonoscopy. This procedure has the distinct advantage of being both diagnostic and therapeutic. Advantages of CTC over fiberoptic colonoscopy include complete evaluation of the colonic mucosa in all patients, patient safety, and the ability of the patient to return to work the same day. Lieberman et al. reported an overall complication rate of fiberoptic colonoscopy of 0.3% (3). Significant problems related to gastrointestinal perforation and problems related to conscious sedation occur in approximately 0.2% of examinations (51). While these complications do have a low rate, the number of affected patients would rise rapidly if fiberoptic colonoscopy were used for population screening. Colonoscopy also fails to examine the proximal colon in 10% to 15% of cases. A study by Morrin et al. demonstrated the efficacy of CTC in evaluating these nonvisualized segments after incomplete colonoscopy (8). Additional advantages of CTC include decreased exam time and the ability to examine both sides of the bowel wall without sedation. Disadvantages include the need for very thorough bowel cleansing, problems of spasm and retained debris, resolution for flat neoplasms, and the fact that the exam is diagnostic only.

Computed-tomography colonography has lower morbidity than fiberoptic colonoscopy. However, at this point in time, the true sensitivity of CTC in a screening population has not been established. The diagnosis of flat neoplasms with CTC is problematic and must be evaluated further. A major barrier to the implementation of CTC for population screening is cost effectiveness. A comprehensive study into this question by Sonnenberg et al. concluded that in order for CTC to be cost effective, it must have a compliance rate 15% to 20% better than, or procedural costs 54% less than, fiberoptic colonoscopy (52).

GASTROENTEROLOGIST'S PERSPECTIVE ON CT COLONOGRAPHY

In general, CTC has been embraced by gastroenterologists as a promising research area, although several important clinical issues remain unresolved. Most gastroenterologists recognize that CTC is evolving rapidly into a technique that may offer a safe and accurate means of detecting colon polyps. The use of advanced technology and a less-invasive method than fiberoptic colonoscopy is seen as an attraction for patients, with the hope that this may encourage otherwise-unwilling patients to undergo colorectal-cancer screening. It is safe and relatively noninvasive. Both 2D sections and 3D endoluminal images can be reviewed for interpretation. Forward and rear-view 3D visualization allows viewing behind haustral folds, which is not possible with conventional colonoscopy. Furthermore, the entire colon usually can be visualized with CTC, even areas proximal to obstructing lesions (8,53,54). As detailed in Table 19.1, multiple studies have shown acceptable sensitivity and specificity for the detection of polyps 10 mm or larger, but the sensitivity is substantially less for smaller polyps (6).

Despite the seemingly obvious advantages of CTC, there are a number of controversies that still need to be addressed. Some studies have shown poor sensitivity and specificity for polyps of all sizes (55–57). Potential explanations for these results include suboptimal bowel preparation,

presence of flat lesions, lack of experience with the technique, and differences in data acquisition and image interpretation. Until a consensus is reached regarding the optimal technique for image acquisition and interpretation, there will be variability in performance and results.

Questions regarding the relatively high cost of CTC and patient acceptance may affect negatively the potential use of CTC as a screening method. Surprisingly, a patient's tolerability appears to favor conventional colonoscopy over virtual colonoscopy in a number of studies (58). Another important controversy is what constitutes a clinically significant polyp. Because there is a low likelihood of finding malignant changes in polyps less than 1 cm, some believe a polyp 1 cm or larger should be the target size for detection. However, there is no evidence to date that performance of CTC every 10 years, while ignoring polyps less than 1 cm, will be as effective as complete colonoscopic polyp removal in reducing colorectal-cancer incidence (2). The data supporting conventional colonoscopy in reducing the incidence of colorectal cancer are predicated upon completely clearing all polyps, regardless of size (2). Until this controversy is resolved, CTC may not be accepted by patients and clinicians as a screening method.

Finally, CTC needs to be tested in a large population of asymptomatic patients with average risk for colon polyps. The majority of studies published to date have included populations at high risk for polyps, such as male veterans and patients with a history of gastrointestinal bleeding or personal history of polyps (33,42,43). Such studies may suffer from suspicion bias, in which tests are reviewed carefully and aggressively when there is a higher clinical suspicion for a finding. If CTC is to impact patient screening, it must detect accurately polyps in average-risk populations.

FUTURE DEVELOPMENTS

One major factor limiting patient compliance with traditional and virtual colonoscopy is the arduous bowel preparation required. False-positive and -negative results in CTC have been attributed to inadequate bowel preparation or adherent stool. In addition, the false-positive examination rate has not been established in a true screening population, and training issues related to interpretation and interobserver variations need to be understood (59). Research has focused on contrast material to label stool, which then can be subtracted from the images to eliminate bowel preparation. In this technique, the patient ingests high-density contrast material 24 hours to 48 hours prior to imaging, which fully opacifies the colon (16). A single CT acquisition is performed after colonic insufflation, and computer software is used to subtract the ingested colonic contents and stool, leaving the colorectal mucosa unaffected. Promising early results were published by Zalis et al. (19). A larger study was published subsequently and suggested that sensitivity for polyp detection using this technique approaches that achieved in prepared colons (16). This technique has the added potential of being performed in a single acquisition, rather than standard supine and prone scanning, reducing radiation by 50%. Elimination of the bowel preparation is expected to improve greatly patient compliance, and it would improve significantly the cost effectiveness of CTC for population screening.

Interpretation time also has a significant impact on the cost effectiveness of CTC. This has prompted the development of several techniques for computer-aided detection of polyps (60–66). Initial work indicates that several automated polyp detectors can achieve a high sensitivity for detection of clinically significant lesions, but many suffer from an excess of false-positive detections. Integration of viewing modes for CTC facilitates ease of interpretation (Figure 19-9).

The diagnostic ability of CTC has been shown comparable to traditional colonoscopy, and future developments such as computer-aided detection and fecal tagging promise to improve significantly its efficacy, patient compliance, and image interpretation time. These improvements, combined with the inherent safety of the examination, have the potential to establish CTC as a viable population screening method

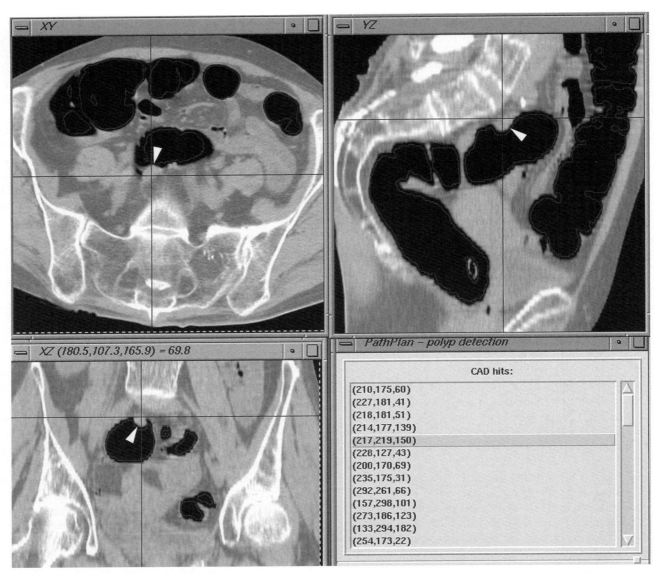

FIG. 19–9. Computer-aided-detection (CAD) software interface. Computer-aided-detection algorithm has been run on CTC data, highlighting suspicious areas, or "hits," indicated by the list in the lower-right corner. User clicks on a location and is taken to the hit, then uses 2D and 3D images to determine if lesion is a true polyp or not. Accurate CAD and similar user interface have the potential to reduce the amount of time required for interpretation of CTC data. Computed-tomography data courtesy of Elizabeth G. McFarland, M.D., Mallinckrodt Institute of Radiology.

within the next decade. Radiologists, gastroenterologists, and other physicians need to work together to improve screening compliance and patient education.

REFERENCES

1. Podolsky DK. Going the distance—the case for true colorectal cancer screening. *N Engl J Med* 2000;343(3):207–208.
2. Winawer SJ, Zauber AG, Ho MN, et al. Prevention of colorectal cancer by colonoscopic polypectomy. The National Polyp Study Workgroup. *N Engl J Med* 1993;329(27):1977–1981.
3. Lieberman DA, Weiss DG, Bond JH, et al. Use of colonoscopy to screen asymptomatic adults for colorectal cancer. Veterans Affairs Cooperative Study Group 380. *N Engl J Med* 2000;343(3):162–168.
4. Coin CG, Wollett FC, Coin JT, et al. Computerized radiology of the colon: a potential screening technique. *Comput Radiol* 1983;7(4):215–221.
5. Vining DJ, Gelfand DW. Noninvasive colonoscopy using helical CT scanning, 3D reconstruction and virtual reality. In: *Meeting of the Society of Gastrointestinal Radiologists*. 1994. Maui, Hawaii.
6. Johnson CD, Dachman AH. CT colonography: the next colon screening examination? *Radiology* 2000;216(2):331–341.
7. Galia M, Midiri M, Carcione A, et al. Usefulness of CT colonography in the preoperative evaluation of patients with distal occlusive colorectal carcinoma. *Radiol Med (Torino)* 2001;101(4):235–242.
8. Morrin MM, Kruskal JB, Farrell RJ, et al. Endoluminal CT colonography after an incomplete endoscopic colonoscopy. *AJR Am J Roentgenol* 1999;172(4):913–918.
9. Fletcher JG, Johnson CD, Welch TJ, et al. Optimization of CT colonography technique: prospective trial in 180 patients. *Radiology* 2000;216(3):704–711.
10. McFarland EG, Brink JA. Helical CT colonography (virtual colonoscopy): the challenge that exists between advancing technology and generalizability. *AJR Am J Roentgenol* 1999;173(3):549–559.
11. Yee J. Virtual colonoscopy (CT and MR colonography). *Gastrointest Endosc* 2002;55(7 Pt 2):S25–S32.
12. Macari M. Virtual colonoscopy: clinical results. *Semin Ultrasound CT MR* 2001;22(5):432–442.
13. Rogalla P, Meiri N, Ruckert JC, et al. Colonography using multislice CT. *Eur J Radiol* 2000;36(2):81–85.
14. Hara AK, Johnson CD, MacCarty RL, et al. CT colonography: single-versus multi-detector row imaging. *Radiology* 2001;219(2):461–465.
15. Macari M, Lavelle M, Pedrosa I, et al. Effect of different bowel preparations on residual fluid at CT colonography. *Radiology* 2001;218(1):274–277.
16. Callstrom MR, Johnson CD, Fletcher JG, et al. CT colonography without cathartic preparation: feasibility study. *Radiology* 2001;219(3):693–698.
17. Sheppard DG, Iyer RB, Herron D, et al. Subtraction CT colonography: feasibility in an animal model. *Clin Radiol* 1999;54(2):126–132.
18. Pochaczevsky R. Digital subtraction bowel cleansing in CT colonography. *AJR Am J Roentgenol* 2002;178(1):241.
19. Zalis ME, Hahn PF. Digital subtraction bowel cleansing in CT colonography. *AJR Am J Roentgenol* 2001;176(3):646–648.
20. Vining DJ. Virtual colonoscopy. *Semin Ultrasound CT MR* 1999;20(1):56–60.
21. Yee J, Hung RK, Akerkar GA, et al. The usefulness of glucagon hydrochloride for colonic distention in CT colonography [see comments]. *AJR Am J Roentgenol* 1999;173(1):169–172.
22. van Gelder RE, Venema HW, Serlie IW, et al. CT colonography at different radiation dose levels: feasibility of dose reduction. *Radiology* 2002;224(1):25–33.
23. Chen SC, Lu DS, Hecht JR, et al. CT colonography: value of scanning in both the supine and prone positions. *AJR Am J Roentgenol* 1999;172(3):595–599.
24. Dachman AH, Kuniyoshi JK, Boyle CM, et al. CT colonography with three-dimensional problem solving for detection of colonic polyps. *AJR Am J Roentgenol* 1998;171(4):989–995.
25. Fletcher JG, Johnson CD, MacCarty RL, et al. CT colonography: potential pitfalls and problem-solving techniques [see comments]. *AJR Am J Roentgenol* 1999;172(5):1271–1278.
26. Macari M, Megibow AJ. Pitfalls of using three-dimensional CT colon-

27. Beaulieu CF, Jeffrey RB Jr, Karadi C, et al. Display modes for CT colonography. Part II. Blinded comparison of axial CT and virtual endoscopic and panoramic endoscopic volume-rendered studies. *Radiology* 1999;212(1):203–212.
28. Karadi C, Beaulieu CF, Jeffrey RB Jr, et al. Display modes for CT colonography. Part I. Synthesis and insertion of polyps into patient CT data. *Radiology* 1999;212(1):195–201.
29. Paik DS, Beaulieu CF, Jeffrey RB Jr, et al. Visualization modes for CT colonography using cylindrical and planar map projections. *J Comput Assist Tomogr* 2000;24(2):179–188.
30. Rogalla P, Bender A, Bick U, et al. Tissue transition projection (TTP) of the intestines. *Eur Radiol* 2000;10(5):806–810.
31. Wang G, McFarland EG, Brown BP, et al. GI tract unraveling with curved cross sections. *IEEE Trans Med Imaging* 1998;17(2):318–322.
32. Haker S, Angenent S, Tannenbaum A, et al. Nondistorting flattening maps and the 3-D visualization of colon CT images. *IEEE Trans Med Imaging* 2000;19(7):665–670.
33. Fenlon HM, Nunes DP, Schroy PC 3rd, et al. A comparison of virtual and conventional colonoscopy for the detection of colorectal polyps [see comments] [published erratum appears in N Engl J Med 2000;17;342(7):524]. *N Engl J Med* 1999;341(20):1496–1503.
34. Macari M, Milano A, Lavelle M, et al. Comparison of time-efficient CT colonography with two- and three-dimensional colonic evaluation for detecting colorectal polyps. *AJR Am J Roentgenol* 2000;174(6):1543–1549.
35. Hara AK, Johnson CD, MacCarty RL, et al. Incidental extracolonic findings at CT colonography. *Radiology* 2000;215(2):353–357.
36. Glick SN. Comparison of colonoscopy and double-contrast barium enema. *N Engl J Med* 2000;343(23):1728; discussion 1729–1730.
37. Glick SN. Virtual colonoscopy [letter; comment]. *N Engl J Med* 2000;342(10):737–738; discussion 738–739.
38. Kudo S, Kashida H, Tamura T. Early colorectal cancer: flat or depressed type. *J Gastroenterol Hepatol* 2000;15 Suppl:D66–D70.
39. Muto T, Bussey HJ, Morson BC. The evolution of cancer of the colon and rectum. *Cancer* 1975;36(6):2251–2270.
40. Chantereau MJ, Faivre J, Boutron MC, et al. Epidemiology, management, and prognosis of malignant large bowel polyps within a defined population. *Gut* 1992;33(2):259–263.
41. Hara AK, Johnson CD, Reed JE, et al. Detection of colorectal polyps with CT colography: initial assessment of sensitivity and specificity. *Radiology* 1997;205:59–65.
42. Yee J, Akerkar GA, Hung RK, et al. Colorectal neoplasia: performance characteristics of CT colonography for detection in 300 patients. *Radiology* 2001;219(3):685–692.
43. Macari M, Bini EJ, Xue X, et al. Colorectal neoplasms: prospective comparison of thin-section low-dose multi-detector row CT colonography and conventional colonoscopy for detection. *Radiology* 2002;224(2):383–392.
44. Lees WR, Gillams AR. Is CT colography a reliable method for detecting colorectal cancer in symptomatic patients? *Radiology* 2001;221(P):307.
45. Morrin MM, Farrell RJ, Kruskal JB, et al. Utility of intravenously administered contrast material at CT colonography. *Radiology* 2000;217(3):765–771.
46. Saito K, Mori M. Rate of progression to advanced stage in depressed-type colorectal adenoma. *Oncol Rep* 2000;7(3):615–619.
47. Laghi A, Iannaccone R, Carbone I. Detection of colorectal lesions with virtual computed tomographic colonography. *Am J Surg* 2002;183:124–131.
48. Johnson CD, Toledano A, Herman B, et al. CT Colonography: performance evaluation in a multicenter setting (American College of Radiology Imaging Network Study 6653). *Radiology* 2001;221 (P):308.
49. Belloni GM, Clarizia FA, Ballarati C, et al. Virtual colonography vs. conventional colonoscopy in polypectomy surveillance: a prospective blinded study. *Radiology* 2001;221(P):308.
50. Imperiale TF, Wagner DR, Lin CY, et al. Risk of advanced proximal neoplasms in asymptomatic adults according to the distal colorectal findings. *N Engl J Med* 2000;343(3):169–174.
51. Rankin GB. Indications, contraindications, and complications of colonoscopy. In: Sivac MV, ed. *Gastrointestinal endoscopy*. Philadelphia; WB Saunders, 1987;873–878.
52. Sonnenberg A, Delco F, Bauerfeind P. Is virtual colonoscopy a cost-

effective option to screen for colorectal cancer? *Am J Gastroenterol* 1999;94(8):2268–2274.

53. Royster AP, Fenlon HM, Clarke PD, et al. CT colonoscopy of colorectal neoplasms: two-dimensional and three-dimensional virtual-reality techniques with colonoscopic correlation. *AJR Am J Roentgenol* 1997; 169(5):1237–1242.

54. Macari M, Berman P, Dicker M, et al. Usefulness of CT colonography in patients with incomplete colonoscopy. *AJR Am J Roentgenol* 1999; 173(3):561–564.

55. Miao YM, Amin Z, Healy J, et al. A prospective single centre study comparing computed tomography pneumocolon against colonoscopy in the detection of colorectal neoplasms. *Gut* 2000;47(6):832–837.

56. Pescatore P, Glucker T, Delarive J, et al. Diagnostic accuracy and interobserver agreement of CT colonography (virtual colonoscopy). *Gut* 2000;47(1):126–130.

57. Rex DK, Vining D, Kopecky KK. An initial experience with screening for colon polyps using spiral CT with and without CT colography (virtual colonoscopy). *Gastrointest Endosc* 1999;50(3):309–313.

58. Akerkar GA, Yee J, Hung R, et al. Patient experience and preferences toward colon cancer screening: a comparison of virtual colonoscopy and conventional colonoscopy. *Gastrointest Endosc* 2001;54(3): 310–315.

59. McFarland EG, Brink JA, Pilgram TK, et al. Spiral CT colonography: reader agreement and diagnostic performance with two- and three-dimensional image-display techniques. *Radiology* 2001;218(2): 375–383.

60. Paik DS, Beaulieu CF, Rubin GD, et al. A computer aided detection algorithm for colonic polyps and lung nodules in helical CT. *Med Phys* 2002;Submitted.

61. Paik DS, Beaulieu CF, Mani A, et al. Evaluation of computer-aided detection in CT colonography: potential applicability to a screening population. *Radiology* 2001;221 (P):332.

62. Yoshida H, Nappi JJ, MacEneaney PM. High performance automated detection of colonic polyps in CT colonography. *Radiology* 2001; 221(P):306.

63. Summers RM, Beaulieu CF, Pusanik LM, et al. Automated polyp detector for CT colonography: feasibility study. *Radiology* 2000;216(1): 284–290.

64. Summers RM, Johnson CD, Pusanik LM, et al. Automated polyp detection at CT colonography: feasibility assessment in a human population. *Radiology* 2001;219(1):51–59.

65. Gokturk SB, Tomasi C, Acar B, et al. A statistical 3-D pattern processing method for computer-aided detection of polyps in CT colonography. *IEEE Trans Med Imaging* 2001;20(12):1251–1260.

66. Acar B, Beaulieu CF, Gokturk SB, et al. Edge displacement field based classification for improved detection of polyps in CT colonography. *IEEE Trans Med Imaging* 2002;In Press.

67. Hara AK, Johnson CD, Reed JE, et al. Detection of colorectal polyps by computed tomographic colography: feasibility of a novel technique. *Gastroenterology* 1996;110(1):284–290.

SECTION IV

Genitourinary Applications

CHAPTER 20

Multidetector CT of the Urinary Tract

Lawrence C. Chow, F. Graham Sommer

INTRODUCTION

The advent of spiral computed-tomography (CT) scanners in the early 1990s was a major milestone in renal imaging. Computed-tomography scanning of the kidneys within a single breathhold became practical, making it a relatively simple matter to acquire data without respiratory misregistration. Spiral CT also allowed, for the first time, acquisition of volumetric datasets rather than individual axial sections, making possible three-dimensional (3D) processing for depicting the normal kidney and renal pathology in new and often more useful ways. With the introduction of multidetector CT (MDCT), a second revolution in renal-CT scanning is taking place, with significantly increased scan speed and higher longitudinal spatial resolution being major benefits. This chapter will describe techniques for the application of this new technology for the improved diagnosis of pathologic processes involving the urinary tract.

APPLICATIONS OF MDCT IN THE URINARY TRACT

Renal CT has evolved to the point where a number of different protocols may be employed fruitfully to investigate a wide range of known or suspected pathologic conditions affecting the kidneys. These include the evaluation of possible renal colic, characterization of a known or suspected renal mass, staging or follow up of renal cell carcinoma, renal CT angiography, and MDCT urography. Each of these applications benefits from MDCT technology.

Following the seminal work of Smith et al. (1–4), the use of noncontrast CT for the evaluation of possible renal colic has become widespread, largely replacing the excretory urogram for this application. Images should be acquired with 2.5-mm nominal section thickness reconstructed to no greater than 5-mm thick sections. Such an examination is rapid and performed in a single breath hold, requiring only about 17 seconds in the average patient. Computed tomography has proved extremely effective as an alternative to excretory urography (EU) for the detection of renal colic, with reported sensitivities and specificities in the high 90s (5) in several large reported studies. Advantages of the noncontrast renal colic CT examination include not only its high accuracy, but also its very rapid performance, requiring only one pass through the abdomen, no need for any patient preparation or iodinated-contrast material, and the ability to diagnose accurately unsuspected disease processes mimicking renal colic in at least 10% of cases in a large reported series (6).

The diagnosis of renal colic by noncontrast CT is made on the basis of both the primary finding of a stone within the ureter and the presence of a number of associated secondary findings that include perinephric stranding (82%/94%), hydronephrosis (83%/94%), hydroureter (90%/93%), periureteral stranding, and unilateral nephromegaly (71%/89%) on the affected side (2) (reported sensitivity/specificity). Several signs to aid in the differentiation of ureteral calculi from pelvic phleboliths have been described. The presence of a halo of soft tissue representing the inflamed ureter encompassing the calcification known as the *tissue rim sign* is perhaps the most useful with a reported sensitivity of 76% to 77% and specificity of 92% to 98% (7,8). Other signs include a central lucency and the *comet tail sign* (eccentric, tapered soft tissue leading to the calcification representing the noncalcified pelvic vein), both of which are highly specific for phleboliths, albeit insensitive (8).

Specific advantages of MDCT over earlier spiral-CT technology include the possibility of reconstructing thinner axial sections (e.g., 2.5 mm with the protocol described above) if desired to evaluate better a calcification as a possible intraureteral stone, and the ability to reconstruct overlapping thin sections for optimization of further 3D-reformatted images that may be valuable in demonstrating the course of the ureters (9).

For a renal CT examination specifically designed to characterize a renal mass, 5-mm thick unenhanced images through the kidneys (generally from the diaphragm to the iliac crest level) are obtained with parameters similar to those described above for the renal-colic examination. Ninety seconds to 120 seconds after the intravenous (IV) administration of contrast agent (120 cc of nonionic contrast, 300 mg I/mL, at 2 cc per second using a power injector), an enhanced acquisition through both kidneys in nephrographic phase is obtained. Advantages of MDCT in this application include the possibility of scanning with thinner sections more rapidly in a breath-held time frame. Again, the selection of imaging parameters depends upon the capabilities of the CT scanner being used. Most MDCT scanners should be able to image the kidneys in 2.0-mm to 2.5-mm mode within a single breath hold. Data can be reconstructed into overlapping 5-mm thick sections for primary interpretation with the option to reconstruct thinner 2.0-mm to 2.5-mm thick images if desired. Such thin sections are advantageous for optimally characterizing very small renal masses by minimizing partial volume-averaging artifacts. On the precontrast images, the presence of calcification within a renal mass is characteristic of renal cell carcinoma, whereas the presence of fat within a mass is diagnostic of a benign angiomyolipoma. Most importantly, however, postcontrast enhancement greater than 10 Hounsfield units (HU) to 15 HU within a mass indicates a vascularized lesion, generally a tumor.

In some situations, the precontrast phase may be deferred. When a scan is being performed simply to stage a known renal cell carcinoma, for example, rather than to characterize the mass, nonenhanced images generally contribute no clinically relevant information. Similarly, follow-up examinations after nephrectomy for renal cell carcinoma also are scanned in this manner. In other instances, scanning during additional phases may be indicated. For example, corticomedullary or vascular phase images may be helpful to distinguish a vascular abnormality such as a renal artery aneurysm or parenchymal pseudoaneurysm from an enhancing renal mass. Delayed images obtained during excretory phase can be useful for differentiating peripelvic cysts from hydronephrosis. While scanning the kidneys in every phase of enhancement is neither practical nor indicated, scans may be tailored individually to answer the clinical question at hand while keeping radiation dose to a minimum.

Renal CT angiography (CTA), another important renal application, has benefited greatly by the improved speed and resolution of MDCT; the use of this technique is discussed in Chapter 24. In recent years, efforts have been made to exploit the excellent contrast resolution and 3D-display capabilities of CT scanning to create an examination capable of demonstrating the renal parenchyma, collecting structures, and ureters in a single examination termed *CT urography* (CTU) (10–12) as a replacement for conventional excretory urography, primarily to investigate patients presenting with painless hematuria. Computed-tomography urography is emerging as a very valuable clinical tool that has only become truly practical with the advent of MDCT, and this technique will be the primary focus of this chapter.

CTU: RATIONALE AND INDICATIONS

The replacement of conventional excretory urography (EU) with CT in recent years for the evaluation of urinary-tract calculi and renal parenchymal masses has left EU with a single major indication: the evaluation of asymptomatic hematuria; yet even the claim to this final indication now is coming under direct challenge from CT. One of the greatest weaknesses of CT regarding this application has been its relatively poor depiction of the renal-collecting structures and ureters, resulting from multiple factors including poor longitudinal resolution, poor distention of the collecting system, and obscuration of the urothelium by dense intraluminal contrast. Of course, hematuria may arise from any point along the urinary tract, but the role of imaging has centered largely on the upper tracts including the kidneys and ureters. While CT has excelled in the detection of urinary tract calculi and renal masses, its ability to depict small urothelial lesions has been of question historically, with reported sensitivities ranging from 50% to 90% (13–15). It is this shortcoming that previously has precluded the application of CT in the evaluation of asymptomatic hematuria because transitional cell carcinoma represents a potentially life-threatening etiology.

In the American Urological Association Best Practice Policy Recommendations for the evaluation of painless hematuria in adults, both CT and EU were suggested as being appropriate imaging modalities (16). Even before the publication of these recommendations, many institutions already had adopted the policy of supplementing EU with cross-sectional imaging in order to complement the sensitivity of EU for urothelial lesions with the sensitivity of cross-sectional modalities for renal parenchymal disease, as well as its greater overall efficacy in identifying the various potential etiologies that may cause hematuria. Clearly, a new paradigm for the imaging evaluation of asymptomatic hematuria is emerging, and while several approaches have been suggested, no clear consensus currently exists. Hybrid strategies of following EU with immediate CT (17) or following contrast-enhanced CT with immediate plain films (18) may be effective, but they are hampered by logistical issues of transferring patients rapidly between CT scanner and conventional radiography rooms. Similarly, an auxiliary CT tabletop that allows the acquisition of plain radiographs with a patient on the CT table has been developed and described (19), but this hardware is not available widely.

The introduction of MDCT finally has provided a tool that combines improved spatial resolution to image better the urothelium and the contrast resolution and cross-sectional information inherent to CT for the best evaluation of the renal parenchyma. The goal of MDCT urography is to provide a single examination capable of diagnosing the most important etiologies of hematuria involving the upper urinary tracts, which include calculi, renal-parenchymal tumors, and transitional cell carcinoma. By taking specific measures to distend the urinary tract, manipulating the timing of contrast administration to allow imaging during desired phases of enhancement, and using various reconstruction techniques, it is possible to obtain MDCT urograms capable of providing the information that previously required both EU and cross-sectional imaging. In fact, by reducing the complexity and duration of the diagnostic work up, the evaluation of patients with painless hematuria could be the genitourinary tract application upon which MDCT technology will have the greatest impact.

MULTIPHASIC MDCT UROGRAPHY— PROTOCOL CONSIDERATIONS

The role of the various phases of renal contrast enhancement in detecting and characterizing renal parenchymal lesions with spiral CT has been studied well (20–24). While each phase of enhancement contributes certain information, the value of multiple acquisitions through the same scan volume must be balanced against the potential deleterious effects of the increased radiation exposure imparted to the patient. Whereas the most straightforward strategy for MDCT urography would entail scanning in each of these four phases (11,25,26), a more tailored approach should allow evaluation of these structures with only two scan passes through the abdomen and pelvis (once pre- and once postcontrast), thus approximately halving the radiation dose delivered to the patient. It also would limit the total number of axial images obtained with each study. This technique should result in a total radiation dose less than that imparted by conventional EU combined with CT.

Clearly, nonenhanced images are necessary for the detection of urinary tract calculi, one of the most common of all etiologies of hematuria. Delayed excretory-phase images are critical for optimal depiction of the urothelium-lined collecting structures and ureters. Nephrographic-phase images are best for evaluation of the renal parenchyma, while it has been shown repeatedly that corticomedullary-phase images offer little in terms of added sensitivity for parenchymal lesions (20–23). Early phase imaging (scan delay of less than 45 seconds after start of contrast administration), while critical for assessing for renal arterial pathology, is of limited usefulness in evaluating patients with hematuria as it contributes significant additional information only in instances when an obstructed system may demonstrate subtle delayed renal enhancement or when a renal artery aneurysm may simulate a parenchymal mass.

With this in mind, it becomes apparent that three phases of renal enhancement must be imaged routinely—precontrast, nephrographic, and excretory phases. Conversely, the ureters need be imaged only during nonenhanced and excretory phases. In an effort to reduce radiation dose, tailored administration of IV contrast material in two sequential boluses separated by a set delay time allows simultaneous imaging of synchronous nephrographic and excretory phases

(12) (Figure 20-1). This arrangement allows the entire protocol to be completed with just two imaging passes through both abdomen and pelvis.

Another major consideration with MDCT urography is achieving sufficient distension of the urinary tract to allow complete visualization of the urothelium. Several strategies have been suggested that can be used in isolation or jointly. The first of these simply is applying abdominal compression with a balloon device inflated after administration of IV contrast material, resulting in distension of the abdominal ureters and renal collecting structures. Subsequent release of compression allows pooled contrast to pass inferiorly into the pelvic ureters (Figure 20-2). This is an effective time-tested strategy that has been used for decades with EU, for which it was described originally (27). While its advantages are simplicity, familiarity, and economy, imaging of the distended renal collecting structures during compression and of the distended pelvic ureters immediately after release of compression cannot be performed in one continuous acquisition, thus precluding a single volumetric dataset of the entire urinary tract. For this reason, 3D reconstructions depicting the urinary tract in its entirety are impractical with this technique and separate reconstructions of the abdomen and pelvis must be generated. In addition, one must be cognizant of the contraindications to abdominal compression that include abdominal aortic aneurysm, recent abdominal surgery, abdominal pain, urinary tract diversions, severe ascites, horseshoe kidney, and inferior vena cava filters.

Nolte-Ernsting and colleagues have suggested the administration of diuretic agents such as furosemide as another method of achieving urinary tract distension for MDCT urography (28) (Figure 20-3). They studied 21 patients with MDCT urography using a four-detector CT scanner and compared the use of 10 mg of intravenously administered furosemide 3 minutes to 5 minutes prior to contrast material injection in 16 patients versus a 250 cc bolus of saline in addition to contrast material in 5 patients on urinary tract visualization. In this limited number of patients, they found that there was more consistent uniform visualization of the upper urinary tract with the diuretic technique, and also that patients who had not received furosemide had 4 to 5 times higher attenuation values within the enhanced collecting structures. Highly concentrated excreted intraluminal contrast agent can diminish the quality of a CT urogram by leading to linear streak artifacts, as well as a loss of fine calyceal detail (10), both of which theoretically could obscure small urothelial lesions or intraluminal-filling defects. An added benefit of pharmacologic diuresis appears to be relative dilution of excreted contrast material within the collecting structures, thus minimizing or preventing these adverse consequences (28).

Imaging of patients in the prone position in an effort to provide greater distension of the urinary tract also has been described, but it has been shown that although prone imaging provides similar distension of the upper urinary tract compared to abdominal compression, distension of the distal

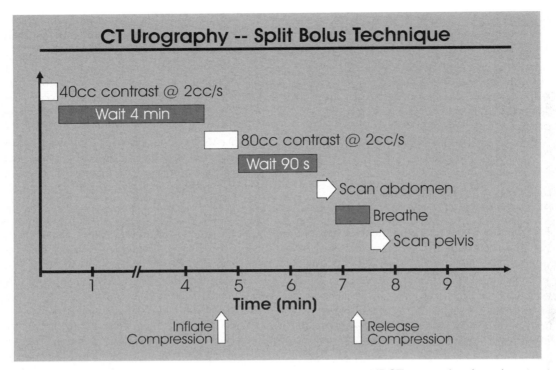

FIG. 20–1. Technique for contrast-enhanced phases of split-bolus MDCT urography. A total contrast dose of 120 cc (300 mg I/mL) is divided into two boluses separated by a delay of at least 2 minutes. Abdominal scan is performed 2 minutes after injection of the second bolus during synchronous nephrographic and excretory phases. The pelvis is scanned immediately after release of compression to allow pooled contrast in the collecting system to distend the mid-to-distal ureters.

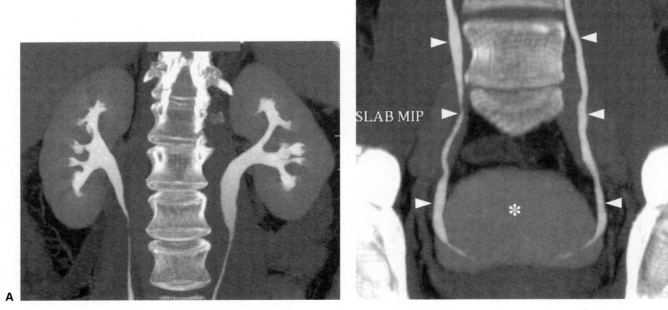

FIG. 20–2. Normal CT urogram. **A:** Coronal thick-slab MIP of the kidneys and upper ureters from a MDCT urography [8-detector row CT, 1.25-mm nominal section thickness (NST), 0.6-mm interval] provides high contrast between the collecting system and renal parenchyma. Notice the superimposition of various portions of the collecting system. **B:** Coronal MIP of the lower ureters in the same patient. The normal ureters vary in width throughout their course (*arrowheads*).

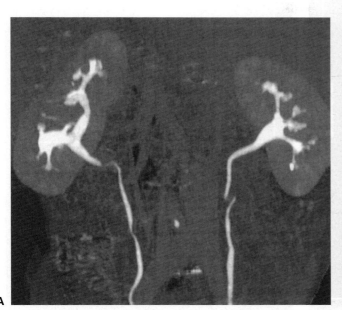
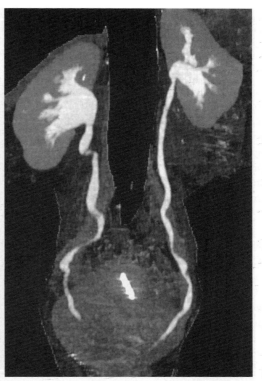

A

B

FIG. 20–3. Normal diuretic CT urogram. **A:** Coronal MIP image of the kidneys and proximal ureters from a MDCT urography (4-detector row CT, 4-mm × 2.5-mm mode, 3-mm slice thickness, 1-mm interval) obtained approximately 5 minutes after the intravenous administration of 10 mg of furosemide shows good opacification of all segments of the renal collecting system, renal pelvises, and proximal ureters. **B:** Coronal MIP image from a MDCT urography using the same technique in another patient depicts one of the advantages of diuretic MDCT urography—the possibility of acquiring a single continuous dataset that includes the entire urinary tract. Osseous elements were edited manually from the dataset prior to generation of MIP images. (Courtesy of Claus Nolte-Ernsting and Joachim E. Wildberger, Department of Radiology, University of Technology, Aachen, Germany)

ureter is superior after release of compression than with prone CTU (10). Additionally, prone CT imaging generally is tolerated less well by patients and is limited by the same contraindications as abdominal compression.

Finally, hydration prior to scanning, either orally or intravenously, is a strategy that can and should be used in conjunction with either abdominal compression or pharma-cologic diuresis. Adequate hydration prior to imaging helps to ensure a natural diuresis with all of its attendant benefits, including urinary tract distension and dilution of excreted contrast material. Additionally, proper hydration prior to contrast administration helps to protect against the nephro-toxic effects of iodinated contrast material (29,30).

At the authors' institution, the MDCT urography proto-col begins with the oral administration of approximately 900 cc of water 15 minutes to 20 minutes prior to scanning, while the patient is in the waiting area. The scan is performed with the patient supine in three distinct phases as follows (Figure 20-4):

I. Precontrast
   a. Compression balloon in place, not inflated
   b. Digital scout view abdomen/pelvis
   c. Scan abdomen/pelvis, 4-mm × 5-mm or 8-mm × 2.5-mm mode
II. Postcontrast with compression
   a. 40 cc nonionic contrast (300 mg I/mL) at 2 cc/sec
   b. 4-minute delay
   c. 80 cc nonionic contrast (300 mg I/mL) at 2 cc/sec
   d. Inflate compression balloon
   e. 90-second delay
   f. Scan abdomen, 4-mm × 2.5-mm, 8-mm × 1.25-mm, or 16-mm × 1.25-mm mode
   g. Scout view abdomen/pelvis
III. Postcontrast, postrelease of compression
   a. Release compression
   b. Scan pelvis, 4-mm × 2.5-mm, 8-mm × 1.25-mm, or 16-mm × 1.25-mm mode
   c. Scout view abdomen/pelvis

Relatively high pitch values of approximately 1.5 pro-vide more rapid scanning for the same anatomic volume with little loss in image quality. With a MDCT scanner, each phase of the study can be performed with a breathhold of

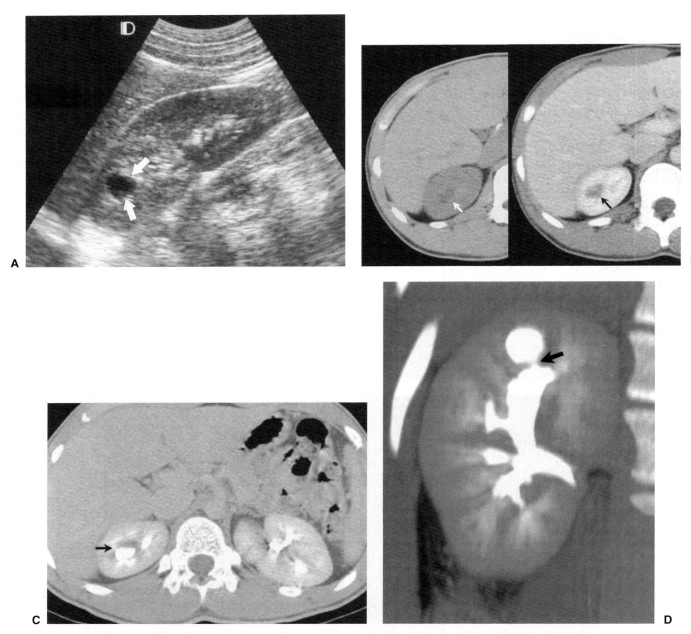

FIG. 20–6. Patient referred for evaluation of hematuria and solid lesion identified on US and CT at another institution. **A:** Longitudinal sonogram of the right kidney from outside institution shows a 1.3 cm nearly anechoic upper-pole lesion with posterior acoustic enhancement and a question of mural nodularity (*arrows*). **B:** Pre- and postcontrast-enhanced CT from same institution demonstrated apparent enhancement of this lesion (*arrows*) from 8 HU to 39 HU, suggesting a solid renal mass. **C:** Axial image from CTU shows dependent layering of contrast agent (*arrow*) within this structure, indicating a nonsolid nature and implying communication with the collecting system. **D:** Double-oblique MIP image of the right kidney from CTU shows a calyceal diverticulum and its communication with the collecting system (*arrow*). [Reprinted with permission from the *American Journal of Roentgenology* (2001;177(4): 849–855). Copyright 2001, American Roentgen Ray Society.]

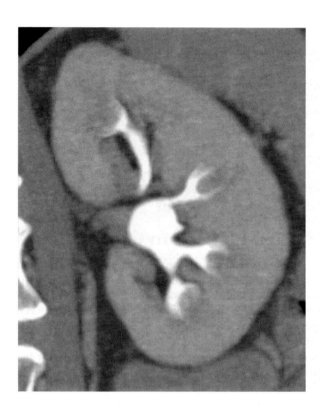

FIG. 20–7. Normal CT urogram (8-detector row CT, 1.25-mm NST, 0.6-mm interval). Coronal oblique thin-slab MIP of the right kidney (truly coronal to the kidney) allows evaluation of each portion of the collecting system without problems of obscuration by superimposition. Sharp calyces and normal papillae are depicted clearly.

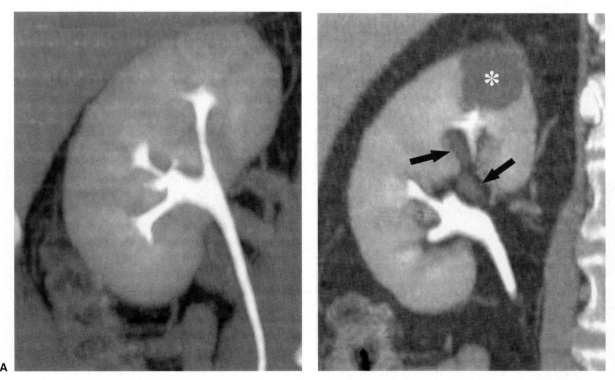

A   B

FIG. 20–8. Simple cysts. Thick-slab MIP image from MDCTU (4-detector row CT, 2.5-mm NST, 1.25-mm interval) **(A)** should not be interpreted in isolation as low-attenuation lesions are obscured by brightly enhancing parenchyma or collecting structures. **B:** Thin-slab MIP clearly depicts a 3-cm simple cyst in the upper pole (*) and several small peripelvic cysts (*arrows*) that are absent from the thick-slab MIP image.

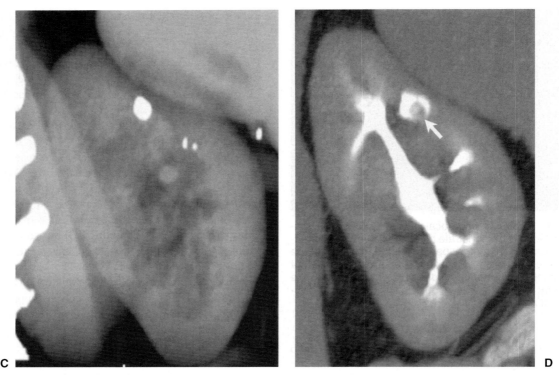

FIG. 20–12. *Continued.* Coronal oblique MIP images from CTU (4-detector row, 2.5-mm NST, 1.25-mm interval) before **(C)** and after **(D)** contrast demonstrate three upper-pole calculi, one of which is within an upper-pole calyceal diverticulum (*arrow*). Stone analysis revealed urate composition, consistent with their radiolucent nature on conventional EU. [Reprinted with permission from the *American Journal of Roentgenology* (2001;177(4):849–855). Copyright 2001, American Roentgen Ray Society.]

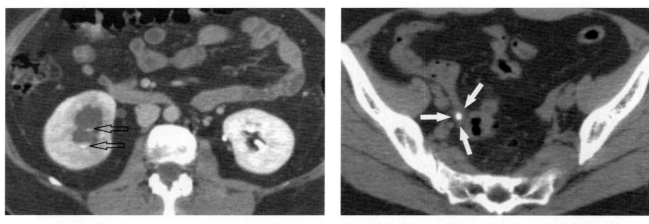

FIG. 20–13. Obstructing distal ureteral calculus. Axial image **(A)** through the kidneys from CTU (4-detector row CT, 2.5-mm NST, 1.25-mm interval) shows moderate right-sided hydronephrosis with delayed enhancement of the right kidney. Layering excreted contrast agent is seen within dependent portions of the dilated collecting system (*arrows*). Distal ureteral calculus is seen on an axial image through the pelvis **(B)** and is differentiated from a phlebolith by a rim of surrounding soft tissue (*arrows*) representing inflamed ureteral wall. *(continued)*

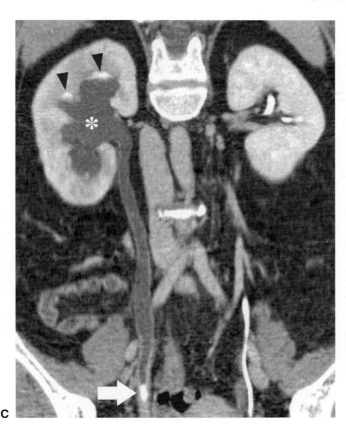

C

FIG. 20–13. *Continued.* A curved planar reformation (C) through the right renal pelvis and ureter clearly demonstrates the dilated urinary tract to the level of the obstructing calculus (*arrow*). Delayed enhancement of the right kidney and excreted contrast (*arrowheads*) in the dilated collecting system (***) also are depicted on this single image.

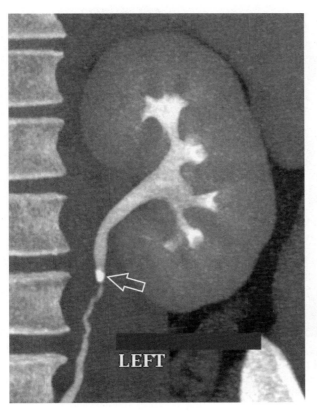

LEFT

FIG. 20–14. Coronal MIP image from MDCTU (8-detector row, 1.25-mm NST, 0.6-mm interval) demonstrates a stone lodged in the proximal left ureter (*arrow*) without hydronephrosis or other evidence of obstruction. Although many stones will be denser than intraluminal contrast, as in this example, precontrast images should be used for the identification of urinary tract calculi, as the potential exists for stones to be isoattenuating with and obscured by intraluminal contrast.

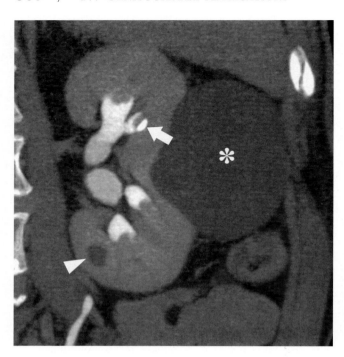

FIG. 20–15. Intrarenal calculi also can be depicted clearly with CTU (8-detector row, 1.25-mm NST, 0.6-mm interval), as in this case of a stone in an upper-pole calyx (*arrow*) depicted on a thin-slab MIP image. A large simple cyst (*) exerts substantial mass effect upon the interpolar portion of the kidney. A smaller cyst is present in the lower pole (*arrowhead*).

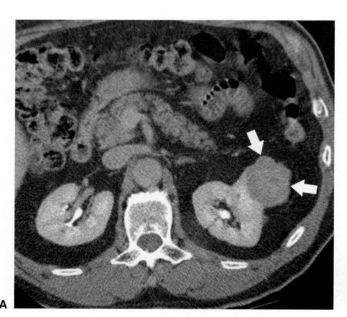

A

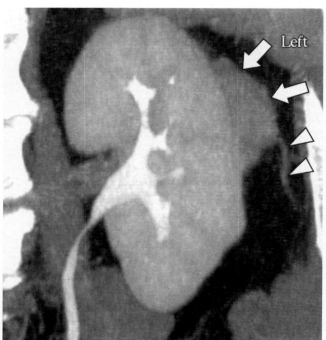

B

FIG. 20–16. Renal cell carcinoma. A 3-cm exophytic mass projects off the anterior surface of the left kidney upper pole (*arrows*) on an axial image from CTU (8-detector-row CT, 1.25-mm NST, 1.25-mm interval) **(A)**. Thick-slab coronal MIP **(B)** image again depicts this mass (*arrows*) with a feeding vessel (*arrowheads*) and a normal appearance of the collecting system.

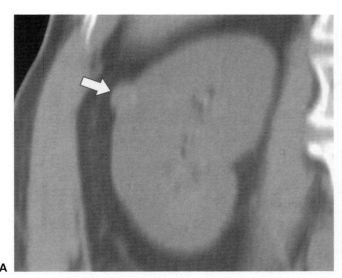

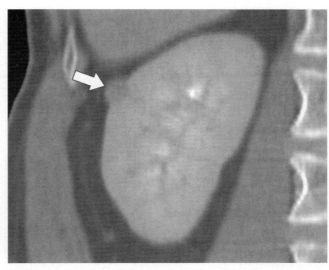

A   B

FIG. 20–17. Renal cell carcinoma. **A:** Coronal MIP image from MDCT urogram (4-detector row CT, 2.5-mm NST, 1.25-mm interval) shows small round exophytic mass along the lateral aspect of the right kidney that is hyperattenuating to kidney (40 HU), simulating a hemorrhagic cyst. **B:** Postcontrast MIP image shows this lesion to be hypoattenuating to renal parenchyma, again simulating a complex cyst, but ROI interrogation reveals enhancement of the lesion to 70 HU, indicating a solid mass. Pathology revealed grade-III papillary renal cell carcinoma.

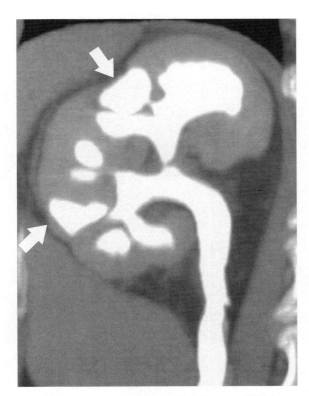

FIG. 20–18. Chronic pyelonephritis. Coronal MIP image of the right kidney in a 57-year-old woman from CTU (2.5-mm NST, 4-detector row CT) demonstrates markedly dilated calyces that protrude beyond the interpapillary line where there is overlying cortical thinning. [Reprinted with permission from the *American Journal of Roentgenology* (2001;177(4): 849–855). Copyright 2001, American Roentgen Ray Society.]

such findings by dense intraluminal contrast material (Figure 20-19). While bone windows are a useful first approximation for this purpose, settings unfortunately must be tailored individually in many cases, as the concentration of intraluminal contrast material will vary from patient to patient. Similarly, axial images obtained through the pelvis after release of abdominal compression should be viewed with the same window-to-level settings. Occasionally, because of peristalsis, a segment of ureter may not be distended at the time of acquisition. Digital scout images obtained at each phase of the study serve as a second chance at visualizing these nondistended segments, although with good hydration and compression, it is unusual for this to become necessary (32).

Transitional cell carcinomas may be detected on the noncontrast images, particularly when obstruction is present. The attenuation values of transitional cell carcinoma on enhanced scans typically are slightly greater than that of adjacent water-density urine but less than that of other potential filling defects such as blood clot and stones (33,34) and enhance only minimally after contrast is given (34,35) (Figure 20-20). Obstruction will occur earlier or later in the natural history of a given tumor depending upon its anatomic location and pattern of growth. Three specific gross morphologies have been described with CT: focal intraluminal mass, ureteral wall thickening, and infiltrating mass (36). Certainly, tumors located in strategically narrow locations, such as the infundibula and ureters (Figure 20-21), and those with more profuse intraluminal growth will obstruct earlier.

It must be emphasized that, while it often is possible to diagnose masses involving the urinary bladder (Figure 20-22), this protocol is not optimized for the evaluation of

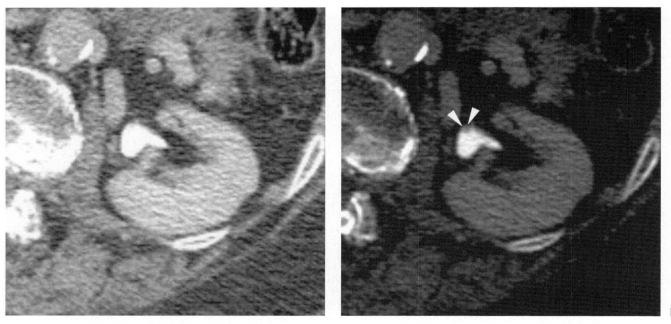

FIG. 20–19. Transitional cell carcinoma. Very small urothelial lesions such as this renal pelvis transitional cell carcinoma may be identified by MDCT urogram, as long as the proper window-level settings are used. The lesion is virtually invisible when viewing standard abdominal settings of 400 and 40 **(A)**, but becomes visible as a 3-mm filling defect (*arrowheads*) when wider windows (900 and 425) are used **(B)**. This lesion likely would be difficult to detect on EU given its small size and location, which would result in its being imaged en face rather than in profile.

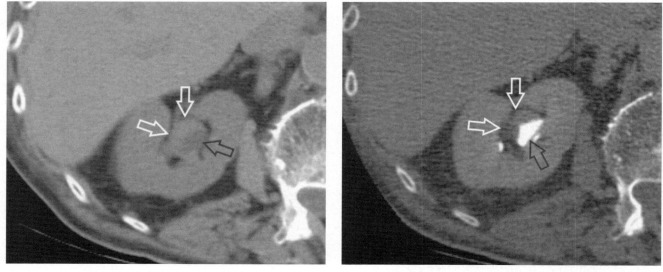

FIG. 20–20. Infundibular transitional-cell carcinoma on CTU (8-detector row CT, 1.25-mm NST, 0.6-mm interval). Precontrast axial-CT image through the upper pole of the left kidney **(A)** shows thickening of the urothelium (*white arrows*) within the collecting system, clearly separate from the renal parenchyma and slightly higher in attenuation than intraluminal urine (*black arrow*). *(continued)*

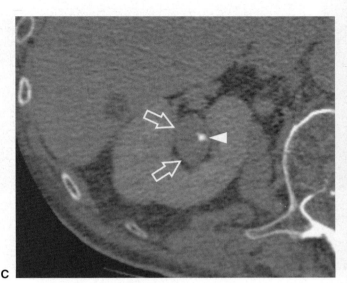

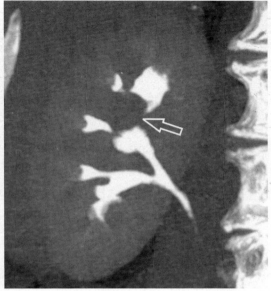

C   D

FIG. 20–20. *Continued.* Enhanced axial-CT images through the same level **(B)** and at a level slightly more caudal **(C)** demonstrate the urothelial mass and collecting system that is narrowed markedly (*arrowhead*) to better advantage. The full extent of this lesion and narrowing of the upper-pole infundibulum (*arrow*) by this mass is demonstrated better on a coronal MIP image from CTU **(D)**.

the bladder. Although virtual cystoscopy with MDCT certainly is feasible (37), patients with painless hematuria are evaluated best with conventional cystoscopy that can be performed rapidly and that has the benefit of offering a tissue diagnosis.

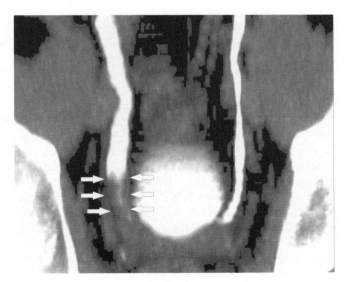

FIG. 20–21. Distal ureteral transitional cell carcinoma in a 45-year-old man with asymptomatic hematuria. Coronal MIP image from MDCT urogram (4-detector row CT, 2.5-mm NST, 1.25-mm interval) demonstrates a concentric mass involving the distal right ureter. Note the relative distension of the right ureter when compared to the left. [Reprinted with permission from the *American Journal of Roentgenology* (2001;177(4): 849–855). Copyright 2001, American Roentgen Ray Society.]

MDCT UROGRAPHY—ADVANTAGES AND DISADVANTAGES

A prospective study directly comparing the efficacy of MDCT urography versus that of EU in individual patients with asymptomatic hematuria poses an ethical dilemma given that it would require that patients undergo two studies, applying ionizing radiation and iodinated contrast material. Two studies have compared the ability of CTU with abdominal compression and EU to depict clearly various segments of the urinary tract—one with single-detector spiral CT and one with MDCT. Both have found that CTU is equivalent or superior to EU in this endeavor (10,25). Similarly, early work has demonstrated the ability of diuretic MDCT urography to depict complete or near-complete opacification of the ureters and pelvicaliceal systems in 94% and 100% of cases respectively (28). An additional advantage of CTU is that there is no need for bowel preparation prior to the study and that the presence of enteric contents (other than intraluminal contrast) has no bearing on the quality of the study obtained. In fact, oral contrast material should be avoided as it may complicate the generation of 3D reformations by obscuring the kidneys and ureters.

A major advantage of CTU over EU is the ability to stage disease. Computed tomography has been used widely for the staging of renal cell carcinoma and is able to depict extrarenal extension, venous invasion, and lymph-node involvement with even single-detector axial CT providing 91% accuracy (38), failing primarily when microscopic invasion goes undetected. The ability of CT to stage upper-tract transitional cell cancers has been somewhat more controver-

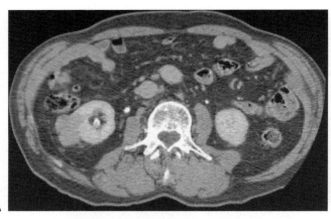

A

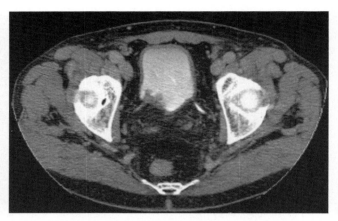

B

FIG. 20–22. Seventy-nine-year-old man on warfarin sodium for atrial fibrillation with gross painless hematuria. Multidetector CT urogram (8-detector row CT, 1.25-mm NST, 0.6-mm interval) demonstrates an exophytic 3-cm right-renal mass **(A)** and a polypoid mass at the bladder orifice **(B)** of the right ureter. Pathology revealed synchronous renal cell and transitional cell carcinoma.

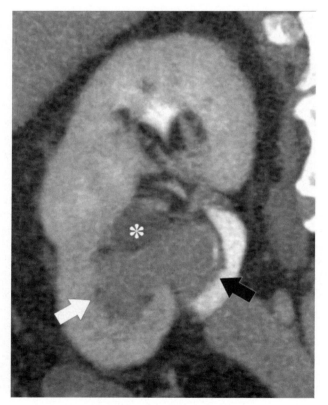

FIG. 20–23. Transitional cell carcinoma. Coronal thin-slab MIP image of the right kidney from CTU (8-detector row, 1.25-mm NST, 0.6-mm interval) of a woman with 2-week history of intermittent gross painless hematuria. A soft tissue mass (*white arrow*) fills a lower-pole calyx and infundibulum. Its medial margin is irregular (*black arrow*) and bulges into the renal pelvis. A fluid-attenuation triangular structure (*) represents an obstructed calyx. No clear fat plane is evident between the mass and renal parenchyma, and medullary invasion was present at pathologic examination.

sial with staging accuracies ranging from 36% to 83% (13,14,36,39,40). Neither CT nor any other imaging modality has been able to distinguish Stage-I tumors (limited to the urothelium and lamina propria layers) from Stage II (involving but not beyond the muscularis layer) (36). A more clinically pertinent question, however, is the ability to differentiate early (Stage I and Stage II) from advanced (Stage III and Stage IV) disease where there is invasion into the peripelvic or periureteral fat, frank renal-parenchymal invasion (Figure 20-23), lymph-node involvement, or distant metastases. Once again, microscopic nodal involvement has been the weak point of CT staging, with multiple studies demonstrating both under- and overstaging of nodal involvement (13,14,36,39,40). Importantly, however, all of these studies were conducted on older-generation single-row detector CT equipment, some even before the advent of spiral CT. It remains to be seen if MDCT will improve upon these numbers.

Critics of CTU have cited the inferior inherent spatial resolution of CT when compared with EU as a disadvantage. With current 16-slice MDCT scanners able to provide truly isotropic voxel sizes of approximately 0.7 mm, however, spatial resolution hardly can be considered a limitation of the technique. Even with 4- and 8-detector row scanners, near isotropic resolution is possible with nominal section thicknesses of 1 mm to 1.25 mm. Moreover, when the superior contrast resolution, ability to provide cross-sectional information with reconstruction in any plane, and added depiction of nonurinary-tract organs by CT are considered, it seems clear that MDCT urography is the study best suited for the detection and characterization of the myriad potential etiologies underlying hematuria.

REFERENCES

1. Smith RC, Rosenfield AT, Choe KA, et al. Acute flank pain: comparison of non-contrast-enhanced CT and intravenous urography. *Radiology* 1995;194(3):789–794.

2. Smith RC, Verga M, Dalrymple N, et al. Acute ureteral obstruction: value of secondary signs of helical unenhanced CT. *AJR Am J Roentgenol* 1996;167(5):1109–1113.
3. Smith RC, Coll DM. Helical computed tomography in the diagnosis of ureteric colic. *BJU Int* 2000;86 Suppl 1:33–41.
4. Smith RC, Levine J, Dalrymple NC, et al. Acute flank pain: a modern approach to diagnosis and management. *Semin Ultrasound CT MR* 1999;20(2):108–135.
5. Dalrymple NC, Verga M, Anderson KR, et al. The value of unenhanced helical computerized tomography in the management of acute flank pain. *J Urol* 1998;159(3):735–740.
6. Katz DS, Scheer M, Lumerman JH, et al. Alternative or additional diagnoses on unenhanced helical computed tomography for suspected renal colic: experience with 1000 consecutive examinations. *Urology* 2000;56(1):53–57.
7. Heneghan JP, Dalrymple NC, Verga M, et al. Soft-tissue ''rim'' sign in the diagnosis of ureteral calculi with use of unenhanced helical CT. *Radiology* 1997;202(3):709–711.
8. Bell TV, Fenlon HM, Davison BD, et al. Unenhanced helical CT criteria to differentiate distal ureteral calculi from pelvic phleboliths. *Radiology* 1998;207(2):363–367.
9. Sommer FG, Jeffrey RB Jr, Rubin GD, et al. Detection of ureteral calculi in patients with suspected renal colic: value of reformatted noncontrast helical CT. *AJR Am J Roentgenol* 1995;165(3):509–513.
10. McNicholas MM, Raptopoulos VD, Schwartz RK, et al. Excretory phase CT urography for opacification of the urinary collecting system. *AJR Am J Roentgenol* 1998;170(5):1261–1267.
11. Caoili EM, Cohan RH, Korobkin M, et al. Urinary tract abnormalities: initial experience with multi-detector row CT urography. *Radiology* 2002;222(2):353–360.
12. Chow LC, Sommer FG. Multidetector CT urography with abdominal compression and three-dimensional reconstruction. *AJR Am J Roentgenol* 2001;177(4):849–855.
13. McCoy JG, Honda H, Reznicek M, et al. Computerized tomography for detection and staging of localized and pathologically defined upper tract urothelial tumors. *J Urol* 1991;146(6):1500–1503.
14. Planz B, George R, Adam G, et al. Computed tomography for detection and staging of transitional cell carcinoma of the upper urinary tract. *Eur Urol* 1995;27(2):146–150
15. Badalament RA, Bennett WF, Bova JG, et al. Computed tomography of primary transitional cell carcinoma of upper urinary tracts. *Urology* 1992;40(1):71–75.
16. Grossfeld GD, Litwin MS, Wolf JS Jr, et al. Evaluation of asymptomatic microscopic hematuria in adults: the American Urological Association best practice policy—part II: patient evaluation, cytology, voided markers, imaging, cystoscopy, nephrology evaluation, and follow-up. *Urology* 2001;57(4):604–610.
17. Perlman ES, Rosenfield AT, Wexler JS, et al. CT urography in the evaluation of urinary tract disease. *J Comput Assist Tomogr* 1996;20(4):620–626
18. The Society of Uroradiology CT. Urography Committee Draft Protocol. In: Society of Uroradiology Annual Meeting, 2000. Kauai, Hawaii; 2000
19. McCollough CH, Daly TR, King BF Jr, et al. An auxiliary CT tabletop for radiography at the time of CT. *J Comput Assist Tomogr* 2001;25(6):876–880.
20. Cohan RH, Sherman LS, Korobkin M, et al. Renal masses: assessment of corticomedullary-phase and nephrographic-phase CT scans. *Radiology* 1995;196(2):445–451.
21. Birnbaum BA, Jacobs JE, Ramchandani P. Multiphasic renal CT: comparison of renal mass enhancement during the corticomedullary and nephrographic phases. *Radiology* 1996;200(3):753–758.
22. Kopka L, Fischer U, Zoeller G, et al. Dual-phase helical CT of the kidney: value of the corticomedullary and nephrographic phase for evaluation of renal lesions and preoperative staging of renal cell carcinoma. *AJR Am J Roentgenol* 1997;169(6):1573–1578.
23. Szolar DH, Kammerhuber F, Altziebler S, et al. Multiphasic helical CT of the kidney: increased conspicuity for detection and characterization of small (< 3-cm) renal masses. *Radiology* 1997;202(1):211–217.
24. Zeman RK, Zeiberg A, Hayes WS, et al. Helical CT of renal masses: the value of delayed scans. *AJR Am J Roentgenol* 1996;167(3):771–776.
25. Heneghan JP, Kim DH, Leder RA, et al. Compression CT urography: a comparison with IVU in the opacification of the collecting system and ureters. *J Comput Assist Tomogr* 2001;25(3):343–347.
26. Lang EK, Macchia RJ, Thomas R, et al. Computerized tomography tailored for the assessment of microscopic hematuria. *J Urol* 2002;167(2 Pt 1):547–554.
27. Ziegler J. Significance and technique of compression of the ureter in elimination pyelography. *Dtsch Med Wochenschr* 1930;56:1772–1775
28. Nolte-Ernsting CC, Wildberger JE, Borchers H, et al. Multi-slice CT urography after diuretic injection: initial results. *Rofo Fortschr Geb Rontgenstr Neuen Bildgeb Verfahr* 2001;173(3):176–180.
29. Eisenberg RL, Bank WO, Hedgock MW. Renal failure after major angiography can be avoided with hydration. *AJR Am J Roentgenol* 1981;136(5):859–861.
30. Gerlach AT, Pickworth KK. Contrast medium-induced nephrotoxicity: pathophysiology and prevention. *Pharmacotherapy* 2000;20(5):540–548.
31. Napel S, Rubin GD, Jeffrey RB Jr. STS–MIP: a new reconstruction technique for CT of the chest. *J Comput Assist Tomogr* 1993;17(5):832–838.
32. Chow LC, Sommer FG. Multidetector CT urography with abdominal compression and reconstruction by sliding thin-slab maximum intensity projection (abstract). *Radiology* 2001;221(P):251
33. Urban BA, Buckley J, Soyer P, et al. CT appearance of transitional cell carcinoma of the renal pelvis: Part 1. Early-stage disease. *AJR Am J Roentgenol* 1997;169(1):157–161.
34. Gatewood OM, Goldman SM, Marshall FF, et al. Computerized tomography in the diagnosis of transitional cell carcinoma of the kidney. *J Urol* 1982;127(5):876–887.
35. Leder RA, Dunnick NR. Transitional cell carcinoma of the pelvicalices and ureter. *AJR Am J Roentgenol* 1990;155(4):713–722.
36. Baron RL, McClennan BL, Lee JK, et al. Computed tomography of transitional-cell carcinoma of the renal pelvis and ureter. *Radiology* 1982;144(1):125–130.
37. Conrad LK, Kirsh EJ, Steinberg G, et al. Comparative viewing modalities for CT cystography. *Abdom Imaging* 2001;26(1):92–97.
38. Johnson CD, Dunnick NR, Cohan RH, et al. Renal adenocarcinoma: CT staging of 100 tumors. *AJR Am J Roentgenol* 1987;148(1):59–63.
39. Buckley JA, Urban BA, Soyer P, et al. Transitional cell carcinoma of the renal pelvis: a retrospective look at CT staging with pathologic correlation. *Radiology* 1996;201(1):194–198.
40. Scolieri MJ, Paik ML, Brown SL, et al. Limitations of computed tomography in the preoperative staging of upper tract urothelial carcinoma. *Urology* 2000;56(6):930–934.

CHAPTER 21

CT of the Female Pelvis

Harpreet K. Pannu

INTRODUCTION

The introduction of multidetector computed tomography (MDCT) is changing the way the pelvis is scanned. The multiple-detector rows in scanners allow simultaneous acquisition of multiple slices, each with reduced slice thickness, to give high-resolution scans of the entire pelvis in seconds. The timing of the scan can be optimized to arterial or venous phases, and the images can be reconstructed using three-dimensional (3D) volume rendering or multiplanar reconstruction (MPR). Pelvic anatomy is not always visualized optimally in the axial plane, and display in the sagittal and coronal planes similar to magnetic resonance imaging (MRI) may prove valuable in detecting and defining disease.

The role of computed tomography (CT) in the pelvis up to the present time has been mainly in staging advanced malignancies and diagnosing inflammatory conditions of the gastrointestinal and genitourinary systems. This has been due to technical limitations with nonspiral and, subsequently, spiral single-detector row scanners. In general, the pelvis is scanned after the abdomen as part of one examination. Owing to limitations of tube heating and scan times with single-detector row CT, the emphasis has been on obtaining optimal studies of the abdominal viscera with lesser detail on the pelvic study. Thicker slices after longer scan delays typically were obtained of the pelvis. Consequently, the value of CT in staging early malignancies or detecting early tumor recurrences has not been optimal. These limitations may be reduced by obtaining thin slices and multiplanar and 3D reconstruction with MDCT. Although initial examination of the gynecologic organs generally is performed with ultrasound and MRI, the ready availability of CT and short examination times have given CT a role in patient management.

In this chapter, some of the common indications for CT of the pelvis and the technique for the study will be reviewed. The focus will be on imaging of the female pelvis. Areas where the technological advances of MDCT may have a clinical impact also will be explored.

CT TECHNIQUE

Since pelvic pathology can extend into the abdomen due to continuity of the peritoneal cavity, both the abdomen and pelvis are included in the scan (Table 21.1). The scan direction can be caudal to cranial or cranial to caudal. In patients with gynecologic malignancies, thin slices during bolus-contrast injection are obtained from the pubic symphysis to the iliac crest on a single-detector scanner. This is followed by a scan from the iliac crest to the diaphragm. For inflammatory conditions, since slice thickness and contrast bolus are not as critical, the scan direction is usually from the diaphragm to the symphysis pubis on a single-detector scanner. With MDCT, the scan direction also can be tailored depending on the clinical problem, however timing is not as critical and most scans are done cranial to caudal.

Positive oral contrast is given to opacify bowel loops that can mimic cystic-gynecologic masses such as hydrosalpinx, ovarian lesions, and necrotic tumors. Oral contrast (750 mL to 1000 mL) is given starting 90 minutes prior to the study. Oral contrast also can be given the night before to opacify the sigmoid colon. Oral water is helpful in cases of calcified metastatic-ovarian implants, where distinction from bowel is easier with negative oral contrast. Intravenous (IV) contrast is injected to distinguish normal branches of the internal iliac vessels from nodes, and to distinguish bladder diverticula from cystic-gynecologic masses. One-hundred-and-twenty milliliters of nonionic contrast is injected intravenously at 2 mL to 3 mL per second.

The scan typically is started 50 seconds after initiating the contrast injection. A second scan after a delay of 5 minutes also can be obtained after the distal ureters and bladder are opacified to assess for ureteral encasement in patients with gynecologic malignancies such as cervical cancer. If true arterial- and venous-phase imaging is desired for vascular mapping, a delay of 30 seconds is used for the arterial phase and 60 seconds for the venous phase with MDCT. Three-dimensional mapping of the relationship of masses to pelvic vessels and vascular anatomy for invasive procedures can be generated using these images.

TABLE 21–1. *CT technique*

Parameter	SDCT	MDCT
Scan direction	Caudal cranial	Caudal cranial or cranial caudal
Oral contrast	Positive contrast	Positive contrast or water
IV contrast	2–3 mL/sec, 120 mL	2–3 mL/sec, 120 mL
Scan delay	1) 50 sec 2) 5 min-delayed images for bladder enhancement as indicated	1) Arterial- and venous-phase imaging if indicated 2) 50 sec 3) 5 min delayed images for bladder enhancement as indicated
Slice thickness	5 mm	1) 3 mm for gynecologic malignancies 2) 5 mm for inflammatory disease
Slice-reconstruction interval	5 mm	1) 2 mm for gynecologic malignancies 2) 5 mm for inflammatory disease
Detector collimation	—	2.5 mm
Postprocessing	—	Multiplanar reconstruction and volume rendering

The slice thickness with a single-detector scanner is typically 5-mm slices at 5-mm intervals. If 3-mm slices are obtained, the scan times may increase to where they are limited by patient breath hold. With MDCT, 3-mm to 5-mm slices can be reconstructed every 3 mm. If additional detail is needed, 1.00-mm to 1.25-mm sections can be acquired. Thin slices are obtained for determining local extension of gynecologic malignancies into the parametrium or invasion of the bladder and rectum. The pelvis is a common site for peritoneal implants, and thin slices may be used to evaluate for subcentimeter implants. Artifact on sagittal and coronal reconstructed slices also is reduced with thinner slices.

In summary, a sample technique for single-detector scanners is administration of oral and IV contrast, and 5-mm slices at 5-mm intervals from symphysis pubis to diaphragm with a scan delay of 50 seconds. A sample protocol for a 4-detector row multidetector scanner (Somatom Volume Zoom scanner, Siemens Medical Solutions, Iselin, NJ) is detector collimation of 2.5 mm, slice thickness of 3 mm, and reconstruction interval of 2 mm. Postprocessing of data into coronal or sagittal multiplanar or volume-rendered images will depend on the clinical application and the questions to be answered.

NORMAL FEMALE PELVIC ANATOMY

The uterus can be anteflexed with the fundus anterior and superior to the bladder, or it can be retroflexed with the

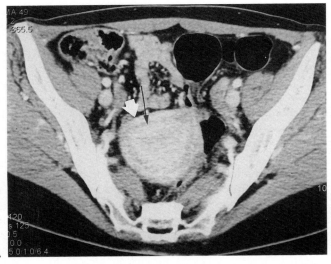

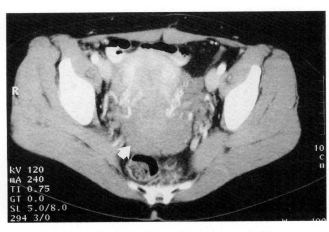

FIG. 21–1. Normal enhancement patterns of the uterus and cervix. **A:** Axial CT of the pelvis with IV contrast in a 40-year-old woman. There is enhancement of the inner and outer myometrium (*arrows*). **B:** Axial CT of the pelvis with IV contrast in a different patient. The cervix (*arrow*) is hypodense to the enhancing outer myometrium on this relatively early scan.

fundus posterior adjacent to the rectosigmoid colon and the cervix lying anterior to the uterine body. The uterus is homogeneous and of soft-tissue attenuation on unenhanced CT scans. It has a variable pattern of enhancement with contrast injection (1). Initially, the junction of the endometrium and myometrium may enhance, the outer myometrium may enhance, or the entire myometrium may enhance diffusely (Figure 21-1). The endometrium is seen as a hypodense area on these early scans and this appearance may mimic endometrial fluid. On scans delayed by several minutes, the endometrium and myometrium both enhance and cannot be distinguished. Similar to the uterine body, the cervix also enhances initially in the inner layer. It can appear hypodense to the myometrium on early scans. On delayed scans, there is more homogeneous enhancement of the cervix.

The parametrium is the soft tissue surrounding the uterus. It contains arterial and venous branches of the internal iliac vessels, the cardinal and uterosacral ligaments, the ureters, and the lymph nodes. The ovaries also lie lateral to the uterus and are seen as soft-tissue-density structures with cystic areas, depending on the age of the patient.

There are three lymphatic pathways for the spread of disease: along the external iliac vessels, internal iliac vessels, and presacral tissues (Figure 21-2) (2). In the external iliac route, the nodes lie posterior to the external iliac vein, between the external iliac artery and vein, or lateral to the external iliac artery (2). Tumor also can spread retrograde into the inguinal nodes. In the internal iliac route, the nodes are adjacent to the branches of the internal iliac artery and the junctional node between the internal and external iliac

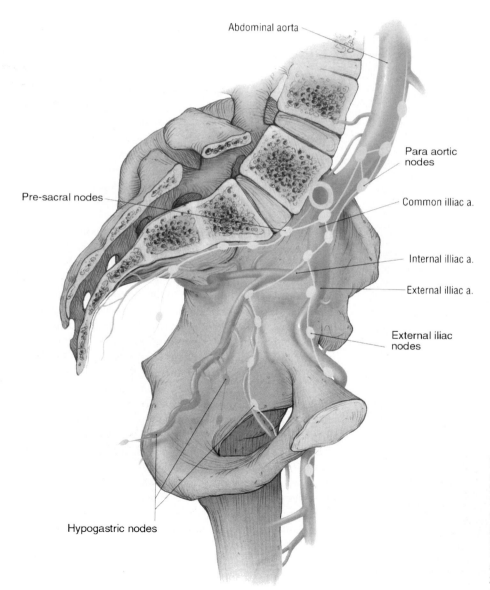

Abdominal aorta

Pre-sacral nodes

Para aortic nodes

Common illiac a.

Internal illiac a.

External illiac a.

External iliac nodes

Hypogastric nodes

FIG. 21–2. Nodal pathways of gynecologic disease. Sagittal illustration of the pelvis shows the three routes of lymphatic drainage for the gynecologic organs: the external iliac nodes, hypogastric nodes, and presacral nodes. (From Pannu HK, Corl FM, Fishman EK. CT evaluation of cervical cancer: spectrum of disease. *Radiographics* 2001;21:1155–1168, with permission.) (See color plate)

vessels can be enlarged (2). Common iliac nodes lie in the area between the common iliac arteries, between the common iliac vessels and psoas muscle and spine, or lateral to the common iliac artery (2). All three routes of spread lead to the paraaortic nodes (3,4). Normal short-axis diameter is less than or equal to 10 mm for the external iliac nodes, less than or equal to 7 mm for the internal iliac nodes, and less than or equal to 9 mm for the common iliac nodes (5).

GYNECOLOGIC NEOPLASMS

Single-Detector CT versus MDCT

The scan time is reduced with MDCT to 0.5 seconds compared with 0.75 seconds to 2.00 seconds for single-detector scanners. Slice thickness is typically 5 mm to 7 mm with a single-detector scanner and 3 mm to 5 mm with MDCT. The entire abdomen and pelvis can be scanned in approximately 35 seconds, even with thinner slices of 3 mm, with 4-row MDCT. Scan times are shorter with 16 row MDCT. For imaging gynecologic malignancies, there is improved spatial resolution on axial slices and the flexibility to reconstruct the images in various planes for detecting lesions and problem solving (Table 21.2, Figure 21-3). Since the data are acquired as a volume, images can be generated in multiple-user-defined planes after the patient has left the department.

Potential benefits of thin slices and multiplanar imaging lie in detecting small abdominal and/or pelvic implants and local extrauterine extension of tumor. Implants from ovarian, and occasionally endometrial, cancers can be few millimeters in size and difficult to detect with thick slices due to partial volume averaging. Thin slices over the relatively large area of the abdomen and pelvis are not routinely feasible with single-detector CT. Multiplanar reconstruction also is not optimal, owing to stair-step artifact from using thick slices. Therefore, curved structures such as the diaphragm and cul de sac are difficult to evaluate. Sagittal and coronal reconstructions using the thinner-slice MDCT dataset result in more optimal visualization of these areas. These images

TABLE 21–2. *Advantages of thin section CT with 3D reconstruction in gynecologic malignancy*

Region	CT display
Diaphragm	Surface of diaphragm displayed in coronal and sagittal planes for detection of plaquelike implants and minimal nodularity
Liver/spleen	Localization of surface implants in coronal plane as seen at surgery
Bowel	Multiplanar review to detect small lesions near bowel surfaces
Pelvic viscera	Generation of coronal and sagittal images similar to MR to assess for invasion of adjacent organs

can be used to confirm diaphragmatic, bowel, paracolic gutter, and pelvic implants, and to assess for additional lesions after review of the axial images (Figure 21-4).

Sagittal reconstructions also can demonstrate the planes between the uterus, bladder, and rectum, similar to magnetic resonance (MR). Since the uterus can be anteflexed or retroflexed, it may be tilted anteriorly or posteriorly on the axial images, obscuring the planes between the uterus and adjacent viscera. Distinction between normal parametrial vessels and ligaments from tumor also is difficult on thick slices, and restriction to the axial plane hinders assessment of the cranial–caudal extension of cervical-tumor volume (6,7). Thin slices and multiplanar images can be used to demonstrate the relationship of the gynecologic malignancy to adjacent pelvic viscera, cul de sac, vasculature, and pelvic sidewall, as well as to determine tumor size (Figure 21-5). Dual-phase imaging after IV contrast allows assessment of tumor enhancement (Figure 21-6).

Ovarian Cancer

Ovarian cancer is the second most common gynecologic malignancy to occur in women, but is the most common gynecologic cause of cancer-related death (8,9). Overall, it is the fifth most common malignancy in women (10), usually affecting postmenopausal women. There is no good screening method, owing to the low incidence of disease and lack of highly sensitive and specific screening tests (11,12). Symptoms also are nonspecific and include pain, bloating, and vaginal bleeding. Consequently, most patients have advanced disease at presentation (13).

The stages of ovarian cancer are tumor confined to the ovaries (Stage I), local extension into the pelvis (Stage II), tumor in the abdomen and pelvis or adenopathy (Stage III), and distant or parenchymal liver metastases (Stage IV) (14). The tumor can spread locally to the uterus and contralateral ovary through peritoneal fluid, lymphatics along the gonadal vessels, and hematogenously (15). The peritoneal route is the most common (15). Ovarian cancer cells slough off the surface of the ovary and spread via the peritoneal fluid that circulates from the pelvis to the diaphragm (16,17). Lower subdiaphragmatic pressure compared to pelvic pressure pulls fluid up into the abdomen from the pelvis (17). The left paracolic gutter is shallower than the right and the majority of fluid flows into the right gutter and around the liver. Common sites of implants are the cul de sac, right lower quadrant, sigmoid colon, and right paracolic gutter. The bowel, omentum, and diaphragm also can be seeded (18). Loculated ascites suggests the presence of peritoneal carcinomatosis.

The initial treatment of ovarian cancer consists of surgical debulking to reduce tumor deposits to less than 1 cm, which affords the patient the best prognosis (9). The role of CT is to detect metastatic implants, particularly at sites that are difficult to explore at surgery, such as the diaphragm, splenic hilum, stomach, lesser sac, liver, mesenteric root,

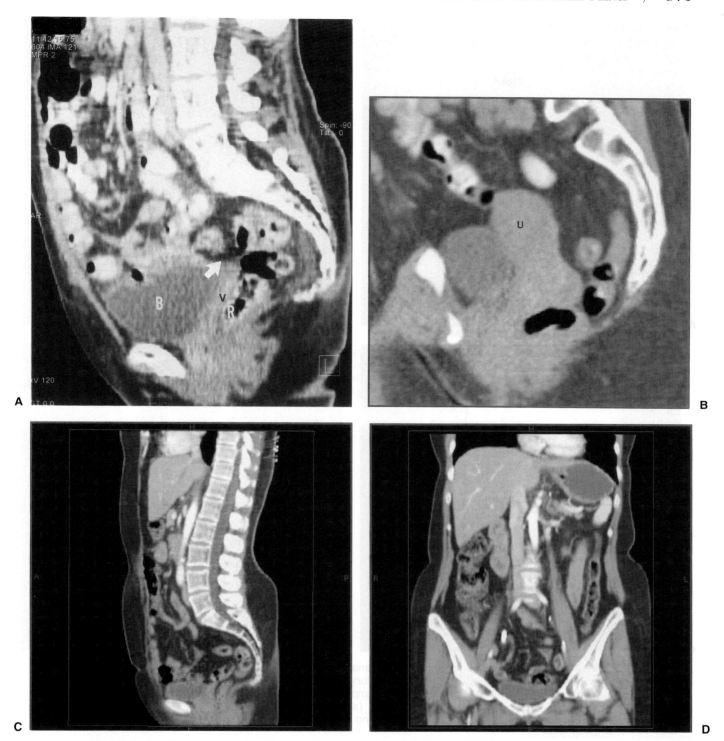

FIG. 21–3. Multiplanar reconstructions (MPR) of MDCT data. **A:** Sagittal MPR of the pelvis. The bladder (*B*), vagina (*V*), rectum (*R*) and cul de sac (*arrow*) are defined well. The uterus is surgically absent. **B:** Sagittal MPR of the pelvis shows the uterus (*U*) along its long axis. **C:** Sagittal MPR of the abdomen and pelvis. Abdominal wall, surface of the liver, and pelvic viscera are visualized. **D:** Coronal MPR of the abdomen and pelvis demonstrating length of paracolic gutters, diaphragm, and liver surface.

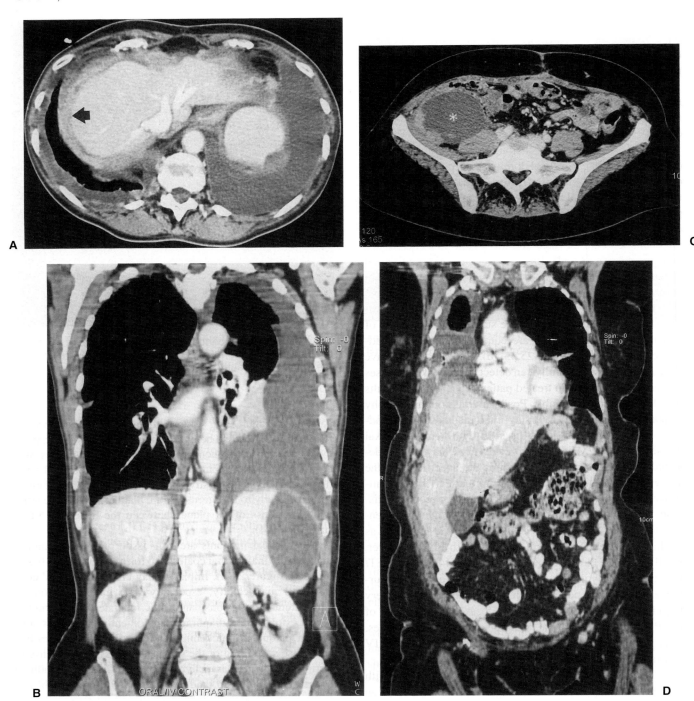

FIG. 21–8. Carcinomatosis from ovarian cancer. Axial image **(A)** shows soft-tissue implants (*arrow*) on surface of the liver. There also are bilateral pleural effusions. Coronal MPR image **(B)** shows scalloping of the spleen by an implant and pleural effusion. **C:** Axial image shows cystic implant (*asterisk*) near cecum. **D:** Coronal MPR image shows normal surface of liver and omentum. Disease is confined to the thorax with a right pleural effusion.

tissue thickening, masses. and loculated fluid suggest the presence of disease in these areas. Primary peritoneal carcinoma is in the differential for carcinomatosis in cases where an ovarian mass is absent (15,49).

Ovarian Teratomas and Cysts

Ovarian teratomas are tumors in young women that usually are benign (50). Cells from three germ-cell layers are present, and fat, bone, teeth, and hair can be formed (50,51). The presence of fat and calcification within a cystic ovarian mass allows for the diagnosis of teratoma (51,52). Fat is present in over 90% of cases, occasionally with a fat–fluid level (50). Calcification tends to be globular or along the periphery of the lesion (47). A soft-tissue-mural nodule of hair and teeth, called a dermoid plug, also may be present. The differential diagnosis for fatty pelvic tumors includes benign and malignant teratoma, lipomatous tumors of the uterus, pelvic lipomas, and pelvic liposarcomas (53).

Complications of cystic teratomas include torsion in 16% of patients, malignant degeneration in 2% of patients, and rupture in 1% to 2% of patients (54). Cystic ovarian teratomas are the most common ovarian neoplasm causing ovarian torsion (55,56). Malignant transformation of a teratoma is suspected when the soft-tissue component of the mass is greater than 10 cm in size (50). This tends to occur in the sixth or seventh decade (51).

Adnexal masses such as functional ovarian cysts are common and may be seen incidentally on CT. In a search of radiology reports in 3448 women, 5% of women had incidental adnexal lesions detected on CT (57). The lesions were seen in both pre- and postmenopausal women. The nature of 30% of lesions was unknown, but of the remaining 70%, 69% were benign and 1% were due to metastatic disease. Functional cysts tend to be less than 3 cm in size and have a wall thickness of less than 3 mm (8). Occasionally, an ovarian cyst can rupture and result in hemoperitoneum (Figure 21-9) (58). Multiple large cysts, ascites, and pleural effusions occur with the ovarian-hyperstimulation syndrome (59). The cysts tend to be peripheral and surround the ovarian stroma (60).

Cervical Cancer

Invasive cervical cancer is the third most common gynecologic malignancy (61). Eighty percent to 90% of cancers are squamous-cell carcinomas, and presenting symptoms include vaginal bleeding and pelvic pain (62). The tumors are exophytic or endocervical and spread to the lower uterine segment, vagina, and parametrium (Figure 21-10) (62). More extensive disease involves the pelvic sidewall, bladder, and rectum. If disease is confined to the cervix without parametrial involvement (Stage IIA), surgery is performed. If there is parametrial invasion (Stage IIB), patients receive radiation therapy (63).

Currently, the role of CT in cervical cancer is to stage

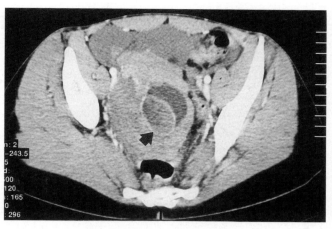

FIG. 21–9. Peritoneal hemorrhage from ruptured ovarian cyst. Computed tomograph of the pelvis with IV contrast in a 24-year-old woman with acute abdominal pain shows complex cystic structure in right adnexa (*arrow*) and free intraperitoneal fluid. The patient's hematocrit had fallen 17 points and there was no evidence of infection or pregnancy.

advanced disease. Initial studies on the accuracy of CT using older nonhelical scanners demonstrated limited accuracy in staging early disease (64). Early cervical cancer is hypodense-to-normal cervical tissue, but can be isodense in 50% of cases (61). Misinterpretation of normal parametrial vessels and ligaments as tumor and the inability to distinguish inflammatory from neoplastic parametrial stranding result in a low accuracy, approximately 55%, of nonhelical CT for detection of Stage IIB disease (6,64,65). There is a lack of definitive staging data for helical or MDCT. The accuracy of MR for determining parametrial invasion is higher than CT, on the order of 80% to 92% (36).

Computed-tomography staging has high accuracy (92%) for disease that is Stage IIIB to Stage IVB (66). Disease is Stage III when there is hydronephrosis, pelvic sidewall extension, and tumor involving the distal third of the vagina. Disease is Stage IV when there is bladder or rectal invasion or distant metastases. Ureteral obstruction on CT obviates the need for intravenous urography because hydronephrosis, hydroureter, and site of obstruction are detected with a single examination (67). Gross bladder and rectal invasion also are detected on CT, although subtle bladder invasion requires cystoscopy. The negative predictive value of MR and CT for bladder invasion is reported as 100% (68). Invasion was diagnosed by biopsy in 57% of cases suspected on imaging. Proctoscopy usually is not performed, as rectal invasion is uncommon without other evidence of locally advanced disease.

Thin axial slices with 3D reconstruction are feasible with MDCT, and these improvements may enhance visualization of the primary tumor, estimation of tumor volume, and detection of extracervical spread. The American College of Radiology Imaging Network (ACRIN) trial is evaluating the accuracy of spiral CT for staging cervical cancer.

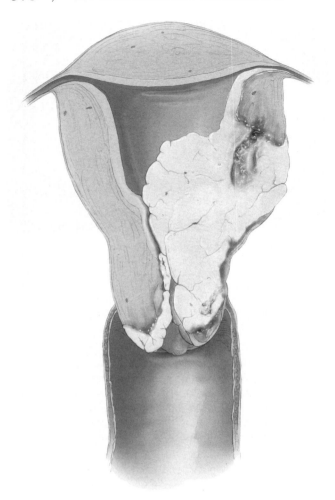

FIG. 21–10. Schematic drawing of cervical cancer. Coronal drawing of the uterus shows extension of the cervical cancer into the myometrium. (From Pannu HK, Corl FM, Fishman EK. CT evaluation of cervical cancer: spectrum of disease. *Radiographics* 2001;21:1155–1168, with permission.) (See color plate)

As in other areas of the body, there is overlap in the size and enhancement of malignant and hyperplastic nodes (69–71). Nodes can be enlarged from infection and metastases, and distinction cannot be made by size alone. Conversely, normal-sized nodes may contain microscopic tumor (61). However, the positive predictive value of malignancy is 100% if the node is necrotic (71). A meta-analysis of the literature on the utility of CT in identifying malignant lymph nodes showed that the presence of normal-sized nodes reduces the probability of metastases, and the probability of tumor is increased only moderately if the nodes are enlarged (72). The results are similar for CT, MR, and lymphangiography. Overall accuracy of CT is 65% to 80% for detecting malignant nodes, and therefore biopsy is necessary for confirmation (69,72). Positron-emission tomography may play a role in the future, but can be limited by normal activity in the urinary system (73,74).

Percutaneous biopsy of enlarged pelvic nodes can be performed with CT guidance. Computed tomography also can be used for radiation therapy-planning and patient follow up (69,70). The sensitivity and specificity are high for detecting recurrent tumor (64). In one study of 39 patients with recurrent disease, 85% of local recurrences were diagnosed correctly on CT (75).

When the primary tumor mass of cervical cancer is visualized on CT, it usually appears as a hypodense mass on contrast-enhanced scans. The tumor is hypodense-to-normal cervical stroma due to necrosis, ulceration, or reduced vascularity (69). Gas occurs within the mass from necrosis or prior biopsy (Figure 21-11) (6). The cervix can be enlarged with an anterior-posterior (AP) diameter greater than 3.5 cm. Anterior-posterior size of the cervix greater than 6 cm on CT correlates with a poorer outcome (64,66). A smooth and well-defined margin to the cervix suggests the absence of extracervical extension of tumor (6). The cervical mass can obstruct the endometrial canal and cause the cavity to dilate with blood, serous fluid, or pus (64,76). The myometrium also can be invaded directly by cervical cancer, and the abnormal areas appear hypodense on contrast-enhanced scans (62). Inferiorly, cervical cancer invades the vagina or is exophytic into it. Superior and inferior extension of tumor can be visualized on sagittal- and coronal-reconstructed images (Figure 21-12).

Local extension of cervical cancer into the parametrium results in soft-tissue masses and ureteral encasement because the ureter normally lies 2 cm lateral to the cervix (Figure 21-13). These two findings are specific for parametrial invasion on CT (6,61,69). Soft-tissue strands in the parametrium are not reliable for diagnosing tumor invasion because they may be due to normal ligaments or inflammatory changes. Normal parauterine and paracervical ligaments are thinner than tumor or inflammatory strands that are greater than 3 mm to 4 mm in thickness (6,69). Visceral branches of the

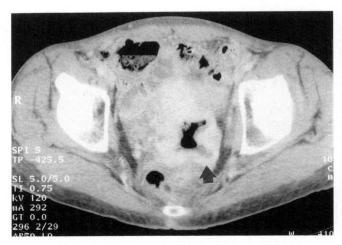

FIG. 21–11. Primary mass of cervical cancer. Computed tomograph of the pelvis with IV contrast shows an enhancing necrotic mass (*arrow*) that enlarges the cervix.

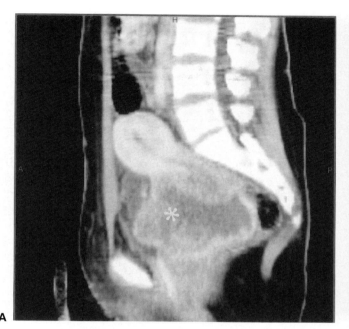
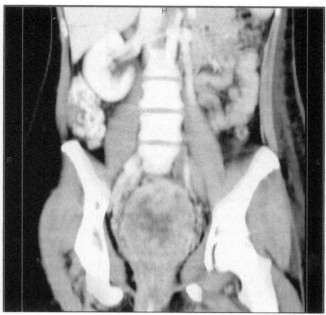

A   B

FIG. 21–12. Extension of cervical cancer into vagina. Sagittal **(A)** and coronal **(B)** volume-rendered images show large cervical mass exophytic into vagina (*asterisk*). Note gross invasion of parametrium on coronal image.

internal iliac vessels also can appear as soft-tissue strands on unenhanced scans. Computed tomography with intravenous contrast and thin slices can be used to distinguish normal structures from tumor (77). However, inflammatory changes secondary to the tumor or instrumentation remain a confounding factor when assessing for parametrial invasion. Both inflammatory changes and tumor can cause stranding and increased density of the parametrial fat and an irregular

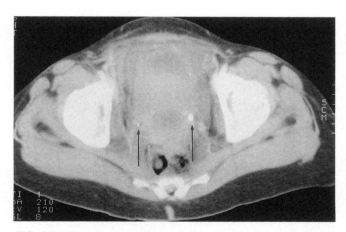

FIG. 21–13. Parametrial invasion by cervical cancer. Computed-tomography image of the pelvis with IV contrast shows stranding of the parametrium and encasement of the contrast-filled ureters by tumor (*arrows*). (From Pannu HK, Corl FM, Fishman EK. CT evaluation of cervical cancer: spectrum of disease. *Radiographics* 2001;21:1155–1168, with permission.)

cervical margin (6,66,69). The inflammation is due to instrumentation, ulceration, and infection of the cervical tumor and prior pelvic surgery (6). Nodularity of the soft tissues also can occur in patients with endometriosis and mimic tumor (78).

When tumor in the pericervical soft tissues extends to within 3 mm of the pelvic sidewall, invasion of the sidewall is diagnosed on CT (61). More extensive invasion results in enlargement and heterogeneity of the piriformis and obturator internus muscles, encasement of the iliac vessels, and lytic lesions in the pelvic bones (3,61,69). Involvement of the bladder and rectum is diagnosed when there is asymmetric nodular thickening of the wall, intraluminal mass, and fistula formation (64). The fat planes between the cervix and these viscera can be assessed on sagittal and axial images of the pelvis.

For the diagnosis of adenopathy, nodal short-axis diameter greater than 1 cm is considered abnormal on CT (61,72). Disease spreads along the external iliac, internal iliac, and presacral nodal chains to the paraaortic nodes, which may result in adjacent bony invasion of the spine (Figure 21-14) (2,3,4). Therefore, lytic osseous lesions usually occur in lumbar vertebrae secondary to direct extension from paraaortic nodes (4).

Distant metastases from cervical cancer occur to the liver, lung, and extrapelvic nodes (4). Liver metastases are solid masses with variable enhancement, and lung metastases occur as multiple pulmonary nodules in 33% to 38% of patients (4,79). Diffuse interstitial lung disease due to lymphangitic carcinomatosis occurs in fewer than 5% of pa-

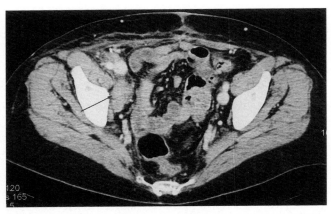

FIG. 21–14. Pelvic adenopathy in a patient with gynecologic malignancy. Axial-CT image shows an enlarged node posterior (*arrow*) to the external iliac vessels.

necessary to distinguish radiation fibrosis from recurrent tumor (64).

Endometrial Cancer

Endometrial cancer is the most common gynecologic malignancy and usually occurs in postmenopausal women (83). It usually is diagnosed while confined to the uterus since women present early with vaginal bleeding (36). Stage-I tumors are confined to the corpus of the uterus, Stage-II tumors invade the cervix, Stage-III tumors extend beyond the uterus but are confined to the pelvis, and Stage-IV tumors have distant metastases or involve the bladder and rectum (84). Important factors for treatment are the depth of myometrial invasion, cervical invasion, and lymph-node metastases (84). Hysterectomy is performed for surgical staging because it is the most reliable method to determine the depth of myometrial invasion (64).

tients, and mediastinal adenopathy and pleural effusions are present in approximately one-third of patients with thoracic metastases (79,80). Thoracic metastases are more common with adenocarcinoma than with squamous-cell carcinoma of the cervix (79).

Adrenal metastases also occur in approximately 15% of patients and usually are from cervical adenocarcinomas (4). Peritoneal carcinomatosis similar to ovarian cancer metastases and necrotic psoas masses are other manifestations of distant metastases (4). The psoas masses can simulate large abscesses, and usually are seen in women infected with the human-immunodeficiency virus (81).

Local recurrence of cervical cancer is defined as tumor that develops more than 6 months after regression of the treated tumor (4). It can be at the vaginal cuff or the pelvic sidewall, as a soft-tissue mass with a variable degree of necrosis, or a primarily cystic mass (4,64,82). Biopsy may be

Computed tomography, ultrasound, and MR have been used to assess for myometrial invasion. A retrospective review of CT reports in 54 patients scanned between 1990 and 1998 found that the sensitivity of CT for myometrial invasion was 61%, but the depth of invasion (less than 50% or greater than 50%) was underestimated in 90% of patients (85). A meta-analysis of six CT studies comprising 203 patients scanned with nonhelical scanners found that the sensitivity of CT for myometrial invasion was between 40% and 86% for five of the six studies (84). The specificity was 75% and accuracy was 61% in a study of 10 patients with deep myometrial invasion (86). For helical CT, the sensitivity and specificity were 83% and 42% for deep myometrial invasion in a study of 25 patients (87). The sensitivity and specificity were 25% and 70% for cervical invasion. The authors felt that restriction to the axial plane was a limiting factor when assessing for myometrial or cervical invasion due to the vari-

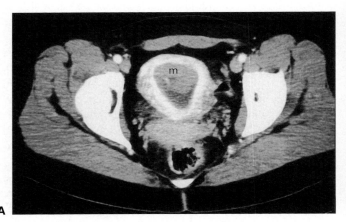

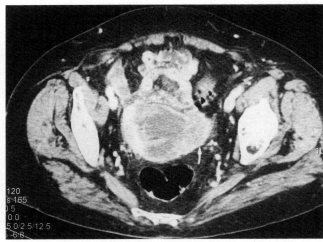

A   B

FIG. 21–15. Endometrial cancer. **A:** Axial-CT image of the pelvis with IV contrast shows soft-tissue mass (*m*) and fluid distending endometrial cavity. **B:** Axial image in a different patient shows hypodense myometrium (*arrow*) secondary to tumor infiltration.

able position of the uterus in the pelvis (87). Magnetic resonance, especially with gadolinium, has a higher sensitivity, ranging from 85% to 100% for detecting invasive endometrial cancer (84,88). Images along the long axis of the uterus and oblique axial images have been suggested to aid in the detection of invasion on MR (89). In the same way, reformatting of thin-section MDCT data in multiple planes may improve visualization of invasion on CT.

Currently, CT is used to stage tumors with a high histologic grade, for radiation-therapy planning, and for follow up (69,84). Lymph-node metastases are 6 to 7 times more common when the depth of myometrial invasion is greater than 50%, and lymphadenectomy is performed in these cases (88). Enlarged nodes greater than 10 mm are suspicious for metastatic disease, but microscopic disease can be present in normal-sized nodes (85). Sensitivity and specificity for nodal disease are 57% and 92%, respectively (90). There is a high likelihood of peritoneal spread of tumor in patients who have ascites on CT (85). In treated patients who are symptomatic, CT can be used to assess for recurrence (90,91). Almost 80% of recurrences occur within the first 3 years (91).

The endometrium normally is hypodense to the myometrium on contrast-enhanced scans. In patients with endometrial cancer, the endometrium may appear thickened, or the cavity may be dilated with fluid with an intraluminal soft-tissue mass (Figure 21-15) (77). Scans delayed by a few minutes show enhancement of the normal myometrium with hypodense areas suggestive of tumor infiltration. Parametrial- and pelvic-sidewall invasion from endometrial cancer are similar to that with cervical cancer (47,69).

A few reports have described the appearance of gestational-trophoblastic disease on CT (92). The uterus is enlarged and adnexal cysts usually are present (93). Hyperdense lesions surrounding hypodense foci suggest the diagnosis of a mole on contrast-enhanced scans (Figure 21-16)

(94). Local extension within the pelvis, as well as pulmonary metastases, can be detected (95).

NONNEOPLASTIC CONDITIONS OF THE FEMALE PELVIS

Pelvic Inflammatory Disease (PID)

Pelvic inflammatory disease is an ascending polymicrobial infection from the vagina and cervix that spreads through the fallopian tubes to the ovaries and paraovarian tissues (96). In cases where the clinical diagnosis is uncertain, or to differentiate between right-sided PID and appendicitis, CT may be performed instead of sonography. The role of CT also includes assessing the extent of disease in patients who do not respond to therapy (60).

With uncomplicated salpingitis, the CT can be normal or there can be a small amount of pelvic fluid (60). Computed-tomography findings of PID include fallopian-tube dilatation, abscess, and adenopathy. The fallopian tubes appear as tubular-fluid-filled structures lateral to the uterus and posterior to the mesosalpinx (Figure 21-17) (47,96). The mesosalpinx is thickened and can be followed laterally from the uterus. Small bowel and dilated appendix usually are anterior to the mesosalpinx. Oral contrast in the adjacent small bowel also is helpful in distinguishing bowel loops from the fallopian tubes. Dilated tubes can be caused by prior infection or obstructing tumor and are not specific for acute inflammation (96). Patients may develop a thick-walled multiloculated tuboovarian abscess with thick septations (60). Although the presence of gas in the adnexal mass is specific for infection, it is rarely present (77).

The infection can spread posteriorly along the uterosacral ligaments with thickening and stranding of the perirectal fat (96). Pelvic stranding also results in an indistinct margin

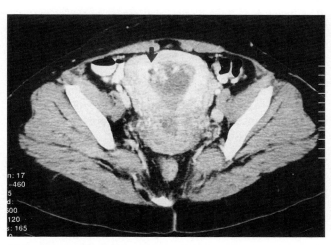

FIG. 21–16. Gestational trophoblastic disease. Axial-CT image shows peripherally enhancing foci in the endometrium with central hypodensity (*arrow*).

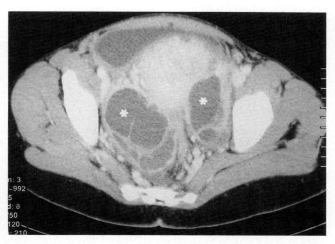

FIG. 21–17. Tuboovarian abscesses. Computed-tomography image of the pelvis with IV contrast in a 49-year-old woman with pain and elevated white-blood-cell count. Bilateral dilated fallopian tubes are present (*asterisk*), and there is minimal free fluid.

to the uterus and bowel loops (60). The rectum can be narrowed extrinsically. Superior extension to the paraaortic nodes results in retroperitoneal adenopathy, and contiguous or lymphatic spread to the liver results in perihepatitis (97). The latter also is called the Fitz-Hugh–Curtis syndrome and a loculated fluid collection near the liver is seen on CT. Anterior enhancement of the liver surface may represent another sign of perihepatitis (98). The differential diagnoses for PID on CT include ovarian cancer, missed appendiceal abscess, and endometriosis.

Endometriosis

Endometriosis is a common condition that affects 15% of menstruating women (99). Ectopic endometrial tissue responds to hormonal stimulation similar to uterine endometrium, and patients may have pain that is worse during menstruation (99,100). The disorder occasionally is seen in postmenopausal women on hormone-replacement therapy (60). Endometriomas usually are in the parauterine soft tissues and bowel implants usually are on the rectosigmoid colon (99,101). The ovary is the most common site (102). Endometriosis also can occur in an abdominal-wall scar from cesarean section and in the pleural cavity (100,103). Pleural involvement is right sided in 95% of cases, and hemothorax or pneumothorax may occur (103,104).

The appearance of endometriomas on CT is variable. They can appear as a simple cyst, a thick-walled cyst, a mixed solid and cystic mass, or as a solid mass (99). In approximately 15% of cysts, a hyperdense crescent-shaped or round focus is seen near the inner cyst wall, which corresponds to a blood clot and is suggestive of an endometrioma (60,105). Solid masses can enhance and there may be an associated hydrosalpinx (60,100,102). Fibrosis secondary to endometriosis can result in hydroureter and bowel obstruction (102). Rarely, there is malignant transformation of endometriosis to endometrioid adenocarcinoma (102,106). Solid components, extensive infiltration of the soft tissues, and bone destruction are seen with malignancy (102,107).

Fibroids

Fibroids are common benign-smooth-muscle masses occurring in 30% to 40% of women of childbearing age (52). They can be submucosal deforming the endometrial cavity, intramural, or subserosal. Exophytic fibroids may be misinterpreted as adnexal masses.

Fibroids are a common incidental finding on CT. They are isodense to the myometrium on unenhanced scans unless there is calcification or necrosis within the fibroid (108,109). Rarely, a lipoleiomyoma is present and appears as a fatty uterine mass (110). The uterus can be lobulated and enlarged if there are multiple fibroids (47). On contrast-enhanced scans, fibroids can be hypo-, iso-, or hyperdense to the myo-

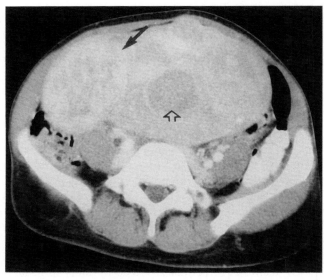

FIG. 21–18. Fibroids. Computed-tomography image of the abdomen with IV contrast shows enlarged heterogeneous uterus with hyperdense (*closed arrow*) and hypodense (*open arrow*) fibroids.

metrium (Figure 21-18) (47,77). Large fibroids may enhance heterogeneously due to areas of reduced vascularity (108). Retroperitoneal edema surrounding the gonadal vein has been described with large benign fibroids (111).

Fibroids can be symptomatic, causing excessive vaginal bleeding, pain, and compression of adjacent pelvic organs. Treatment options include hormonal therapy, myomectomy, hysterectomy, and uterine-artery embolization (112). Hormonal therapy with progestins or gonadotropin-releasing hormone agonists causes reduction in fibroid size while on therapy. However, a few months after treatment is stopped, fibroids may enlarge (112). Side effects such as osteoporosis and menopausal symptoms limit long-term use of hormones. Percutaneous embolization is an alternative to surgical resection (113–115). Bilateral uterine-artery embolization with polyvinyl-alcohol particles results in decreased uterine and dominant fibroid volumes, as well as symptomatic improvement in the majority of patients (112,116). The clinical failure rate is approximately 10%, and may be due to adenomyosis and presence of collateral blood supply (117,118). Complications such as infection and uterine ischemia are uncommon (116).

Imaging before and after embolization, if performed, usually is done with ultrasound or MR to determine fibroid size, location, and enhancement. A small study in four patients who had CT after embolization found that there is contrast retention in fibroids on scans performed within a few hours of the procedure (108). This retention is felt to be due to reduction of arterial inflow with stasis of blood in the fibroid and decreased washout of contrast. The fibroids appear as hypodense masses with gas due to necrosis on scans performed after a few months. Rim calcification also has been described in treated fibroids (119).

Ovarian Torsion

Ovarian torsion in adult women usually is associated with the presence of a large ovarian mass, often a cystic teratoma (56). The ovary twists on its pedicle causing venous obstruction and subsequent arterial obstruction (120). The ovary is edematous and enlarged, often five times the size of the contralateral ovary. On unenhanced CT, a soft-tissue hyperdense mass is identified relative to the contralateral normal ovary. Prominent peripheral hypodense follicles also have been noted (121). This hyperdensity is due to hemorrhage in the ovary and fallopian tube (56,120). An associated ovarian mass, usually cystic, is seen in adults (56). The wall of the cystic mass demonstrates smooth, concentric, or eccentric wall thickening (greater than 3 mm) (56). Wall thickness greater than 10 mm is suggestive of hemorrhagic infarction. The mass may rotate to the contralateral side of the pelvis when compared with images obtained prior to torsion (60).

The fallopian tube also is thickened to greater than 10 mm and appears as a masslike structure between the ovary and uterus (55,56). The tube can appear to drape over the cystic mass. Thickening of the tube due to an edematous vascular pedicle is a specific sign of torsion (56). Other findings that have been described include lack of enhancement in cases of infarction and gas in a branching pattern within the ovary (120,122). Free intraperitoneal fluid secondary to venous congestion or intraperitoneal hemorrhage also is seen in most patients (55,56,121). As a secondary sign, the uterus is deviated toward the abnormal ovary (56,120).

VASCULAR CONDITIONS

Ovarian Vein Varices

Varices of the ovarian vein are seen commonly on imaging. In a study of 273 female renal donors who underwent conventional angiography, 27 patients (9.9%) were noted to have varices (123). When 22 of these 27 patients were asked to complete a questionnaire, 59% reported chronic pelvic pain. A CT study of 34 female renal donors found that 47% had dilated and incompetent ovarian veins (124). Dilated veins are detected incidentally in asymptomatic women and are also associated with pelvic congestion syndrome. This syndrome causes chronic pelvic pain in multiparous women that is exacerbated by prolonged standing (124,125). Varicose dilatation of the ovarian vein is a differential diagnosis for chronic pelvic pain (more than 6 months) (126), as are endometriosis and pelvic adhesions.

Incompetence or absence of valves in the ovarian veins allows retrograde flow of blood and dilatation of the ovarian veins (124). The left ovarian vein is affected most commonly. Other causes of pelvic varices are obstruction of the inferior vena cava and portal hypertension (127).

Proposed criteria for diagnosis of varices on CT are i) four or more ipsilateral tortuous parauterine veins, ii) diameter of at least one parauterine vein greater than 4 mm, iii) ovarian-vein diameter greater than 7 mm to 8 mm, and iv) complete opacification of the ovarian vein on early images before pelvic-venous enhancement (Figure 21-19) (124,127). If symptomatic, varices can be ligated surgically or embolized with coils (125,128). In the renal donors who were found to have varices on angiography, symptoms resolved in most cases after left nephrectomy and ovarian-vein ligation (123).

Ovarian Vein Thrombosis

Thrombosis of the ovarian vein is seen most commonly in postpartum women (129). Patients have nonspecific symptoms such as fever and pain. In untreated cases, pulmonary emboli and uterine necrosis may develop (130). The right ovarian vein is affected in 80% to 90% of cases, possibly due to compression by the gravid uterus (130). Thrombosis of the gonadal veins also can occur with pelvic inflammatory disease following gynecologic surgery and malignancy (129,131,132). Occasionally, ovarian vein thrombosis may be a sequela of appendicitis or diverticulitis.

On unenhanced scans, the ovarian vein is dilated, and the thrombus may be hyperdense or isodense to the vessel wall (133). On contrast-enhanced scans, the venous wall enhances and the lumen is hypodense (130). Perivascular edema may be present (133). A heterogeneous adnexal mass, possibly representing pelvic-vein thrombophlebitis, also has been described (134). Computed tomography is highly sensitive, detecting the thrombosis in all 12 patients in one study (133).

PREGNANCY AND POSTPARTUM IMAGING WITH CT

CT During Pregnancy

Computed tomography typically is not performed during pregnancy owing to concerns regarding radiation exposure for the fetus. However, the scan may be performed to screen patients rapidly for life-threatening injuries after trauma and for pelvimetry (135). Other possible indications are suspected pulmonary embolism, appendicitis, and urinary-tract calculi (136).

For thromboembolic disease, the initial diagnostic evaluation can begin with a lower-extremity ultrasound since the presence of deep venous thrombosis indicates the need to initiate treatment. If negative, a nuclear-medicine-ventilation-perfusion scan usually is performed with reduction of the perfusion dose (136,137). However, a recent study suggested that the fetal dose with spiral thoracic CT is low if a technique of 100 mAs is used and a topogram is not obtained (138). Iodinated contrast agents are used during pregnancy if indicated (136,138).

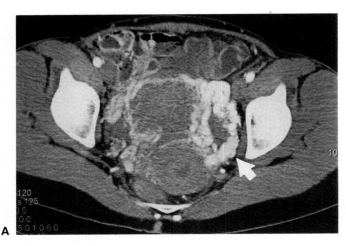

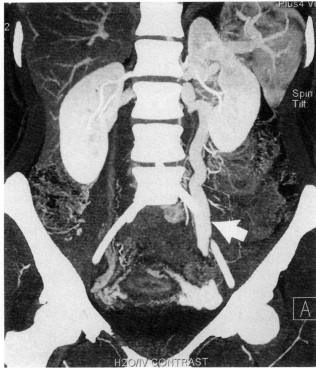

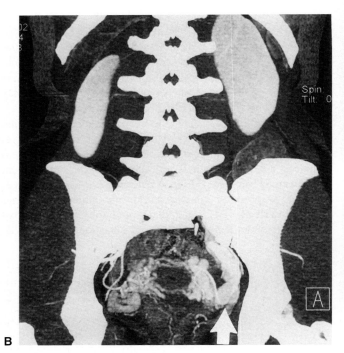

FIG. 21–19. Ovarian vein varices. Computed-tomography image of the pelvis with IV contrast in an asymptomatic woman. Axial image **(A)** and coronal images **(B)** and **(C)** show dilated left adnexal veins and ovarian vein (*arrows*).

Appendicitis has an incidence of approximately 0.38 to 1.69 per 1000 pregnancies, and urinary-tract calculi have an incidence of 0.7 per 1000 pregnancies (139). The work up usually starts with ultrasound for suspected cases (136,139,140). The appendix can be difficult to visualize by ultrasound late in pregnancy, and limited CT has been performed for diagnosis (141). On the scan, the position of the appendix may be altered due to displacement by the enlarging uterus (139). For ureteral calculi, a limited excretory urogram is part of the algorithm if ultrasound is nondiagnostic (139,140).

Radiation exposure on CT can be reduced by obtaining thicker sections, decreasing the mAs, increasing the scan pitch, and limiting the scan area (135,136). Radiation risks relate primarily to childhood leukemia and central nervous system abnormalities (136,139,142,143). Patient counseling is suggested if the dose to the fetus is greater than 10 mGy (142). The risk of adverse effects in the fetus is increased if the exposure is greater than 100 mGy (143). The central nervous system is susceptible during weeks 8 through 25 of pregnancy, and mental development can be affected with doses greater than 200 mGy (143). However, adverse events may occur spontaneously unrelated to radiation. In a pregnant woman not exposed to medical radiation, the incidence of major malformations in the fetus is 2% to 4%, intrauterine-growth retardation occurs in 4%, and spontaneous abortion in 15% (143).

On CT, a central low-attenuation area initially is present

in the uterus with pregnancy. The fetus is first visualized first late in the first trimester or early in the second trimester (135). Initially, it appears as an area of high attenuation in the amniotic fluid. The fetal skeleton is seen towards the end of the second trimester, and viscera are identified in the third trimester (135).

Placental enhancement is seen in the second trimester of pregnancy (135). The placenta is heterogeneous, with low-attenuation areas surrounded by higher-attenuation areas (135). Enhancement of the placenta is greater than the myometrium. The placenta enhances more homogeneously in the third trimester (144). In third-trimester patients, dynamic scanning of the placenta with MR shows greater enhancement than the myometrium immediately following contrast injection, enhancement equal to the myometrium at 45 seconds, and less enhancement than the myometrium at 90 seconds (144). Late in pregnancy, avascular areas of placental infarction may occur normally (135). With trauma, the placenta can infarct, the myometrium can be disrupted, and there can be pelvic hemorrhage (Figure 21-20) (135).

CT Pelvimetry

Pelvimetry occasionally is performed to assess the dimensions of the bony pelvis prior to vaginal delivery in patients with suspected small pelvic size or breech presentation of the fetus (145). Conventional or digital radiography, CT, or MR can be used for pelvimetry. Computed tomography and digital radiography are the most commonly used methods (145,146). Computed tomography and radiography are similar in accuracy and radiation dose, but CT takes less

time (146,147). The radiation dose is reduced with CT if only a lateral topogram is done, or if a PA topogram is done instead of an AP view (145,148).

The three images obtained with CT are a lateral topogram, a PA or AP topogram, and a single axial slice (148,149). In some cases, only the lateral topogram is obtained in pregnant patients, with the complete series being done prior to pregnancy (145). The axial slice is obtained at the level of the ischial spines. If the spines are difficult to identify on the AP topogram, the fovea of the femur are used as a landmark. However, spines can be inferior to this level (149).

The transverse pelvic inlet is measured on the AP view, the anterior–posterior pelvic inlet is measured on the lateral view, and the interspinous distance is measured on the axial slice (150). The interspinous distance also can be measured on the AP view if the spines are identified and the diameter corrected for magnification (147). This eliminates the need for the axial slice. The transverse diameter is most accurate at the isocenter of the gantry (148,150). The bony pelvis is considered to be small for vaginal delivery if the AP diameter of the pelvic inlet is less than 11 cm, the transverse diameter is less than 12 cm, and the interspinous distance is less than 10 cm (149).

Postpartum Uterus

Computed tomography is performed after delivery to evaluate for complications such as abscess, ovarian vein thrombosis, and pelvic hematoma (151–153). After an uncomplicated vaginal delivery, intrauterine blood and gas, gas

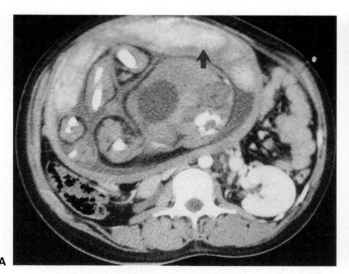
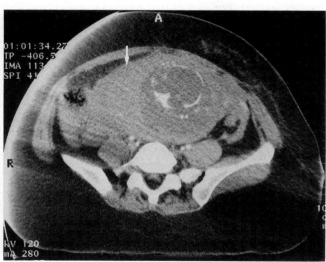

FIG. 21–20. Computed tomograph of the placenta. **A:** Axial image with IV contrast a 21-year-old woman in the third trimester of pregnancy shows dense enhancement of the placenta (*arrow*). The fetus clinically was viable. **B:** Axial image with IV contrast in a 35-year-old woman in the second trimester of pregnancy and recent trauma. There is no enhancement of the placenta (*arrow*), and there was disruption of the myometrium at surgery. Fetal heart tones were absent.

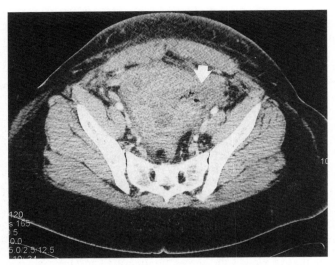

FIG. 21–21. Endometritis. Computed-tomography image with IV contrast in a 27-year-old woman with postpartum sepsis after caesarean section shows fluid and gas in the endometrium and myometrium (*arrow*) compatible with clinical diagnosis of endometritis.

in the symphysis pubis and sacroiliac joints, and widening of the symphysis pubis are normal findings on CT (154). Intrauterine gas may be seen up to 3 weeks after an uncomplicated delivery and the diagnosis of endometritis is made based on clinical findings of fever and pain (151). Computed tomography, if performed, is used to exclude an extrauterine abscess (Figure 21-21) (60). Acute endometrial blood and retained products of conception both appear hyperdense on CT and are distinguished by ultrasound (151).

After cesarean section, the myometrium appears discontinuous along the vertical or transverse incision through the uterus (155). The incision may have an irregular edge and does not necessarily imply dehiscence (155). Other normal findings are parametrial and endometrial fluid and gas, and a hematoma in the bladder flap anterior to the uterus.

HELLP Syndrome

The HELLP syndrome occurs when there is hemolysis, elevation of liver function tests, and a low platelet count (152,156). It is a complication of preeclampsia-eclampsia (156). On CT, the liver is enlarged and has peripheral low-attenuation areas of infarction and intraparenchymal or subcapsular hematomas (152,157). Ascites also can be present and the liver may rupture (152,158).

MISCELLANEOUS CONDITIONS

Pelvic Organ Prolapse

Pelvic organ prolapse is a relatively common condition that typically affects middle-aged and older multiparous women (159). It is a global problem affecting the bladder,

uterus, and rectum, with organ descent occurring when there is an increase in abdominal pressure. Prolapse occurs due to connective-tissue tears or deficient muscular support in the pelvic floor. Position of the pelvic organs below the pubococcygeal line that is drawn from the inferior pubic symphysis to the last coccygeal joint is abnormal (Figure 21-22) (159). This low position of the viscera may be detected incidentally on axial CT images and can be confirmed with sagittal reconstructions.

Surgical Reconstruction

In patients treated with anterior exenteration and reconstruction for cancer, the bladder and uterus are removed and the anterior pelvis is reconstructed with omentum (Figure 21-23). A bulging mass in the perineum on physical examination may be due to recurrent tumor or prolapse of omental fat and bowel. The two entities can be distinguished on CT.

Vaginal reconstruction is performed in patients with congenital atresia of the vagina or scarring secondary to radiation and surgery (160). Cecum or sigmoid colon, skin, bladder, and omental or musculocutaneous flaps are among the sources of tissue that are used to create the neovagina. The normal vagina appears flat on axial images and the mucosa can enhance with intravenous contrast. A neovagina formed from bowel has a round appearance (Figure 21-24). The soft-tissue bowel is in the center and there is surrounding mesenteric fat.

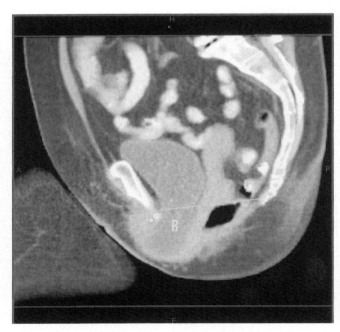

FIG. 21–22. Cystocele. Sagittal volume-rendered image shows bladder (*B*) descent below the pubococcygeal line compatible with cystocele.

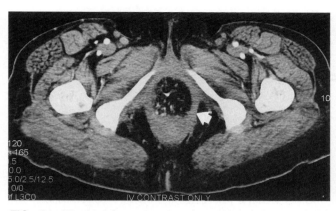

FIG. 21–23. Anterior reconstruction with omentum. Axial image with IV contrast in a woman with anterior pelvic exenteration and reconstruction for cervical cancer. Omental flap with fat and vessels (*arrow*).

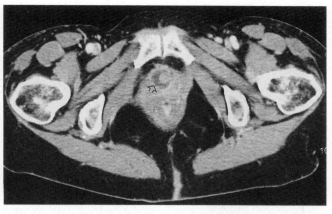

FIG. 21–25. Urethral diverticulum. Computed-tomography image of the pelvis with IV contrast shows a C-shaped low-attenuation area in the wall of the urethra surrounding the lumen compatible with urethral diverticulum (*arrow*).

Urethral Diverticula

Urethral diverticula usually are acquired after infection of the periurethral glands (161). The diverticula are out-pouchings from the urethral lumen into the wall that may or may not communicate with the lumen. Diverticula usually are detected with fluoroscopy during voiding cystography or during injection through a double-balloon catheter and also can be detected noninvasively by ultrasound or MR. On cross-sectional imaging, diverticula are cystic structures within the urethral wall (Figure 21-25) that follow the contour of the urethral lumen encircling it. Diverticula may be complicated by stones and carcinoma.

Uterine Anomalies

Congenital uterine anomalies occur in 0.5% of women (162). Arrested development of the Mullerian ducts results in absence of one or both uterine horns. Uterine didelphys occurs when there is complete failure of fusion of the Mullerian ducts (163). Two uterine horns, two cervices, and two vaginas are formed. This makes up 10% of uterine anomalies, occurring in approximately one in a thousand women (163). A longitudinal vaginal septum usually is present and patients may have an obstructed hemivagina. On cross-sectional imaging, two uterine bodies and cervices are identified.

Partial failure of fusion of the Mullerian ducts results in a bicornuate uterus (Figure 21-26). Two uterine horns and one vagina are formed. In the bicornis-bicollis type, there are two cervices; in the bicornis-unicollis type, there is one cervix (162). Uterus bicornis bicollis is the most common uterine anomaly that is associated with renal agenesis (162).

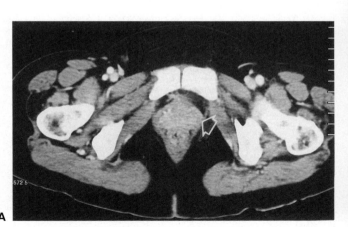

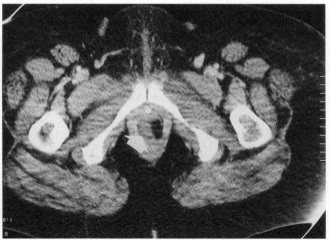

FIG. 21–24. Vaginal reconstruction. **A:** Computed-tomography image of the pelvis with IV contrast shows flat morphology and enhancement of a normal vagina (*arrow*). **B:** Computed-tomography image of the pelvis with IV contrast in a 46-year-old woman with a history of vaginal reconstruction for stenosis. A neovagina was created using cecum, which appears as a soft-tissue density (*arrow*) surrounded by mesenteric fat.

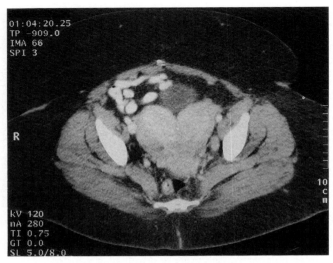

FIG. 21–26. Uterine duplication. Computed-tomography image of the pelvis with oral and IV contrast shows two uterine horns and probable single cervix. Left kidney was absent (*not shown*).

REFERENCES

1. Kaur H, Loyer EM, Minami M, et al. Patterns of uterine enhancement with helical CT. *Eur J Radiol* 1998;28:250–255.
2. Park JM, Charnsangavej C, Yoshimitsu K, et al. Pathways of nodal metastasis from pelvic tumors: CT demonstration. *Radiographics* 1994;14:1309–1321.
3. Kim RY, Weppelmann B, Salter MM, et al. Skeletal metastases from cancer of the uterine cervix: frequency, patterns, and radiotherapeutic significance. *Int J Radiat Oncol Biol Phys* 1987;13:705–708.
4. Fulcher AS, O'Sullivan SG, Segreti EM, et al. Recurrent cervical carcinoma: typical and atypical manifestations. *Radiographics* 1999; 19:S103–S116.
5. Vinnicombe SJ, Norman AR, Nicolson V, et al. Normal pelvic lymph nodes: evaluation with CT after bipedal lymphangiography. *Radiology* 1995;194:349–355.
6. Vick CW, Walsh JW, Wheelock JB, et al. CT of the normal and abnormal parametria in cervical cancer. *AJR Am J Roentgenol* 1984; 143:597–603.
7. Hawnaur JM. Staging of cervical and endometrial carcinoma. *Clin Radiol* 1993;47:7–13.
8. Jeong YY, Outwater EK, Kang HK. Imaging evaluation of ovarian masses. *Radiographics* 2000;20:1445–1470.
9. Bristow RE, Duska LR, Lambrou NC, et al. A model for predicting surgical outcome in patients with advanced ovarian carcinoma using computed tomography. *Cancer* 2000;89:1532–1540.
10. National cancer institute website. http://www.nci.nih.gov. Accessed 4/01.
11. Ozols RF, Schwartz PE, Eifel PJ. Ovarian cancer, fallopian tube carcinoma, and peritoneal carcinoma. In: Devita VT, Hellman S, Rosenberg SA, eds. *Cancer—Principles and practice of oncology*, 6th ed. Philadelphia, PA: Lippincott Williams & Wilkins, 2001:1597.
12. NIH Consensus Conference. Ovarian cancer: screening, treatment, and follow-up. *JAMA* 1995;273:491–497.
13. Forstner R, Chen M, Hricak H. Imaging of ovarian cancer. *J Magnet Resonan Imag* 1995;5:606–613.
14. Kawamoto S, Urban BA, Fishman EK. CT of epithelial ovarian tumors. *Radiographics* 1999;19:S85–S102.
15. Coakley FV. Staging ovarian cancer: role of imaging. *Radiol Clin North Am* 2002;40:609–636.
16. Amendola MA. The role of CT in the evaluation of ovarian malignancy. *Crit Rev Diagn Imaging* 1985; 24:329–368.
17. Meyers MA. Distribution of intra-abdominal malignant seeding: dependency on dynamics of flow of ascitic fluid. *AJR Am J Roentgenol* 1973;119:198–206.
18. Meyers MA. The spread and localization of acute intraperitoneal effusions. *Radiology* 1970;95:547–554.
19. Forstner R, Hricak H, Occhipinti KA, et al. Ovarian cancer: staging with CT and MR imaging. *Radiology* 1995;197:619–626.
20. Meyer JI, Kennedy AW, Friedman R, et al. Ovarian carcinoma: value of CT in predicting success of debulking surgery. *AJR Am J Roentgenol* 1995;165:875–878.
21. Calkins AR, Stehman FB, Wass JL, et al. Pitfalls in interpretation of computed tomography prior to second-look laparotomy in patients with ovarian cancer. *Br J Radiol* 1987;60:975–979.
22. Pectasides D, Kayianni H, Facou A, et al. Correlation of abdominal computed tomography scanning and second-look operation findings in ovarian cancer patients. *Am J Clin Oncol* 1991; 14:457–462
23. Shiels RA, Peel KR, Macdonald HN, et al. A prospective trial of computed tomography in the staging of ovarian malignancy. *Br J Obstet Gynecol* 1985;92:407–412.
24. Buy JN, Moss AA, Ghossain MA, et al. Peritoneal implants from ovarian tumors: CT findings. *Radiology* 1988;169:691–694.
25. Kurtz AB, Tsimikas JV, Tempany CMC, et al. Diagnosis and staging of ovarian cancer: comparative values of doppler and conventional US, CT, and MR imaging correlated with surgery and histopathologic analysis—report of the radiology diagnostic oncology group. *Radiology* 1999;212:19–27.
26. Coakley FV, Choi PH, Gougoutas CA, et al. Peritoneal metastases: Detection with spiral CT in patients with ovarian cancer. *Radiology* 2002;223:495–499.
27. Brenner DE, Shaff MI, Jones HW, et al. Abdominopelvic computed tomography: evaluation in patients undergoing second-look laparotomy for ovarian carcinoma. *Obstet Gynecol* 1985;65:715–719.
28. Simon A, Fields S, Schenker JG, et al. Computed tomography prior to surgery for ovarian carcinoma. *Aust N Z J Obstet Gynaecol* 1986; 26:199–202.
29. Guidozzi F, Sonnendecker EWW. Evaluation of preoperative investigations in patients admitted for ovarian primary cytoreductive surgery. *Gynecol Oncol* 1991;40:244–247.
30. Megibow AJ, Bosniak MA, Ho AG, et al. Accuracy of CT in detection of persistent or recurrent ovarian carcinoma: correlation with second-look laparotomy. *Radiology* 1988;166:341–345.
31. Prayer L, Kainz C, Kramer J, et al. CT and MR accuracy in the detection of tumor recurrence in patients treated for ovarian cancer. *J Comput Assist Tomogr* 1993;17:626–632.
32. Fultz PJ, Jacobs CV, Hall WJ, et al. Ovarian cancer: comparison of observer performance for four methods of interpreting CT scans. *Radiology* 1999;212:401–410.
33. Sella T, Rosenbaum E, Edelmann DZ, et al. Value of chest CT scans in routine ovarian carcinoma follow-up. *AJR Am J Roentgenol* 2001; 177:857–859.
34. Dachman AH, Visweswaran A, Battula R, et al. Role of chest CT in the follow-up of ovarian adenocarcinoma. *AJR Am J Roentgenol* 2001; 176:701–705.
35. Tempany CMC, Zou KH, Silverman SG, et al. Staging of advanced ovarian cancer: Comparison of imaging modalities-report from the radiological diagnostic oncology group. *Radiology* 2000; 215:761–767.
36. Ascher SM. Staging of gynecologic malignancies. *Top Magnet Reson Imaging* 2001;12:105–129.
37. Low RN, Saleh F, Song SYT, et al. Treated ovarian cancer: comparison of MR imaging with serum CA-125 level and physical examination—A longitudinal study. *Radiology* 1999;211:519–528.
38. Low RN, Semelka RC, Worawattanakul S, et al. Extrahepatic abdominal imaging in patients with malignancy: comparison of MR imaging and helical CT, with subsequent surgical correlation. *Radiology* 1999; 210:625–632.
39. Fenchel S, Grab D, Nuessle K, et al. Asymptomatic adnexal masses: Correlation with FDG PET and histopathologic findings. *Radiology* 2002;223:780–788.
40. Grab D, Flock F, Stohr I, et al. Classification of asymptomatic adnexal masses by ultrasound, magnetic resonance imaging, and positron emission tomography. *Gynecol Oncol* 2000;77:454–459.
41. Rieber A, Nussle K, Stohr I, et al. Preoperative diagnosis of ovarian tumors with MR imaging: comparison with transvaginal sonography, positron emission tomography, and histologic findings. *AJR Am J Roentgenol* 2001;177:123–129.
42. Rose PG, Faulhaber P, Miraldi F, et al. Positive emission tomography

for evaluating a complete clinical response in patients with ovarian or peritoneal carcinoma: correlation with second-look laparotomy. *Gynecol Oncol* 2001;82:17–21.

43. Cho SM, Ha HK, Byun JY, et al. Usefulness of FDG PET for assessment of early recurrent epithelial ovarian cancer. *AJR Am J Roentgenol* 2002;179:391–395.

44. Nakamoto Y, Saga T, Ishimori T, et al. Clinical value of positron emission tomography with FDG for recurrent ovarian cancer. *AJR Am J Roentgenol* 2001;176:1449–1454.

45. Torizuka T, Nobezawa S, Kanno T, et al. Ovarian cancer recurrence: Role of whole-body positron emission tomography using 2-[fluorine-18]-fluoro-2-deoxy-D-glucose. *Eur J Nucl Med Mol Imaging* 2002; 29:797–803.

46. Makhija S, Howden N, Edwards R, et al. Positron emission tomography/computed tomography imaging for the detection of recurrent ovarian and fallopian tube carcinoma: a retrospective review. *Gynecol Oncol* 2002;85:53–58.

47. Sawyer RW, Walsh JW. CT in gynecologic pelvic diseases. *Semin Ultrasound CT MR* 1988;9:122–142.

48. Dvoretsky PM, Richards KA, Angel C, et al. Survival time, causes of death, and tumor/treatment-related morbidity in 100 women with ovarian cancer. *Hum Pathol* 1988;19:1273–1279.

49. Chopra S, Laurie LR, Chintapalli KN, et al. Primary papillary serous carcinoma of the peritoneum: CT–pathologic correlation. *J Comput Assist Tomogr* 2000;24:395–399.

50. Lee JKT, Willms AB, Semelka RC. Pelvis. In: Lee JKT, Sagel SS, Stanley RJ, Heiken JP, eds. *Computed body tomography with MRI correlation.* Philadelphia, PA: Lippincott–Raven, 1998:1209–1274.

51. Outwater EK, Siegelman ES, Hunt JL. Ovarian teratomas: tumor types and imaging characteristics. *Radiographics* 2001;21:475–490.

52. Hamm B, Kubik-Huch RA, Fleige B. MR imaging and CT of the female pelvis: radiologic–pathologic correlation. *Eur Radiol* 1999; 9:3–15.

53. Dodd GD, Budzik RF. Lipomatous tumors of the pelvis in women: spectrum of imaging findings. *AJR Am J Roentgenol* 1990; 155:317–322.

54. Fibus TF. Intraperitoneal rupture of a benign cystic ovarian teratoma. *AJR Am J Roentgenol* 2000;174:261–262.

55. Kim YH, Cho KS, Ha HK, et al. CT features of torsion of benign cystic teratoma of the ovary. *J Comput Assist Tomogr* 1999;23:923–928.

56. Rha SE, Byun JY, Jung SE, et al. CT and MR imaging features of adnexal torsion. *Radiographics* 2002;22:283–294.

57. Slanetz PJ, Hahn PF, Hall DA, et al. The frequency and significance of adnexal lesions incidentally revealed by CT. *AJR Am J Roentgenol* 1997;168:647–650.

58. Hertzberg BS, Kliewer MA, Paulson EK. Ovarian cyst rupture causing hemoperitoneum: imaging features and the potential for misdiagnosis. *Abdom Imaging* 1999;24:304–308.

59. Jung BG, Kim H. Severe spontaneous ovarian hyperstimulation syndrome with MR findings. *J Comput Assist Tomogr* 2001;25:215–217.

60. Bennett GL, Slywotzky CM, Giovanniello G. Gynecologic causes of acute pelvic pain: Spectrum of CT findings. *Radiographics* 2002; 22:785–801.

61. Hricak H, Yu KK. Radiology in invasive cervical cancer. *AJR Am J Roentgenol* 1996;167:1101–1108.

62. Eifel PJ, Berek JS, Thigpen JT. Cancer of the cervix, vagina, and vulva. In: DeVita VT, Hellman S, Rosenberg SA, eds. *Cancer: Principles and practice of oncology.* Philadelphia: Lippincott-Raven, 1997:1433–1475.

63. Subak LL, Hricak H, Powell CB, et al. Cervical carcinoma: computed tomography and magnetic resonance imaging for preoperative staging. *Obstet Gynecol* 1995;86:43–50.

64. Walsh JW. Computed tomography of gynecologic neoplasms. *Radiol Clin North Am* 1992;30:817–830.

65. Soper JT. Radiographic imaging in gynecologic oncology. *Clin Obstet Gynecol* 2001;44:485–494.

66. Ogino I, Okamoto N, Andoh K, et al. Analysis of prognostic factors in stage IIB–IVA cervical carcinoma treated with radiation therapy: value of computed tomography. *Int J Radiat Oncol Biol Phys* 1997; 37:1071–1077.

67. Goldman SM, Fishman EK, Rosenshein NB, et al. Excretory urography and computed tomography in the initial evaluation of patients with cervical cancer: are both examinations necessary? *AJR Am J Roentgenol* 1984;143:991–996.

68. Chung H, Ahn HS, Kim YS, et al. The value of cystoscopy and intravenous urography after magnetic resonance imaging or computed tomography in the staging of cervical carcinoma. *Yonsei Med J* 2001; 42:527–531.

69. Hricak H. Role of imaging in the evaluation of pelvic cancer. *Important Adv Oncol* 1991:103–133.

70. Lewis E. The use and abuse of imaging in gynecologic cancer. *Cancer* 1987;60:1993–2009.

71. Yang WT, Lam WWM, Yu MY, et al. Comparison of dynamic helical CT and dynamic MR imaging in the evaluation of pelvic lymph nodes in cervical carcinoma. *AJR Am J Roentgenol* 2000;175:759–766.

72. Scheidler JJ, Hricak H, Yu KK, et al. Radiological evaluation of lymph node metastases in patients with cervical cancer: a meta-analysis. *JAMA* 1997;278:1096–1101.

73. Williams AD, Cousins C, Soutter WP, et al. Detection of pelvic lymph node metastases in gynecologic malignancy: a comparison of CT, MR imaging, and positron emission tomography. *AJR Am J Roentgenol* 2001;177:343–348.

74. Grigsby PW, Siegel BA, Dehdashti F. Lymph node staging by positron emission tomography in patients with carcinoma of the cervix. *J Clin Oncol* 2001;19:3745–3749.

75. Heron CW, Husband JE, Williams MP, et al. The value of CT in the diagnosis of recurrent carcinoma of the cervix. *Clin Radiol* 1988; 39:496–501.

76. Aartsen EJ. Fluid detection in the uterus during and after irradiation for carcinoma of the cervix – clinical implications. *Eur J Surg Oncol* 1990;16:42–46.

77. Urban BA, Fishman EK. Helical (spiral) CT of the female pelvis. *Radiol Clin North Am* 1995;33:933–948.

78. Walker JL, Manetta A, Mannel RS, et al. The influence of endometriosis on the staging of cervical cancer. *Obstet Gynecol* 1990; 75:543–545.

79. Shin MS, Shingleton HM, Partridge EE, et al. Squamous cell carcinoma of the uterine cervix: patterns of thoracic metastases. *Invest Radiol* 1995;30:724–729.

80. Perez-Lasala G, Cannon DT, Mansel JK, et al. Case report: Lymphangitic carcinomatosis from cervical carcinoma – an unusual presentation of diffuse interstitial lung disease. *Am J Med Sci* 1992; 303:174–176.

81. McDermott VG, Langer JE, Schiebler ML. Case report: HIV-related rapidly progressive carcinoma of the cervix (AIDS) – CT and MRI findings. *Clin Radiol* 1994;49:896–898.

82. Eising EG, Reiser MF, Vassallo P, et al. Cystic pelvic mass in a patient having recurrent carcinoma of the cervix. *Invest Radiol* 1990; 25:205–208.

83. DeVita VT, Hellman S, Rosenberg SA, eds. *Cancer: Principles and practice of oncology.* Philadelphia: Lippincott-Raven, 1997:1433–1539.

84. Kinkel K, Kaji Y, Yu KK, et al. Radiologic staging in patients with endometrial cancer: a meta-analysis. *Radiology* 1999;212:711–718.

85. Zerbe MJ, Bristow R, Grumbine FC, et al. Inability of preoperative computed tomography scans to accurately predict the extent of myometrial invasion and extracorporal spread in endometrial cancer. *Gynecol Oncol* 2000;78:67–70.

86. Kim SH, Kim HD, Song YS, et al. Detection of deep myometrial invasion in endometrial carcinoma: Comparison of transvaginal ultrasound, CT, and MRI. *J Comput Assist Tomogr* 1995;19:766–772.

87. Hardesty LA, Sumkin JH, Hakim C, et al. The ability of helical CT to preoperatively stage endometrial cancer. *AJR Am J Roentgenol* 2001;176:603–606.

88. Frei KA, Kinkel K, Bonel HM, et al. Prediction of deep myometrial invasion in patients with endometrial cancer: clinical utility of contrast-enhanced MR imaging – A meta-analysis and Bayesian analysis. *Radiology* 2000;216:444–449.

89. Shibutani O, Joja I, Shiraiwa M, et al. Endometrial carcinoma: efficacy of thin-section oblique axial MR images for evaluating cervical invasion. *Abdom Imaging* 1999;24:520–526.

90. Connor JP, Andrews JI, Anderson B, et al. Computed tomography in endometrial carcinoma. *Obstet Gynecol* 2000;95:692–696.

91. Reddoch JM, Burke TW, Morris M, et al. Surveillance for recurrent endometrial carcinoma: development of a follow-up scheme. *Gynecol Oncol* 1995;59:221–225.

92. Sanders C, Rubin E. Malignant gestational trophoblastic disease: CT findings. *AJR Am J Roentgenol* 1987;148:165–168.

93. Davis WK, McCarthy S, Moss AA, et al. Computed tomography of gestational trophoblastic disease. *J Comput Assist Tomogr* 1984; 8:1136–1139.

94. Miyasaka Y, Hachiya J, Furuya Y, et al. CT evaluation of invasive trophoblastic disease. *J Comput Assist Tomogr* 1985;9:459–462.

95. Green CL, Angtuaco TL, Shah HR, et al. Gestational trophoblastic disease: A spectrum of radiologic diagnosis. *Radiographics* 1996; 16:1371–1384.

96. Wilbur AC, Aizenstein RI, Napp TE. CT findings in tuboovarian abscess. *AJR Am J Roentgenol* 1992;158:575–579.

97. Romo LV, Clarke PD. Fitz-Hugh–Curtis syndrome: pelvic inflammatory disease with an unusual CT presentation. *J Comput Assist Tomogr* 1992;16:832–833.

98. Tsubuku M, Hayashi S, Terahara A, et al. Fitz-Hugh–Curtis syndrome: linear contrast enhancement of the surface of the liver on CT. *J Comput Assist Tomogr* 2002;26:456–458.

99. Fishman EK, Scatarige JC, Saksouk FA, et al. Computed tomography of endometriosis. *J Comput Assist Tomogr* 1983;7:257–264.

100. Coley BD, Casola G. Incisional endometrioma involving the rectus abdominis muscle and subcutaneous tissues: CT appearance. *AJR Am J Roentgenol* 1993;160:549–550.

101. Nardi PM, Ruchman RB. CT appearance of diffuse peritoneal carcinomatosis. *J Comput Assist Tomogr* 1989;13:1075–1077.

102. Gougoutas CA, Siegelman ES, Hunt J, et al. Pelvic endometriosis: various manifestations and MR imaging findings. *AJR Am J Roentgenol* 2000;175:353–358.

103. Im JG, Kang HS, Choi BI, et al. Pleural endometriosis: CT and sonographic findings. *AJR Am J Roentgenol* 1987;148:523–524.

104. Volkart JR. CT findings in pulmonary endometriosis. *J Comput Assist Tomogr* 1995;19:156–159.

105. Buy JN, Ghossain MA, Mark AS, et al. Focal hyperdense areas in endometriomas: a characteristic finding on CT. *AJR Am J Roentgenol* 1992;159:769–771.

106. Weinfeld RM, Johnson SC, Lucas CE, et al. CT diagnosis of perihepatic endometriosis complicated by malignant transformation. *Abdom Imaging* 1998;23:183–184.

107. Stringfellow JM, Hawnaur JM. CT and MR appearances of sarcomatous change in chronic pelvic endometriosis. *Br J Radiology* 1998; 71:90–93.

108. Vott S, Bonilla SM, Goodwin SC, et al. CT findings after uterine artery embolization. *J Comput Assist Tomogr* 2000;24:846–848.

109. Casillas J, Joseph RC, Guerra JJ. CT appearance of uterine leiomyomas. *Radiographics* 1990;10:999–1007.

110. Prieto A, Crespo C, Pardo A, et al. Uterine lipoleiomyomas: US and CT findings. *Abdom Imaging* 2000;25:655–657.

111. Smith AK, Coakley FV, Jackson R, et al. CT and MRI of retroperitoneal edema associated with large uterine leiomyomas. *J Comput Assist Tomogr* 2002;26:459–461.

112. Goodwin SC, McLucas B, Lee M, et al. Uterine artery embolization for the treatment of uterine leiomyomata midterm results. *J Vasc Interv Radiol* 1999;10:1159–1165.

113. Siskin GP, Englander M, Stainken BF, et al. Embolic agents used for uterine fibroid embolization. *AJR Am J Roentgenol* 2000; 175:767–773.

114. Katsumori T, Nakajima K, Mihara T, et al. Uterine artery embolization using gelatin sponge particles alone for symptomatic uterine fibroids: midterm results. *AJR Am J Roentgenol* 2002; 178:135–139

115. Spies JB, Roth AR, Jha RC, et al. Leiomyomata treated with uterine artery embolization: Factors associated with successful symptom and imaging outcome. *Radiology* 2002;222:45–52.

116. Spies JB, Scialli AR, Jha RC, et al. Initial results from uterine fibroid embolization for symptomatic leiomyomata. *J Vasc Interv Radiol* 1999;10:1149–1157.

117. Smith SJ, Sewall LE, Handelsman A. A clinical failure of uterine fibroid embolization due to adenomyosis. *J Vasc Interv Radiol* 1999; 10:1171–1174.

118. Nikolic B, Spies JB, Abbara S, et al. Ovarian artery supply of uterine fibroids as a cause of treatment failure after uterine artery embolization: a case report. *J Vasc Interv Radiol* 1999;10:1167–1170.

119. Nicholson TA, Pelage JP, Ettles DF. Fibroid calcification after uterine artery embolization: Ultrasonographic appearance and pathology. *J Vasc Interv Radiol* 2001;12:443–446.

120. Kimura I, Togashi K, Kawakami S, et al. Ovarian torsion: CT and MR imaging appearances. *Radiology* 1994;190:337–341.

121. Zissin R. Torsion of a normal ovary in a post-pubertal female: unenhanced helical CT appearance. *Br J Radiol* 2001;74:762–763.

122. Kawahara Y, Fukuda T, Futagawa S, et al. Intravascular gas within an ovarian tumor: a CT sign of ovarian torsion. *J Comput Assist Tomogr* 1996;20:154–156.

123. Belenky A, Bartal G, Atar E, et al. Ovarian varices in healthy female kidney donors: incidence, morbidity, and clinical outcome. *AJR Am J Roentgenol* 2002;179:625–627.

124. Rozenblit AM, Ricci ZJ, Tuvia J, et al. Incompetent and dilated ovarian veins: a common CT finding in asymptomatic parous women. *AJR Am J Roentgenol* 2001;176:119–122.

125. Tazarov PG, Prozorovskij KV, Ryzhkov VK. Pelvic pain syndrome caused by ovarian varices: treatment by transcatheter embolization. *Acta Radiol* 1997;38:1023–1025.

126. Harris RD, Holtzman SR, Poppe AM. Clinical outcome in female patients with pelvic pain and normal pelvic US findings. *Radiology* 2000;216:440–443.

127. Coakley FV, Varghese SL, Hricak H. Pictorial essay: CT and MRI of pelvic varices in women. *J Comput Assist Tomogr* 1999;23:429–434.

128. Mathis BV, Miller JS, Lukens ML, et al. Pelvic congestion syndrome: a new approach to an unusual problem. *Am Surg* 1995;61:1016–1018.

129. Jacoby WT, Cohan RH, Baker ME, et al. Ovarian vein thrombosis in oncology patients: CT detection and clinical significance. *AJR Am J Roentgenol* 1990;155:291–294.

130. Kubik-Huch RA, Hebisch G, Huch R, et al. Role of duplex color doppler ultrasound, computed tomography, and MR angiography in the diagnosis of septic puerperal ovarian vein thrombosis. *Abdom Imag* 1999;24:85–91.

131. Yassa NA, Ryst E. Ovarian vein thrombosis: a common incidental finding in patients who have undergone total abdominal hysterectomy and bilateral salpingo-oophorectomy with retroperitoneal lymph node dissection. *AJR Am J Roentgenol* 1999;172:45–47.

132. Quane LK, Kidney DD, Cohen AJ. Unusual causes of ovarian vein thrombosis as revealed by CT and sonography. *AJR Am J Roentgenol* 1998;171:487–490.

133. Twickler DM, Setiawan AT, Evans RS, et al. Imaging of puerperal septic thrombophlebitis: prospective comparison of MR imaging, CT, and sonography. *AJR Am J Roentgenol* 1997;169:1039–1043.

134. Savader SJ, Otero RR, Savader BL. Puerperal ovarian vein thrombosis: evaluation with CT, US, and MR imaging. *Radiology* 1988; 167:637–639.

135. Lowdermilk C, Gavant ML, Qaisi W, et al. Screening helical CT for evaluation of blunt traumatic injury in the pregnant patient. *Radiographics* 1999;19:S243–S255.

136. Kalbhen CL. CT of pregnant women for urinary tract calculi, pulmonary thromboembolism, and acute appendicitis. *AJR Am J Roentgenol* 2002;178:1285–1286.

137. Boiselle PM, Reddy SS, Villas PA, et al. Pulmonary embolus in pregnant patients: survey of ventilation-perfusion imaging policies and practices. *Radiology* 1998;207:201–206.

138. Winer-Muram HT, Boone JM, Brown HL, et al. Pulmonary embolism in pregnant patients: fetal radiation dose with helical CT. *Radiology* 2002;224:487–492.

139. Kennedy A. Assessment of acute abdominal pain in the pregnant patient. *Semin Ultrasound CT MR* 2000;21:64–77.

140. Boridy IC, Maklad N, Sandler CM. Suspected urolithiasis in pregnant women: imaging algorithm and literature review. *AJR Am J Roentgenol* 1996;167:869–875.

141. Castro MA, Shipp TD, Ouzounian J, et al. The use of helical computed tomography in pregnancy for the diagnosis of acute appendicitis. *Am J Obstet Gynecol* 2001;184:954–957.

142. Mann FA, Nathens A, Langer SG, et al. Communicating with the family: The risks of medical radiation to conceptuses in victims of major blunt-force torso trauma. *J Trauma* 2000;48:354–357.

143. Timins J. Pregnancy and medical radiation, part I. *J Women's Imaging* 2002;4:31–32.

144. Marcos HB, Semelka RC, Worawattanakul S. Normal placenta: gadolinium-enhanced, dynamic MR imaging. *Radiology* 1997; 205:493–496.

145. Thomas SM, Bees NR, Adam EJ. Trends in the use of pelvimetry techniques. *Clin Radiol* 1998;53:293–295.

146. Raman S, Samuel D, Suresh K. A comparative study of x-ray pelvimetry and CT pelvimetry. *Aust N Z J Obstet Gynecol* 1991;31:217–220.

147. Morris CW, Heggie JCP, Acton CM. Computed tomography pelvime-

try: accuracy and radiation dose compared with conventional pelvimetry. *Australas Radiol* 1993;37:186–191.

148. Wiesen EJ, Crass JR, Bellon EM, et al. Improvement in CT pelvimetry. *Radiology* 1991;178:259–262.

149. Aronson D, Kier R. CT pelvimetry: The foveae are not an accurate landmark for the level of the ischial spines. *AJR Am J Roentgenol* 1991;156:527–530.

150. Smith RC, McCarthy S. Improving the accuracy of digital CT pelvimetry. *J Comput Assist Tomogr* 1991;15:787–789.

151. Zuckerman J, Levine D, McNicholas MMJ, et al. Imaging of pelvic postpartum complications. *AJR Am J Roentgenol* 1997;168:663–668.

152. Urban BA, Pankov BL, Fishman EK. Postpartum complications in the abdomen and pelvis: CT evaluation. *Crit Rev Diag Imag* 1999; 40:1–21.

153. Rooholamini SA, Au AH, Hansen GC, et al. Imaging of pregnancy-related complications. *Radiographics* 1993;13:753–770.

154. Garagiola DM, Tarver RD, Gibson L, et al. Anatomic changes in the pelvis after uncomplicated vaginal delivery: a CT study in 14 women. *AJR Am J Roentgenol* 1989;153:1239–1241.

155. Twickler DM, Setiawan AT, Harrell RS, et al. CT appearance of the pelvis after cesarean section. *AJR Am J Roentgenol* 1991; 156:523–526.

156. Barton JR, Sibai BM. Hepatic imaging in HELLP syndrome (hemolysis, elevated liver enzymes, and low platelet count). *Am J Obstet Gynecol* 1996;174:1820–1827.

157. Zissin R, Yaffe D, Fejgin M, et al. Hepatic infarction in preeclampsia as part of the HELLP syndrome: CT appearance. *Abdom Imaging* 1999;24:594–596.

158. Casillas VJ, Amendola MA, Gascue A, et al. Imaging of nontraumatic hemorrhagic hepatic lesions. *Radiographics* 2000;20:367–378.

159. Pannu HK, Kaufman HS, Cundiff GW, et al. Dynamic MR imaging of pelvic organ prolapse: spectrum of abnormalities. *Radiographics* 2000;20:1567–1582.

160. Niazi ZBM, Kutty M, Petro JA, et al. Vaginal reconstruction with a rectus abdominis musculoperitoneal flap. *Ann Plast Surg* 2001; 46:563–568.

161. Siegelman ES, Banner MP, Ramchandani P, et al. Multicoil MR imaging of symptomatic female urethral and periurethral disease. *Radiographics* 1997;17:349–365.

162. Salem S. The uterus and adnexa. In: Rumack CM, Wilson SR, Charboneau JW, eds. *Diagnostic ultrasound*, 2nd ed. St. Louis: Mosby-Year Book, 1998:519–573.

163. Heinonen PK. Clinical implications of the didelphic uterus: long-term follow-up of 49 cases. *Eur J Obstet Gynecol Reprod Biol* 2000; 91:183–190.

SECTION V

Vascular Applications

CHAPTER 22

Angiography of the Aorta and Its Branches

Geoffrey D. Rubin

INTRODUCTION

Multidetector computed tomography (MDCT) has expanded substantially the role of computed tomography (CT) for imaging the arterial system over single-detector computed tomography (SDCT). The benefits of MDCT allow acquisitions to be performed substantially faster and with thinner sections than SDCT. Moreover, anatomic coverage encompassing the entire arterial tree is made possible by higher table speeds. This chapter focuses on the important technical principles for optimizing computed-tomography angiography (CTA) acquisition and the range of clinical applications that CTA effectively addresses. Although CTA can be performed satisfactorily using SDCT, this chapter will focus exclusively on MDCT. Readers interested in performing CTA examinations using SDCT scanners are referred to the second edition of this book.

TECHNICAL CONSIDERATIONS

Detector Rows

The rapid pace of MDCT development has resulted in a wide spectrum of CT-scanner capabilities. Current scanning design incorporates from 2 to 16 rows of detectors and gantry rotations from 0.5 to 1.0 second; difference in the speed of MDCT acquisition can vary by 16-fold. This has a tremendous impact on the types of clinical applications to which the scanner may be directed and the amount of iodinated contrast medium required to perform the examination. In general, there is no advantage to having fewer detector rows or slower maximal gantry rotation speed. When considering the inverse relationship between MDCT cost and the number of detector rows, an important point to consider is the optimal number of rows for a given clinical application. While there is little doubt that the quality of cardiac CT images is improved greatly with 16 rows, there has been no documentation of improved image quality when imaging the abdominal aorta, for example, using 16 rows versus 8 rows or even 4 rows. Thus, one might argue that a 4-row scanner may be

perfectly adequate for abdominal aortic imaging (Figure 22-1). However, when imaging of lower extremity arterial inflow and run-off is desired, there are substantial advantages to 8 rows over 4 rows, as a 1.00-mm to 1.25-mm acquisition is only practical with 8 or more rows. The 30 seconds required to acquire 1000 mm of coverage from the diaphragm through the toes when acquiring an 8-mm × 1.25-mm acquisition at a pitch of 1.7 and a rotation of 0.5 seconds may be entirely satisfactory. Completing the scan in 15 seconds using similar acquisition parameters on a 16-row scanner might seem unnecessary unless noise reduction is required to image a 400-kg patient. The added "headroom" of 16 rows allows the gantry rotation to increase to 1.0 seconds, allowing the scan to be acquired in 30 seconds with 40% less noise. The patient who requires thoracic aortic assessment in addition to abdominal and lower extremity arterial assessment poses a challenge. Is an 8-row scanner satisfactory to image 1500 mm if 45 seconds are required and the contrast injection must be extended by reducing the flow rate from 5.0 to 3.3 mL per second? Unfortunately, answers to these questions are not available through carefully designed hypothesis-driven investigations published in the peer-reviewed literature. Recently, the pace of CT development has overwhelmed the ability to study these issues formally. Perhaps, in time, formalized investigations of these issues will appear in the peer-reviewed literature; however, in the interim, this chapter will present some guiding principles used to consider how to select acquisition parameters for performing CTA. In general, not every clinical situation requires a 16-row scanner to achieve diagnostic images; the flexibility in acquisition-parameter selection afforded by a 16-row scanner over 8-row, 4-row, or 2-row scanners means that more patient scans will be diagnostic, particularly at the extremes of patient size, iodinated contrast limitations, and anatomic coverage or small vessel detail requirements.

Three factors determine the difference between a high-quality CTA and a nondiagnostic examination: section thickness, image noise, and consistent arterial opacification. If

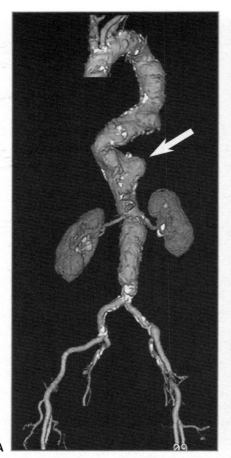

A

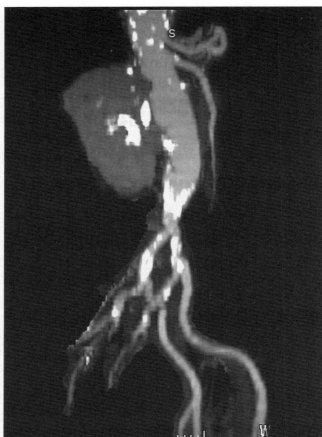

B

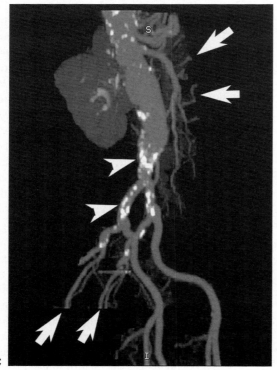

C

FIG. 22–1. A: Anterior volume-rendered images of 4-row MDCT angiogram obtained in a 73-year-old subject with a thoracic aortic aneurysm (*arrow*) assessed prior to endoluminal repair. This examination was compared to a SDCT angiogram obtained 11 months prior. Scan coverage was 534 mm and 580 mm; scan duration was 71 seconds and 31 seconds; contrast medium volume was 306 mL and 124 mL; and the mean aortoiliac attenuation was 329 HU and 376 HU, for SDCT and MDCT, respectively. Steep right anterior oblique MIPs of the abdominal aorta and iliac arteries from the SDCT angiogram **(B)** and the MDCT angiogram **(C)**. Improved distinction of calcified plaque (*arrowheads*) and greater visualization of superior mesenteric and internal iliac artery branches (*arrows*) are demonstrated. *(continued)*

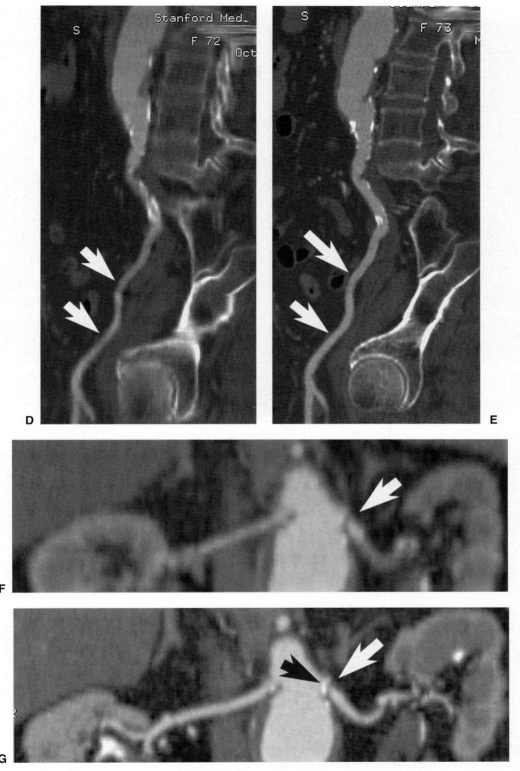

FIG. 22–1. *Continued.* Curved sagittal **(D,E)** reformations of the distal abdominal aorta, right common and external iliac arteries from SDCT and MDCT angiograms, respectively. Substantially better longitudinal spatial resolution on the MDCT scan is seen in the lumbar spine and regions of attenuation dropout are seen in obliquely oriented regions of the external iliac artery on the SDCT scan (*arrows*). Curved coronal reformations **(F,G)** from SDCT and MDCT angiograms, respectively, demonstrate a left renal-artery stenosis (*short white arrows*). Calcification at the origin of the left renal artery is seen only on the 4CCT examination (*black arrow*). The obliquely oriented right renal artery is visualized substantially better on the MDCT examination. *(continued)*

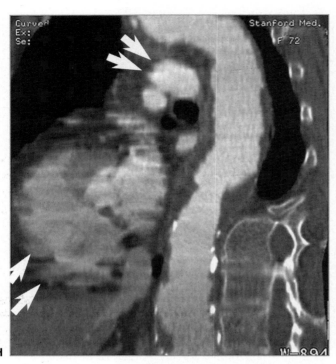

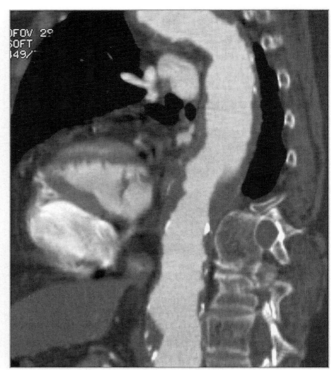

FIG. 22–1. *Continued.* Curved sagittal reformations through the descending aorta from the SDCT **(H)** and the MDCT angiograms **(I)** demonstrate substantially less pulsation artifact in the myocardium, pericardial and epicardial fat, and the left pulmonary artery (*arrows*).

any one of these factors is inadequate, the entire examination will be compromised. The following sections discuss these issues and their interdependence with each other and with the principle acquisition variables of scan duration, table speed, gantry rotation speed, number of detector rows, and X-ray-tube current.

Scan Duration

Because CTA requires intense and reasonably homogeneous arterial enhancement with minimal venous enhancement, scan durations typically should not exceed 50 seconds, and preferably should not exceed 30 seconds. One notable exception to this occurs when imaging the lower extremity arterial run-off, which is discussed specifically later in this chapter. When imaging occurs in the chest and abdomen, breathing will induce motion-related artifacts. In the thorax and abdomen, the scan duration typically is governed by the patient's breathholding ability. Virtually all patients without severe respiratory dysfunction will maintain a 30-second breath hold, provided it is preceded by a period of hyperventilation. In fact, many patients will be capable of a 40-second breath hold. Fortunately, this rarely is necessary when using MDCT, and breath-hold durations are substantially shorter. Although the iliac arteries always are included in scans of the abdominal aorta, breathing-induced artifacts are negligible below the iliac crests. Unlike SDCT, even with the narrowest

detector groups, the relatively high table speeds of 8-row and 16-row MDCT allow approximately 400 mm of longitudinal coverage needed for the adult chest and abdomen to be imaged with a 30-second breath hold. When scanning with 4-row CT scanners, thicker sections are required to allow imaging of the chest and abdomen during a breath hold. Table 22.1 typically presents a comparison of detector configurations and scan durations for thoracoabdominal-aortic and iliac-arterial CTA.

TABLE 22–1. *Detector configurations and scan durations*

Detector configuration	Gantry rotation (sec)	Scan duration for 500-mm scans (sec)	Scan duration for 1000-mm scan (sec)
1 × 3	.8	78	156
4 × 1.25		47	94
4 × 2.5		24	48
4 × 1.25	.5	30	60
4 × 2.5		15	30
8 × 1.25		15	30
16 × 1.25		7	15

Scan durations relative to detector configuration and gantry rotation for a typical 500-mm CTA of the thoracoabdominal aorta and iliac arteries and a typical 1000-mm CTA of the abdominal aorta and lower-extremity inflow and run off. A pitch of 1.7 is assumed for all scans. A typical 3-mm collimated SDCTA is included in the first row for perspective.

Section Thickness

Fundamental to MDCT is the consideration of section thickness as a reconstruction parameter, rather than an acquisition parameter. Nevertheless, the narrowest section thickness that can be reconstructed is dependent upon the width of the detector groups (see Chapter 14). Moreover, CTA always should be performed with the narrowest section thickness that can be reconstructed. Therefore, for CTA, it is reasonable to think of the width of the individual detector groups that are defined when prescribing the acquisition as the primary determinant of section thickness.

With 8-row and 16-row MDCT, the nominal section thickness is usually 1.00 mm to 1.25 mm. The only exception to this rule is when thinner sections are desired and a 16-row scanner is being used. Images with 0.625 to 0.750 nominal section thickness can be obtained for true isotropic voxels, but at a substantial cost in image noise. In our practice outside of the central nervous system and coronary circulation, only submillimeter-thick sections are acquired in pediatric patients only when imaging the upper extremity, the renal and mesenteric arteries in very thin adults. While 1.25-mm-thick sections are desirable with 4-row scanners, the scan duration may be unacceptably long. The greatest determinant of the use of 1.25-mm or 2.5-mm section thickness for a 4-row acquisition that covers 500 mm to 1000 mm will be gantry rotation speed. A 0.5 second per rotation gantry rotation will allow acquisitions of 1.25-mm section thickness over a longer distance than if the maximum gantry rotation speed is 0.8 seconds per rotation.

Image Noise

Image noise can have a profoundly adverse effect on three-dimensional (3D) visualization, particularly with volume rendering and maximum-intensity projection (MIP). Although a noisy scan may yield unsatisfactory 3D renderings, transverse sections may be diagnostic. Depending on the purpose of the scan, the exclusive assessment and presentation of transverse sections may be satisfactory; however, for many applications and, in particular, for referring physicians, the absence of diagnostic-quality 3D renderings may limit the usefulness of CTA.

The visibility of any structure in the body is dependent on the ratio of the contrast difference of that structure and its immediate background to the noise, or the "contrast-to-noise difference." During CTA, this ratio is influenced by the amount of arterial opacification and the degree of image noise. As section thickness is halved, the image noise increases by approximately 40%. Thus, there is a conflicting relationship between the desire to reduce section thickness in order to see smaller blood vessels and better detail in larger vessels and the desire to reduce noise. Fortunately, image noise also is influenced by factors that do not affect the spatial resolution of the scan. These factors include the X-ray current and potential and the reconstruction algorithm or kernel. For some scanners, pitch can indirectly influence the noise of the scan. This occurs because greater tube current is required to compensate for reconstruction strategies that avoid an increase in the effective section thickness as the pitch is increased. While for many acquisitions an increase in pitch will not affect noise, if the maximum tube current is selected for a scan with a given pitch value and that pitch value is increased, no more current can be supplied to compensate and noise will increase.

With respect to the reconstruction algorithms, a soft reconstruction kernel is best for CTA. Although there is some loss of transverse spatial resolution when using a soft kernel over standard or high-resolution bone algorithms, the resulting noise reduction substantially improves 3D renderings.

For most patients weighing less than 125 kg, 1.25-mm nominal section-thickness images have sufficiently low noise when combined with a soft reconstruction kernel and a high tube current [= 50 milliamperes (mA)]. If thinner submillimeter sections are desired, or in patients larger than 125 kg, noise becomes a substantial hindrance to achieving diagnostic results. An additional strategy to consider when tube current has been maximized is to slow the gantry rotation. While this approach will result in longer acquisition time, it will reduce noise proportional to the decrease in rotation speed. It is important to be aware, however, that the longer acquisition time required by the slower rotation speed will put greater demands on the X-ray tube, and thus may necessitate a reduction in the tube current to avoid overheating. When this happens, a decrease in gantry speed may do more harm than good. Consequently, various gantry rotations should be employed to assess which one allows the highest mAs product, thus maximizing the ability of this strategy to reduce noise. Slowing the gantry rotation is a useful strategy for imaging obese patients, but it has limited applicability for acquiring sections with submillimeter-section thickness because the table speed may be slowed to an unacceptable level, resulting in an acquisition that takes too long. This strategy for noise reduction when acquiring submillimeter sections is reserved for limited coverage, such as scans of the hands, feet, or renal arteries.

One final strategy that may be necessary for very obese patients is a shift to thicker sections. Even with a 16-row CT scanner, the loss of longitudinal spatial resolution from 1.25-mm to 2.5-mm-thick sections may mean the difference between a nondiagnostic and a diagnostic CT scan. Fortunately for both 8-row and 16-row CT scanners, the decision to assess 2.5-mm-thick sections can be made during image reconstruction; thus, as long as the raw data are saved, both 1.25-mm and 2.5-mm sections can be reconstructed and compared to select the image set that yields the greatest diagnostic value.

Radiation Safety

As with any application of CT scanning, radiation exposure is a consequence of CTA. Two points about radiation safety and MDCT germane to CTA are worth noting. First, because CTA relies on low-noise thin-section imaging, the radiation exposure is higher than some applications, such as thoracic CT, but typically less than CT-imaging strategies that require multiple phases of acquisition through the same region of anatomy. Moreover, the demand for speed, which typically necessitates using the fastest gantry rotation speeds and highest pitches available, tends to keep radiation exposure in check. It is important to remember that the increased radiation exposure with MDCT compared to SDCT decreases substantially when the number of detector rows is increased from four to eight or sixteen.

Most relevant to any discussion of radiation safety is the consideration of risk stratification, or assessing the risk associated with the procedure versus the risk of not performing the procedure. While the risk of not performing the procedure is difficult to quantify, the risk of radiation exposure has been quantified using some basic assumptions about the interaction of low levels of radiation and biological tissues. Moreover, the radiation exposure of CTA can be related to that of conventional angiography, with CTA typically being lower. When the radiation exposure of a 4-row MDCT protocol for an aortogram was compared to a run-off study, it was found that the radiation exposure was one quarter of the standard conventional angiographic protocol. In spite of favorable comparisons such as this, and the consideration that most patients undergoing CTA have life expectancies impacted by advanced manifestations of cardiovascular disease and are over 50 years of age with a lesser likelihood of radiation-induced morbidity, radiation risk should be considered carefully in children and young adults in whom gonadal or female breast irradiation will occur. For these latter patients, magnetic resonance imaging (MRI) may be preferable.

Spiral-Scan Reconstruction

Maximal longitudinal spatial resolution and optimized multiplanar and 3D visualization of CTA data requires generation of overlapping transverse reconstructions. In general, a reconstruction interval of one half the effective section thickness is a satisfactory compromise between an unwieldy number of reconstructed sections and improved longitudinal resolution. Sections generated with a low-noise reconstruction kernel ("standard" or "soft") will result in 3D renderings superior to reconstructions using higher spatial-frequency kernels ("bone"), which tend to be degraded unacceptably by image noise. A targeted field of view of 18 cm to 25 cm results in improved in-plane resolution, compared to larger fields of view used for routine thoracic or abdominal applications.

CONTRAST ADMINISTRATION

Computed-tomography angiography is performed with nonionic iodinated contrast (300–400 mgI/mL) injected into a peripheral vein. Nonionic contrast is used to minimize idiosyncratic reactions that might jeopardize patient immobility during CTA acquisition and to diminish morbidity if extravasation occurs. The goal of intravenous (IV) contrast-medium delivery is to achieve consistently high arterial enhancement with minimal venous enhancement. The first step toward achieving this goal is to ensure that MDCT acquisition is synchronized to the appearance of iodinated contrast medium in the target arteries. With bolus duration equivalent to the scan duration, the likelihood of "wasting" contrast medium prior to imaging is minimized.

To ensure that the contrast bolus duration is equivalent to the scan duration, one of two related equations are solved after the acquisition parameters have been selected:

$$\text{Contrast Medium Volume (mL)} = \text{Contrast Medium Flow Rate (mL/s)} \cdot \text{Scan Duration (s)} \quad (1)$$

or

$$\text{Contrast Medium Flow Rate (mL/s)} = \frac{\text{Contrast Medium Volume (mL)}}{\text{Scan Duration (s)}} \quad (2)$$

In general, and for a specific iodine concentration, the flow rate of contrast medium dictates arterial opacification. Therefore, for most CTAs, Eq. (1) is used to calculate the volume of contrast medium required. For normal adults weighing between 60 kg and 120 kg, a flow rate of 4 mL per second should opacify reliably the thoracic aorta to a level greater than 200 Hounsfield units (HU) for CTA of at least 20-seconds duration (1). Patients with very abnormal hemodynamics associated with sepsis (high cardiac output, low systemic vascular resistance) may opacify the systemic arteries unpredictably; however, this is rarely a problem for CTA applications in the aorta. For adults weighing less than 60 kg or more than 120 kg, flow rates of 3.5 mL per second and 5 mL per second, respectively, typically are satisfactory. When the injection duration is less than 20 seconds, higher flow rates are required to achieve the same level of opacification as a lower flow rate extended over a longer period of time. Thus, although CTA performed using MDCT substantially reduces the amount of iodine required to complete a diagnostic study compared to SDCT, the allowable reduction in contrast utilization does not have a linear relationship to the scan duration. In other words, halving the scan duration does not imply that halving the contrast dosage will provide the same level of arterial enhancement.

Flow rates of up to 4 mL per second can be administered comfortably through a 3-cm, 22-gauge IV catheter, and up to 7 mL per second can be administered comfortably through a 3-cm, 20-gauge IV catheter. In children or patients whose iodine dosage must be limited because of azotemia, Eq. (2) is used to calculate the flow rate required to deliver the dose of contrast medium in a bolus of equivalent length to scan duration. When a patient is azotemic and the calculated flow rate from Eq. (2) is too low to achieve sufficient arterial enhancement, the scan duration may be reduced to maintain opacification with less contrast medium at the expense of scan coverage or longitudinal spatial resolution. For children, 2 mL to 3 mL of 300 mgI per mL solution per kilogram typically is delivered. In performing CTA on children as small as 3 kg, it was found that power injection always is preferable to hand injection for controlling the bolus duration, particularly when flow rates as low as 0.2 mL per second are required.

Equations (1) and (2) both assume the use of a fixed monophasic contrast-medium injection. Some investigators have found that tailored biphasic injections (2) or exponentially decaying flow rates (3) can provide greater uniformity of contrast enhancement within the aorta from beginning to end of the CTA. A monophasic injection tends to result in a lesser degree of enhancement during the early portion of CTA, with enhancement rising throughout the scan (2). Although less uniform than the aforementioned multiphasic approaches, monophasic injections are the norm for CTA because of their simplicity and tend to give satisfactory results. Nevertheless, IV iodinated-contrast dynamics are complex and can be highly unpredictable without a formal assessment. The association between patient weight, iodine dose, and maximal arterial enhancement depends on physiologic factors that can be modeled and used to achieve more predictable and consistent levels of arterial enhancement (2,3). While currently unavailable on clinical CT systems, these approaches for patient-specific ''bolus shaping'' likely are to become more important in the future for optimizing contrast-medium utilization, particularly as CTA scan times commonly fall below 10 seconds with increasing numbers of detector-rows.

One other important refinement to contrast-medium administration that has been available in Europe for several years and should be available in the United States at the time of this publication, is the use of a dual-chamber injector to inject a saline flush immediately following iodinated-contrast injection. The use of a saline flush can diminish the total iodine dose while providing an equal degree of enhancement by clearing the veins from the injection site to the heart of contrast media that normally is pooled and unavailable for useful arterial enhancement during CTA (4). Effective bolus shaping also depends upon this technology.

While some authors have suggested that aortic CTA may be performed adequately with a fixed delay time, it is believed that scan-delay determination is a key element to achieving consistent CTA results and avoiding nondiagnostic exams due to insufficiently opacified blood vessels.

The optimal delay time between initiation of the IV-contrast bolus and commencement of spiral scanning cannot be predicted from the patient's blood pressure, heart rate, or other noninvasive physiologic measures; rather, it must be determined individually for the selected target anatomy.

There are two ways to ensure synchronization of contrast-medium bolus with scan acquisition: a preliminary contrast injection may be used to test the time required from injection initiation to aortic opacification (5,6) or the scan can be triggered based upon near real-time monitoring of the CTA contrast injection.

When using a preliminary test injection to determine scan delay, 10 mL or 15 mL of iodinated-contrast medium is sufficient for the thoracic or abdominal aorta, respectively. For children, approximately 1 mL per 5 kg of body weight is used, up to 10 mL. The injection is administered at the same rate as CTA, typically 4 mL per second. Five-millimeter collimated sections (80 kV to 100 kV, 80 mA) are acquired every 2 seconds at the anticipated initiation point of CTA, for a total of 20 images. In adults, imaging commences eight seconds after the injection begins. Shorter delays are required in children and depend upon the site of IV access. A time–density curve is generated from a region of interest drawn within the main artery imaged, usually the aorta, to determine accurately appropriate scan-delay time for individual patients (Figure 22-2). While the circulation time to the aorta will be 20 ± 8 seconds in 80% of adult patients, it typically is impossible to predict which patients will have substantially delayed circulation, which can be caused by elevated cardiac-filling pressures, poor cardiac output, tricuspid regurgitation, and stenoses in the veins between the injection site and the heart. When present, these lesions can prolong the arrival of contrast to the aorta by up to 45 seconds. Once the images are acquired, visual inspection typically identifies the time of greatest opacification; however, for some patients, the creation of a time–density curve is the most reliable means for finding this peak. The time to greatest opacification was selected as the delay for CTA acquisition.

An alternative to the use of a test bolus to determine scan delay is to trigger the CTA acquisition directly while monitoring a target blood vessel for the appearance of enhancement following initiation of the primary contrast injection. The use of scan triggering typically requires selection of an option on the scanner prescription page. The name and operation of this option vary with the CT manufacturer. Common to all is the selection of a transverse level for bolus monitoring. A single unenhanced section is acquired and a region of interest is positioned graphically within the artery to be monitored. This typically is the aorta at the level where CTA is to begin, but it may be positioned either further proximal in the arterial system if the initiation point is in the head or neck or further distal in the arterial system if there is concern that the bolus may be overrun, as can be the case with 16-row scanners when imaging arteries of the extremities. A preliminary delay between the initiation of contrast-medium injection and the beginning of the monitoring phase is selected. For most systemic arterial applications, eight seconds is a conservative value for this delay. For the monitoring phase, an interscan delay of approximately 1 second to 3 seconds is selected. This value should be minimized to avoid overly prolonging the time from arterial enhancement to CTA initiation. Finally, the scan is triggered either manually or automatically depending on the manufacturer's

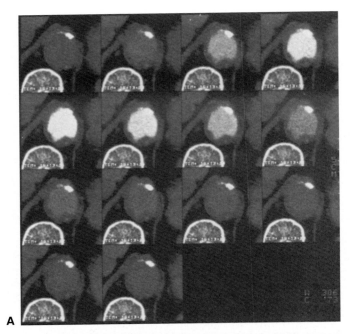

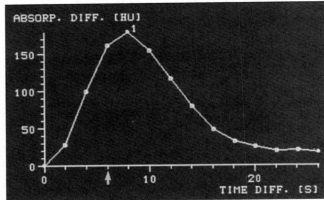

FIG. 22–2. A: Axial-CT sections obtained at the level of the supraceliac aorta every 2 seconds. The first image was obtained 8 seconds following initiation of a 20-mL contrast bolus injected at 5 mL per second. **B:** Time–density curve generated by placing a region of interest within the aorta. Time zero on the curve represents the point where imaging began (8 seconds after initiation of the 20-mL bolus). Due to a 4-second bolus duration, a 4-second window is centered about the peak of the curve. Eight seconds is added to the time to reach this window, and this value used as the CTA-injection delay, 14 seconds in this case.

implementation. Automatic triggering occurs once enhancement within the region of interest rises above a specified level, usually 150 HU to 250 HU Manual triggers rely upon operator observation, either on reconstructed transverse sections or from a graphical output of enhancement over time. Both approaches yield satisfactory results and, although an automated trigger may seem preferable, manual intervention still is necessary if the region of interest encompasses unenhancing portions of the target vessel or was placed inadvertently on a structure that is not an artery. If the operator is not attuned to these possibilities, the bolus may pass without triggering of CTA.

Although the use of bolus monitoring can save time and is a more direct way to trigger CTA than a separate test injection, there is an important pitfall to this approach. The overall time from arrival of contrast in the target artery to triggering of CTA ranges from 2 seconds to 8 seconds, depending upon the CT manufacturer. Consequently, the length of injection must be prolonged to allow for this delay. With injection flow rates that typically range from 5 mL to 7 mL per second, an increase in the contrast-medium dosage of up to 40 mL to 60 mL may be required.

For thoracic aortic CTA, injection into the right antecubital vein is preferable to the left, as left antecubital injection results in opacification of the left brachiocephalic vein and resultant perivenous artifact can degrade substantially visualization of the brachiocephalic artery origins. While the majority of injections is performed via the right antecubital vein, if a catheter is present within the superior vena cava, injection into the superior vena cava results in a tighter bolus and greater arterial opacification because of less contrast medium pooling within the veins.

Although it has found that dilution of 300 mgI per mL solutions of contrast medium to near isoosmolar levels (150 mgI/mL) results in significantly greater arterial enhancement and less perivenous artifact than the same dosage of iodine delivered in 300 mg I per mL solution (7), dilute solutions are used for aortic CTA. This study focused only upon performance of routine thoracic spiral CT where required vascular opacification is much less than for CTA. Additional investigation is required to establish whether relationships between iodine concentration, perivenous artifact, and arterial enhancement determined for low iodine dosages (15 gm to 22.5 gm) similarly are applicable at the higher doses required for CTA. Furthermore, the typical capacity of power injectors is 200 mL, making delivery of typical CTA doses of 40 g I to 50 g I in a 150 mg I per mL solution impossible. For this reason, 300 mg I per mL nonionic-contrast medium is used for all aortic CTA.

Alternative Visualization

A detailed discussion of the various methods for alternative two-dimensional (2D) and 3D visualization of CTA data is presented elsewhere, and salient advantages and disadvantages of the most commonly used visualization techniques are summarized in Table 22.2. Specific applications of these visualization techniques are included in the subsequent discussions of the various lesions assessed with CTA. It is important to stress, however, that the quality of multiplanar reformations and 3D renderings is influenced primarily by the quality of the CT data. A thorough understanding of CT principles is required for optimal creation of multiplanar and 3D renderings, and no amount of sophisticated rendering and image segmentation can resurrect a poor acquisition.

TABLE 22–2. *Visualization techniques*

	Multiplanar or curved-planar reformation	MIP	VR
Advantages	"Slices" through the center of the vessel to show lumen, useful with arterial stents or eccentric calcifications	Best visualization of small or poorly enhancing blood vessels, particularly within parenchymal organs or where background attenuation is high	Displays complex anatomic relationships in regions of vessel overlap or tortuosity
Disadvantages	Inaccurate curve drawing can falsely imply lesions not present	Confusion in regions of vessel overlap Cannot image interior of metallic stents Limited in regions of heavy calcification	Incorrect opacity-transfer function can falsely imply or exclude lesions

Artifacts

Common sources of artifacts in CTA scans include breathing-induced misregistrations, cardiac motion-induced misregistration, metallic artifacts, perivenous streaks, and the helical artifact. The majority of breathing-related artifacts are prevented easily with patient coaching. As long as the patient is aware of the importance of the breath hold, the required breath hold is within patient capability, and instructions are given to hyperventilate and then suspend ventilation at the point of maximal inspiration, respiration-induced artifacts will be minimal. It also is important when scanning long distances, such as assessing lower extremity arterial inflow and run-off, to remind the patient to breathe, but otherwise remain motionless after the abdomen has been scanned.

Misregistration due to cardiac motion and arterial pulsation is most relevant to assessments of the heart and great vessels, particularly the ascending aorta. While cardiac gated acquisitions will eliminate the majority of these artifacts, the penalties of prolonged scan time and increased radiation exposure associated with gated acquisition may not be tolerable. While there is little else that can be done to reduce artifacts caused by cardiac pulsation during image acquisition, it is interesting to note that these artifacts are reduced substantially as the number of detector rows increases (8). This phenomenon is attributed to the fact that the higher table speeds associated with higher numbers of detector rows result in less heartbeats imaged during the time of cardiac scanning, effectively spreading the motion out over a greater longitudinal distance. Arterial pulsation can create a diagnostic challenge when it is suggestive of ascending aortic dissection. Though the increasing acquisition speed of spiral CT has reduced substantially the prevalence of this artifact, there is an intervention that can be applied retrospectively to the raw scan data to minimize further these artifacts. "Segmented" or "weighted half-scan" reconstruction is an alternative interpolation technique that minimizes the amount of projection data required to generate a cross section. As implemented by General Electric, this results in a

reduction of projection data required to reconstruct a cross section from the standard 360 degrees to 225 degrees. For a 0.5-second gantry rotation period, segmented reconstruction effectively improves the temporal resolution of the scan from 0.5 seconds to 0.3 seconds. This has been shown to eliminate artifacts that might be misconstrued as intimal flaps on CT scans (9).

Metallic artifacts, while ubiquitous from vascular clips, indwelling catheters, cardiac leads, joint prostheses, and orthopedic-fixation hardware, may be reduced using the strategies discussed previously for increasing photon flux in situations of high image noise, but usually improve only minimally. In general, metallic artifacts do not hinder substantially CTA diagnosis.

Perivenous streaks likely are caused by a combination of beam hardening and motion caused by transmitted pulsation to veins carrying undiluted contrast medium to the heart. Strategies designed to minimize this artifact include the use of diluted contrast-medium solutions (7,10), caudal-to-cranial scan direction, femoral venous access (11), and a saline "chaser" bolus immediately following the iodinated contrast-medium injection (4). Perivenous streaks from the superior vena cava tend to have their greatest influence on visualization of the ascending aorta, and therefore are particularly important to bear in mind when assessing patients suspected of aortic dissection. In practice, perivenous streaks rarely are confused with intimal dissection in the ascending aorta, as their orientation varies from section to section and they typically extend beyond the confines of the aortic wall. The most problematic region for perivenous artifacts is the origin of the supraaortic branches adjacent to an opacified left brachiocephalic vein. Perivenous streaks in this region can mask extension of intimal flaps into these branches and occlusive disease caused by atherosclerotic plaque. If detected at initial section reconstruction (within 2 minutes of bolus initiation), delayed sections can be prescribed rapidly to enable reimaging during a second pass of arterial contrast prior to the equilibrium phase. Other than this rapid intervention and reinjection at another site, there

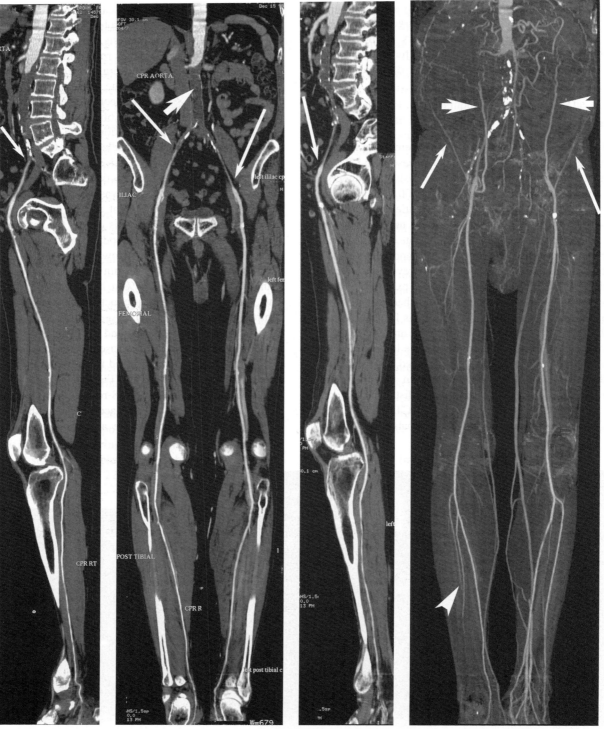

B,C **D,E**

FIG. 22–22. *Continued.* Four-millimeter × 2.5-mm MDCT angiogram: **(B)** Curved-sagittal reformation through the aorta and right lower extremity run off, **(C)** curved-coronal reformation, and **(D)** curved-sagittal reformation through the aorta and left lower extremity run off demonstrate atheroma and thrombus filling the infrarenal aorta, resulting in a complete aortic occlusion (*large arrows*) with reconstitution of flow in the right proximal external iliac and the left proximal femoral arteries (*long arrows*). **E:** Frontal MIP following manual removal of the bones demonstrates the patent inferior epigastric arteries (*short arrows*) and the patent deep-lateral circumflex iliac arteries (*long arrows*) that form critical collateral pathways to supply arterial blood to the lower extremities. With the exception of a mid-right anterior tibial artery occlusion (*arrowhead*), the run off is excellent.

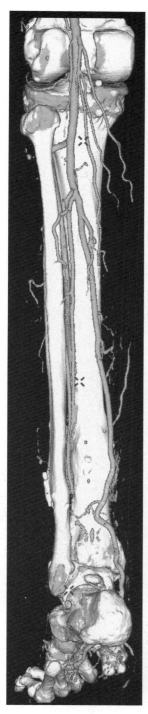
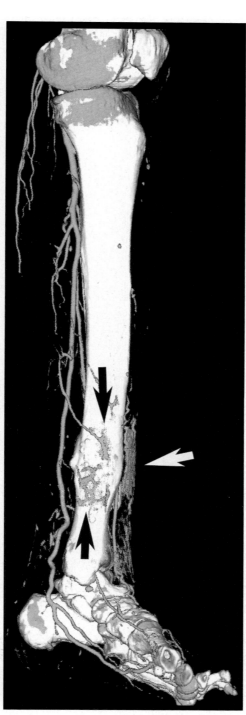

FIG. 22–23. Right lower extremity CTA acquired with 4.00-mm × 1.25-mm acquisition. **A:** Posterior volume rendering, **(B)** left lateral volume rendering. *(continued)*

A,B

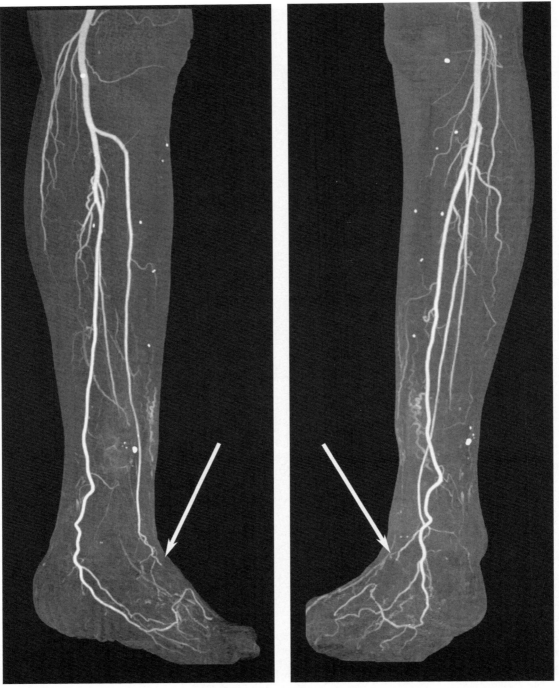

C

D

FIG. 22–23. *Continued.* **C:** Left lateral MIP following bone removal, and **(D)** right anterior oblique MIP following bone removal demonstrate the major arteries of the lower leg in this patient with chronic osteomyelitis of the distal tibia. Hyperemic regions are evident (*short arrows*) over the region of osteomyelitis. The dorsal pedis artery is occluded (*long arrows*); however, the posterior tibial artery is large and fills the pedal arch, which can be observed to supply individual digital arteries. The combination of bony and arterial visualization can be very useful to plastic surgeons planning a wide excision and arterial anastomosis to a free myocutaneous graft. (See Color Fig. 22–23)

Pitch was increased to 1.7 from 1.5, with a scan duration of approximately 36 seconds. The contrast-medium-injection protocol was similar to that described with a 4-mm × 2.5-mm acquisition and 0.5-second gantry rotation as discussed above. With 16-row MDCT, scan times are halved again to 18 seconds. This is a remarkable technical achievement and one that creates a dilemma for lower extremity CTA acquisition. While the fastest acquisition of the thinnest possible sections is the typical credo for a CT angiographer, this acquisition is too fast to image the lower extremity arterial system, given typical circulation times from aorta to feet of 30 seconds to 40 seconds. With 16-row MDCT, 1.00-mm to 1.25-mm detector thickness, 0.5-second gantry rotation, and 1.7 pitch, the CT scanner travels faster than arterial blood. One potentially desirable way to slow down the scan and improve the longitudinal spatial resolution would be to shift to a submillimeter section thickness in a 16-mm × 0.5-mm to 0.75-mm mode. Unfortunately, our experience is that only the thinnest of patients can tolerate this without an excessively noisy scan. This challenge has been approached in two ways. First, the pitch was reduced to 1.3 and gantry rotation increased to 0.6 second, increasing scan time by 29%, to 28 seconds. Next, the scan is triggered in the proximal superficial femoral arteries in the upper thigh. It is important to watch the bolus-monitoring images carefully in case the superficial femoral arteries are occluded and manual trigger is needed once the profunda femoral arteries opacify. By triggering the scan at a lower point along the arterial system, it was found that the likelihood of overrunning the contrast-medium injection decreases substantially, and foot opacification is more consistent. For the 16-row MDCT angiograms, 120 mL to 150 mL of 350 mg I per mL contrast medium was injected at 5 mL per second.

Because lower extremity arterial CTAs result in over 1000 transverse sections, 3D visualization is mandatory. Both MIP and VR make excellent survey tools and may be sufficient for the entirety of the interpretation if there is minimal calcium in the arterial walls. If MIP is to be used, bone removal is required prior to rendering. Recently developed algorithms automatically or semiautomatically remove the bones from the data set, making this operation substantially less cumbersome than in the past, when only manual techniques were available. With VR, the bones need not be removed, provided that real-time manipulation of the volume allows quick and intuitive control to the both rotation, zoom, pan, and clipping planes. When the vessel walls are laden with calcified plaque, transverse sections and CPR allow lumen analysis, which will be obscured on MIP and VR views.

Rarely, early venous opacification can complicate interpretation. While this is uncommon with 4-row scanners, it is even more rare with 8-row and 16-row scanners, owing to faster scan times. When it does occur, venous opacification is usually less than arterial opacification, allowing structures to be separated easily when assessing volume renderings, as different colors can be applied to attenuation values corresponding to arterial and venous enhancement. The presence of venous opacification on a properly timed CTA usually indicates ipsilateral accelerated capillary transit or arteriovenous shunting. In a study of 24 patients with 0.8-second rotation 4-row MDCT, seven patients had early venous filling. In five of these patients, ipsilateral inflammation was documented clinically as ischemic foot ulceration or infected iliofemoral bypass graft (87).

In addition to assessing occlusive disease of the lower-extremity inflow and run off, CTA is useful for assessing femoropopliteal aneurysms, determining whether arterial injury has occurred in penetrating trauma or adjacent to fractures, mapping arterial anatomy, and assessing for anomalies when planning fibular or myocutaneous transfer grafts. Computed-tomography angiography also is very useful for establishing graft patency, allowing visualization of both patent and occluded bypass grafts.

TRAUMA

Aortic injury occurs most commonly in the thoracic aorta at the aortic isthmus. The majority of patients with aortic transections never survive to be transported to a medical center for diagnosis and treatment. A small minority of patients has a contained rupture and present to the emergency department alive. In these patients, accurate diagnosis and triage to the operating room must be rapid.

The use of CT for detection of aortic injury has become a controversial topic (88–90). The principal application of conventional CT is the detection of mediastinal hemorrhage. A recently published meta-analysis of 18 previously published series of posttraumatic thoracic CT revealed that mediastinal hemorrhage had a specificity of 87.1% and a sensitivity of 99.3% for predicting aortic injury (89). Furthermore, reliance on CT for triaging patients to angiography only when CT was suspicious resulted in an overall cost savings of over $365,000.00 in a series conducted by Mirvis et al. of 677 trauma patients with chest radiographic abnormalities warranting aortic imaging (89). While these results are impressive, some have argued that confident identification of mediastinal hematoma, particularly on unenhanced CT, is extremely difficult (88).

The application of spiral CTA to suspected aortic trauma offers a new and important dimension to CT studies in these patients (Figures 22–24 and 22–25). Although initial reports have not relied upon the use of high-resolution spiral acquisitions coupled with high-flow iodinated-contrast injections, results are encouraging. Gavant and colleagues published the first spiral-CTA series of aortic injury. Using 7-mm collimation and contrast-medium flow rate of 1.5 mL to 2.0 mL per second, they found that CT sensitivity was greater than that of conventional arteriography (100% versus 94.4%), but specificity and positive predictive values were less than those of conventional arteriography (81.7% and 47.4%, respectively for CT, versus 96.3% and 81% for arteriography) in a subset of 127 of 1518 patients with non-

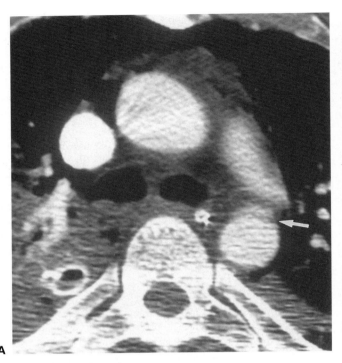

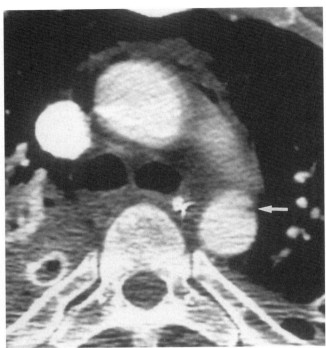

A   B

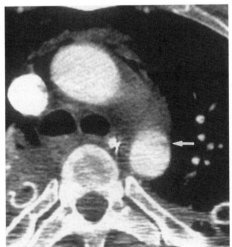

FIG. 22–24. Status post high-speed motor-vehicle accident—subtle aortic injury. **A–C:** Consecutive transverse helical CTA reconstructions obtained with 3-mm collimation, 2.0 pitch, and 2-mm reconstruction intervals demonstrate a subtle intimal injury of the aortic isthmus (*arrow*). Because of other injuries and skeptical trauma surgeons, an aortogram was not obtained until 3 months later. No abnormality was detectable on the standard LAO view (**D**); however, based upon the CT appearance, a true lateral view (**E**) was obtained that revealed the development of a small pseudoaneurysm (*arrow*). The injury was confirmed in the operating room. (From Rubin GD. Helical CT angiography of the thoracic aorta. *J Thorac Imaging* 1997;12:128–142, with permission.)

C

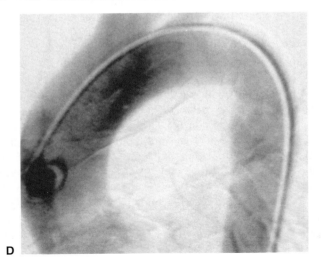

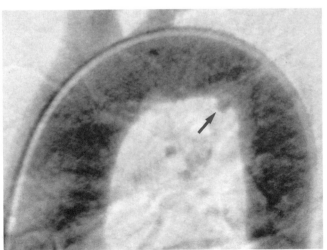

D   E

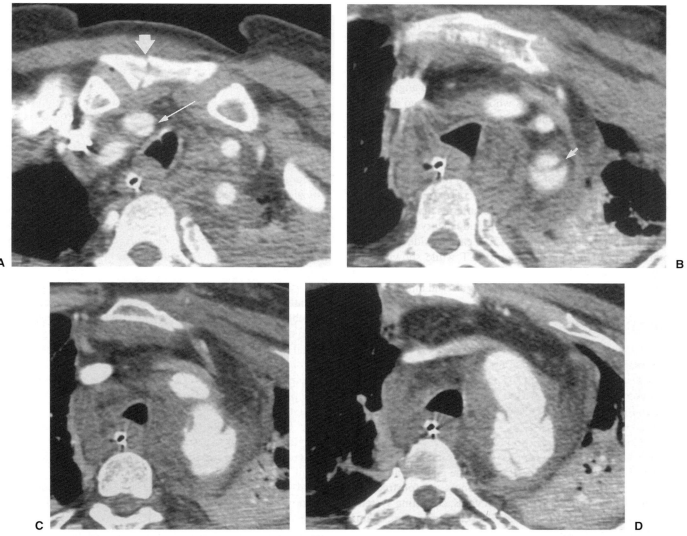

FIG. 22–25. Status post high-speed motor-vehicle accident—gross aortic injury. **A–D:** Transverse helical-CTA sections every 1 cm demonstrate aortic injury with pseudoaneurysm formation at the aortic isthmus. An intimal injury extends into the left subclavian artery (*short arrow*). An isolated intimal dissection in the right common carotid artery (*long arrow*) also is demonstrated deep to a vertical fracture of the manubrium (*wide arrow*). There is extensive mediastinal hematoma. The findings were confirmed in the operating room. (From Rubin GD. Helical CT angiography of the thoracic aorta. *J Thorac Imaging* 1997;12:128–142, with permission.)

trivial blunt thoracic trauma who underwent both CT and aortography. Perhaps the most encouraging result of this study was that no false-negative results occurred in the 21 patients with aortic injury (91). This remains the only published comparative series of spiral CTA of blunt thoracic-aortic trauma to date.

Gavant subsequently described the CT appearance of 38 thoracic aortic or great vessel injuries in 36 patients identified with spiral CT and confirmed with aortography or surgery. Six (17%) of these cases had no readily discernible paraaortic or mediastinal hematoma. Transverse sections showed either an intimal flap or thrombus protruding into the aortic lumen in all cases. Of 28 injuries to the descending

aorta, 23 (82%) were associated with a pseudoaneurysm. In subjectively comparing the value of reconstructed transverse sections to multiplanar reformations and 3D renderings, the authors felt that transverse sections were best for depicting the proximal and distal extent of the lesion and, aside from the fact that multiplanar reformations and 3D renderings "portray the thoracic aortic lumen in a familiar light," did not contribute substantially to identification and characterization of aortic injury (92).

Some caution should be exercised when interpreting the very impressive reported sensitivity of spiral CT for aortic injury. In the aforementioned study, iodinated-contrast medium was administered only to patients with evidence

CHAPTER 24

CT Angiography: Renal Applications

Elliot K. Fishman, Karen M. Horton

INTRODUCTION

The development of subsecond spiral computed tomography (CT), and more recently multidetector CT (MDCT), has provided the radiologist with unparalleled capability to acquire high-quality images of the kidneys and renal vasculature (1–2). It is now possible to obtain ultrathin section images (0.50 mm–1.25 mm), reconstruct data at narrow interscan intervals (0.5 mm–1.0 mm), and acquirese these data in the arterial, corticomedullary, venous, and/or excretory phases. However, the most significant advantage of the newest scanners is the ability to obtain volumes of data rather than thinner axial slices.

With a volume-acquisition system, that is MDCT, a volume of interest (i.e., the entire abdomen, liver, kidney, etc.) is imaged and can be displayed as a true volume, rather than as individual slices. Therefore, a CT scan now consists of three-dimensional (3D) volume display of information in a format that is easier and faster to analyze and has unique display capabilities. For example, the renal artery can be displayed as a series of 100 to 200 axial slices or a single coronal 3D image can be created in which the vessel is viewed in its entirety, similar to a catheter-based angiogram. However, the CT angiogram is faster, less invasive, less expensive, and safer than conventional angiograms, and it can be viewed in any plane or orientation for optimal diagnosis (3–5). In addition, with CT angiography (CTA) there are no geometric constraints of a C-arm, as used in classic angiography.

Although the techniques used for acquiring data for CTA are critical, they are not the focus of this presentation. Specific protocols are manufacturer specific and scanner specific (4-slice versus 16-slice MDCT). Specific scan protocols can be found on our Web site at http://www.ctisus.com. However, a few basic principles are discussed below.

TECHNIQUE

Oral- and Intravenous-Contrast Agents

Positive oral-contrast agents are never used in patients undergoing CTA, as they interfere with 3D imaging and require extensive editing. The use water as an oral-contrast agent is preferred to distend the stomach and intestines. In imaging the kidney, up to 1000 cc of water is administered routinely over a 15-minute to 20-minute period before the study. Water also provides a fluid bolus, which helps provide increased urine output, which is valuable for obtaining CT urograms.

A volume of 120 cc of oral contrast is used routinely for most renal applications. The volume can be decreased to 70 cc to 80 cc, if necessary, in patients with decreased renal function. In patients with borderline renal function, Visapaque-320 (Amersham Health, Princeton, NJ) is the preferred contrast agent owing to its better profile in patients with compromised renal function. Intravenous contrast typically is injected at 3 mL to 4 mL per second. Although several articles have suggested using injection rates of 5 mL per second, these high injection rates may not be necessary. Use of a saline chaser of 25 mL to 30 mL also may be helpful to limit contrast volumes in patients with compromised renal function. New dual-head injectors should make this easier to perform in routine clinical practice (6).

Data Acquisition and Protocols

Although timing of the arterial, corticomedullary, and/or venous phases can be done with either a timing bolus or computer-assisted software, preset delays also can be used with high-quality results. Typical scan delays are 25 seconds to 30 seconds for arterial-phase imaging, and 50 second to 60 seconds for corticomedullary phase imaging. In patients with a known history of cardiac disease, older patients, or patients with cardiomegaly on the topogram (scout view), an additional 10 seconds can be added to the scan delay. A recent article by Macari et al. demonstrated that successful CTA in the abdomen could be done with uniform preset scan delays (7).

Although many of the renal applications can be performed on single-detector CT (SDCT) scanners, the ability to use shorter scan times, higher resolution, and thinner sections makes MDCT the technique of choice. Sixteen-slice MDCT has obvious advantages over 4-slice MDCT in angiographic applications, providing a combination of faster data acquisition and isotropic datasets. With 16-slice MDCT, a typical acquisition through the kidneys, even with 0.75-mm scan thickness, is under 10 seconds. Short scan-acquisition times allows easier timing of data acquisition and phase-of-contrast enhancement.

For detailed vascular anatomy, slice thickness should be between 1.00 mm and 1.25 mm with data reconstruction at 1-mm intervals using 4-slice MDCT, and 0.50-mm to 0.75-mm slice thickness with 0.50-mm to 0.75-mm interscan intervals using 16-slice MDCT. All data are sent to the workstation in the original resolution (512×512) for postprocessing. Several systems now have 3D software on the satellite-scanner consoles, allowing even more convenience for data processing. Both multiplanar reconstruction (MPR) (coronal and sagittal imaging) and 3D imaging are used routinely for image analysis. Currently available commercial software may provide a complete integration of the axial, multiplanar, and 3D capabilities in a single display.

Image Display

Although discussion of the various workstations and the importance of specific rendering algorithms are critical, they are discussed in the literature and in several other chapters in this book and will not be addressed at length in this chapter (8–11). However, several recurring themes will be highlighted for completeness.

Creation of 3D angiograms usually is performed best on a freestanding workstation separate from the actual point of scanning. This allows consultation with referring physicians without interfering with the scanner's core scanning functions. As noted previously, the availability of postprocessing capabilities near the scanners is valuable in providing rapid feedback to referring physicians. Although there is strong argument for a central 3D lab, this functionality needs to be available clinically for referring physicians. Referring physicians are becoming more interested in the 3D volume display than the original axial displays alone. It is believed that this current trend will become an increasingly important method of visualization in the future.

A 3D imaging system allowing direct interaction with the CT volume is preferred over a system creating select preset views for the user. The radiologist must take an active role in image analysis, as he or she alone can select the best optimal plane and orientation for demonstrating the extent and presence of renal pathology. Unsuspected pathology also is more likely to be detected when the radiologist interactively views the data volume. This typically is referred to as real-time rendering and currently is available on select workstations, but it is becoming available more commonly.

Volume rendering is the preferred 3D rendering technique for CTA. Its specific advantages in vascular imaging include a more accurate visualization of vascular patency and stenosis, as well as detection of vascular anomalies. Numerous articles have shown volume rendering to be ideal for abdominal CTA. However, maximum intensity projection (MIP) rendering also is valuable as an adjunct display, especially for smaller vessels within an enhancing organ such as the kidney. However, MIP has several disadvantages in the presence of vascular calcification, which may result in an overestimation of the degree of vessel stenosis. In general, both volume rendering and MIP are used in most cases of renal CTA to optimize detection of any possible pathology.

Alternative visualization techniques including stereoscopic display are valuable when viewing complex vascular anatomy such as in the renal transplant donor (10,11), in cases of partial-nephrectomy planning, or in renal-cancer surgery patients when vascular invasion is present. Presurgical planning using 3D imaging is becoming increasingly important in genitourinary imaging.

CLINICAL APPLICATIONS IN RENAL IMAGING

Numerous articles have been published documenting the value of 3D CT imaging of the kidneys and renal vasculature. Please note that many of the early articles used single-slice CT and not the newer multislice systems, which yield superior results. Articles reporting on the experience with 4-slice MDCT now are appearing in the literature, while articles on the value of 16-slice scanners should begin to appear over the next 6 months to 12 months. Personal experience with 16-slice MDCT has shown that it is ideal for renal imaging and quickly has become the gold standard in this practice.

There are numerous clinical applications for CTA of the kidney documented in the literature. The most common applications include evaluation of potential renal-transplant donors; detection, classification, and staging of renal masses; determining whether a patient with renal cancer is eligible for nephron-sparing surgery; and evaluation of suspected renal-artery stenosis (11–14). Other applications include evaluation of ureteropelvic-junction (UPJ) obstruction and renal-trauma evaluation. Although many of these applications can be done with a single-detector spiral CT scanner, MDCT has significant advantages, especially when viewing the main renal artery and its branches. The increased speed of data acquisition, in addition to elimination of artifacts due to patient motion or breathing, allows thinner slice collimation even when larger volumes are to be imaged. The use of 0.50-mm to 1.25-mm thick sections is essential when evaluating vessel stenosis and identifying small branch vessels. As noted previously, the faster acquisition times of 4-, 8-, 10-, and now 16-slice MDCT allow for superior timing of contrast delivery and data acquisition, especially for arterial-phase imaging.

Potential Renal Donors

In the past, most renal transplants were from cadavers. Few living-related transplants were performed owing to the major surgery required to harvest a living kidney. Therefore, the waiting list for renal transplant continues to grow, and now it is greater than 4 years in many states. Many patients will die before a kidney becomes available. Recently, the widespread use of laparoscopic nephrectomy has helped increase the number of living-related donors. No longer does a classic nephrectomy with all its potential complications and postoperative recovery times have to be performed. Laparoscopic nephrectomy has been shown to decrease the length of hospital stays, recovery times, and return-to-work times for the donor. Ratner et al. have shown that, with laparoscopic nephrectomy, the average hospital stay decreases from 5.7 days ± 1.7 days to 2.7 days ± 1.0 days, return to full activity decreases from 4.2 weeks ± 2.4 weeks to 2.3 weeks ± 1.1 weeks, and the return-to-work time decreases from 6.4 weeks ± 3.1 weeks to 3.9 weeks ± 1.6 weeks when compared to a classic renal nephrectomy (15,16).

Although laparoscopic surgery has tremendous advantages, it also provides additional challenges to the transplant surgeon. Vascular mapping of the arterial and venous systems, as well as the pelvocalyceal systems and ureters, must be defined accurately. Aberrant or anomalous vessels, including lumbar and gonadal veins, need to be identified to avoid potential vascular injury. Renal-arterial anatomic variations are common, with 32% of individuals having multiple renal arteries (Figures 24–1 to 24–4). Venous anatomic

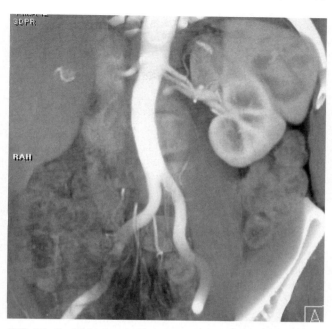

FIG. 24–2. Multiple renal arteries in a potential renal donor. Three-dimensional mapping demonstrates two left renal arteries with a discrete branch off the upper renal artery to the upper pole of the kidney.

variations also are common, with up to 28% of patients having multiple right renal veins. Left-sided variants include a single retroaortic renal vein in 3% of patients, a circumaortic renal vein in 17% of patients, and lumbar veins joining the left renal vein in up to 75% of patients (Figure 24-5) (12). Similarly, with the increased age of renal donors, it is not surprising that incidental renal-cell carcinomas will be detected. The presence of renal-artery stenosis will be more common if the age of the donor pool continues to increase and must be excluded preoperatively. Finally, a key advantage of CT is the global nature of the exam, meaning that nearly the entire abdomen is visualized during the routine renal-CT angiogram.

As with all clinical applications for CTA, the design of the study protocol for a renal-transplant donor must be optimized to answer all of the needs of the urologic surgeon. Minimizing the radiation dose to renal donors, who in many cases are in their 20s or 30s, also must be considered. Optimal study protocol requires dual phase acquisitions at 25 seconds and 60 seconds after contrast injection begins, representing an arterial dominant phase and a late cortical–medullary phase. Noncontrast studies and excretory-phase scanning are not necessary; rather, a delayed topogram can be obtained approximately 4 minutes after the study to obtain a classic intravenous pyelography- (IVP) style film using the topogram mode (scout view) on the scanner (17). A routine scan protocol on a 4-slice multidetector scanner uses 120 kilovolts peak (kVp) and 150 miliamperes (mAs) with 1.25-mm-thick slices (1-mm collimation) and a pitch of 6. Typical scan protocols will take under 30 seconds per acqui-

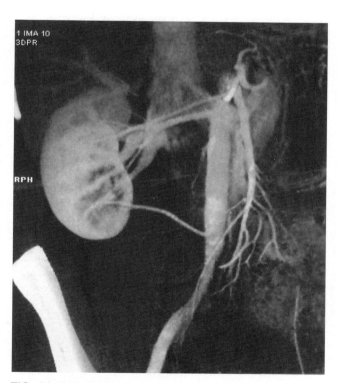

FIG. 24–1. Multiple renal arteries in potential renal donor. Three-dimensional mapping demonstrates three right renal arteries. The patient's left kidney was removed as the donor kidney.

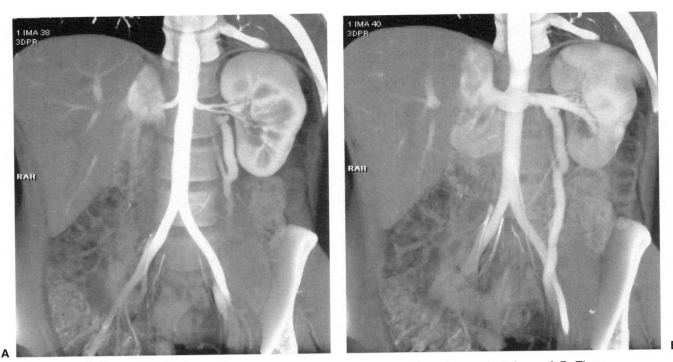

FIG. 24–3. Prehilar branching of the left renal artery in a potential renal-transplant donor. **A,B:** Three-dimensional mapping demonstrates prehilar branching of the left renal artery. The patient also has a prominent left gonadal vein.

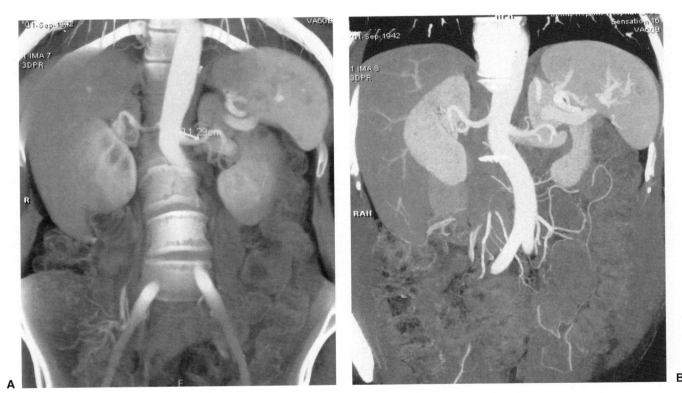

FIG. 24–4. Prehilar branching of the left renal artery in a potential renal donor. **A,B:** Three-dimensional mapping demonstrates prehilar branching (1.3 cm from origin) in a potential renal donor, in both volume rendering and MIPs.

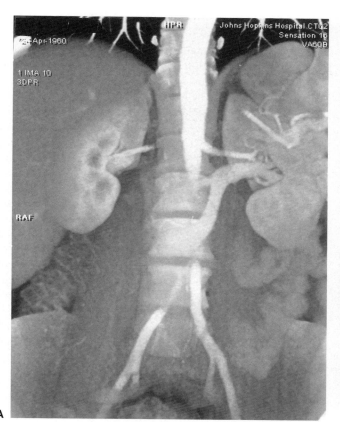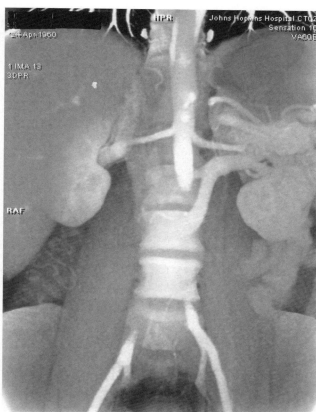

A   B

FIG. 24–5. Retroaortic renal vein in a potential renal-transplant donor. **A,B:** The CT angiogram demonstrates a bifurcating left renal vein with both branches extending in a retroaortic configuration.

sition. With a 16-slice system, 0.75-mm detectors are used to acquire 0.75-mm-thick scans, which are reconstructed at 0.5-mm intervals. Table speed is 24 mm per second and data acquisition is under 10 seconds. The new 16-slice scanners process data at approximately 6 slices per second (versus 5 seconds to 9 seconds per scan on a 4-slice MDCT), and the entire arterial and venous phase can be reconstructed in 3 minutes or less.

The axial scans initially are reviewed to identify any gross renal or extrarenal pathology, and 3D vascular maps then are generated (18–20). For renal imaging, volume rendering is used routinely for 3D display and supplemented with MIP images. The arterial dominant images are viewed with real-time display and the individual renal arteries defined. Care is taken to view the entire aorta through the bifurcation and iliac vessels to detect any accessory renal arteries. The renal arteries then are followed from their origin off the aorta into the renal hilum and parenchyma. Perihilar branching, when present, is defined best on the 3D images, as this can be missed easily on axial-CT images alone. The renal arteries also are studied to rule out renal-artery stenosis or aneurysms. On the venous-phase images, the renal veins are outlined carefully to determine any variations, including retroaortic or circumaortic renal arteries. Definition of the left adrenal vein, as well as the gonadal vein, also is defined

for vascular mapping. Many transplant surgeons believe that depiction of the left adrenal vein facilitates dissection at the time of laparoscopic harvesting. Dissection medial to the upper pole of the left kidney and along the superior margin of the left renal vein is difficult, and it is hindered by poor visibility. The left adrenal vein must be defined, clipped, and ligated (Figure 24-6). Scatarige et al. reported that, in over 92% of cases, the left adrenal vein could be identified, on average, 5.2 mm from the left lateral wall of the aorta (21).

All vessels are defined systematically, and select images documenting their appearance are sent to the transplant surgeon (14,15). Single-detector CT has been shown to be nearly as accurate as classic angiography, and personal experience with MDCT has shown that it provides excellent correlation with surgery. The small polar vessels missed with single-detector CT now are viewed routinely with MDCT. Kawamoto et al. reviewed a series of 74 consecutive patients who underwent 4-slice MDCT and found that the CT findings and surgical findings agreed in up to 97% of patients for identification of renal arteries. The two missed accessory renal arteries were deemed insignificant by the surgeons involved. Early branching of the renal artery had CT and surgical agreement in 96% of patients. Renal-vein anomalies showed a 99% agreement with surgical findings.

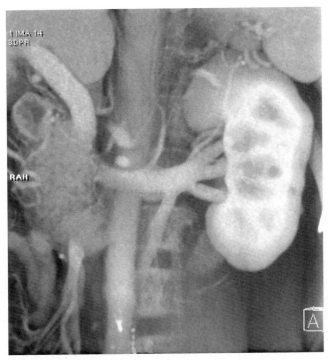

FIG. 24–6. Three-dimensional mapping of left adrenal vein in potential renal donor. Volume rendering in venous phase demonstrates the left adrenal vein arising off the left renal vein. This is an important landmark during laparoscopic nephrectomy.

The dual-phase CT angiogram also may define the presence of other pathology that may exclude the patient from being a donor. These include polycystic kidney disease, horseshoe kidney with a thick isthmus, or an occult renal-cell carcinoma (Figure 24-7). Multiple bilateral renal stones, as well as evidence of loss of cortex due to infarction or infection, also may exclude the patient. Therefore, CT provides a single comprehensive examination answering all of the questions that previously required several examinations.

In addition to being a fast and efficient single examination for evaluation of potential renal donors, CT is also more economical. Cochran et al. found that ''use of CT angiography plus conventional radiography instead of excretory urography and conventional arteriography can result in a 35–50% reduction in cost of the imaging studies in potential renal donors'' (22). Several articles also have noted the specific successes of this noninvasive imaging in this patient population. Using SDCT, Lerner et al. found that ''the enhanced 3-D computerized tomography reformation and reconstruction process appears to be as accurate as renal angiography for arterial anatomy, and more sensitive than renal angiography and IVP in evaluating venous and parenchymal anatomy'' (23).

Renal-cell Carcinoma

Computed tomography has become the study of choice for the evaluation of a suspected renal mass. The important clinical issues to be addressed when a mass is detected are its Bosniak classification and, if an obvious renal tumor is

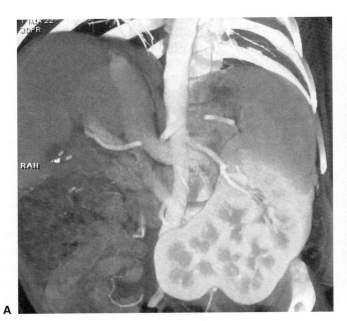

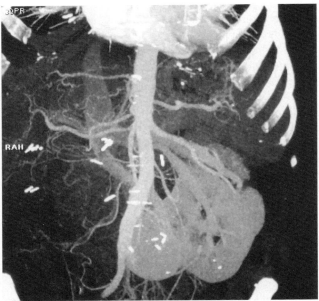

FIG. 24–7. Pancake kidney. **A,B:** The patient was evaluated for hepatitis C. Three-dimensional mapping demonstrates a complex left renal mass that is a pancake kidney due to fusion of the two kidneys. Multiple renal arteries were defined in the volume-rendering techniques (VRT) and MIP images.

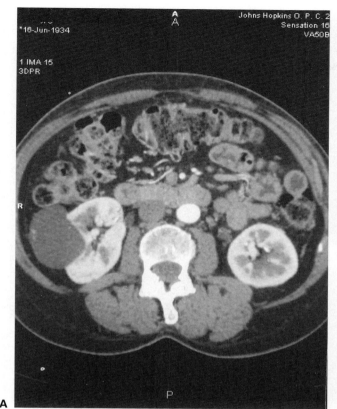

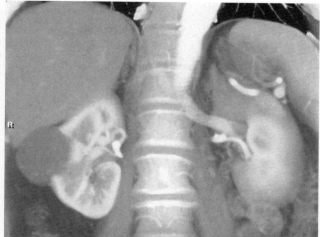

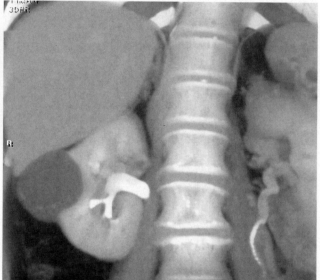

FIG. 24–8. Renal cyst of Bosniak-II classification. **A–C:** Axial and volume-rendered 3D images demonstrate well-defined nonenhancing cystic lesion in the right kidney. Faint calcification also is seen in the cyst wall. Note the lack of lesion enhancement between early phase (**A,B**) corti-comedullary and late-phase (**C**) excretory-phase images.

present, its accurate staging. Computed tomography has become the accepted gold standard to address all of these questions. Computed-tomography angiography builds on prior imaging success in CT and completes the full circle to provide "single stop shopping" for renal pathology (Figure 24-8). Computed-tomography angiography with dual-phase acquisition provides the needed detail of the renal artery and vein and allows excellent preoperative planning. Since over 80% of renal-cell carcinomas are hypervascular, these tumors typically are defined well on the arterial phase of acquisition (Figure 24-9). Please note that one pitfall of arterial-phase imaging is that if the lesion is small (less than 2 cm) and totally intrarenal, it easily may be overlooked on these early phase images. In these cases, the mass may be defined best on the venous-phase or excretory-phase images.

The late corticomedullary or venous phase especially is valuable to determine the presence of renal-vein thrombus and potential extension of clot into the intrahepatic inferior vena cava (IVC) or right atrium. Tumor thrombus often will

be hypervascular on the arterial-phase images. A 3D volume display is ideal for this application. Real-time rendering especially is valuable for determining the presence and extent of clot in vessels such as the renal vein, which run obliquely (Figure 24-10). The presence of extensive collateralization in the perirenal and pararenal spaces is not uncommon in hypervascular renal-cell carcinomas. The presence and extent of these collaterals is defined well on these dual-phase angiographic maps. Computed-tomography angiography also is ideal for other aspects of tumor staging, such as detection of liver metastases, adenopathy, and detection of muscle metastases. Arterial-phase imaging especially is valuable for detecting liver or pancreatic metastases, which typically are hypervascular in metastatic renal-cell carcinoma. Lesions may become isodense by the time venous-phase images are acquired. Contralateral tumors also may be detected with dual-phase imaging (Figure 24-11).

Although CT angiography with 3D reconstruction optimally defines the extent of disease, there has been no study

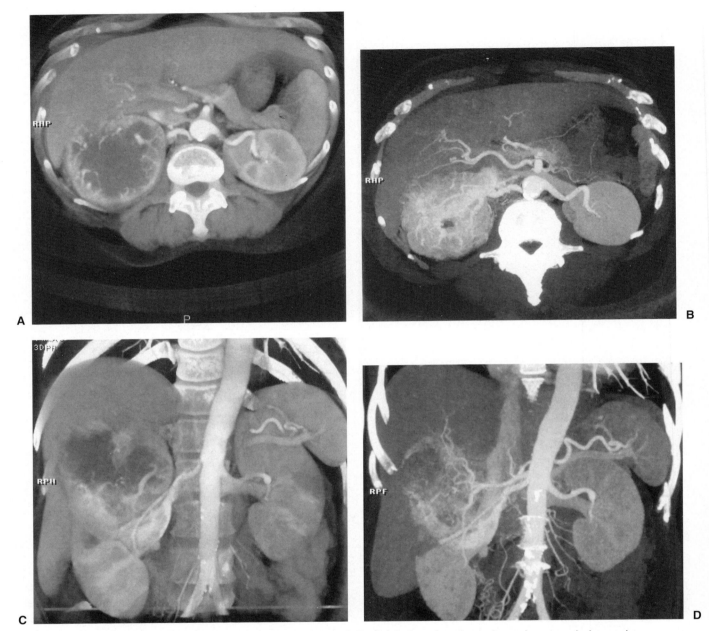

FIG. 24–9. Hypervascular renal-cell carcinoma. **A,B:** Axial-plane imaging using volume rendering and MIP demonstrates a large hypervascular right renal-cell carcinoma. **C,D:** Coronal display using volume rendering and MIP demonstrates the large upper-pole renal tumor with hypervascularity.

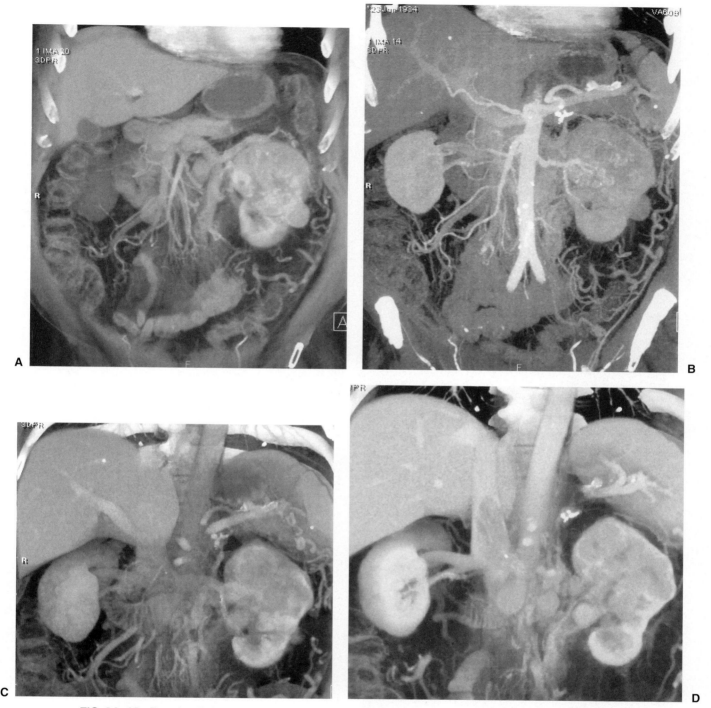

FIG. 24–10. Renal-cell carcinoma with vascular invasion. **A,B:** Three-dimensional mapping with volume rendering and MIP demonstrates an infiltrating tumor of the left kidney involving most of the upper two-thirds of the kidney. Neovascularity is seen. **C,D:** Tumor extension into renal vein and IVC is detected on these venous-phase images using VRT.

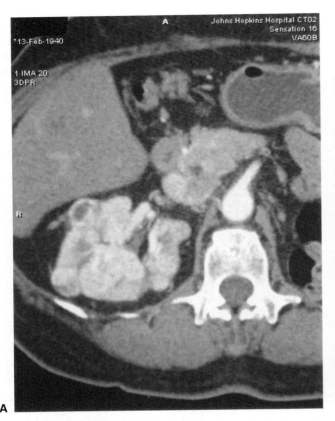

A

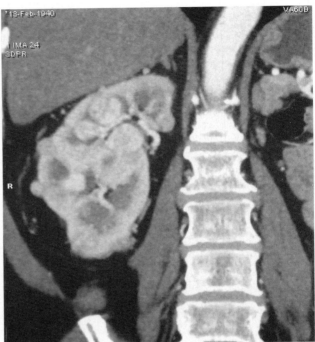

B

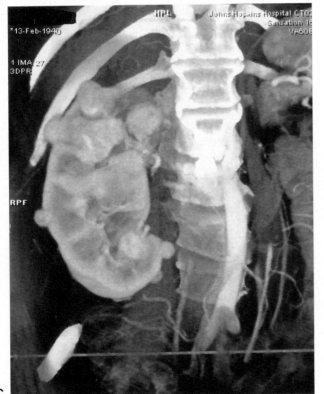

C

FIG. 24-11. Multifocal metastatic renal-cell carcinoma. The patient had a nephrectomy 10 years earlier for malignant renal-cell carcinoma and now presented with flank pain. **A-C:** Computed-tomography angiography demonstrates multiple hypervascular masses in the kidney consistent with metastatic tumor from the contralateral kidney. The multidimensional display of lesions with two-dimensional (2D) axial, coronal, and 3D volume rendering demonstrate true extent of tumor masses.

to date that suggests that it improves the staging of tumor. Rather, it guides appropriate patient management, including whether to perform a classic nephrectomy or a nephron-sparing surgery (partial nephrectomy) in a specific patient (23,24). Sheth et al. nicely summarized the use of CT angiography and 3D imaging for renal masses in a recent article: "Three-dimensional CT provides the urologist with an interactive road map of the relationships among the tumor, the major vessels, and the collecting system. This information is particularly critical if the tumor extends into the inferior vena cava or if nephron-sparing surgery is being planned" (24). Herts et al. emphasized the value of the multiple phases of data acquisition in patients before planned surgery: "Triphasic renal CT better reveals the artery and vein anatomy of the kidney than does parenchymal phase imaging only. Triphasic helical CT is indicated in patients undergoing planning for urologic surgery when vascular anatomy is clinically important"(25).

Nephron-sparing Surgery

One of the key applications for 3D CT angiography is in the selection of patients with renal tumors who are candidates for nephron-sparing surgery or a partial nephrectomy. With well over half of all renal-cell carcinomas now being detected incidentally, smaller tumors (less than 4 cm) are identified more frequently in younger patients. Unlike the typical patient in the past who presented with symptoms of flank pain, hematuria, or metastases, tumor in these patients typically is detected on an ultrasound, CT, or MRI ordered for reasons other than suspected renal pathology.

In the past, partial nephrectomy was only an option for patients in whom a total nephrectomy would leave the patient dependent on dialysis for survival. This included patients with a mass in a solitary kidney, patients with bilateral renal masses, patients with borderline renal function where nephrectomy would result in renal failure, or patients with a syndrome predisposing the patient for future renal tumors.

With advances in surgical technique and increased clinical experience, urologic surgeons are opting for partial nephrectomy in a new group of patients. The ideal candidate for a partial nephrectomy should have a mass of less than 4 cm, exophytic in location. The mass should not be in close proximity to the renal pelvis and cortical vessels. Additionally, there should be no evidence of adenopathy or tumor spread. Three-dimensional angiography is ideal for providing this information. On a single dual-phase examination, all of the information needed by the urologic surgeon can be provided in a single comprehensive examination. Coll et al. reviewed a total of 97 renal masses in 60 cases and found that 3D volume-rendered CT integrated "essential information from angiography, venography, excretory urography and conventional 2D CT into a single imaging modality" (26). At their institution, this became the preferred means of data display (Figure 24-12).

Several different studies have looked carefully at this subgroup of patients with similarly encouraging results. For example, Smith et al. noted that "the 3D helical CT uniquely assists the urologist by providing preoperative information in a flexible display that aids in determining whether nephron sparing surgery is possible and planning the surgical procedure" (27). With an ever-increasing number of patients presenting with incidentally detected tumors, the use of 3D CTA for this application will continue to grow (28).

Catalano et al. recently reported their results using a 4-slice MDCT scanner with multiphase CT (arterial, nephrographic, and urographic phases) (29). The authors analyzed the axial images, MPRs, and 3D images (using mainly MIP techniques) to determine the accuracy of staging and patient selection for partial nephrectomy. The authors found that

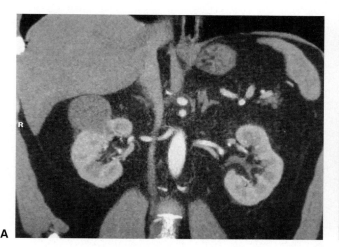
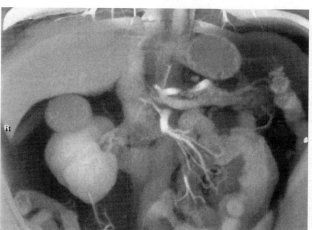

FIG. 24–12. Renal-cell carcinoma treated with partial nephrectomy. **A,B:** Coronal **(A)** and 3D volume rendering **(B)** of 4-cm solitary hypervascular mass arising off the upper pole of the right kidney. Based on mass location and the exophytic nature of the mass, a partial nephrectomy was performed successfully.

the presence and size of all lesions were defined accurately. In Robson Stage-I lesions, they were able to diagnose fat infiltration with 96% sensitivity, 93% specificity, and 95% accuracy, with positive and negative predictive values of 100% and 93%, respectively. In higher-grade lesions, the authors found 100% accuracy (29).

Radiofrequency Ablation

Three-dimensional rendering also is helpful in cases where radiofrequency ablation is used for treatment of small renal neoplasms. Three-dimensional mapping is critical in both patient selection and follow-up to determine ultimate procedure success. Farrell et al. reviewed a series of 35 tumors in 20 patients and found that their initial experience showed no residual or recurrent tumor or major side effect in any of the patients (30). However, the authors caution that follow up ranged from 1 month to 23 months and further follow up was needed to determine long-term efficacy. Roy-Choudhury et al. similarly found that percutaneous radiofrequency ablation could play a major role in the treatment of small renal masses, especially in the elderly patient (31). Both authors did note that CT could be used to guide radiofrequency ablation, particularly on scanners equipped with CT fluoroscopy for real-time guidance of the procedure.

Renal-artery Stenosis

Another renal application for CT angiography is the evaluation of suspected renal-artery stenosis. Although there

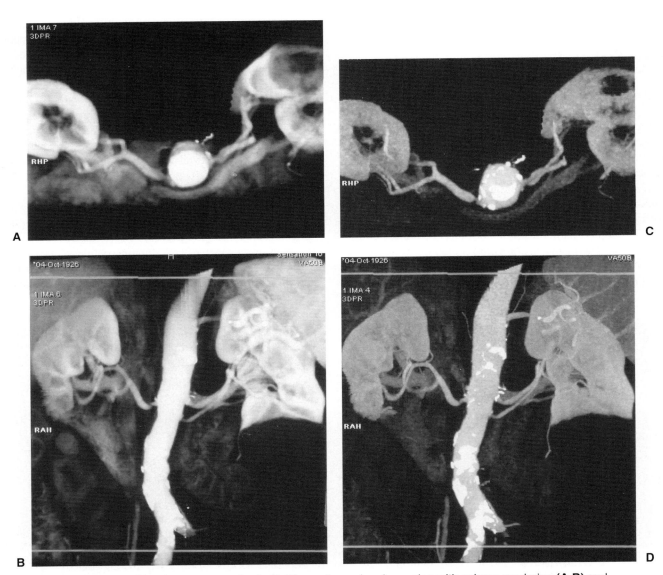

FIG. 24-13. Renal-artery stenosis. **A–D:** Three-dimensional mapping with volume rendering **(A,B)** and **(C,D)** MIP demonstrates significant stenosis of the right renal artery of approximately 70%. Mild narrowing of origin of both left renal arteries was noted as well.

has been much debate concerning the ideal imaging modality for renal-artery stenosis, there is little doubt that MDCT can play a major role, especially with MDCT. Previous articles by Brink et al. have shown that thin-section CT with maximum thickness of 2 mm is necessary for accurately determining renal-artery stenosis (32). With single-detector scanners, the ability to use thin sections and cover a large enough volume was often a challenge. Multidetector CT, with its rapid acquisition, thin collimation, and long data acquisition, optimally displays even small renal vessels. Computed tomography clearly can define the presence of single or multiple renal arteries and accurately define the presence of stenosis in any of these vessels. For this application, 1.00-mm to 1.25-mm slice thickness is used on a 4-slice MDCT scanner, and isotropic datasets of 0.75 slice thickness reconstructed at 0.50-mm intervals are used on a 16-slice MDCT scanner. Isotropic datasets are ideal when trying to detect and quantify the presence and degree of vessel stenosis.

Once an adequate CT dataset has been acquired, postprocessing of the dataset is critical to detect the presence of stenosis and to grade its extent. Articles by Kuszyk and Ebert have shown that 3D CT with volume rendering is accurate for determining degree of stenosis as long as correct rendering parameters are selected (33,34). The potential of interobserver variation and some of its causes were addressed in these articles. An article by Addis et al. compared a range of postprocessing techniques and found that "all five CT angiography display techniques (axial, MIP, MPR, shaded surface display and volume rendering) accurately display vessels and stenosis greater than 4 mm in diameter. However, volume rendering tends to be more accurate for stances of 2–4 mm and was statistically better in the measurement of diameters of 0.5–1.0 mm." (35)

Volumetric rendering supplemented with MIP is used routinely to image the renal arteries. The MIP technique can be problematic in the presence of calcification and can overestimate the degree of stenosis present. Volume rendering clearly defines vessel lumen from calcification; consequently, this problem does not exist. Please note that one can err in setting the parameters of volume rendering, resulting in over- or underestimating the degree of stenosis present. However, with careful attention to detail and experience, this becomes less of an issue. However, owing to the inherent limitations of the MIP technique, the presence of calcification on a vessel wall easily can stimulate total or extensive stenosis when none may be present. Therefore, care must be taken when performing 3D rendering techniques for this application (Figures 24–13 and 24–14).

Endoluminal imaging also can be used for evaluation of renal-artery stenosis, although current experience is limited with this technique. Neri et al. found that "virtual endoscopy enables the creation of endoluminal views of the aorta and its branches by processing spiral computed tomographic (CT) images, thereby allowing the preoperative and postoperative evaluations of abdominal aortic aneurysms, aneurysms of the splenic, celiac, and common iliac arteries, and renal artery stenoses" (36).

Postrenal Transplant

Computed-tomogrpahy angiography also can be used in postrenal-transplant patients to evaluate for vessel patency. Although ultrasound is used commonly in this application, CT has proven valuable in difficult cases. Hofmann et al. found that "three-dimensional helical CT angiography of renal transplant recipients presenting with hypertension, graft dysfunction, or both after transplantation yields valuable information that can be used to guide further therapy" (37). With MDCT, the contrast load can be decreased to 70 cc to 80 cc and still provide a diagnostic study. The recent

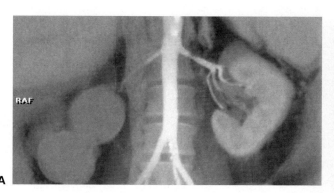
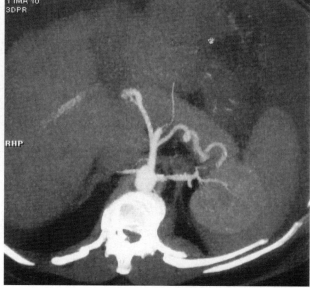

FIG. 24–14. Renal-artery stenosis. **A,B:** Three-dimensional mapping demonstrates marked narrowing of proximal left renal artery. The patient was developing worsening renal dysfunction. The right kidney is nonfunctioning from prior UPJ obstruction.

introduction of dual-head CT injectors, which allow a second bolus with saline, may help reduce the needed contrast load for CTA. Hooper et al. previously described the use of a saline-chaser technique to reduce contrast volumes in thoracic CT. Dorio et al. recently reported the use of saline chaser for liver evaluation. They found that 100 mL of contrast and a 50-mL saline chaser provided little difference in lesion conspicuity compared to 150 mL of contrast alone. The authors concluded that this technique could both reduce costs and decrease the risk of contrast-induced nephropathy.

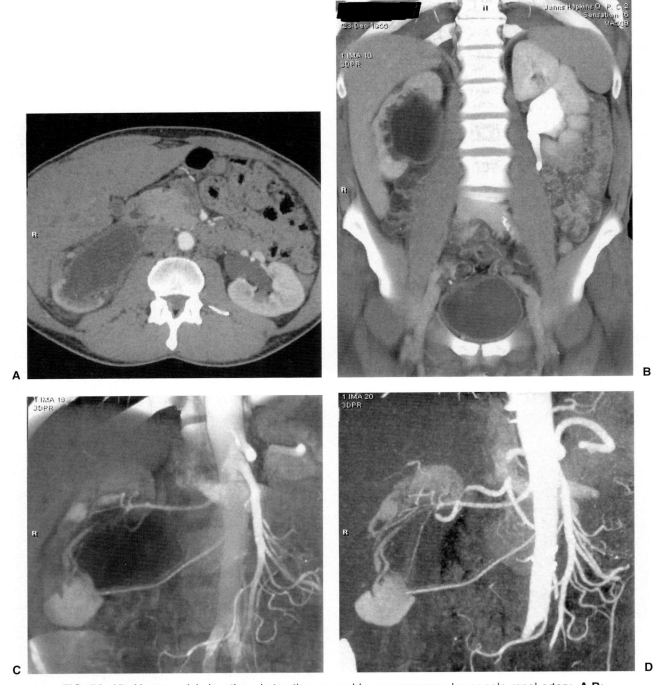

FIG. 24–15. Ureteropelvic-junction obstruction caused by an accessory lower-pole renal artery. **A,B:** Axial **(A)** and coronal volume display **(B)** demonstrate the patient's right hydronephrosis with thinning of cortex of the right kidney. **C,D:** Computed-tomography angiogram with volume rendering **(C)** and MIP **(D)** define the crossing vessel that was a lower-pole accessory renal artery. Note that relationship to the dilated pelvis is seen best on the volume-rendered image.

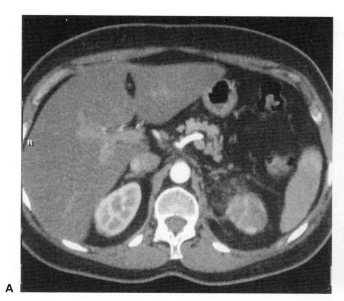
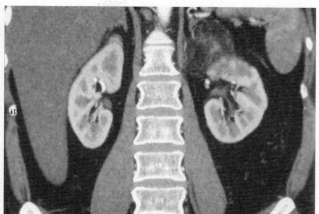

FIG. 24–16. Renal angiomyolipoma. **A,B:** Three-dimensional mapping demonstrates a fatty tumor arising off the upper pole of the left kidney consistent with a renal angiomyolipoma.

URETEROPELVIC JUNCTION OBSTRUCTION (UPJ OBSTRUCTION)

There are many potential causes of UPJ obstruction, including an impacted stone, scarring from prior stone passage, transitional cell carcinoma, or the presence of a crossing vessel, which may be either an accessory renal artery or venous anomaly. Preoperative detection of the cause of UPJ obstruction is critical, not only to help determine the etiology of obstruction, but also to plan surgical repair, including determining whether laparoscopic or open surgery will be performed. Computed-tomography angiography can detect the presence of arterial or venous causes of UPJ obstruction, including duplicated vessels, aberrant arteries, and venous

anomalies. The presence of other causes of UPJ obstruction also can be detected routinely with CTA (Figure 24-15).

Miscellaneous Applications

Although the goal of this chapter is not to define every application for CT angiography, a few brief comments should be made regarding other applications seen in daily practice. Computed-tomography angiography does play a role in detection and staging of other renal tumors, including Wilm's tumor in children, as well as angiomyolipomas and transitional-cell carcinomas in adult patients (Figures 24–16–24–18). For angiomyolipomas, CTA may help de-

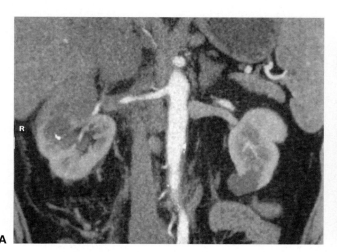
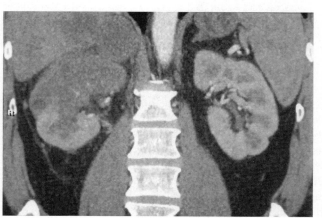

FIG. 24–17. Transitional-cell carcinoma of the kidney. **A,B:** The patient presented with a history of hematuria. Three-dimensional mapping demonstrate an infiltrating tumor in the upper pole of the right kidney that subsequently was proven to be an infiltrating transitional-cell carcinoma.

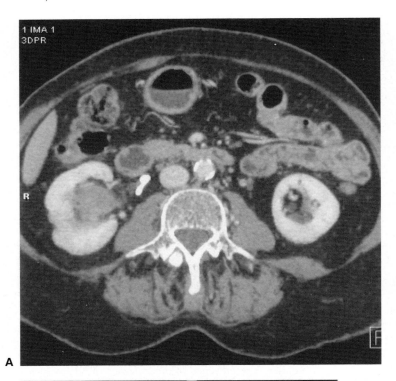

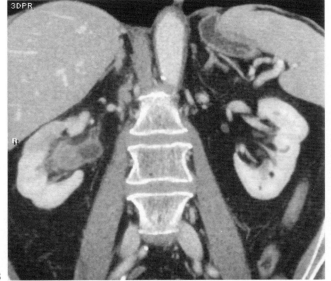

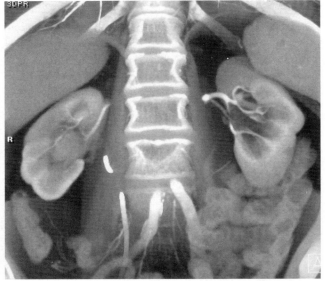

FIG. 24–18. Transitional-cell carcinoma of the renal pelvis. **A–C:** Axial, coronal, and 3D mapping demonstrates a tumor infiltrating the right renal pelvis without evidence of vascular invasion.

tect small aneurysms within the tumor that may be prone to bleeding and suggest early resection or embolization when possible. Similarly, CTA is ideal in the patient with spontaneous renal hemorrhage to determine the underlying cause, whether tumor, aneurysm, or vasculitis. Computed-tomography angiography is valuable in the trauma patient to assess vascular pedicle injuries. In a patient with penetrating trauma, the presence of pseudoaneurysms may be detected, especially on arterial-phase imaging. Delayed scans in these patients may be ideal for detecting contrast extravasation on CT urograms (Figure 24-19).

Investigation of the cause of renal infarction is also a strong indication for CT angiography. Focal emboli or renal stenosis may be identified as the underlying cause (Figures 24–20 and 24–21). In the course of CT angiography for evaluation of endovascular stent-graft placement or aortic aneurysm repair, the relationship of the aneurysm to the renal arteries will play a major role in determining patient eligibility. Computed-tomography angiography also is valuable following aneurysm resection or stent placement for evaluation of renal-artery patency.

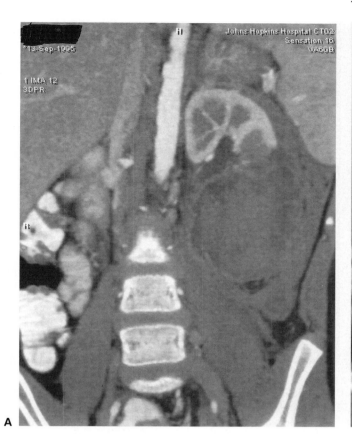
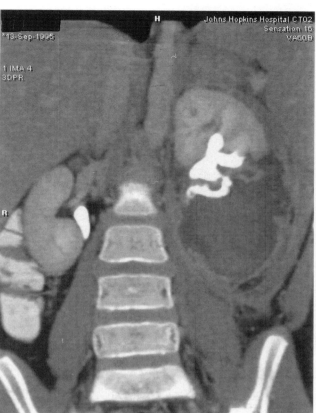

FIG. 24–19. Renal laceration with contrast extravasation on excretory phase. **A,B:** Renal laceration with perirenal hematoma is seen on early phase imaging at 4 minutes postinjection; contrast extravasation is seen from the renal pelvis.

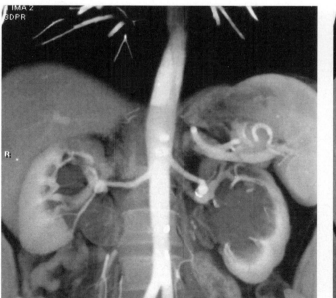
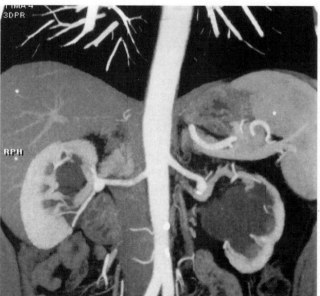

FIG. 24–20. Bilateral renal-artery aneurysms. **A,B:** Computed-tomography angiogram was done for evaluation of the patient's hepatitis C. Three-dimensional mapping with volume rendering and MIP demonstrates bilateral renal-artery aneurysms.

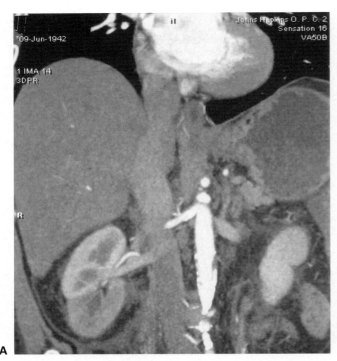
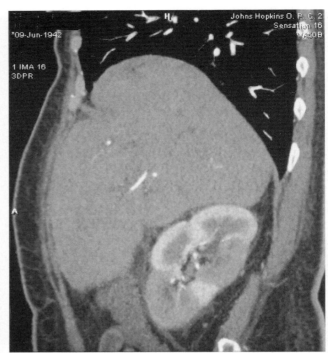

A **B**

FIG. 24–21. Acute pyelonephritis. The patient has a history of primary sclerosing cholangitis and diabetes and was undergoing pretransplant evaluation. **A,B:** Computed-tomography scan demonstrated multiple low-density zones in the kidney consistent with the diagnosis of acute polynephritis that was treated medically.

CONCLUSION

The advances from single-detector spiral CT to MDCT have provided the radiologist with unique imaging capabilities and revolutionized how patients with a wide range of renal pathology are imaged and evaluated. The ability to provide a noninvasive exam, which may cost 25% to 33% less than a more invasive study, with equal or greater accuracy and greater ease of use is truly an exciting development.

The development of faster workstations, coupled with better user interfaces and investigative tools, promises to help improve the clinical practice of CT. The introduction over the last 12 months of multidetector scanners with 8 to 16 detectors and acquisition speeds in the 500 millisecond range, coupled with routine slice collimation of 0.50 mm to 0.75 mm resulting in isotropic datasets, will continue to advance the field of CT (38–39). Changes in workflow are occurring and are needed in order to take full advantage of technological advances.

REFERENCES

1. Foley WD, Mallisee TA, Hohenwalter MD, et al. Multiphase hepatic CT with a multirow detector CT scanner. *AJR Am J Roentgenol* 2000; 175:679–685.
2. Hu H, He HD, Foley WD, et al. Four multidetector-row helical CT: image quality and volume coverage speed. *Radiology* 2000; 215:55–62.
3. Johnson PT, Heath DG, Kuszyk BS, et al. CT angiography with volume rendering: advantages and applications in splanchnic vascular imaging. *Radiology* 1996;200:564–568.
4. Kuszyk BS, Heath DG, Ney DR, et al. CT angiography with volume rendering: imaging findings. *AJR Am J Roentgenol* 1995; 165:445–448.
5. Rieker O, Duber C, Pitton M, et al. CT angiography versus intraarterial digital subtraction angiography for assessment of aortoiliac occlusive disease. *AJR Am J Roentgenol* 1997;169:1133–1138.
6. Dorio PJ, Lee FT Jr, Henseler KP, et al. Using a saline chaser to decrease contrast media in abdominal CT. *AJR Am J Roentgenol* 2003; 180:929–934.
7. Macari M. Infrarenal abdominal aortic aneurysms at multi-detector row CT angiography: intravascular enhancement without a timing acquisition. *Radiology* 2001;220:519–523.
8. Drebin RA, Carpenter L, Hanrahan P. Volume rendering. *Comput Graph* 1988;22:65–74.
9. Ney DR, Drebin RA, Fishman EK, et al. Volumetric rendering of computed tomographic data: principles and techniques. *IEEE Comput Graph Applic* 1990;10:24–32.
10. Johnson PT, Heath DG, Duckwall JR, et al. Enhanced display of vascular anatomy with stereoscopic viewing. *J Diagn Radiogr Imaging* 1999; 2(1):25–28.
11. Smith PA, Marshall FF, Urban BA, et al. Three-dimensional CT stereoscopic visualization of renal masses: impact on diagnosis and patient treatment. *AJR Am J Roentgenol* 1997;169:1331–1334.
12. Rubin GD, Dake MD, Semba CP. Current status of three-dimensional spiral CT scanning for imaging the vasculature. *Radiol Clin North Am* 1995;33:51–70.
13. Rubin GD, Dake MD, Napel S, et al. Spiral CT of renal artery stenosis: comparison of three-dimensional rendering techniques. *Radiology* 1994;190:181–189.
14. Chernoff DM, Silverman SG, Kininis R, et al. Three-dimensional imaging and display of renal tumors using spiral CT: a potential aid to partial nephrectomy. *Urology* 1994;43:125–129.
15. Ratner LE, Cisek L, Moore R, et al. Laparoscopoic live donor nephrectomy. *Transplantation* 1995;60:1047–1049.

16. Ratner LE, Kavoussi L, Sroka M, et al. Laparoscopic assisted live donor nephrectomy: comparison with the open approach. *Transplantation* 1997;63:229–233.
17. Smith PA, Ratner LE, Lynch FC, et al. Role of CT angiography in the preoperative evaluation for laparoscopic nephrectomy. *Radiographics* 1998;18:589–601.
18. Platt JF, Ellis JH, Korobkin M, et al. Potential renal donors: comparison of conventional imaging with helical CT. *Radiology* 1996; 198:419–423.
19. Rubin GD, Alfrey EJ, Dake MD, et al. Spiral CT for the assessment of living renal donors. *Radiology* 1995;195:457–462.
20. Platt JF, Ellis JH, Korobkin M, et al. Helical CT evaluation of potential kidney donors: findings in 154 subjects. *AJR Am J Roentgenol* 1997; 169:1325–1330
21. Scatarige JC, Horton KM, Ratner LE, Fishman EK. Left adrenal vein localization by 3D real-time volume-rendering CTA before laparoscopic nephrectomy in living renal donors. *Abdom Imag* 2001; 26:553–556.
22. Cochran ST, Krasny RM, Danovitch GM, et al. Helical CT angiography for examination of living renal donors. *AJR Am J Roentgenol* 1997; 168:1569–1573.
23. Lerner LB, Henriques HF, Harris RD. Interactive 3-dimensional computerized tomography reconstruction in evaluation of the living renal donor. *Urology* 1999;161;403–407.
24. Sheth S, Scatarige JC, Horton KM, et al. Current concepts in the diagnosis and management of renal cell carcinoma: role of multidetector CT and three-dimensional CT. *Radiographics* 2001;21:234–237.
25. Herts BR. Triphasic helical CT of the kidneys: contribution of vascular phase scanning in patients before urologic surgery. *AJR Am J Roentgenol* 1999;173:1273–1277.
26. Coll DM, Uzzo RG, Herts BR, et al. 3-Dimensional volume rendered computerized tomography for preoperative evaluation and intraoperative treatment of patients undergoing nephron sparing surgery. *J Urol* 1999;161:1097–1102.
27. Smith PA, Marshall FF, Corl FM, et al. Planning nephron-sparing renal surgery using 3D helical CT angiography. *J Comput Assist Tomogr* 1999;23:649–654.
28. Polascik TJ, Pound CR, Meng MV, et. Partial nephrectomy: technique, complications and pathological Findings. *J Urol* 1995; 154:1312–1318.
29. Catalano C, Fraioloi F, Laghi A, et al. High-resolution multidetector CT in the preoperative evaluation of patients with renal cell carcinoma *AJR Am J Roentgenol* 2003;180:1271–1277.
30. Farrell MA, Charboneau WJ, DiMarco DS, et al. Imaging-guided radiofrequency ablation of solid renal tumors. *AJR Am J Roentgenol* 2003; 180:1509–1513.
31. Roy-Choudhury SH, Cast JEI, Cooksey G, et al. Early experience with percutaneous radiofrequency ablation of small solid renal masses. *AJR Am J Roentgenol* 2003;180:1055–1061.
32. Brink JA, Lim JT, Wang G, et al. Technical optimization of helical CT for depiction of renal artery stenosis: in vitro analysis. *Radiology* 1995;194:157–163.
33. Kuszyk BS, Heath DG, Johnson PT, et al. CT angiography with volume rendering for quantifying vascular stenoses: in vitro validation of accuracy. *AJR Am J Roentgenol* 1999;173:449–455.
34. Ebert DS, Heath DG, Kuszyk BS, et al. Evaluating the potential and problems of three-dimensional computed tomography measurements of arterial stenosis. *J Digit Imag* 1998;11:151–157.
35. Addis KA, Hopper KD, Iyriboz TA, et al. CT angiography: in vitro comparison of five reconstruction methods. *AJR Am J Roentgenol* 2001; 177:1171–1176.
36. Neri E, et al. Spiral CT virtual endoscopy of abdominal arteries: clinical applications. *Abdom Imag* 2000;25:59–61.
37. Hofmann LV, Smith PA, Kuszyk BS, et al. Three-dimensional helical CT angiography in renal transplant recipients: a new problem-solving tool. *AJR Am J Roentgenol* 1999;173:1085–1089.
38. Gupta AK, Nelson RC, Johnson GA, et al. Optimization of eight-element multi-detector row helical CT technology for evaluation of the abdomen. *Radiology* 2003;227:739–745.
39. Kawamoto S, Montgomery RA, Lawler LP, et al. Multidetector CT angiography for preoperative evaluation of living laparoscopic kidney donors. *AJR Am J Roentgenol* 2003;180:1633–1638.

SECTION VI

Miscellaneous Applications

images when higher pitches were used. This was due not only to the scan-reconstruction algorithms available, but also to the method used to obtain single spiral scans. With higher pitches, slice profile might increase up to 27% (i.e., 5.0-mm collimation may actually be 6.5 mm), and the mAs actually would decrease on the higher pitches, resulting in poor image quality. With MDCT, the selected slice thickness is achieved without any blooming artifact. In addition, the mAs are constant across the scan volume regardless of the pitch selected. However, these assumptions can vary among individual scanners, depending on the manufacturer and system model. It therefore is important to be aware of the scanner capabilities in order to optimize protocol design.

Other key decisions for musculoskeletal-CT imaging include whether to use intravenous (IV) contrast; whether 3D or MPR will be required; the area to be scanned; the reconstruction algorithm; and which rendering technique will be used for 3D imaging.

IV-Contrast Considerations

In cases of pelvic trauma, a noncontrast study usually is satisfactory for identification of pelvic fractures (Figure 25-1). In cases where a potential vascular injury is suspected, a CT angiogram may be done concurrently. Numerous articles have documented a high accuracy for CT angiography (CTA) in this setting. In addition, soft-tissue pathology (i.e., abscess, tumor, myositis) is demonstrated optimally with IV contrast. Protocol design for CT angiograms varies, but typically includes rapid injection of iodinated contrast material (120 cc of contrast at 3 cc per second), a 25-second to 30-second delay, thin collimation, and close interscan spacing (1.25-mm slice thickness reconstructed at 1.00-mm intervals or 0.75-mm slice thickness at 0.50-mm intervals, for 4-slice or 16-slice MDCT, respectively). Generally, only arterial-phase acquisition is required to depict arterial anatomy. Identification of soft-tissue abnormalities often requires venous-phase acquisition as well (4).

3D or MPR Considerations

Multiplanar reconstruction and 3D imaging require thin collimation and close interscan spacing. Image postprocessing is a routine part of skeletal imaging, particularly for evaluation of fractures or congenital deformities. Data postprocessing may be done with scanner-based software or on independent 3D workstations. Although freestanding workstations usually have several advantages, such as superior user interfaces, functionality, and reconstruction algorithms, they are not mandatory for basic 3D mapping. With the advent of routine isotropic datasets on 16-slice MDCT scanners, musculoskeletal-CT scans now can be interpreted with real-time volume displays. This subject is discussed in greater detail in Chapter 2 (5–7).

Anatomic Area to Be Scanned

Scan protocols are determined by both the area and volume to be scanned (i.e., wrist versus entire upper extremity). When a large volume is to be scanned, slice collimation of 2.5 mm or 1.5 mm usually is selected with 4-slice and 16-slice MDCT scanners, respectively, to limit the scan time required. With 4-slice, 8-slice, or 16-slice MDCT, data can be reconstructed at 1.0-mm intervals even with 2.5-mm collimation (Figure 25-2).

Reconstruction Algorithm

The selected reconstruction algorithm will depend on the clinical application. For soft-tissue or muscle imaging, a standard soft-tissue algorithm is used; if bony detail is needed, a high-resolution algorithm is required. The ideal reconstruction algorithm also will depend on whether 3D rendering is needed. Some high-resolution algorithms create images with too much noise, resulting in 3D images of suboptimal quality. Trial and error may be necessary to optimize scanning protocols and 3D reconstruction algorithms. In selected cases, the data may need to be reconstructed with two different algorithms (Figure 25-3).

Rendering Techniques for 3D Imaging

The use of 3D imaging requires a basic understanding of the available rendering techniques and their implementation. Many facilities routinely use only volume-rendering technique (VRT) for bone and soft-tissue protocols. Volume rendering has proven to be the most flexible technique, as well as the most accurate. Using a trapezoid-based rendering system, bone and soft tissue can be displayed easily and accurately in a range of presentations by adjusting display parameters such as opacity and brightness (Figure 25-4). Shaded-surface-rendering technique also can be used to display bone in 3D, but image quality suffers due to the use of a binary-classification technique that uses less than 10% of the dataset to create the images. Volume-rendered images of bone can be displayed in several different presentations that can vary the bone opacity or transparency depending on clinical application or physician preference. These images are reviewed routinely in real time to optimize selection of the ideal image display and view the images in stereo mode. Preset 3D-imaging protocols may not be as effective as real-time review of the images by the radiologist or referring physician. In cases where iodinated contrast is used, images also can be reviewed with maximum-intensity-projection technique (MIP); however, this technique is not useful for bone imaging (7,8).

CLINICAL APPLICATIONS

Trauma

One of the most common applications for CT and 3D imaging is the evaluation of musculoskeletal trauma. Even

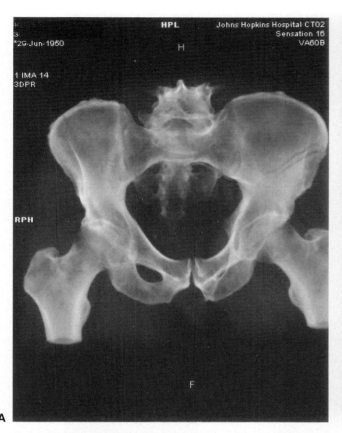

A

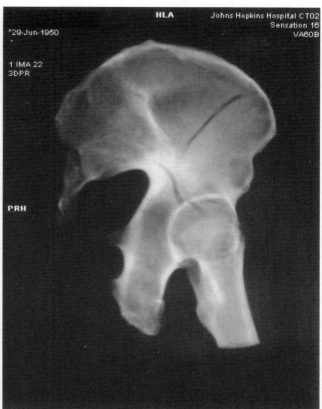

B

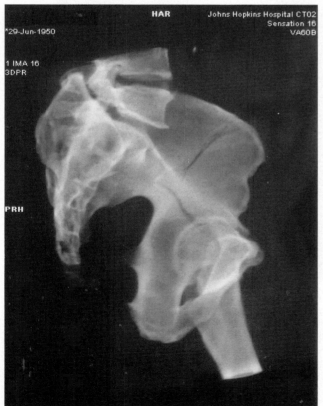

C

FIG. 25–1. Left acetabular-fractures status—post motor-vehicle accident as pedestrian. **A–C:** Three-dimensional CT scans demonstrate fracture of left acetabulum involving anterior column, medial wall, and extending into iliac crest. Three-dimensional mapping demonstrates the extensive fracture and involvement of weight-bearing surface. This was repaired with percutaneous screw fixation.

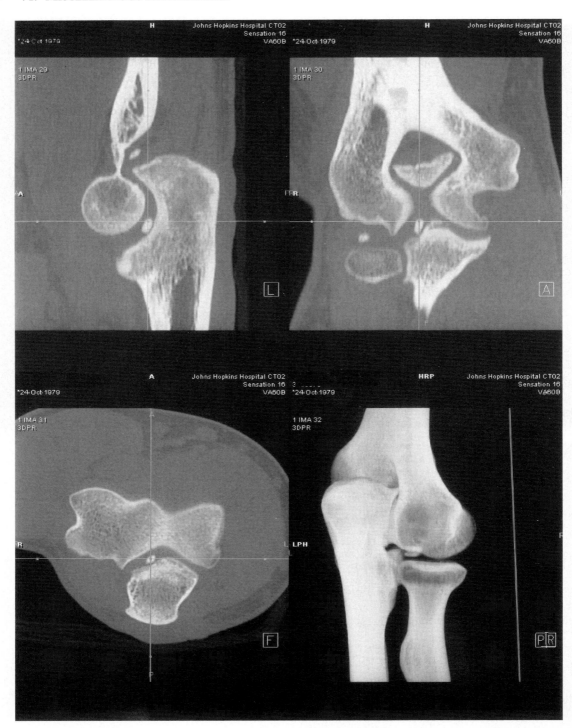

FIG. 25–2. Multiple loose bodies in the elbow joint. Twenty-one-year-old patient with a history of remote trauma to elbow and persistent pain. A composite image of 2D and 3D images shows multiple osteochondral loose bodies in the anterior compartment of the elbow. These bony fragments were removed arthroscopically. Please note that this dataset was isotropic, which allows for the exquisite resolution in all planes and perspectives.

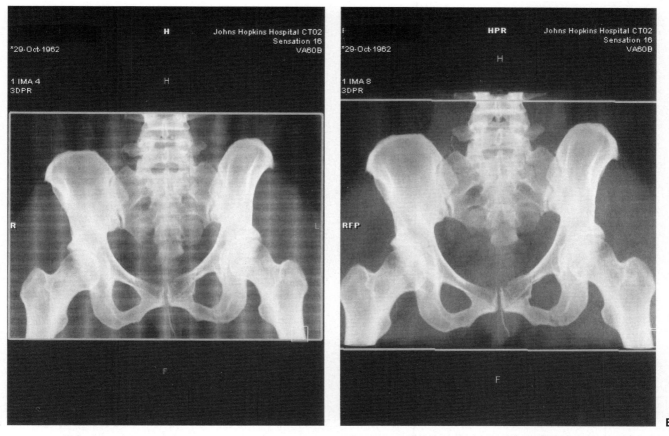

FIG. 25–3. Impact of algorithm selection on 3D rendering. Reconstruction using two different algorithms shows the increased noise on the high-resolution algorithm **(A)** compared to the standard algorithm **(B)**. This is very important for doing 3D imaging as two reconstructions of a single dataset may be necessary for review of high-resolution bone in axial or multiplanar mode and standard reconstructed algorithm for 3D mapping.

in the earliest days of CT scanning, numerous articles highlighted the advantages of CT and 3D imaging as both a diagnostic and clinical-management tool. Patients commonly were referred for CT either as a result of plain films indeterminate for fracture or in cases of extensive fracture to define the true extent of injury for clinical management (Figures 25–5 and 25–6). The addition of 3D imaging in these cases changed patient management in up to 30% of cases. Over the past two decades, referral patterns for many trauma applications have not changed (9,10). What has changed, however, is the increased availability and speed of CT scanners, placement of CT scanners in or near the emergency room, the need for rapid triage of emergency-room patients, and increased use of CT across a wide range of emergency-room applications. The increased use of CT early in the clinical evaluation provides a more rapid triage and diagnosis, which is practically important with the increasing patient volume in emergency departments. For example, some centers equipped with a CT scanner in the emergency room perform CT of the cervical spine instead of plain films. Similarly, many centers are beginning to use similar

triage algorithms for pelvic and complex upper-extremity trauma (11–15).

The use of MDCT, especially 16-slice systems, is ideal in all trauma applications. Computed tomography can limit the need for sedation and provide a single comprehensive exam that combines imaging of the solid organs, vascular anatomy, and skeletal structures. This especially is true in pediatric patients, where sedation nearly is eliminated with the use of MDCT. The potential exists for single-volume acquisition with MDCT to replace plain radiographs in the emergency department over the next 3 years to 5 years (Figure 25–7).

The importance of high-quality MDCT datasets especially is evident in small-part imaging, such as the wrist (Figures 25–8 and 25–9). Goldfarb et al., in their recent review, noted, ''We prefer not to use reconstructed images for a second plane, unless prior use of a scanner shows that the machine can produce excellent quality reconstructed images that equal the quality of directly acquired images'' (6). The use of 0.50-mm to 0.75 mm slice thickness and isotropic datasets are ideal for this application. Supplemented by 3D

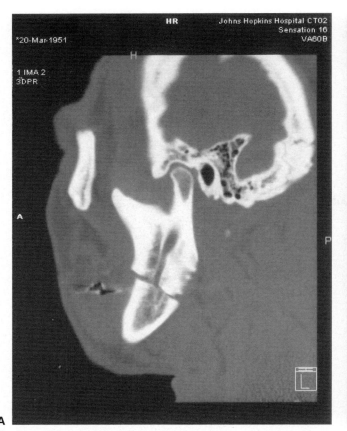

A

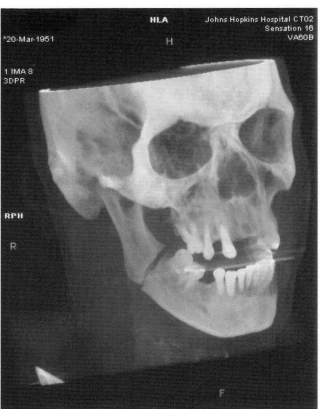

B

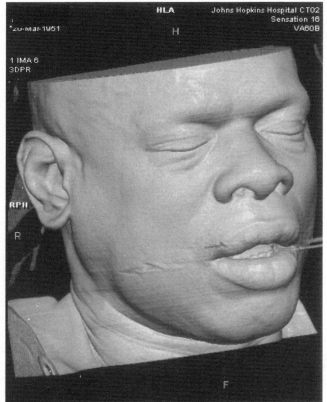

C

FIG. 25–4. Mandibular fracture. **A–C:** The patient had a recent physical altercation following alcohol intoxication. Two-dimensional and 3D mapping demonstrate the mandibular fracture with minimal displacement. Three-dimensional volume rendering also allows visualization of the overlying soft tissues and skin.

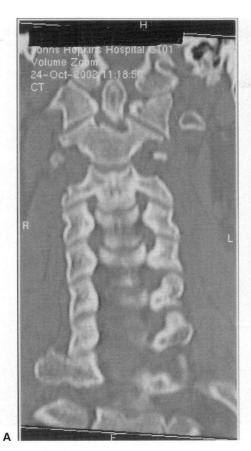

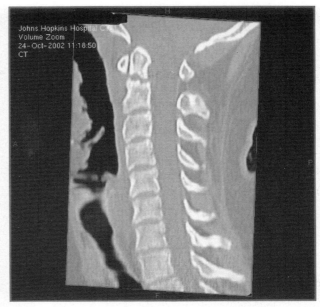

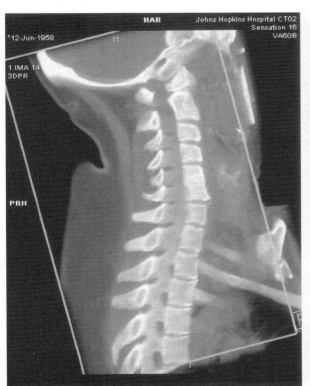

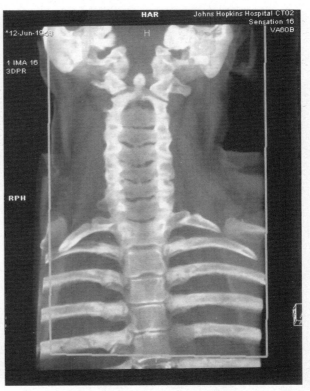

FIG. 25–5. Odontoid fracture. **A,B:** Three-dimensional mapping demonstrates evidence of a prior odontoid fracture. The 3D visualization demonstrates the fracture and the sclerotic changes along the fracture line with no evidence of fusion.

FIG. 25–6 A,B. Successful C5–C6 cervical fusion. Three-dimensional mapping in this patient with persistent pain following fusion and subsequent MVA demonstrates satisfactory fusion without evidence of narrowing of canal or other complication. No acute fracture was seen.

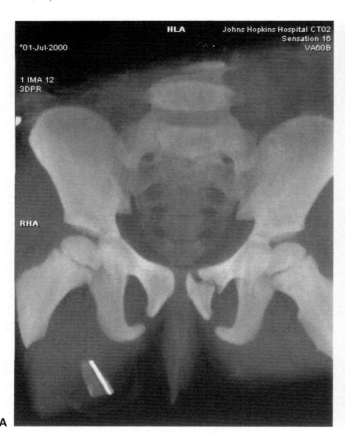

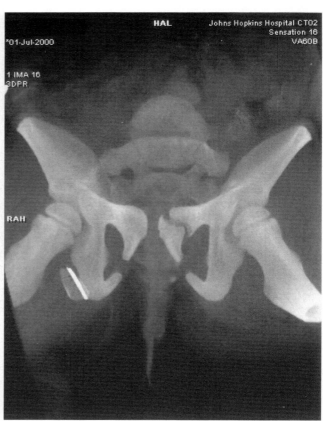

A

B

FIG. 25–7. Fracture of superior pubic ramus. **A,B:** Two-and-a-half-year-old patient was in a motor-vehicle accident. Three-dimensional mapping demonstrates an isolated superior left pubic-ramus fracture without any associated injuries.

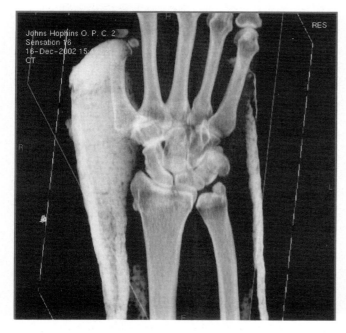

FIG. 25–8. Impacted radial fracture. The patient fell and landed on her wrist. Three-dimensional mapping demonstrates evidence of fracture of distal radius that extends intraarticularly. No dislocation was seen. The patient was treated conservatively.

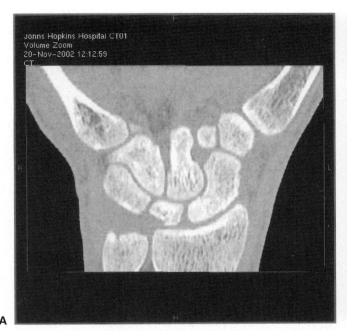
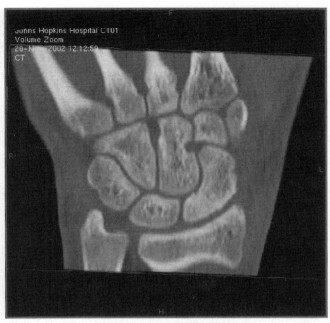

FIG. 25–9. Nonunion of right scaphoid fracture. **A,B:** The patient has a history of a scaphoid fracture approximately 1 year earlier. Coronal and 3D CT demonstrates the fracture line through the scaphoid with lack of healing consistent with nonunion. No evidence of avascular necrosis was seen. The patient was placed in a short-arm thumb-spica cast and will be using a bone simulator. If this is not satisfactory, then operative intervention will be necessary.

renderings, isotropic datasets permit display of all necessary views for surgical decision making. Isotropic datasets eliminate the need for two views and thereby facilitate the examination without compromising quality. The elimination of the second CT acquisition also reduces the radiation dose to the patient.

In the evaluation of pelvic trauma, MDCT is ideal for combining skeletal imaging with other studies, such as CTA to diagnose vascular injury, or CT cystogram to detect bladder injury. When technically adequate, CT cystograms are as accurate as conventional cystograms for detecting bladder injury. Although opacification of the bladder with IV contrast can distend the bladder to a reasonable degree if delayed scans are obtained, bladder injuries can be overlooked with this protocol. Computed-tomography cystography is a more accurate technique. A typical protocol involves placing a Foley catheter in the bladder and under-gravity-infusing contrast (30 mL of contrast in 500 mL of saline) into the bladder until adequate distention is achieved. A high level of diagnostic accuracy for detection of bladder injury can be achieved using this technique (Figures 25–10 and 25–11).

The use of isotropic datasets and volume visualization can provide unique perspectives that are invaluable in determining the full extent of injury and can be used to guide treatment planning. For example, Scott et al. have demonstrated that 3D imaging alone is all that is required to determine the extent of acetabular fractures, even when adequate plain films are available. Similar results have been shown across a wide spectrum of fractures, such as the craniofacial region, shoulder, and pelvis (9,10,16).

Computed tomography also has proven valuable in lower-extremity trauma, including tibial plateau fracture, ankle fracture or dislocation, and calcaneal injury (Figures 25–12 and 25–13). In the tibial plateau, CT commonly is requested to define extent of injury, particularly to evaluate the articular surface of the tibial plateau for possible depression. In most centers, a depression greater than 4 mm to 5 mm requires surgical intervention. Complex knee injuries, including fracture and/or dislocation of the patella, are diagnosed easily with CT. Associated meniscal injuries also have been diagnosed with CT, but MRI remains the gold standard in these cases. Injuries to the ankle mortise, including fractures and/or dislocations, readily are identified with CT volumetric acquisitions and a combination of multiplanar (coronal, sagittal) and 3D displays. Calcaneal fractures, including injuries to the tarsal bones, are imaged ideally with similar displays even with the patient in cast. Many surgeons require 3D mapping preoperatively on all calcaneal fractures.

In addition to being more time efficient, CT eliminates many of the diagnostic limitations of plain radiographs. Axially oriented fractures may be missed on routine axial CT if the fracture plane parallels the plane of the CT scan, but are identified clearly with volume display. Computed tomography has the added advantage of providing detailed soft-tissue imaging; injury to these regions may be the first sign of significant injury (Figure 25-14).

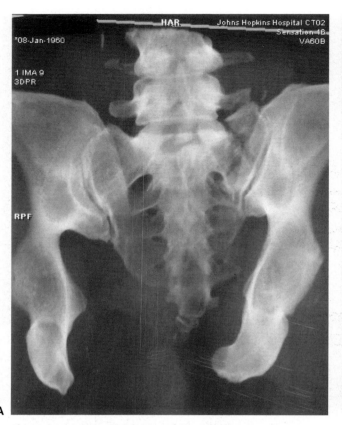

A

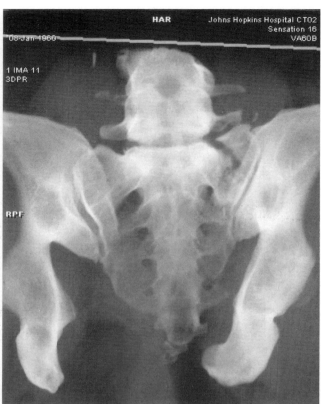

B

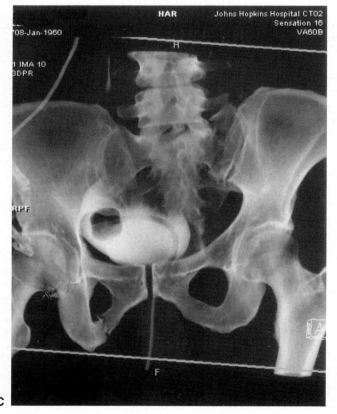

C

FIG. 25–10. Sacral fracture. **A–C:** The patient was hit by a car while under the influence of drugs and dragged several feet. Volume-rendered 3D images demonstrate fracture of left side of sacrum extending through S-2. Associated fracture of the right superior and inferior ramus with diastasis of symphysis is seen. Pelvic hematoma results in bladder displacement.

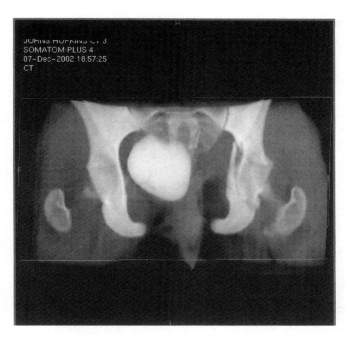

FIG. 25–11. Acetabular fracture with pelvic hematoma. The bladder is distended well and displaced to the right by pelvic hematoma due to the left acetabular fracture. No bladder injury was seen.

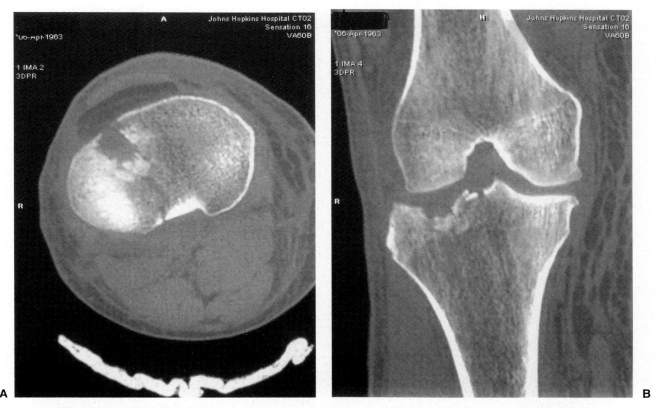

FIG. 25–12. Tibial plateau fracture. **A,B:** Two-dimensional and 3D imaging demonstrates fracture extending through tibial spine, as well as lateral tibial plateau with depression of nearly 10 mm. The fracture mapping with reconstruction demonstrates an extensive fracture with a minimal degree of displacement. *(continues)*

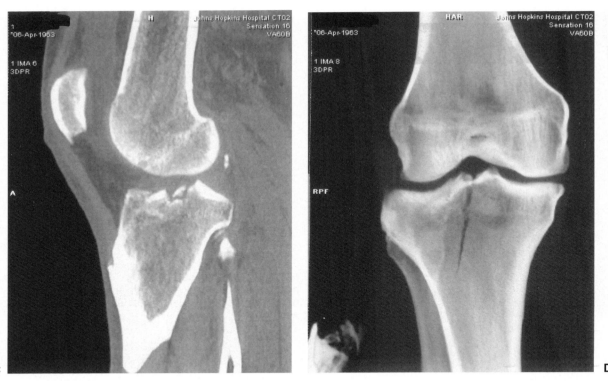

FIG. 25–12. *Continued.* Tibial plateau fracture. **C,D:** Two-dimensional and 3D imaging demonstrates fracture extending through tibial spine, as well as lateral tibial plateau with depression of nearly 10 mm. The fracture mapping with reconstruction demonstrates an extensive fracture with a minimal degree of displacement.

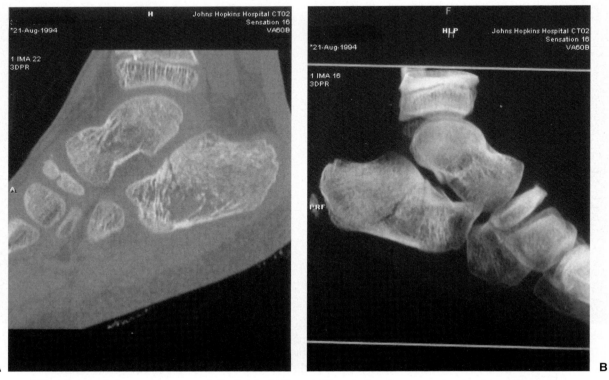

FIG. 25–13. Calcaneal fracture. **A,B:** Sagittal 2D and 3D mapping demonstrates fracture of the calcaneus without disruption of ankle mortise in this pediatric patient. The patient had jumped out of the window. Note the use of volume rendering with low opacity.

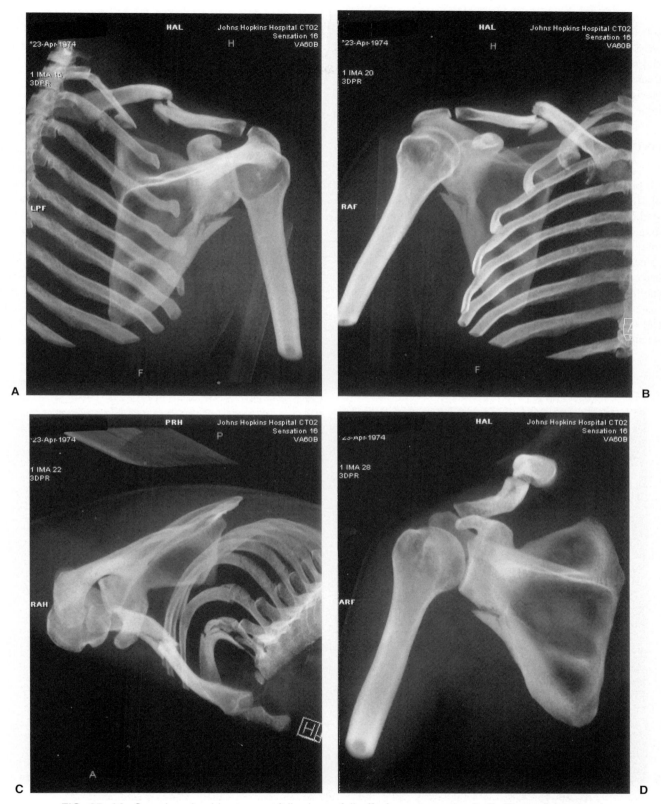

FIG. 25–14. Complex shoulder trauma following a fall off of a motorcycle. **A–D:** Three-dimensional imaging clearly defines the fractures involving the right clavicle and scapula, as well as the first rib. Multiple 3D views with volume rendering demonstrate the extent of the fracture and orientation of the fracture fragments. The patient was treated conservatively without intraoperative intervention based on orientation of the fractures as seen on the 3D mapping.

A new area of interest has been the CT evaluation of soft-tissue structures such as the tendons in the hand and wrist. Sunagawa et al. found that CT aided in the diagnosis and surgical planning of flexor-tendon ruptures (17). Soft-tissue imaging of the paraspinal musculature and the supraclavicular zones may be useful in select applications including infection and localization of nodes for biopsy.

ONCOLOGIC APPLICATIONS

Computed tomography has remained a valued modality for oncologic imaging, in spite of the continuing evolution of MRI, and is used routinely for tumor detection and staging studies in lung, renal, and ovarian cancers. Computed tomography may be the first study to detect musculoskeletal involvement, particularly in the ribs, thoracic and lumbar spine, and the pelvis. Additionally, the detection of unsuspected muscle metastases from such tumors as renal-cell carcinoma and lung cancer is becoming more common as scans tend to be obtained in earlier phases of enhancement and resolution continues to improve in the newest MDCT scanners.

Computed tomography also is used for a number of clinical applications (18–20) (Figures 25–15 and 25–16), including resolving inconsistencies between interpretation of plain radiographs and patient symptoms, or between bone scans and plain radiographs. Computed tomography also may be used to detect tumor infiltration, which is difficult to discern with other studies. Computed tomography also has proven valuable in determining the extent of tumor before planning therapy, including surgery, chemotherapy, or radiation therapy. Tumor volumes can be calculated accurately using volumes determined from MDCT datasets. The use of MPR and 3D imaging plays a crucial role in this application. In addition, CT has been used successfully to define the optimal site of lesions for biopsy. Biopsies can be done with CT guidance and, if necessary, with CT fluoroscopy, allowing biopsy of smaller lesions in more difficult locations. Computed-tomography fluoroscopy also can be used to guide radiofrequency ablation of osteoid osteoma. Newer MDCT scanners are continuing to focus on the interventional use of real-time CT fluoroscopy. The use of positron-emission tomography (PET) and/or CT may be valuable for this application in the future. Computed tomography is effective

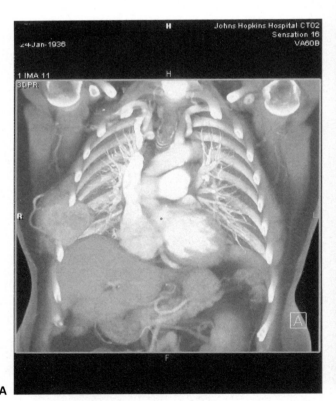
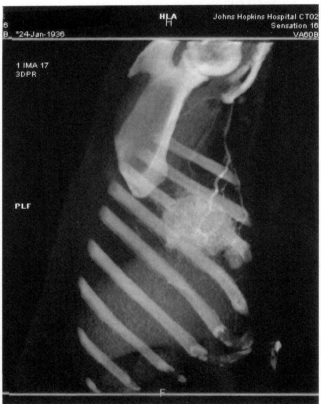

A

B

FIG. 25–15. A,B: Metastatic renal-cell cancer. Sixty-seven-year-old patient presents with chest pain. The patient had a remote history of a renal-cell carcinoma. The images demonstrate a hypervascular mass in the right chest wall with associated rib destruction. Note the vascularity of lesions seen on multiple images in both axial and coronal display. Three-dimensional mapping demonstrates the feeding vessel to the lesion. Biopsy of the lesion was metastatic renal carcinoma. The patient was treated with radiation therapy.

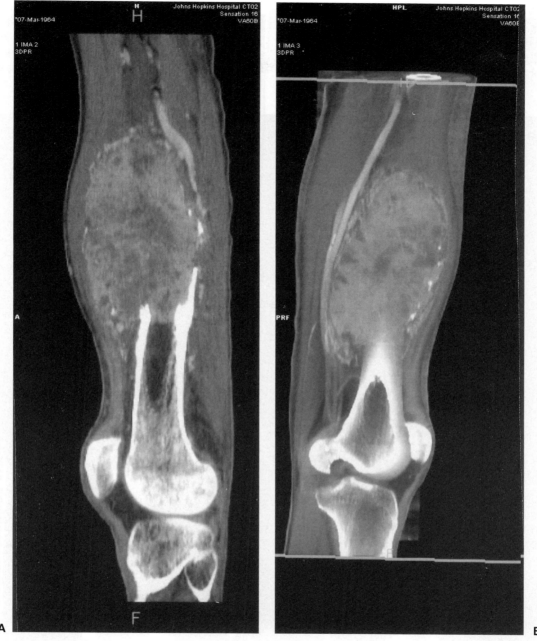

FIG. 25–16. Metastatic lung cancer to muscle and bone. **A,B:** Thirty-eight-year-old male with a history of increasing thigh pain. Computed-tomography scan demonstrates large intramuscular mass that is hypervascular with pathologic fracture of femur. This subsequently was proven to be metastatic lung cancer to muscle. Three-dimensional mapping with volume rendering provides definition of both soft-tissue and bone involvement of lesion.

in defining the presence and extent of disease that may be detected or suggested with bone scanning or PET scanning. Computed tomography, for example, can determine whether increased uptake in a bone scan is Paget's disease or blastic metastases. When combined with PET, CT can be used to define more precisely the site of increased tracer uptake on a FDG study. Computed tomography may clarify PET findings, including differentiating stress fractures from metasta-

ses in cases of increased uptake in the sacrum. Several manufacturers have taken this one step further by combining CT and PET scanning into a single imaging device. This appears to be more accurate than trying to merge images retrospectively from two different datasets acquired at separate times on two different imaging devices.

The use of MDCT with optimal scan protocols is supplemented routinely by 3D reconstructions (Figures 25–9

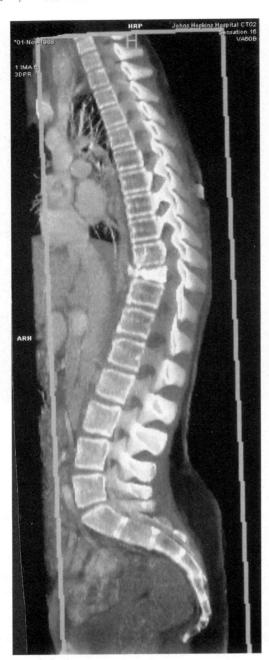

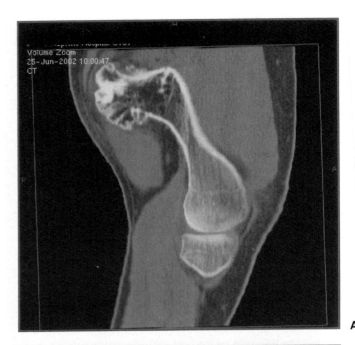

A

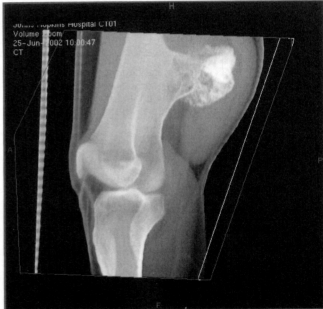

B

FIG. 25–19. Metastatic Ewing sarcoma to thoracic spine. Fourteen-year-old female with a history of Ewing sarcoma of the left proximal humerus that subsequently metastasized to lungs and other bones. Collapse of T10 with sclerotic changes noted. Note how single acquisition allows definition of the entire spine.

FIG. 25–20. Osteochondroma of the distal femur. **A,B:** Nineteen-year-old male with pain in the knee. Three-dimensional mapping demonstrated a large osteochondroma. Note the matrix of the lesion without evidence of malignant degeneration or fracture. The tumor was resected successfully.

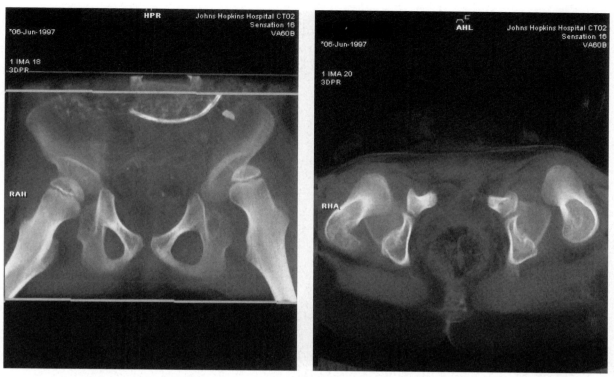

FIG. 25–21. Congenital hip dysplasia. **A,B:** The patient is a 5-year-old with myelodysplasia. The patient has shallow acetabulum bilaterally, left greater than right. The left epiphysis appears smaller than the right. They are both small for the age of the patient. The patient subsequently underwent bilateral femoral osteotomies, as well as a left iliac osteotomy.

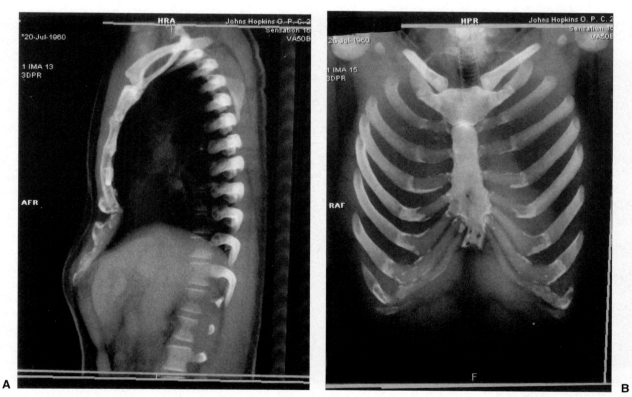

FIG. 25–22. Pectus deformity. **A,B:** Three-dimensional mapping demonstrates the patient's pectus excavatum deformity. Changes in orientation of costocartilage also are well defined on this study.

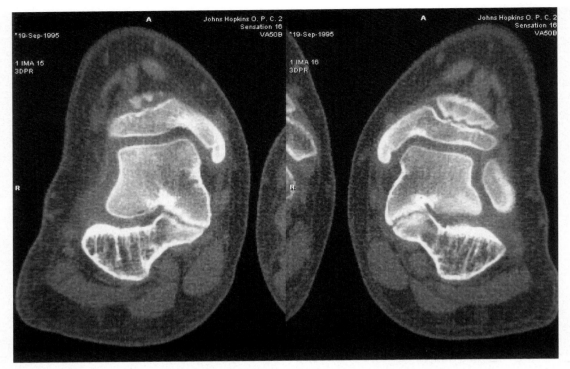

FIG. 25–23. Talocalcaneal coalition. The patient had increasing pain in the foot. Computed tomography demonstrates near fusion of the talocalcaneal joint. This was treated with surgical repair.

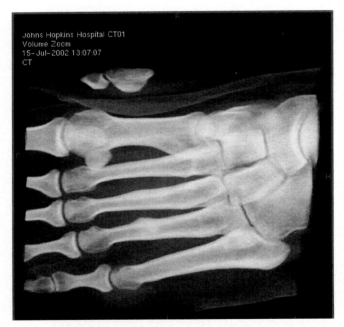

FIG. 25–24. Stress fracture of fourth metatarsal. The patient experienced pain in the foot. Evidence of a stress fracture is seen involving the fourth metatarsal. Three-dimensional mapping demonstrates periosteal reaction.

Up to 90% of tarsal coalitions involve the talocalcaneal or calcaneonavicular joints, both of which occur with near-equal frequency. Other coalitions, including talonavicular coalition, are rare. Although tarsal coalition may be diagnosed on plain radiographs, the use of CT and 3D CT provides a more definitive diagnosis.

POSTOPERATIVE ORTHOPEDIC IMAGING

One of the most challenging clinical scenarios is the patient with prior orthopedic surgery involving insertion of pins, plates, screws, or joint replacement. Although some material generates less artifact than others, axial CT still may be limited by artifact from metal implants. However, image postprocessing can solve this problem. Some scanners provide postprocessing software that can reduce artifact or extend the CT scale to minimize artifact generated from beam hardening.

Multiplanar reconstruction and/or 3D volume rendering with thin collimation and narrow interscan spacing has proven particularly valuable. Because artifact typically is random on each individual CT slice, reconstruction of overlapping CT slices will limit artifact and result in diagnostic-quality CT images (26,27). This technique is effective in assessment of fracture healing or postoperative infection, evaluation of suspected failure of hardware, and follow up of patients with persistent pain following orthopedic implants. When using 3D reconstruction, it has been found that using color for metal (blue works best) against the classic opacifi-

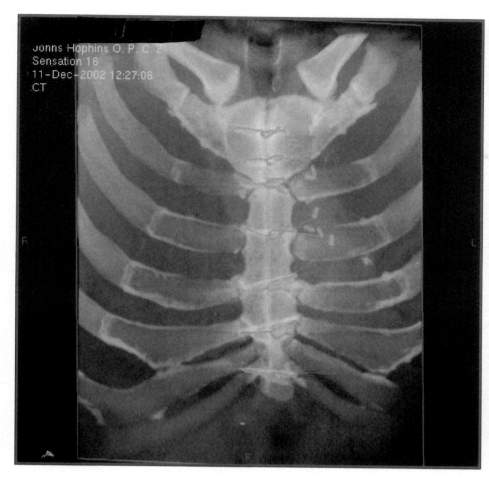

FIG. 25–25. Normal median sternotomy following coronary-artery bypass surgery. Three-dimensional mapping was done in a patient with persistent chest pain. A successful median sternotomy without evidence of complication is seen on this examination. (See Color Fig. 25–25)

cation usually selected for bone is ideal. Slice thickness of 0.50 mm to 1.25 mm is ideal with a 0.5-mm to 1.0-mm reconstruction interval (Figures 25-25 to 25-28). A standard algorithm can help minimize the artifact from metal implants.

SOFT-TISSUE AND MUSCLE IMAGING

One growing application of CT in the emergency room is the evaluation of known or suspected musculoskeletal infection. With the ever-increasing numbers of immunosuppressed patients, there has been a corresponding rise in the number of patients presenting with potential musculoskeletal infection. Multidetector CT is a rapid and accurate technique for evaluating suspected or known musculoskeletal infection. Practical advantages over MRI include scanner availability, location of CT compared to MR, speed of examination, and availability. Intravenous-contrast examination is necessary to accentuate the difference between normal and abnormal soft tissues.

Pathologic processes usually can be detected on noncontrast studies when substantial inflammation is present; however, information regarding extent of inflammation and/or level of involvement is inferior to the contrast-enhanced study. Our protocols for contrast enhancement will vary depending on the body part studied. The use of contrast helps differentiate between normal and abnormal tissue. When muscle becomes edematous or ischemic, it commonly enlarges and has blurred edges due to surrounding edema. With IV contrast, normal musculature will enhance up to 50 Hounsfield units (HU) to 80 HU, whereas abnormal muscle will enhance to a lesser degree. Areas of necrosis do not demonstrate enhancement. Scanning 40 seconds to 50 seconds after contrast injection (100 cc to 120 cc of contrast injected at 2 cc to 3 cc per second) provides optimal differentiation between normal and abnormal muscle. One of the potential limitations is that enhancing muscle abscesses can resemble closely necrotic tumors. However, in most cases, the clinical history is quite different, and thus the radiologic interpretation is not problematic (28).

When evaluating muscle inflammation, it also is important to review bone windows through the appropriate scan levels. Often bony involvement is the primary source of inflammatory process, or it may become involved secondarily. This particularly is true for infection in the chest wall, sternoclavicular joint, sacroiliac joints, and sacrum. Similarly, images may need to be reviewed at lung window settings to exclude the presence of air in processes such as necrotizing

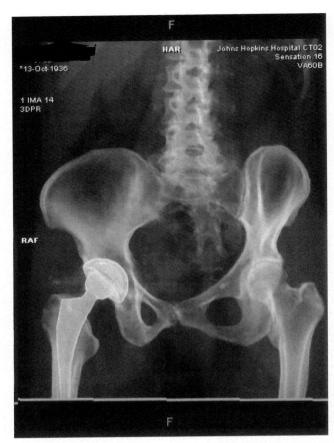

FIG. 25–26. Total hip replacement. Patient had experienced pain, and the study was done to rule out a loose prosthesis. Three-dimensional mapping using color coding demonstrates the prosthesis to be in satisfactory position with no evidence of loosening. (See Color Fig. 25–26)

fasciitis. In these cases, early diagnosis is essential to decrease the high incidence of morbidity and mortality.

In the evaluation of musculoskeletal infection, the patient is scanned with a standard algorithm. High-resolution or bone algorithms create substantial noise, resulting in images suboptimal for soft-tissue assessment. When high-resolution images of bone are desired, reconstruction with both algorithms is ideal. This can be done in mere seconds with 16-slice MDCT.

Most cases of musculoskeletal inflammation do not require 3D or multiplanar imaging to detect the primary disease process. However, they may be valuable in determining the extent of inflammation, which may assist the surgeon in preoperative planning. This especially is true when imaging spinal infection. Defining disc-space involvement is facilitated with sagittal multiplanar or 3D sagittal reconstruction formats. Sternal and sternoclavicular joint involvement also is optimized with 3D volume displays. As with other applications of MDCT datasets, 3D volume display is becoming more routine in primary interpretation, particularly owing to the large number of axial images generated with the newest scanners (Figures 25–29 and 29–30).

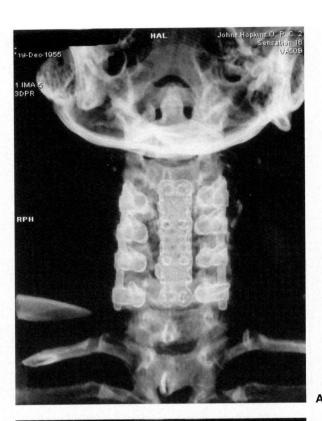

A

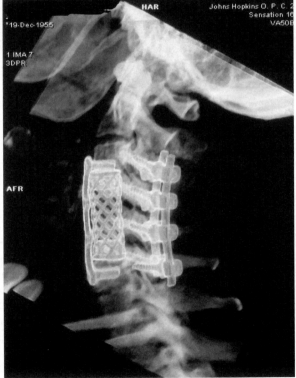

B

FIG. 25–27. Post C4–C5 corpectomy and removal of epidural abscess with spinal fusion. **A,B:** Extensive hardware is in place involving multiple vertebral bodies and posterior elements and shows a good postoperative result. Note how the metal artifact is minimized by the use of 3D mapping with volume rendering. (See Color Fig. 25–27)

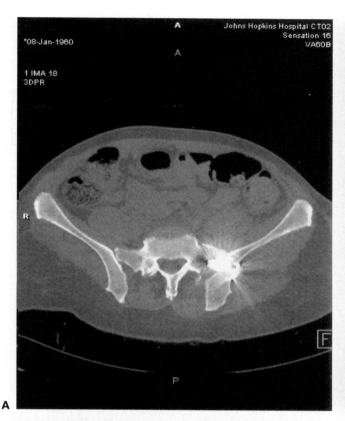

A

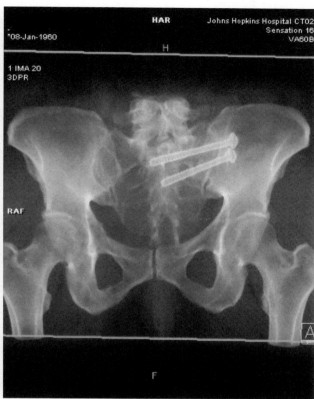

B

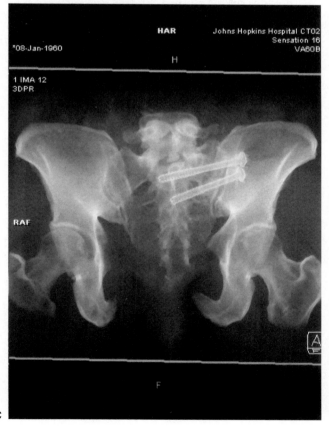

C

FIG. 25–28. Intraoperative repair of sacral fracture. **A–C:** Three-dimensional mapping demonstrates two screws in place across sacroiliac joint to repair the patient's sacral fracture. Note that despite artifact on axial images, 3D reconstructions show no evidence of artifact and demonstrate the satisfactory postoperative reduction.

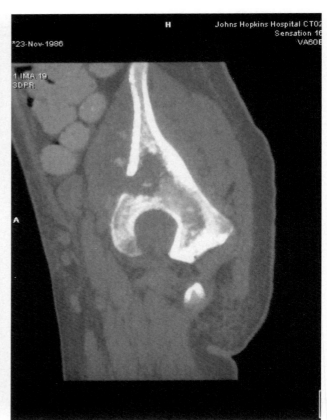

A

B

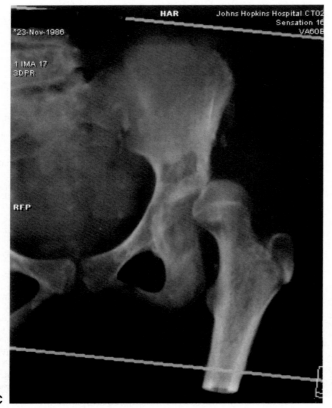

C

FIG. 25–29. Osteomyelitis of the left acetabulum. **A–C:** The patient had a history of sickle-cell anemia and had multiple hospital admissions with transfusions and repeated infections. The patient presented with muscle pain and fever. Computed-tomography scan demonstrates evidence of osteomyelitis involving left superior acetabulum with inflammatory process extending in the hip joint. The femur is displaced laterally out of the joint space, which is seen best on 3D mapping.

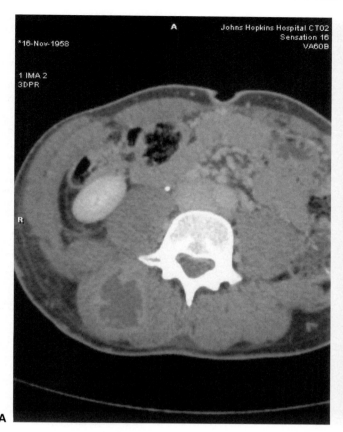
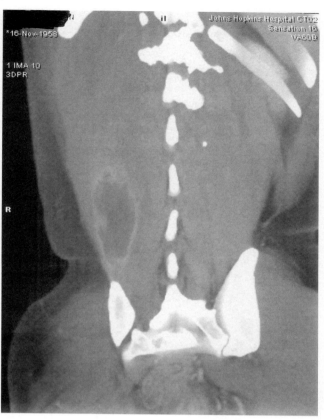

FIG. 25–30. Intramuscular abscess in the right paraspinal muscles. **A,B:** Forty-four-year-old HIV + patient presented with right flank pain felt to be renal in origin. A CT scan was done that demonstrated the unsuspected right paraspinous muscle abscess. This was treated with incision and drainage, followed by antibiotics.

CONCLUSION

The role of CT in evaluation of musculoskeletal pathology will continue to grow and evolve with the continued evolution of MDCT (29). New patient protocols will be developed, especially in the emergency-room setting, where, in many cases, CT will be the initial and only study performed on trauma patients. The use of CT in volume-display mode also will be ideal for rapid screening of the trauma patient and potentially may become a cost-effective and time-effective study technique. The latest generation of MDCT scanners now allows routine use of isotropic datasets of 0.50-mm to 0.75-mm thickness, ideal for the high-resolution imaging necessary in musculoskeletal imaging. With the use of isotropic datasets and 3D volume viewing, it is believed that the role of CT for musculoskeletal imaging will continue to increase in clinical application.

REFERENCES

1. Pretorius ES, Fishman EK. Volume-rendered three-dimensional spiral CT: musculoskeletal applications. *Radiographics* 1999;19:1143–1160.
2. Pretorius ES, Fishman EK. Spiral CT and three-dimensional CT of musculoskeletal pathology—emergency room applications. *Radiol Clin North Am* 1999;37(5):953–974.
3. Tanenbaum LN. Multichannel helical CT of the musculoskeletal system. *Appl Radiol* 2003;32(5):15–24.
4. Beauchamp NJ Jr, Scott WW Jr, Gottlieb LM, et al. CT evaluation of soft tissue and muscle infection and inflammation: a systematic compartmental approach. *Skeletal Radiol* 1995;24(5):317–324.
5. Young JWR, Resnik CS. Fracture of the pelvis: current concepts of classification. *AJR Am J Roentgenol* 1990;155:1169–1175.
6. Goldfarb CA, Yin Y, Gilula LA, et al. Wrist fractures: what the clinician wants to know. *Radiology* 2001;219:11–28.
7. Kuszyk BS, Heath DG, Bliss DF, et al. Skeletal 3-D CT: advantages of volume rendering over surface rendering. *Skeletal Radiol* 1996; 25:207–214.
8. Ney DR, Drebin RA, Fishman EK, et al. Volumetric rendering of computed tomographic data: principles and techniques. *IEEE Comput Graphic Appl* 1990;10:24–32.
9. Scott WW Jr, Fishman EK, Magid D. Acetabular fractures: optimal imaging. *Radiology* 1987;165:537–539.
10. Scott WW Jr, Magid D, Fishman EK, et al. Three dimensional imaging of acetabular trauma. *J Orthop Trauma* 1987;1(3):227–232.
11. Mower WR, Hoffman JR, Zucker ML. Odontoid fractures following blunt trauma. *Emerg Radiol* 2000;7:3–6.
12. Nuñez DB, Zuluaga A, Fuentes-Bernardo DA, et al. Cervical spine trauma: how much more do we learn by routinely using helical CT? *Radiographics* 1996;16:1307–1318.
13. Daffner R. Cervical radiography for trauma patients: a time effective technique? *AJR Am J Roentgenol* 2000;175:1309–1311.
14. Blackmore CC, Emerson SS. Mann FA, et al. Cervical spine imaging in patients with trauma: determination of fracture risk to optimize use. *Radiology* 1999;211:759–765.
15. Berlin L. Malpractice issues in radiology. CT versus radiography for initial evaluation of cervical spine trauma: what is the standard care? *AJR Am J Roentgenol* 2003;180:911–915.

16. Nuñez DB, Quencer RM. The role of helical CT in the assessment of cervical spine injuries. *AJR Am J Roentgenol* 1998;171:951–957.

17. Sunagawa T, Ochi M, Ishida O, et al. Three-dimensional CT imaging of flexor tendon ruptures in the hand and wrist. *J Comput Assist Tomogr* 2003;279(2):169–174.

18. Kuszyk BS, Ney DR, Fishman EK. The current state of the art in 3D oncologic imaging: an overview. *Int J Radiat Oncol Biol Phys* 1995; 33:1029–1039.

19. Llauger J, Palmer J, Amores S, et al. Primary tumors of the sacrum: diagnostic imaging. *AJR Am J Roentgenol* 2000;174:417–424.

20. Blacksin MF, Benevenvia J. Neoplasms of the scapula. *AJR Am J Roentgenol* 2000;174:1129–1135.

21. Murray KA, Crim JR. Radiographic imaging for treatment and follow-up of developmental dysplasia of the hip. *Semin Ultrasound CT MR* 2001;22(4):306–340.

22. Stec AA, Pannu HK, Tadros YE, et al. Evaluation of the bony pelvis in classic bladder extrophy by using 3D-CT: further insights. *Urology* 2001;58(6):1030–1035.

23. Pretorius ES, Haller JA, Fishman EK. Spiral CT with 3D reconstruction in children requiring reoperation for failure of chest wall growth after pectus excavatum surgery: preliminary observations. *Clin Imag* 1998; 22:108–116.

24. Donnelly LF. Use of three-dimensional reconstructed helical CT images in recognition and communication of chest wall anomalies in children. *AJR Am J Roentgenol* 2001;177:441–445.

25. Newman JS, Newberg AH. Congenital tarsal coalition: multimodality evaluation with emphasis on CT and MR imaging. *Radiographics* 2000; 20:321–332.

26. Fishman EK, Magid D, Robertson DD, et al. Metallic hip implants: CT with multiplanar reconstruction. *Radiology* 1986;160:675–681.

27. Link TM, Berning W, Scherf S, et al. CT of metal implants: reduction of artifacts using an extended CT scale technique. *J Comput Assist Tomogr* 2000;24(1):165–172.

28. Pretorius ES, Fishman EK. Helical CT of skeletal muscle metastases from primary carcinoma. *AJR Am J Roentgenol* 2000;174:401–404.

29. Stevens K, Tao C, Lee SU, et al. Subchondral fractures in osteonecrosis of the femoral head: comparison of radiography, CT and MR imaging. *AJR Am J Roentgenol* 2003;180:363–368.

CHAPTER **26**

Pediatric Abdominal Applications

Marilyn J. Siegel

INTRODUCTION

Because computed tomography (CT) allows direct, noninvasive demonstration of normal and abnormal anatomy, it has had a major impact on the evaluation of abdominal diseases in children. With the advent of helical technology, particularly multidetector scanners, diagnostic images with excellent resolution can be obtained even in very small neonates and infants. In this chapter, the techniques, protocols, and common clinical indications for performing multidetector CT (MDCT) in the pediatric abdomen will be discussed. The CT findings in abdominal neoplasms, appendicitis, and blunt trauma are covered.

PATIENT PREPARATION

Sedation

The indications and protocols for sedation are discussed in the prior chapter. The reader is referred to that section for more details.

Bowel Opacification

Opacification of the small and large bowel is necessary for most examinations of the abdomen, as unopacified bowel loops can simulate a mass or abnormal fluid collection. The exceptions are patients with depressed mental status, who are at risk of aspiration, and those with acute blunt abdominal trauma, where there may be insufficient time for contrast administration. A diluted (1%–2%) solution of water-soluble iodine-based oral-contrast agent is given by mouth or through a nasogastric tube if necessary. The oral contrast agent can be mixed with fruit juice if needed to mask the unpleasant taste.

The gastrointestinal tract from stomach to terminal ileum usually can be well opacified if the contrast is given twice: 45 minutes to 60 minutes before the examination, and again 15 minutes prior to scanning. The initial volume should approximate that of an average feeding. The volume

just prior to scanning is one half that of the first. Appropriate volumes of contrast medium versus patient age are shown in Table 26.1.

CT TECHNIQUE

Intravenous-Contrast Material

If intravenous (IV) contrast material is to be administered, an IV line should be in place before the child arrives in the radiology department (1). This reduces patient agitation that otherwise would be associated with a venipuncture performed immediately prior to administration of contrast material. The largest gauge cannula that can be placed is recommended. The volume of contrast is 2 mL per kilogram (not to exceed 4 mL/kg or 125 mL). Nonionic agents are recommended. They have the advantage of decreasing discomfort at site of injection and patient motion during intravenous administration (2).

Contrast media may be injected either by hand or by power injector. Power injection is used when a 22-gauge or larger cannula can be placed into an antecubital vein. Flow rates range from 1.5 mL to 2.0 mL per second for a 22-gauge catheter and from 2.0 mL to 3.0 mL per second for a 20-gauge catheter. A hand injection is used when IV access is through a peripheral access line in the dorsum of the hand or foot. Contrast medium can be injected via a central venous catheter or a 24-gauge catheter by a power injector if the rate of injection is slow (1 mL/sec) and there is proper intravascular positioning of the access line (3,4).

Scan-Delay Times

The optimal scan-delay time depends on the volume of contrast material and the rate of injection. As a general rule, the duration of the contrast bolus should be equivalent or as close as possible to the duration of the CT scan. The goal is to initiate the scan during the portal venous phase of enhancement. In adults, a delay time of 50 seconds to 70 seconds *from the onset of contrast administration* is employed

low attenuation, usually containing some areas of identifiable fat. Occasionally, they coexist with cystic renal disease. Computed-tomography can help in the detection of subtle foci of fat, considered a pathognomonic finding for angiomyolipoma.

ADRENAL TUMORS

Neuroblastoma

Neuroblastoma is the most common extrarenal malignant abdominal tumor in children, followed in frequency by ganglioneuroblastoma and ganglioneuroma (38). Most patients with neuroblastoma are between 1 year and 5 years of age; mean patient age at diagnosis is 2 years. More than half of all neuroblastomas arise in the abdomen, and two-thirds of these originate in the adrenal gland. The extraadrenal neuroblastomas originate in the sympathetic ganglion cells or paraaortic bodies, and they may be found anywhere from the cervical region to the pelvis. Neuroblastomas tend to metastasize early, and more than half of all patients have bone marrow, skeletal, liver, or skin metastases when initially diagnosed. Lung and pleural metastases are rare.

Computed-tomography features of neuroblastoma include a homogeneous or heterogeneous pararenal or paraspinal soft tissue mass with lobulated margins (39,40). The tumor enhances but remains hypodense relative to surrounding tissues (Figure 26-8). Calcifications within the tumor—which may be coarse, mottled, solid, or ring-shaped—are observed in approximately 85% of neuroblastomas on CT.

Local spread of tumor takes the form of prevertebral extension across the midline, vascular encasement, hepatic metastases, intraspinal extension, and renal invasion or infarction (41). Axial images are excellent for demonstrating the midline extent of tumor, lymph nodes, and hepatic metastases. Multiplanar and 3D reconstructions are valuable for delineating the craniocaudal extent of the tumor and vessel encasement (Figure 26-8B). Defining tumor extent is important for treatment planning and prognosis.

Other Adrenal Masses

Adrenocortical Neoplasms

Adrenal lesions other than neuroblastomas are rare in childhood, accounting for 5% or less of all adrenal tumors (22,42). Of the adrenocortical tumors, carcinoma is the most common, followed by adenoma. The mean age at presentation of patients with carcinoma and adenoma is approximately 6 years and 3 years, respectively. Most adrenal carcinomas are hormonally active, producing virilization, feminization, or Cushing's syndrome (40). Adenomas can cause Cushing's syndrome or primary aldosteronism, but also may be detected incidentally.

Adrenal carcinomas typically are large masses at the time of presentation, often greater than 4 cm to 5 cm in diameter, with an attenuation value equal to that of soft tissue (Figure 26-9). These masses enhance minimally after IV-contrast administration. Low-density areas from prior necrosis are common, and some tumors may contain calcifications. Local invasion occurs in approximately 50% of cases,

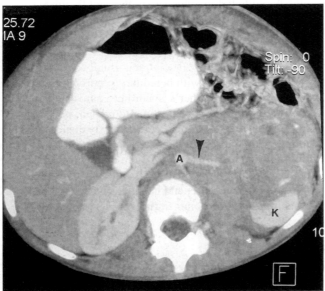
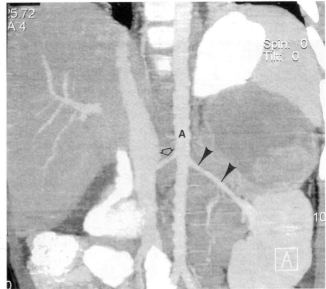

A   B

FIG. 26–8. Neuroblastoma in a 2-year-old girl. **A:** Axial contrast-enhanced CT scan shows a suprarenal low-density mass extending across the midline in the retroperitoneum and displacing the left kidney (*K*) posteriorly. The tumor surrounds the aorta (*A*) and left renal artery (*arrowhead*). **B:** Coronal multiplanar image shows the craniocaudal extent of tumor and encasement of the left renal artery (*arrowheads*), right renal artery (*open arrow*), and aorta (*A*).

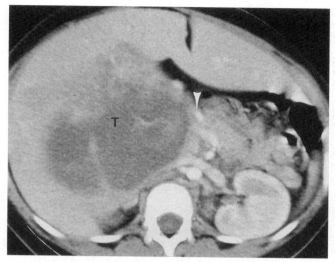

FIG. 26–9. Adrenal carcinoma in a 15-year-old girl with virilization. A large tumor (*T*) with poorly defined borders is present in the right adrenal gland, displacing the superior mesenteric artery (*arrowhead*) and small bowel to the left.

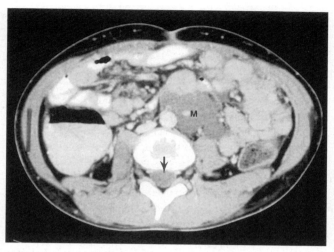

FIG. 26–10. Neurofibroma in a 14-year-old boy. Contrast-enhanced CT scan demonstrates a hypodense mass (*M*) extending anterior to the left psoas muscle and displacing bowel loops anteriorly and to the left. A small neurofibroma (*arrow*) also is noted in the spinal canal.

and distant metastases involve the lung and liver. Cortisol-producing adenomas range between 2 cm and 5 cm in diameter, whereas aldosterone-secreting tumors usually are less than 2 cm in diameter. Both types of adenomas tend to be homogeneous and of low attenuation due to their high lipid content.

Pheochromocytoma

Pheochromocytomas are catecholamine-producing neoplasms of the adrenal medulla that cause paroxysmal hypertension in children. Paragangliomas are catecholamine-secreting tumors arising in an extraadrenal location. Most pheochromocytomas and paragangliomas in children are sporadic; however, they may be associated with multiple endocrine neoplastic (MEN) syndromes and the phakomatoses, including neurofibromatosis, tuberous sclerosis, von Hippel–Lindau disease, and Sturge–Weber disease (42). Approximately 85% of catecholamine-secreting tumors arise in the adrenal medulla; the remainder occurs in the sympathetic ganglia adjacent to the vena cava or aorta, near the organ of Zuckerkandl, or in the wall of the urinary bladder. Up to 70% of tumors are bilateral and about 5% are malignant (42). They are usually at least 3 cm in diameter at the time of diagnosis. On CT, pheochromocytomas are of soft tissue density and frequently enhance after IV administration of contrast medium.

Non-Adrenal Retroperitoneal Soft-tissue Masses

Although rare, both benign and malignant primary tumors occur in the retroperitoneal soft tissues. Benign retroperitoneal tumors include teratoma, lymphangioma, neurofibroma, and lipomatosis. On CT, teratomas usually appear as well-defined fluid-filled masses with variable amounts of fat and calcium (43). Lymphangiomas are well-circumscribed multiloculated fluid-filled masses. Benign neurogenic tumors, such as neurofibromas, often have a homogenous low-attenuation value higher than water, but lower than paraspinal muscle. They typically occur along a nerve and its branches and are situated in a parapsoas or presacral location (Figure 26-10). Lipomatosis appears as a diffuse, infiltrative mass with an attenuation value equal to fat; it grows along fascial planes and may invade muscle.

Rhabdomyosarcoma is the most common malignant tumor of the retroperitoneum, followed by neurofibrosarcoma, fibrosarcoma, and extragonadal germ cell tumors. These tumors demonstrate features similar to those of neuroblastoma. However, malignant retroperitoneal tumors may invade vessels, unlike neuroblastoma, which encases but does not invade vessels.

HEPATIC AND BILIARY MASSES

The primary objectives in imaging patients with focal hepatic neoplasms are accurate tumor detection, characterization, segmental localization, and delineation of adjacent vascular structures. When a malignant tumor is suspected, the presence of tumor in surgically critical areas, such as the porta hepatis, portal vein, and inferior vena cava, and the presence of regional extrahepatic spread and distant metastases need to be determined. These features help to determine whether surgical or medical management is most appropriate.

Tumor Characterization with Multislice CT (Protocol 2—Table 26.4)

The detection of a focal lesion in the liver depends on the relative difference in attenuation between the lesion and the normal liver. Multiphase CT imaging can help optimize this difference. Hypervascular tumors, such as hemangioendothelioma, hepatic adenoma, focal nodular hyperplasia, small hepatocellular carcinomas, and hypervascular metastases are seen best during the hepatic arterial phase of enhancement, appearing as hyperdense masses compared with the surrounding liver. Hypervascular tumors may be obscured during the portal phase because the increased attenuation of the tumors is similar to that of the enhanced liver. Hypovascular tumors, such as hepatoblastoma and large hepatocellular carcinomas, are seen best in the portal venous phase of enhancement, when the difference in attenuation between liver and tumor is maximal. During this phase, they appear hypodense relative to adjacent liver.

Primary Malignant Neoplasms

Primary hepatic tumors account for fewer than 5% of pediatric tumors and are the third most frequent neoplasm after Wilms' tumor and neuroblastoma (44,45). Malignant hepatic tumors are twice as frequent as benign tumors, with hepatoblastoma and hepatocellular carcinoma accounting for the majority. The former occurs in children under the age of 5 years, whereas the latter is more frequent in older children. Malignant hepatic tumors usually present as upper-abdominal masses.

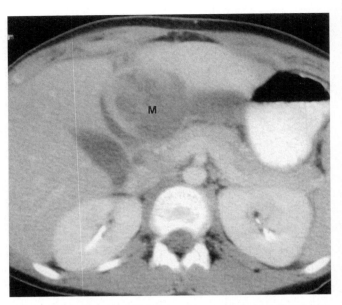

FIG. 26–11. Hepatocellular carcinoma in a 4-year-old boy with a right upper-quadrant mass. Contrast-enhanced CT scan during the portal venous phase shows a well-defined hypoattenuating mass (*M*).

Hepatoblastoma and hepatocellular carcinoma (HCC) have similar CT features. Both tumors usually appear as solitary masses confined to a single lobe. The right lobe is involved twice as often as the left lobe, but these lesions may involve both lobes or be multicentric. They generally have a density lower than that of normal hepatic parenchyma

TABLE 26–4. *Protocol 2*

Indication	Liver dual-phase imaging
	(Hepatic tumor)
Extent	Arterial phase, dome to tip of liver
	Portal-venous phase, diaphragm to pubic symphysis
Scanner settings	kVp, 80 for patients weighing <50 kg; higher kVp for larger patients
	mA, lowest possible based on patient weight
Detector collimation	2.5 mm for 4-row scanner
	1.5 mm for 16-row scanner
Table speed (pitch)	15 mm–20 mm per rotation for 4-row scanner
	36 mm per rotation for 16-row scanner
Slice thickness	3 mm–5 mm for 4-row scanner
	2 mm–5 mm for 16-row scanner
Oral contrast	Water-soluble contrast material given 45 minutes to 60 minutes prior to scan. Additional volume given 15 minutes prior to scan.
Intravenous-contrast volume	2 mL/kg (maximum of 4 mL/kg or 125 mL)
Contrast injection rate	Hand injection, rapid bolus administration
	Power injector
	22 gauge, 1.5 mL to 2.0 mL per sec
	20 gauge, 2.0 mL to 3.0 mL per sec
Scan delay	15-sec to 20 sec delay time for arterial phase in infants and 25-sec to 30-sec delay time in older patients.
	50-sec to 60-sec delay time for portal-venous phase
Miscellaneous	1. Unenhanced scans not routinely acquired.
	2. Delayed scans at 5 minutes to 10 minutes may help to confirm hemangioendothelioma.
	3. If the child is sedated or uncooperative, CT scans are obtained at quiet breathing.

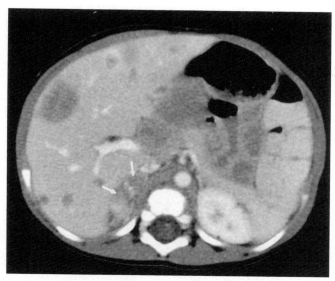

FIG. 26–12. Hepatic metastases in a neonate with neuroblastoma. Contrast-enhanced CT scan shows a small soft tissue tumor (*arrows*) arising in the right adrenal gland and multiple low-density hepatic metastases. (Case courtesy of Fred Hoffer, M.D. Memphis, TN.)

Hepatic Metastases

The malignant tumors of childhood that most frequently metastasize to the liver are Wilms' tumor, neuroblastoma, and lymphoma. Clinically, patients with hepatic metastases present with hepatomegaly, jaundice, abdominal pain or mass, or abnormal hepatic-function tests.

Metastatic disease usually appears as focal, discrete lesions, but diffuse infiltrative involvement can be seen in neuroblastoma (Figure 26-12). Hepatic metastases typically are multiple and hypodense relative to normal liver on contrast-enhanced CT.

Benign Neoplasms

Benign tumors account for about one-third of all hepatic tumors in children. The majority are of vascular origin and usually hemangioendotheliomas (44–46). Hepatic adenomas and focal nodular hyperplasia account for fewer than 2% of hepatic tumors in childhood. Most patients with hemangioendotheliomas are under 6 months of age and present with hepatomegaly or congestive heart failure due to high-output overcirculation. Occasionally, affected patients present with bleeding diathesis secondary to platelet sequestration (Kasabach–Merritt syndrome) or massive hemoperitoneum due to spontaneous tumor rupture. By comparison with adults, cavernous hemangioma is infrequently found in children, although sometimes it is encountered as an incidental finding.

Hemangioendothelioma and cavernous hemangioma have similar appearances on CT. Both may be solitary or multicentric and will demonstrate low density relative to the

on unenhanced scans and during both the arterial and portal venous, phases of contrast enhancement (Figure 26-11), although they may demonstrate small areas of transient hyperattenuation in the arterial phase. Both tumors often are heterogeneous because they contain hemorrhage, necrosis, or focal steatosis. Calcifications are common in both tumors, and they have a tendency to invade the portal vein.

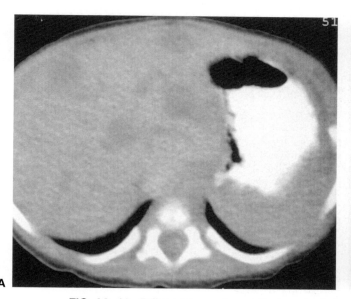

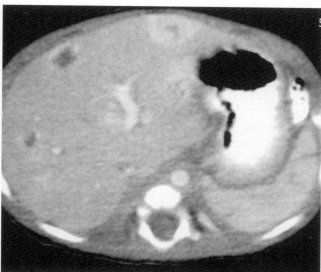

A   B

FIG. 26–13. Diffuse hemangioendotheliomatosis in a neonate. **A:** Precontrast CT scan demonstrates multiple hypodense areas in the liver. **B:** Computed-tomography scan obtained during the late arterial phase of enhancement shows areas of peripheral enhancement around most of the lesions. One lesion anteriorly demonstrates near-complete enhancement.

liver on unenhanced CT scans. Images in the hepatic arterial phase after administration of iodinated contrast demonstrate a characteristic pattern of peripheral nodular enhancement that progresses to central fill-in during the portal venous phase of enhancement (Figure 26-13). Small tumors may rapidly become hyperdense without showing peripheral enhancement, whereas larger lesions may not demonstrate central enhancement on delayed scans, reflecting areas of fibrosis or thrombosis.

After the vascular lesions, mesenchymal hamartoma is the next most common benign hepatic tumor of childhood. This tumor usually is found as an asymptomatic mass in boys under 2 years of age. On CT, the lesion appears as a well-circumscribed multilocular mass containing multiple low-attenuation areas separated by solid tissue (47). After IV contrast administration, the thicker septae may enhance, whereas the central contents do not enhance.

Hepatic cysts are uncommon in children, but occasionally may be detected incidentally on a CT examination performed for other clinical indications. Similar to cysts elsewhere in the body, the CT criteria for diagnosis is a water-attenuation mass with imperceptible or thin walls.

BILIARY MASSES

Choledochal Cyst

Choledochal cyst is the most common mass arising in the biliary ductal tree (48). Classically, patients present with pain, jaundice, and a palpable abdominal mass, although the complete triad is present in only about a third of patients. The CT findings of choledochal cyst are cystic dilatation of the common hepatic and central portions of the left and right hepatic ducts (Figure 26-14). Generalized ductal dilatation with gradual tapering to the periphery, characteristic of acquired obstruction, is absent.

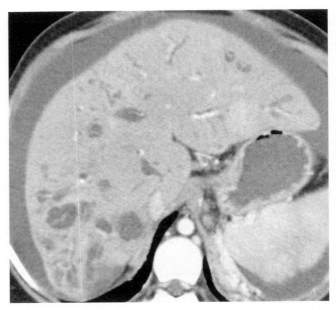

FIG. 26–15. Caroli's disease in a 19-year-old female with hematemesis. Postcontrast CT scan demonstrates multiple near-water-density cystic and tubular-appearing areas in the right lobe of the liver. Also noted is a large amount of ascites due to cirrhosis.

Caroli's Disease

Caroli's disease has two forms. One form is characterized by saccular dilation of the intrahepatic bile ducts, an increased frequency of calculus formation and cholangitis, and the absence of cirrhosis and portal hypertension. The second form is characterized by hepatic fibrosis, cirrhosis, and portal hypertension. Both are associated with renal cystic disease.

CT of Caroli's disease shows multiple dilated intrahe-

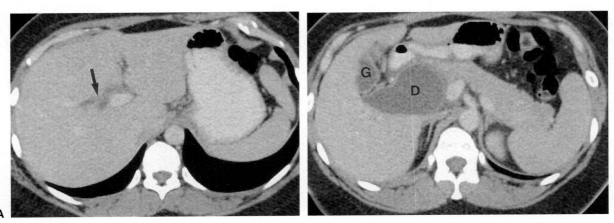

FIG. 26–14. Choledochal cyst in an 18-year-old girl with abdominal pain. A: Postcontrast CT scan demonstrates mildly dilated right hepatic duct (*arrow*). The peripheral branches are not dilated. B: A more caudal scan shows a dilated common bile duct (*D*), representing the choledochal cyst, medial to the gallbladder (*G*).

patic ducts. These are displayed as tubular structures or as round saccular cystic spaces of varying sizes which often communicate with the dilated intrahepatic bile ducts (Figure 26-15). The disease can affect a single segment or lobe of the liver or can be seen diffusely throughout the liver. Other findings include the central dot sign and bridging of the bile duct walls, which causes the cystic dilatations to appear septated. The central dot sign refers to a small dot in the dependent portion of the dilated bile duct, which enhances intensely after IV contrast. It is thought to represent portal-venous radicles that are enveloped by, but not actually inside of, the dilated bile ducts. The extrahepatic bile ducts can be normal, narrowed, slightly dilated, or associated with a choledochal cyst. Patients with cirrhosis may have ascites, hepatosplenomegaly, dilated portal and splenic veins, and collateral vessel formation as a result of portal hypertension.

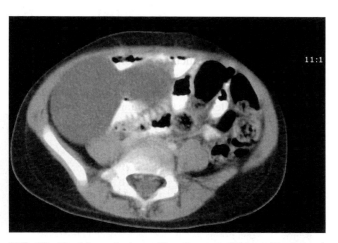

FIG. 26–16. Mesenteric cyst in a 3-year-old boy with abdominal pain. A well-defined near-water-density mass is noted in the right abdomen. The lesion involved the small-bowel mesentery.

PANCREATIC MASSES

Most pancreatic masses in the pediatric population are traumatic pseudocysts (49–51). Neoplasms are rare and usually benign. Pancreaticoblastoma is the most common pancreatic neoplasm in young children (49,50). It is an encapsulated epithelial tumor containing tissue resembling fetal pancreas, usually arises in the pancreatic head, and has a favorable outcome. On contrast-enhanced CT, the tumor appears as a focal mass of homogeneous or heterogeneous soft tissue density. Malignant degeneration is rare, but should be considered when there are hepatic and lymph-node metastases and vascular encasement.

Solid and papillary epithelial neoplasm of the pancreas is the most common tumor in adolescent girls and generally has a favorable prognosis. It is well encapsulated and usually occurs in the tail of the pancreas. On CT, this neoplasm appears as a well-defined thick-walled cystic mass containing papillary projections and occasionally septa (49,51).

SPLENIC MASSES

Focal splenic lesions in children include abscess, neoplasms (most commonly lymphoma and rarely hamartoma), vascular malformations (lymphangioma, hemangioma), and cysts. Abscesses, vascular malformations, and cysts have a low-attenuation value on CT. Solid tumors are of soft tissue density. Vascular malformations enhance after IV contrast administration.

GASTROINTESTINAL AND MESENTERIC MASSES

Lymphangiomatous malformations, also termed mesenteric cysts, and enteric duplications account for most benign gastrointestinal or mesenteric masses. On CT, a mesenteric cyst is a near-water-density mass with a barely discernible wall (Figure 26-16), whereas an enteric duplication appears as a cystic mass with a thick wall. The density of both lesions may be higher if they contain blood or proteinaceous material.

Lymphoma is the most common cause of a malignant mesenteric or bowel wall mass (52). Intraabdominal lymphoma more often is due to non-Hodgkin's lymphoma than to Hodgkin's disease. The CT features of gastrointestinal lymphoma include mural thickening greater than 1 cm in diameter, extraluminal soft tissue mass, and mesenteric invasion (53).

Lymphoma can involve the bowel wall, as well as retroperitoneal and/or mesenteric lymph nodes. The CT appearance of adenopathy varies from individually enlarged lymph nodes of soft tissue attenuation to a large homogeneous mass obscuring normal structures.

PELVIC MASSES

Anterior pelvic masses may be of gynecologic, nodal, or lower urinary tract origin. Posterior pelvic masses may arise in the presacral space and usually originate from either neurogenic or embryonic tissues.

Ultrasonography is employed initially for the evaluation of most suspected gynecologic masses because it does not use ionizing radiation. However, sonography is suboptimal for evaluating the presacral space because of the gas-filled rectum and sigmoid colon. Computed tomography is not degraded by bowel gas and therefore is useful when sonography is indeterminate. The major indications for CT examination of the pediatric pelvis are evaluation of a suspected or known pelvic mass and determination of the presence or absence of a suspected abscess. As a rule, CT is used to evaluate masses arising in reproductive structures and the urinary bladder, and MRI is preferred for evaluation of presacral masses.

injuries to increase the sensitivity for detecting urine leakage from the collecting system or urinary bladder.

The decision to use oral-contrast agent should be made on a case-to-case basis. Oral-contrast agent is not needed to diagnose solid-organ injuries, but can be useful for diagnosing proximal small bowel and pancreatic injuries.

CT Patterns of Abdominal Injury

The CT appearance of intraabdominal injuries depends on whether the injury is to a solid or hollow organ. The spectrum of injuries in solid organs, such as the liver, spleen, and kidney, ranges from small intraparenchymal and subcapsular hematomas to large lacerations or fractures with capsular disruption (84,85). Typically, hematomas appear on CT as round or oval fluid collections. Fractures and lacerations appear as irregular linear areas of low attenuation within an organ (Figures 26–21 and 26–22). Subcapsular hematomas are lenticular or oval in configuration and flatten or indent the underlying parenchyma. Acute blood generally has an attenuation lower than that of surrounding tissue on contrast-enhanced CT scans. A fresh hematoma will have a relatively higher attenuation value on an unenhanced scan. Other CT findings associated with hepatic injuries include subcapsular or intraparenchymal gas due to acute tissue necrosis and periportal areas of low attenuation. Periportal low-attenuation zones, presumably representing edema, have been noted in 65% of children with blunt abdominal trauma, and in 30% of patients, they are the only CT abnormality (86,87).

Intra- or extraperitoneal fluid may be seen with fractures or lacerations extending to the surface of an organ. In fact, a localized fluid collection (i.e., the sentinel clot) may be appreciated more readily than the underlying parenchymal injury, and thus may be a radiologic clue to the diagnosis

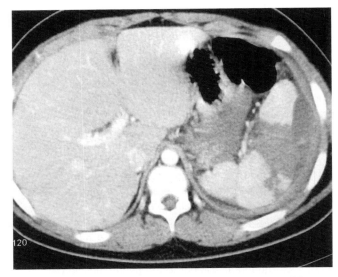

FIG. 26–22. Splenic fracture. Contrast-enhanced CT scan through the upper abdomen demonstrates multiple splenic fractures and blood in the perisplenic space.

(88,89). The attenuation value of clotted blood in the peritoneal cavity usually is 45 HU to 70 HU, whereas the attenuation of free lysed blood is about 30 HU A large intraperitoneal fluid collection suggests a more severe injury (89). Fluid collections in the perirenal and pararenal spaces, interfascial spaces, and psoas space are suggestive of injury to retroperitoneal organs (90).

Computed-tomography findings of pancreatic injury range from diffuse pancreatic enlargement and small peripancreatic fluid collections to intraparenchymal lacerations and fractures, pancreatic disruption, and ascites (91). A fluid collection dissecting between the splenic vein and the poste-

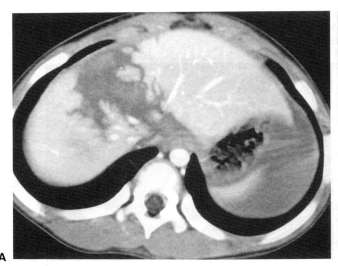
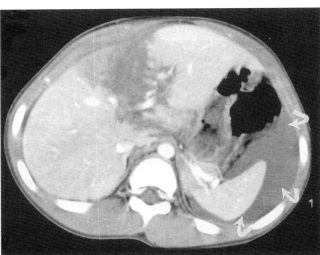

FIG. 26–21. Hepatic fracture in a 14-year-old girl. **A,B:** Two CT scans through the upper abdomen show a complex fracture though the dome of the liver and blood in the perisplenic space (*arrows*). The fracture extends into the porta hepatis.

rior body of the pancreas is highly suggestive of pancreatic injury. Up to 72% of children with pancreatic injury have fluid between the splenic vein and pancreas, whereas fewer than 1% of children without pancreatic injury have similar fluid collections (92,93).

In hollow-organ injuries, such as the intestine, CT findings include bowel wall or mucosal fold thickening, free intra- or retroperitoneal air, peritoneal fluid, and small bowel obstruction due to an acute hematoma or a subsequent stricture (94–96). Fluid from an intestinal injury tends to accumulate between bowel loops (i.e., interloop sign), whereas fluid from hepatic or splenic injuries collects in the paracolic gutters. Lap-belt ecchymosis sign occurs in approximately 70% of children with bowel injuries and is a sensitive clinical indicator of bowel injury (97).

Findings associated with rupture of the urinary bladder include thickening of the bladder wall and leakage of contrast-enhanced urine into the peritoneal or extraperitoneal spaces.

Hypoperfusion Syndrome

Hypoperfusion associated with hypovolemic shock has a characteristic CT appearance, evidenced by diffusely dilated fluid-filled small bowel loops; intense contrast enhancement of the kidneys, bowel wall, and mesentery; a flattened or collapsed inferior vena cava and a small aorta; and intraperitoneal fluid (98) (Figure 26-23). Hypovolemia, vasoconstriction, replacement of a depleted vascular volume with IV contrast, and fluid losses into the bowel lumen and peritoneum are thought to be responsible for the CT appearance. It is critical that the radiologist recognize the CT findings of hypoperfusion, as they are indicative of severe injury and poor prognosis.

Acute Arterial Extravasation

Areas of active bleeding appear as foci of high-attenuation fluid with an attenuation value similar to that of the major arteries. A large hematoma with a variable CT attenuation because of incomplete mixing of contrast-enhanced and nonenhanced blood usually surrounds the area of active arterial extravasation (99). The CT diagnosis of active arterial extravasation is of major clinical importance because it indicates the need for either urgent surgery or embolization.

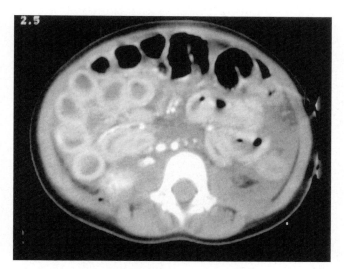

FIG. 26–23. Hypoperfusion syndrome. Computed-tomography scan through the mid-abdomen reveals blood in the right and left paracolic gutters, dilated small bowel loops with intensely enhancing walls, a small aorta (*arrowhead*), and inferior vena cava (*arrow*), as well as a dense right nephrogram, findings diagnostic of hypovolemic shock.

REFERENCES

1. Siegel MJ. Techniques. In: Siegel MJ, ed. *Pediatric body CT*. Philadelphia: Lippincott Williams & Wilkins, 1999:1–41.
2. Stockberger SM, Hickling JA, Liang Y, et al. Spiral CT with ionic and nonionic contrast material: evaluation of patient motion and scan quality. *Radiology* 1998;206:631–636.
3. Kaste SC, Young CW. Safe use of power injectors with central and peripheral venous access devices for pediatric CT. *Pediatr Radiol* 1995; 26:499–501.
4. Herts BR, O'Malley CM, Wirth SL, et al. Power injection of contrast media using central venous catheter feasibility, safety, and efficacy. *AJR Am J Roentgenol* 2001;176:447–453.
5. Frush DP, Donnelly LF, Bisset GS. Effect of scan delay on hepatic enhancement for pediatric abdominal multislice helical CT. *AJR Am J Roentgenol* 2001;176:1559–1561.
6. Cody DD. Image processing in CT. *Radiographics* 2002;2:1255–1268.
7. Rydberg J, Buckwalter KA, Caldmeyer KS, et al. Multisection CT: scanning techniques and clinical applications. *Radiographics* 2002; 20:1787–1806.
8. Ruben GD. Data explosion: the challenge of multidetector CT. *Eur J Radiol* 2000;36:74–81.
9. Silverman PM. *Multislice computed tomography*. Philadelphia: Lippincott Williams & Wilkins, 2002.
10. Donnelly LF, Emery KH, Brody AS, et al. Minimizing radiation dose for pediatric body applications for single-detector helical CT: strategies at a large children's hospital. *AJR Am J Roentgenol* 2001; 176:303–306.
11. Haaga JR. Commentary. Radiation dose management weighing risk versus benefit. *AJR Am J Roentgenol* 2001;177:289–291.
12. Frush DP, Slack CC, Hollingsworth CL, et al. Computer-simulated radiation dose reduction for abdominal multidetector CT of pediatric patients. *AJR Am J Roentgenol* 2002;179:1107–1113.
13. Kamel IR, Hernandez RJ, Martin JE. Radiation dose reduction in CT of the pediatric pelvis. *Radiology* 1994;90:683–687.
14. Patterson A, Frush DP, Donnelly L. Helical CT of the body: arc setting adjusted for pediatric patients. *AJR Am J Roentgenol* 2001; 176:297–301.
15. Roger LF. Taking care of children: check out the parameters used for helical CT (editorial). *AJR Am J Roentgenol* 2001;31:388.
16. Slovis TL. The ALARA concept in pediatric CT: myth or reality. *Radiology* 2002;223:5–6.
17. Siegel MJ, Suess C, Chen X, et al. Radiation doses and image quality for pediatric patients in multi-slice CT: comparison using different tube voltages and varying phantom sizes and shapes. *Radiology*.
18. Geller E, Smergel EM, Lowry PA. Renal neoplasms of childhood. *Radiol Clin North Am* 1997;35:1391–1413.
19. Green DM, Coppes MJ, Breslow NE, et al. Wilms' tumor. In: Pizzo PA, Poplack DG, eds. *Principles and practice of pediatric oncology*. Philadelphia: Lippincott–Raven, 1997:733–759.
20. Julian JC, Merguerian PA, Shortliffe LMD. Pediatric genitourinary tumors. *Curr Opin Oncol* 1995;7:265–274
21. Lowe LH, Isuani BH, Heller RM, et al. Pediatric renal masses: Wilms' tumor and beyond. *Radiographics* 2000;20:1585–1603.

22. Shamberberger RC. Pediatric renal tumors. *Semin Surg Oncol* 1999; 16:105–120.

23. Siegel MJ. The kidney. In: Siegel MJ, ed. *Pediatric body CT*. Philadelphia: Lippincott Williams & Wilkins, 1999:226–252.

24. Rieumont MJ, Whitman GJ. Mesoblastic nephroma. *AJR Am J Roentgenol* 1994;162:76.

25. Charles AK, Vujanic GM, Berry PJ. Renal tumours of childhood. *Histopathology* 1998;32:293–309.

26. Beckwith JB, Kiviat NB, Bonadio JF. Nephrogenic rests, nephroblastomatosis, and the pathogenesis of Wilm tumor. *Pediatr Pathol* 1990; 10:1–36.

27. Bove KE, McAdams AJ. The nephroblastomatosis complex and its relationship to Wilm tumor: a clinicopathologic treatise. *Perspect Pediatr Pathol* 1976;3:185–223.

28. Fernbach SK, Feinstein KA, Donaldson JS, et al. Nephroblastomatosis: comparison of CT with US and urography. *Radiology* 1988; 166:153–156.

29. Lonergan GJ, Martinez-Leon MI, Agrons GA, et al. Nephrogenic rests, nephroblastomatosis, and associated lesions of the kidney. *Radiographics* 1998;18:947–968.

30. Rohrschneider WK, Weirich A, Rieden K, et al. US, CT and MR imaging characteristics of nephroblastomatosis. *Pediatr Radiol* 1998; 28:435–43.

31. Argons GA, Kingsman KD, Wagner BJ, et al. Rhabdoid tumor of the kidney in children: a comparison of 21 cases. *AJR Am J Roentgenol* 1997;168:447–451.

32. Chung CJ, Lorenzo R, Rayder S, et al. Rhabdoid tumors of the kidney in children: CT findings. *AJR Am J Roentgenol* 1995;164:6976–700.

33. Davidson AJ, Choyke PL, Hartman DS, et al. Renal medullary carcinoma associated with sickle cell trait: radiologic findings. *Radiology* 1995;195:83–85.

34. Sheeran SR, Sussman SK. Renal lymphoma: spectrum of CT findings and potential mimics. *AJR Am J Roentgenol* 1998;171:1067–1072.

35. Sacher P, Willi UV, Niggli F, et al. Cystic nephroma: a rare benign renal tumor. *Pediatr Surg Int* 1998;13:197–199.

36. Argons GA, Wagner BJ, Davidson AJ, et al. Multilocular cystic renal tumor in children: radiologic–pathologic correlation. *Radiographics* 1995;15:654–669.

37. Lemaitre L, Robert Y, Dubrulle F, et al. Renal angiomyolipoma: growth followed up with CT and/or US. *Radiology* 1995;197:598–602.

38. Brodeur GM, Castleberry RP. Neuroblastoma. In: Pizzo PA, Poplack DG, eds. *Principles and practice of pediatric oncology*. Philadelphia: Lippincott–Raven, 1997:761–797.

39. Siegel MJ. Adrenal glands, pancreas, and other retroperitoneal structures. In: Siegel MJ, ed. *Pediatric body CT*. Philadelphia: Lippincott Williams & Wilkins, 1999:253–286.

40. Westra SJ, Zaninovic AC, Hall TR, et al. Imaging of the adrenal gland in children. *Radiographics* 1994;14:1323–1340.

41. Siegel MJ, Ishwaran H, Fletcher BD, et al. Staging of neuroblastoma at imaging: report of the radiology diagnostic oncology group. *Radiology* 2002;223:168–175.

42. Hayes WS, Davidson AJ, Grimley PM, et al. Extraadrenal retroperitoneal paraganglioma: clinical, pathologic, and CT findings. *AJR Am J Roentgenol* 1990;155:1247–1250.

43. Davidson AJ, Hartman DS, Goldman SM. Mature teratoma of the retroperitoneum: radiologic, pathologic, and clinical correlation. *Radiology* 1989;172:421–425.

44. Pobiel RS, Bisset GS III. Pictorial essay: imaging of liver tumors in the infant and child. *Pediatr Radiol* 1995;25:495–506.

45. Siegel MJ. Pediatric liver imaging. *Semin Liver Dis* 2001;21:251–269.

46. Kesslar PJ, Buck JL, Selby DM. Infantile hemangioendothelioma of the liver revisited. *Radiographics* 1993;13:657–670.

47. Ros PR, Goodman AD, Ishak KG, et al. Mesenchymal hamartoma of the liver: radiologic–pathologic correlation. *Radiology* 1986; 158:619–624.

48. Kim OH, Chung HJ, Choi BG. Imaging of the choledochal cyst. *Radiographics* 1995;15:69–88.

49. Herman TE, Siegel MJ. CT of the pancreas in children. *AJR Am J Roentgenol* 1991;157:375–379.

50. Lee JY, Kim I, Kim WS, et al. CT and US findings of pancreaticoblastoma. *J Comput Assist Tomogr* 1996;20:370–374.

51. Vaughn DD, Jabra AA, Fishman EK. Pancreatic disease in children and young adults: evaluation with CT. *Radiographics* 1998;18:1171–1187.

52. Ruess L, Frazier AA, Sivit C. CT of the mesentery, omentum, and peritoneum in children. *Radiographics* 1995;15:89–104.

53. Siegel MJ, Evans S, Balfe DM. CT of small bowel and mesenteric disease in children. *Radiology* 1988;169:127–130.

54. Siegel MJ. Pelvic tumors in childhood. *Radiol Clin North Am* 1997; 35:1455–1475.

55. Castleberry RP, Cushing B, Perlman E, et al. Germ cell tumors. In: Pizzo PA, Poplack DG, eds. *Pediatric oncology*, 3rd ed. Philadelphia: Lippincott–Raven, 1997;921–945.

56. Buy JN, Ghossain MA, Moss AA, et al. Cystic teratoma of the ovary: CT detection. *Radiology* 1989;171:697–701.

57. Quillin SP, Siegel MJ. CT features of benign and malignant teratomas in children. *J Comput Assist Tomogr* 1992;16:722–726.

58. Ghossain MA, Buy NJ, Ligneres C, et al. Epithelial tumors of the ovary: comparison of MR and CT findings. *Radiology* 1991;181:863–870.

59. Argons GA, Wagner BJ, Lonergan GJ, et al. Genitourinary rhabdomyosarcoma in children: radiologic–pathologic correlation. *Radiographics* 1997;17:919–937.

60. Wexler LH, Helman LJ. Rhabdomyosarcoma and the undifferentiated sarcomas. In: Pizzo PA, Poplack DG, eds. *Principles and practice of pediatric oncology*. Philadelphia: Lippincott–Raven, 1997:799–829.

61. Kesslar PJ, Buck JL, Suarez ES. Germ cell tumors of the sacrococcygeal region: radiologic–pathologic correlation. *Radiographics* 1994; 14:607–620.

62. Balthazar EJ, Birnbaum BA, Yee J, et al. CT and sonography correlation in acute appendicitis: prospective evaluation of 100 patients. *Radiology* 1994;190:31–35.

63. Garcia-Pena BM, Mandl KD, Kraus SJ, et al. Ultrasonography and limited computed tomography in the diagnosis and management of appendicitis in children. *JAMA* 1999;282:1041–1046.

64. Lowe LH, Perez R, Scheker LE, et al. Appendicitis and alternative diagnoses in children: findings on unenhanced limited helical CT. *Pediatr Radiol* 2001;31:569–577.

65. Siegel MJ, Carel C, Surratt S. Ultrasonography of acute abdominal pain in children. *JAMA* 1991;266:1987–1989.

66. Sivit CJ, Siegel MJ, Applegate KE, et al. When appendicitis is suspected in children. *Radiographics* 2001;21:247–262.

67. Crady SK, Jones JS, Wyn T, et al. Clinical validity of ultrasound in children with suspected appendicitis. *Ann Emerg Med* 1993; 22:1125–1129.

68. Quillin SP, Siegel MJ, Coffin CM. Acute appendicitis in children: value of sonography in detecting perforation. *AJR Am J Roentgenol* 1992; 159:1265–1268.

69. Vignault F, Filiatrault D, Brandt ML, et al. Acute appendicitis in children: evaluation with US. *Radiology* 1990;176:501–504.

70. Sivit CJ, Newman KD, Boenning DA, et al. Appendicitis: usefulness of US in a pediatric population. *Radiology* 1992;185:549–552.

71. Fefferman NR, Roche KJ, Pinkney LP, et al. Suspected appendicitis in children: focused CT technique for evaluation. *Radiology* 2001; 220:691–695.

72. Lane MJ, Katz DS, Ross BA, et al. Unenhanced helical CT for suspected appendicitis. *AJR Am J Roentgenol* 1997;168:465–469.

73. Lane MJ, Liu DM, Huynh MD, et al. Suspected acute appendicitis: nonenhanced helical CT in 300 consecutive patients. *Radiology* 1999; 213:341–346.

74. Raman SS, Lu DSK, Kadell BM, Vodopich DJ, Sayre J, Cryer H. Accuracy of nonfocused helical CT for the diagnosis of acute appendicitis: a 5-year review. *AJR Am J Roentgenol* 2002;178:1319–1325.

75. Kamel IR, Goldberg SN, Keogen MR, et al. Right lower quadrant pain and suspected appendicitis: nonfocused appendiceal CT—review of 100 cases. *Radiology* 2000;217:159–163.

76. Rao PM, Rhea JT. Novelline RA, et al. Helical CT technique for the diagnosis of appendicitis: prospective evaluation of a focused appendix CT examination. *Radiology* 1997;202:139–144.

77. Rao RM, Rhea JT, Novelline RA, et al. Helical CT combined with contrast material administered only through the colon for imaging of suspected appendicitis. *AJR Am J Roentgenol* 1997;169:1275–1280.

78. Friedland JA, Siegel MJ. CT appearance of acute appendicitis in childhood. *AJR Am J Roentgenol* 1997;168:439–442.

79. Siegel MJ. Thoracoabdominal trauma. In: Siegel MJ, ed. *Pediatric body CT*. Philadelphia: Lippincott Williams & Wilkins, 1999:346–371.

80. Neish AS, Taylor GA, Lund DP, et al. Effect of CT information on

the diagnosis and management of acute abdominal injury in children. *Radiology* 1998;206:327–331.

81. Ruess L, Sivit CJ, Eichelberger MR, et al. Blunt abdominal trauma in children: impact of CT on operative and nonoperative management. *AJR Am J Roentgenol* 1997;169:1011–1014.

82. Ruess L, Sivit CJ, Eichelberger MR, et al. Blunt hepatic and splenic trauma in children: correlation of a CT injury severity scale with clinical outcome. *Pediatr Radiol* 1995;25:321–325.

83. Bond SJ, Eichelberger MR, Gotschall CS, et al. Nonoperative management of blunt hepatic and splenic injury in children. *Ann Surg* 1996; 223:386–289.

84. Taylor GA, Sivit CJ. Computed tomography imaging of abdominal trauma in children. *Semin Pediatr Surg* 1992;1:253–359.

85. Stalker HP, Kaufman RA, Towbin R. Patterns of liver injury in childhood: CT analysis. *AJR Am J Roentgenol* 1986;147:1199–1205.

86. Patrick LE, Ball TI, Atkinson GO, et al. Pediatric blunt abdominal trauma: periportal tracking at CT. *Radiology* 1992;183:698–691.

87. Siegel MJ, Herman TE. Periportal low attenuation at CT in childhood. *Radiology* 1992;183:685–688.

88. Hulka F, Mullins RJ, Leonardo B, et al. Significance of peritoneal fluid as an isolated finding on abdominal computed tomographic scans in pediatric trauma patients. *J Trauma* 1998;44:1069–1072.

89. Sivit CJ, Taylor GA, Bulas DI, et al. Blunt trauma in children: significance of peritoneal fluid. *Radiology* 1991;178:185–188.

90. Siegel MJ, Balfe DM. Blunt renal and ureteral trauma in childhood: CT patterns of fluid collections. *AJR Am J Roentgenol* 1989; 152:1043–1047.

91. Siegel MJ, Sivit CJ. Pancreatic emergencies. *Radiol Clin North Am* 1997;35:815–830.

92. Lane MJ, Mindelzun RE, Sandhu JS, et al. CT diagnosis of blunt pancreatic trauma: importance of detecting fluid between the pancreas and the splenic vein. *AJR Am J Roentgenol* 1994;163:833–835.

93. Sivit CJ, Eichelberger MR. CT diagnosis of pancreatic injury in children: significance of fluid separating the splenic vein and the pancreas. *AJR Am J Roentgenol* 1995;165:921–924.

94. Cox TD, Kuhn JP. CT scan of bowel trauma in the pediatric patient. *Radiol Clin North Am* 1996;34:807–818.

95. Jamieson DH, Babyn PS, Pearl R. Imaging gastrointestinal perforation in pediatric blunt abdominal trauma. *Pediatr Radiol* 1996;26:188–194.

96. Strouse PJ, Close BJ, Marshall KW, et al. CT of bowel and mesenteric trauma in children. *Radiographics* 1999;19:1237.

97. Sivit CJ, Taylor GA, Newman KD. Safety-belt injuries in children with lap-belt ecchymosis: CT findings in 61 patients. *AJR Am J Roentgenol* 1991;157:111–114.

98. Sivit CJ, Taylor GA, Bulas DI, et al. Posttraumatic shock in children: CT findings associated with hemodynamic instability. *Radiology* 1992; 182(7):23–726.

99. Taylor GA, Kaufman RA, Sivit CJ. Active hemorrhage in children after thoracoabdominal trauma: clinical and CT features. *AJR Am J Roentgenol* 1994;162:401–404.

whether active bleeding is detected on CT. Many trauma centers now routinely treat patients with Class 3 and 4 hepatic injuries with nonoperative management as long as they are hemodynamically stable and have no active bleeding on CT (6). Splenic lesions continue to be problematic due to their propensity for delayed splenic rupture. Nevertheless, there has been a refinement in the understanding of those types of splenic lesions that may predispose to delayed rupture based on the CT finding of the "contrast blush" within the spleen. These areas likely represent pseudoaneurysms with underlying vascular injury (8,9) (Figure 27-1). Minimally invasive therapies may be directed by the initial CT, most notably the use of subselective catheter embolization of a variety of visceral and pelvic injuries when CT detects active arterial extravasation. In patients with splenic injuries diagnosed by CT, early catheter embolization was noted to improve nonoperative salvage of spleens in 92% of patients (10). This is particularly true in lumbar and pelvic hemorrhage, as angiographic embolization has been recognized for years as the optimal method to control retroperitoneal hemorrhage from lumbar artery or internal iliac arterial bleeding (11,12) (Figure 27-2).

A final trend in the management of blunt-trauma patients has been the steadily increasing role of ultrasound to aid in the initial diagnostic work up (13–16). It is clear from numerous studies that the "FAST" exam (focused abdominal sonogram for trauma), directed toward the identification of free fluid in unstable patients, can replace reliably diagnostic peritoneal lavage (13–16). Studies from trauma centers in Europe and the United States have supported the claim that unstable patients with large amounts of free fluid detected by ultrasound in the resuscitation room are reliable for major parenchymal injuries. A few centers within Europe and the United States have attempted to expand the role of sonography to not just look for free fluid, but also to evaluate critically solid parenchymal organs for underlying injury (14). Some centers have reported successful outcomes using this technique, with a concombinant reduction in the number of CT scans that are required (15,17,18). Therefore, it may be possible to reduce the need for CT in low acuity patients. Larger studies will need to validate this approach, as many of the sonographic findings of parenchymal injury are subtle and require experienced observers. There are, however, some potential drawbacks to this. The identification of free intraperitoneal fluid as the sole criterion for establishing significant trauma with the FAST exam will be of limited value in patients with major retroperitoneal injuries. Retroperitoneal injuries may be associated with high morbidity and mortality. Major injuries to the pancreas, kidney, descending colon, and duodenum require urgent surgical intervention. It has also been noted that some visceral injuries to the liver and spleen, for example, may produce no significant hemoperitoneum; thus, the underlying diagnosis of the parenchymal injury may be falsely negative in a study that focuses purely on the detection of free intraperitoneal fluid (Figure 27-3). A recent retrospective study noted that 57 of 210

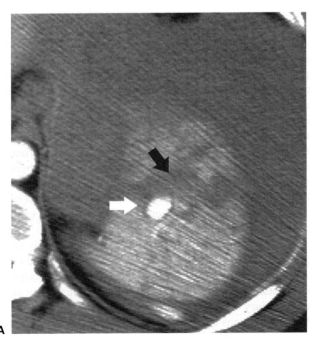
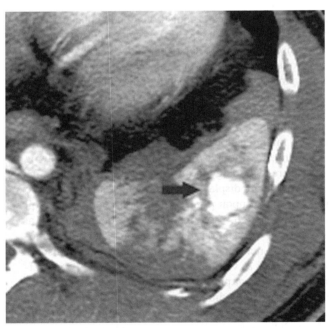

FIG. 27-1. A,B: Splenic fracture with pseudoaneurysm formation in two patients. Note in **(A)** the focal rounded area of high attenuation (*white arrow*) adjacent to a low attenuation fracture through the upper pole of the spleen (*black arrow*, fracture). Note that the pseudoaneurysm is nearly isoattenuating with the adjacent thoracic aorta. A large amount of hemoperitoneum is seen adjacent to the splenic fracture. In another patient **(B)**, note large intrasplenic pseudoaneurysm.

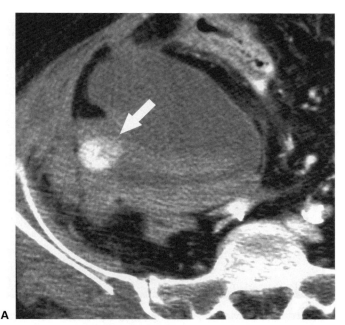

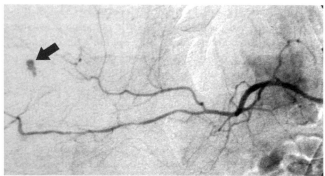

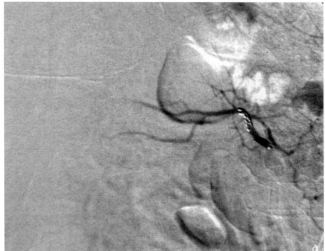

FIG. 27–2. A: Lumbar artery pseudoaneurysm following blunt abdominal trauma. Note focal area of high attenuation in the right iliac fossa from lumbar artery pseudoaneurysm (*arrow*). **B,C:** Selective lumbar artery angiogram reveals pseudoaneurysm (*arrow*). This was embolized successfully with coils **(C)**.

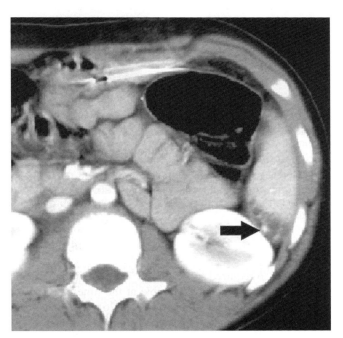

FIG. 27–3. Splenic injury without associated hemoperitoneum. A subcapsular hematoma of the spleen is noted, with areas of active bleeding seen beneath the splenic capsule (*arrow*). No hemoperitoneum is identified.

splenic injuries (27%) on CT had no hemoperitoneum, as did 71 of 206 liver injuries (34%), 30 of 63 renal injuries (48%), 4 of 35 mesenteric injuries (11%), and 2 of 7 pancreatic injuries (29%) (19). Surgery or embolization was required in 26 (17%) of these patients (19). It has also been noted that free fluid alone, in the absence of solid organ injury, is not an indication for surgery (20). Of 90 patients with free fluid on CT and no solid organ injury, only 7 had blunt intestinal injury. The remaining patients had an uneventful outcome (20). This finding also has been corroborated in pediatric patients (21). Despite these limitations, it is clear that ultrasound is playing a larger role in the evaluation of trauma patients, and its ultimate incorporation into diagnostic algorithms is likely to reflect institutional preference and local expertise.

TECHNICAL FACTORS FOR SCAN ACQUISITION IN TRAUMA

Routine Scan for Abdominal and Pelvic Trauma

The use of oral contrast in the evaluation of blunt abdominal trauma continues to generate some controversy, particularly among trauma surgeons. While there have been no known adverse effects of administering water-soluble contrast to trauma patients, there still is some resistance on the

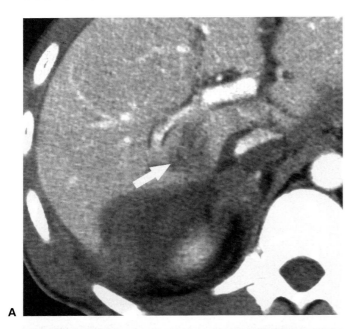

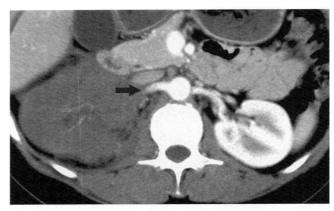

FIG. 27–8. Traumatic renal-artery occlusion. Note absence of perfusion of the right kidney. The right renal artery (*arrow*) is occluded just beyond its origin.

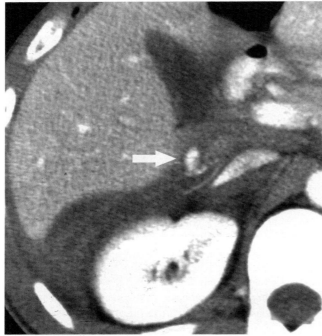

FIG. 27–7. Hepatic laceration with active arterial extravasation. In **(A)**, note hepatic laceration (*arrow*) extending to bare area of the liver, with hemorrhage surrounding the inferior vena cava. In **(B)**, note pseudoaneurysm (*arrow*) and surrounding subhepatic hemorrhage, representing active arterial extravasation.

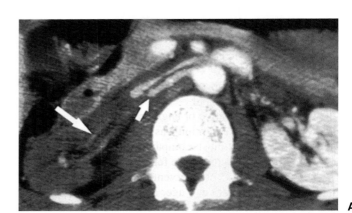

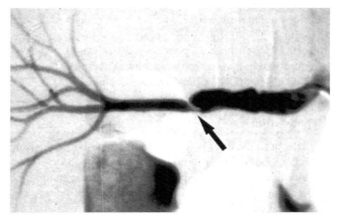

FIG. 27–9. A,B: Traumatic intimal dissection of the renal artery. Note small hypodense right kidney. The right renal artery (*short arrow*) demonstrates a high-grade occlusion with minimal visualization of the distal right renal artery and renal vein (*large arrow*). Selective right renal angiography **(B)** demonstrates high-grade obstruction from intimal dissection (*arrow*).

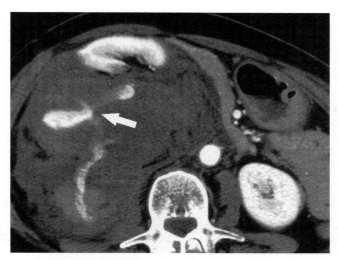

FIG. 27–10. Renal fracture with active arterial extravasation. Note high attenuation focus surrounded by large hematoma, indicating active arterial extravasation (*arrow*). A small fragment of the perfused kidney is displaced markedly anteriorly by the large hematoma.

Renal Injuries

Computed tomography is ideally suited to evaluate renal trauma, as it provides precise information regarding renal perfusion and excretion. Although renal injuries are quite common following blunt trauma, the vast majority can be treated successfully with nonoperative management. In fact, there is a growing trend to treat stable patients with even with grade IV renal injuries. Santucci and McAninch

were able to manage nonoperatively 50% of patients with grade-IV injuries (27).

One advantage of MDCT is improved renovascular assessment with thinly collimated scans. Renal artery dissection from blunt trauma may result in complete or partial thrombosis of the renal artery (Figures 27–8 and 27–9). Renal infarcts may be due to trauma or occlusion of intrarenal vessels. Computed tomography is diagnostic for complete occlusion when no perfusion or excretion is evident. Angiography is unwarranted in this setting, and the patient should undergo urgent renal revascularization. Other renal-vascular lesions, such as pseudoaneurysms, cannot be successfully managed with angiographic embolization (28) (Figures 27–10 to 27–13). Injuries to the main renal vein, although relatively uncommon, may also be diagnosed with MDCT (Figure 27-14).

Other Injuries

Although the liver and spleen are the most common sites of active arterial extravasation following blunt abdominal trauma, numerous other organs and vascular structures may be injured. Quite commonly, pelvic fractures lead to massive bleeding, requiring angiographic embolization. In the setting of a patient with multiple orthopedic and pelvic fractures, it often is difficult to be certain of the site of bleeding. With MDCT, it is now possible to target angiographic embolization to the areas of active arterial extravasation (10). Similarly, other retroperitoneal injuries, such as renal and lumbar artery injuries, are often approached with angio-

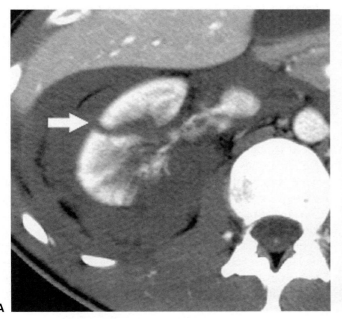 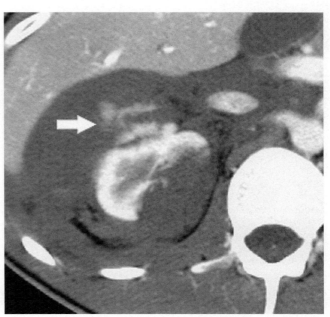

A   B

FIG. 27–11. Renal fracture with active arterial extravasation. Note linear fracture (*arrow*) traversing right kidney in **(A)**. In **(B)**, active arterial extravasation is seen in the perirenal space (*arrow*).

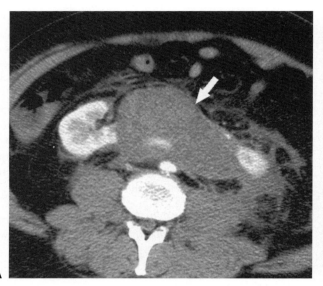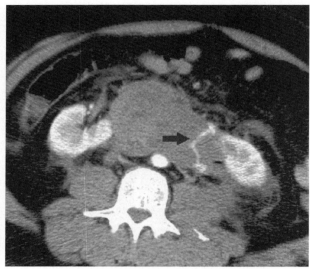

A   **B**

FIG. 27–12. Active arterial extravasation following rupture of the isthmus in a patient with a horseshoe kidney. Note large hematoma in the isthmus of the horseshoe kidney in **(A)** (*arrow*). Active arterial extravasation (*arrow*) is seen in **(B)**.

graphic embolization as the least invasive technique. Computed tomography not only identifies the areas of bleeding, but also actively guides the angiography team to select the vessel most likely injured (11).

AORTIC INJURY

Aortic transection following a deceleration injury is usually is lethal (29). In the small percentage of patients who

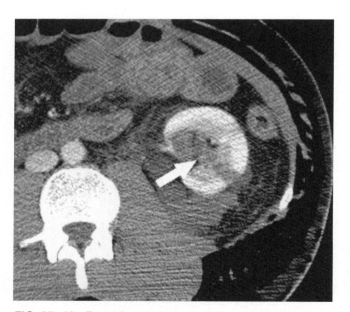

FIG. 27–13. Renal fracture successfully treated with nonoperative management. Note linear fracture extending through the entire renal parenchyma (*arrow*). A small amount of perirenal hematoma is noted, but there is no active arterial extravasation. The patient was managed successfully nonoperatively.

survive the initial injury, it may be exceedingly challenging to establish the diagnosis with plain chest radiographs obtained during resuscitation in the trauma room. In the past, catheter angiography had been used to evaluate patients based on either an abnormal chest X-ray or a highly suggestive mechanism of injury. However, the vast majority of screening aortograms are negative, which increases the level of invasiveness, medical cost, and contrast burden to the patient.

An increasing body of evidence suggests that spiral CT can replace catheter angiography for detection of injuries of the thoracic aorta (29–38). Sensitivities range from 96% to 100%, with excellent specificity and negative predictive value (29–38). In a prospective study by Mirvis et al., contrast-enhanced spiral CT was 100% sensitive and 99.7% specific for aortic injury (36). It had 100% negative predictive value, with an overall diagnostic accuracy of 99.7% (36). Even in patients with normal screening chest radiographs, some trauma surgeons advocate the use of CT if there is a likely major mechanism of injury, such as a high speed motor vehicle accident or a fall from greater than 5 feet. In a study by Exadaktylos and colleagues, 26% of patients with blunt chest trauma confirmed on CT had normal chest radiographs (35). In 13 of 25 patients (52%), there were multiple injuries, including two aortic lacerations, three pleural effusions, and one pericardial effusion (35). It is well known that CT will demonstrate a pneumothorax not visible on a supine chest radiograph, and CT therefore may be extremely valuable in assessing clinically important chest injuries other than major thoracic vascular injury.

There is a substantial reduction in cost in using helical CT, rather than catheter angiography, to screen patients for potential aortic arch injuries. In a study by Parker and col-

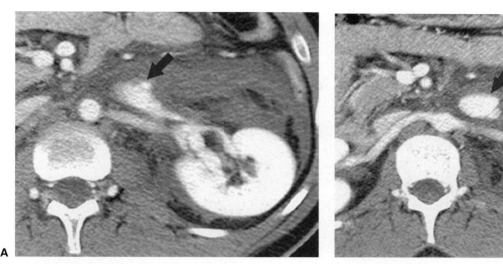

FIG. 27–14. Renal venous injury with active extravasation. In **(A)**, note contrast extravasation from left renal vein (*arrow*). Note pooling of extravasated contrast in **(B)** (*arrow*).

leagues, helical CT with single-slice scanners demonstrated an accuracy and sensitivity equivalent to those of catheter angiography (29). However, the total cost of performing helical CT was one half that of performing catheter angiography (29). Thus, not only can an invasive procedure be avoided, but a major cost savings is realized using CT to evaluate thoracic trauma.

To date there have been few reports of the use of MDCT for thoracic aortic injuries, but it is clear that the improved anatomic depiction through enhanced spatial resolution with thinner collimation inevitably will improve image quality of thoracic aortic studies. The diagnosis of aortic injury is based primarily on direct signs of intimal tear and pseudoaneurysm formation (Figures 27–15 and 27–16). Indirect signs include

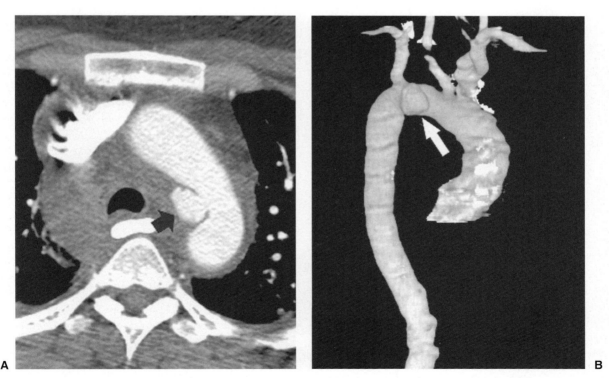

FIG. 27–15. Aortic transection with pseudoaneurysm formation. On axial image **(A)**, note large pseudoaneurysm extending medially from the region of the ligamentum arteriosum. In **(B)**, maximum intensity projection clearly outlines pseudoaneurysm.

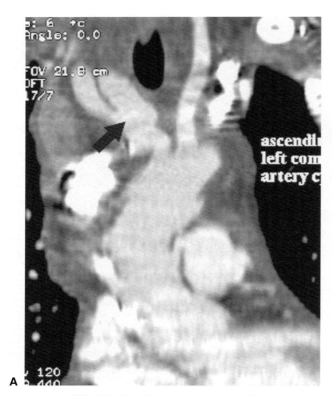

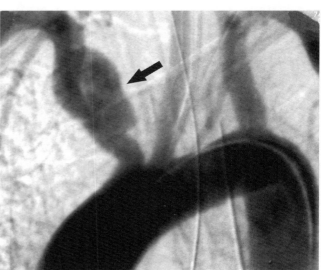

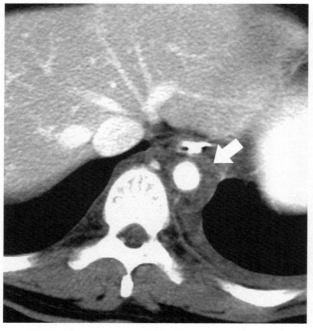

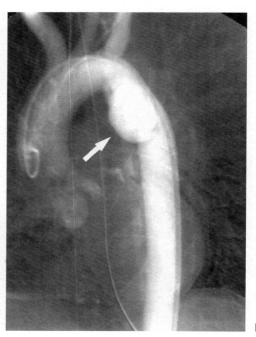

FIG. 27–16. Pseudoaneurysm of the innominate artery following blunt trauma. In **(A)**, which is a CPR, note large pseudoaneurysm extending from the origin of the innominate artery. This was confirmed by arch angiography **(B)** (*arrow*, pseudoaneurysm).

FIG. 27–17. Periaortic hemorrhage on upper abdominal scans as only CT evidence for aortic transection. In **(A)**, note periaortic hemorrhage involving the distal thoracic aorta (*arrow*). Arch aortogram **(B)** revealed large pseudoaneurysm from aortic transection (*arrow*).

periaortic and/or mediastinal hemorrhage. Fishman et al., have emphasized the fact that direct signs of aortic injury are most accurate (31). Indirect signs often may be misleading and due to injuries other than the thoracic aorta (31). It should be noted that periaortic hemorrhage around the upper abdominal aorta, seen on abdominal CT scans for trauma, always should raise the suspicion of an aortic-arch injury (39) (Figure 27-17).

In addition to improving spatial resolution, the speed of scan acquisition with MDCT is likely to reduce motion artifacts and improve overall image quality. In addition, CPR and multiplanar reformations (MPR) are enhanced by the near-volumetric data acquisition.

AREAS OF DIAGNOSTIC DIFFICULTY IN CT FOR BLUNT ABDOMINAL TRAUMA

Pancreatic Injuries

Pancreatic trauma is relatively rare and estimated to occur in no more than 3% to 6% of all abdominal injuries (40–44). However, the mortality from this injury continues to be substantial, with a 20% mortality rate having been reported with complete pancreatic transection. One of the major factors contributing to the relatively high rate of morbidity from this injury is the inability to achieve a prompt and accurate diagnosis. Clinical assessment of patients with possible blunt trauma to the pancreas is often challenging and fraught with difficulty. The serum amylase may be normal, even in patients with complete pancreatic transection, and peritoneal signs are often inconspicuous (40,41).

The surgical classification of pancreatic injury is based on the status of the duct of Wirsung, and whether or not there is an associated duodenal injury. The most severe injuries to the pancreas (category IV) involve transection of the head of the pancreas, with associated duodenal and common bile duct injury. The most common site of injury is the transverse portion of the body of the pancreas, as the pancreas is impaled against the spine via a deceleration injury (Figure 27-18). In patients with mid-body to distal lacerations, splenectomy and distal pancreatectomy have been the traditional

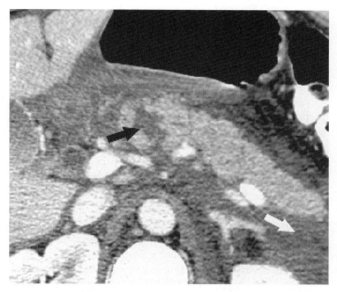

FIG. 27–19. Pancreatic fracture with post traumatic pancreatitis. Patient was scanned 6 hours after motor vehicle accident with mid-epigastric pain. Note fracture plane in the neck of the pancreas (*black arrow*). In **(B)**, there is extensive peripancreatic fluid and hemorrhage, consistent with post traumatic pancreatitis (*white arrow*).

methods of treatment. However, as more experience is gained with emergency endoscopic retrograde cholangiopancreatography (ERCP), stenting of the pancreatic duct may emerge as a minimally invasive alternative to surgical resection.

Subtle pancreatic lacerations may be exceedingly difficult to diagnose, even with MDCT. Therefore, a high level of clinical suspicion should always be maintained in patients with a mechanism of injury suggestive of pancreatic laceration. Typical history includes a blow to the mid-epigastrum with abdominal pain disproportionate to the physical findings. On CT, it has been noted that post-traumatic changes of pancreatitis may be evident (Figure 27-19). However, these findings are time dependent and may not be seen immediately after trauma. Active arterial extravasation has been diagnosed with pancreatic injuries and may be an important observation necessitating emergency surgery. Another important finding is the identification of retropancreatic fluid as a sign of pancreatic ductal disruption. Fluid tracks along the splenic vein between the body and tail of the pancreatic parenchyma. In difficult cases, a dedicated pancreatic protocol, using 1.25-mm collimated scans and a rapid IV bolus technique, similar to the protocol used for staging in pancreatic carcinoma, may be invaluable for detecting subtle pancreatic lacerations. Endoscopic retrograde cholangiopancreatography is emerging as an important imaging modality, along with endoscopic sonography, to evaluate for possible pancreatic injuries.

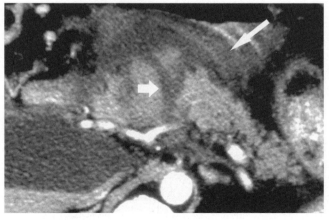

FIG. 27–18. Pancreatic fracture. Note linear fracture plane in the mid-body of the pancreas (*short arrow*). Hemorrhage into the lesser sac is noted (*long arrow*).

Injuries to the Gastrointestinal Tract

Many patients with gastrointestinal lacerations and disruption of the luminal gastrointestinal tract do not undergo CT, but go directly to surgery due to hemodynamic instability. Not infrequently, bowel injuries are seen in the setting of multiple intraperitoneal injuries, and with the increasing use of the FAST exam, patients with large amounts of free intraperitoneal fluid who are hemodynamically stable are sent directly to laparotomy without CT. In a small percentage of patients, isolated injuries to the luminal gastrointestinal (GI) tract may be diagnosed in patients without other associated injuries. A constellation of findings may be noted in luminal GI-tract lesions that often are quite subtle (45–49). There may be focal thickening of the bowel due to intramural hematoma, tiny extraluminal gas bubbles of pneumoperitoneum, or adjacent water-density free fluid (Figure 27-20). Abnormal areas of enhancement of the bowel wall may be noted due to delayed mural transit of contrast from mesenteric hematomas or presumed vasodilatation of injured segments due to local loss of autoregulation. It should be noted that hemoperitoneum may not be seen in patients with small bowel lacerations, and the only finding may be a focal water-density fluid collection often located between the reflected leaves of the mesentery, known as ''intraloop fluid'' (Figures 27–21 and 27–22). High attenuation fluid between the leaves of the mesentery suggests mesenteric vascular injury, such as a mesenteric hematoma (Figure 27-23). These patients should be carefully observed, or undergo laparoscopic or open surgery for presumed mesenteric vascular injury. Water-density fluid [0 Housfield units (HU) to 15 HU] should raise the suspicion of extravasated small bowel contents from a perforation. Focal high attenuation within a thickened segment of bowel is also a sign of bowel injury

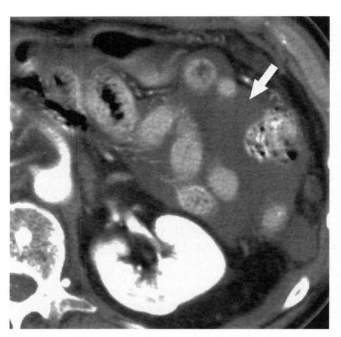

FIG. 27–21. Bowel perforation with intraloop fluid. Note large amount of fluid between the leaves of the mesentery (intraloop) in the left upper quadrant (*arrow*, intraloop fluid).

and may be due to intramural hematoma or intense enhancement of the bowel segment with IV contrast (Figure 27-24).

Diaphragmatic Injuries

Injuries to the diaphragm often are subtle on CT and require careful attention for indirect signs (50,51). Recently,

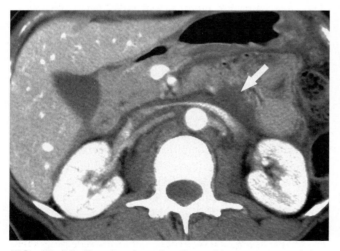

FIG. 27–20. Duodenal perforation with extravasated free fluid. Note water-density (15 HU) fluid collection posterior to the transverse duodenum, adjacent to the left renal vein (*arrow*). At surgery, a laceration of the posterior wall of the transverse duodenum was noted, with extravasated free fluid.

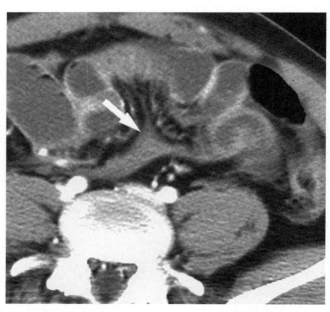

FIG. 27–22. Small bowel injury with subtle intraloop fluid and free air. There is a small intraloop fluid collection (*arrow*) adjacent to distal small bowel loops (*SB*). A small focus of free air is noted (*short arrow*) adjacent to the injury.

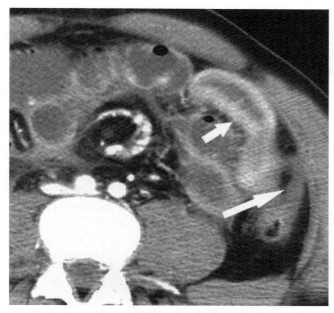

FIG. 27–23. Hypoperfusion syndrome. CT scan through the mid-abdomen reveals dilated small bowel loops with intensely enhancing walls, fluid in the left paracolic gutter, and a small aorta and inferior vena cava.

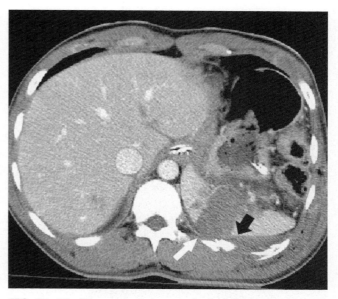

FIG. 27–25. "Dependent viscera sign" of diaphragm rupture. Note large splenic laceration and lack of visualization of the diaphragm posterior to the spleen (*black arrow*). A small portion of the diaphragm is visualized more medially (*arrow*).

observation of the "dependent viscera sign" has been identified by Bergin and associates, who noted in a retrospective study that when there was contact of either the liver or stomach with posterior ribs without visualization of the diaphragm, rupture of the diaphragm was likely (Figure 27-25). Using this dependent viscera sign, 90% of ruptured dia-

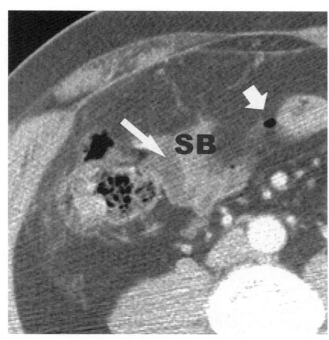

FIG. 27–24. Hyperdense bowel as a sign of bowel injury. Note high attenuation loop of jejunum in left-upper quadrant (*short arrow*), with intense enhancement and mural thickening. An adjacent small amount of free fluid (*long arrow*) is noted in the left pericolic gutter. At surgery, jejunal intramural hematoma with small perforation was noted.

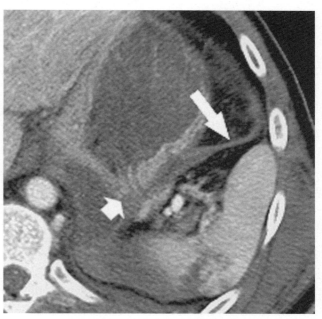

FIG. 27–26. Collar sign of diaphragmatic rupture. Note the constriction of the mid-body of the stomach (*short arrow*) as it herniates through the diaphragm. *Long arrow* indicates diaphragm.

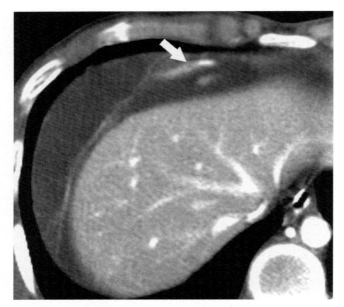

FIG. 27–27. Active arterial extravasation from phrenic artery. Note high-attenuation focus in right subphrenic space (*arrow*) representing arterial extravasation.

phrams could be identified retrospectively. Other findings include the "collar sign," related to constriction of the stomach and/or colon, herniating through a diaphragmatic defect (Figure 27-26). The use of MDCT may aid in identification of the diaphragm and confirm focal areas of diaphragmatic disruption due to the use of routine thinner collimation. In addition, retrospective scans performed at thinner collimation may be helpful to assist in performing MPR. Diaphragmatic injuries may be associated with lacerations of the phrenic artery that also may be diagnosed with MDCT (Figure 27-27).

REFERENCES

1. Crim JR, Moore K, Brodke D. Clearance of the cervical spine in multitrauma patients: the role of advanced imaging. *Semin Ultrasound CT MR* 2001;22(4):283–305.
2. Cornelius RS. Imaging of acute cervical spine trauma. *Semin Ultrasound CT MR* 2001;22(2):108–124.
3. Daffner RH. Helical CT of the cervical spine for trauma patients: a time study. *AJR Am J Roentgenol* 2001;177(3):677–679.
4. Funke C, Funke M, Raab B, Grabbe E. Fractures of the cervical vertebrae: diagnosis with multi-slice spiral CT [in German]. *Rontgenpraxis* 2001;54(2):49–55.
5. Myers JG, Dent DL, Stewart RM, et al. Blunt splenic injuries: dedicated trauma surgeons can achieve a high rate of nonoperative success in patients of all ages. *J Trauma* 2000;48(5):801–805; discussion 805–806.
6. Goan YG, Huang MS, Lin JM. Nonoperative management for extensive hepatic and splenic injuries with significant hemoperitoneum in adults. *J Trauma* 1998;45(2):360–364; discussion 365.
7. Jacobs IA, Kelly K, Valenziano C, et al. Nonoperative management of blunt splenic and hepatic trauma in the pediatric population: significant differences between adult and pediatric surgeons? Am Surg 2001, 67(2):149–154.
8. Schurr MJ, Fabian TC, Gavant M, et al. Management of blunt splenic trauma: computed tomographic contrast blush predicts failure of nonop-
erative management. *J Trauma* 1995;39(3):507–512; discussion 512–513.
9. Omert LA, Salyer D, Dunham CM, et al. Implications of the "contrast blush" finding on computed tomographic scan of the spleen in trauma. *J Trauma* 2001;51(2):272–277; discussion 277–278.
10. Haan J, Scott J, Boyd-Kranis RL, et al. Admission angiography for blunt splenic injury: advantages and pitfalls. *J Trauma* 2001;51(6): 1161–1165.
11. Cook RE, Keating JF, Gillespie I. The role of angiography in the management of haemorrhage from major fractures of the pelvis. *J Bone Joint Surg Br* 2002;84(2):178–182.
12. Dondelinger RF, Trotteur G, Ghaye B, et al. Traumatic injuries: radiological hemostatic intervention at admission. *Eur Radiol* 2002;12(5): 979–993.
13. McGahan JP, Wang L, Richards JR. From the RSNA refresher courses: focused abdominal US for trauma. *Radiographics* 2001;21 Spec No:S191–S199.
14. Richards JR, Schleper NH, Woo BD, et al. Sonographic assessment of blunt abdominal trauma: a 4-year prospective study. *J Clin Ultrasound* 2002;30(2):59–67.
15. Rose JS, Levitt MA, Porter J, et al. Does the presence of ultrasound really affect computed tomographic scan use? A prospective randomized trial of ultrasound in trauma. *J Trauma* 2001;51(3):545–550.
16. McKenney MG, McKenney KL, Hong JJ, et al. Evaluating blunt abdominal trauma with sonography: a cost analysis. *Am Surg* 2001; 67(10):930–934.
17. McGahan JP, Richards J, Gillen M. The focused abdominal sonography for trauma scan: pearls and pitfalls. *J Ultrasound Med* 2002;21(7): 789–800.
18. Richards JR, Knopf NA, Wang L, et al. Blunt abdominal trauma in children: evaluation with emergency US. *Radiology* 2002;222(3): 749–754.
19. Shanmuganathan K, Mirvis SE, Sherbourne CD, et al. Hemoperitoneum as the sole indicator of abdominal visceral injuries: a potential limitation of screening abdominal US for trauma. *Radiology* 1999; 212(2):423–430.
20. Livingston DH, Lavery RF, Passannante MR, et al. Free fluid on abdominal computed tomography without solid organ injury after blunt abdominal injury does not mandate celiotomy. *Am J Surg* 2001;182(1): 6–9.
21. Nastanski F, Cohen A, Lush SP, et al. The role of oral contrast administration immediately prior to the computed tomographic evaluation of the blunt trauma victim. *Injury* 2001;32(7):545–549.
22. Federle MP, Yagan N, Peitzman AB, et al. Abdominal trauma: use of oral contrast material for CT is safe. *Radiology* 1997;205(1):91–93.
23. Hulka F, Mullins RJ, Leonardo V, et al. Significance of peritoneal fluid as an isolated finding on abdominal computed tomographic scans in pediatric trauma patients. *J Trauma* 1998;44(6):1069–1072.
24. Yao DC, Jeffrey RB Jr., Mirvis SE, et al. Using contrast-enhanced helical CT to visualize arterial extravasation after blunt abdominal trauma: incidence and organ distribution. *AJR Am J Roentgenol* 2002; 178:17–20.
25. Willmann JK, Roos JE, Platz A, et al. Multidetector CT: detection of active hemorrhage in patients with blunt abdominal trauma. *AJR Am J Roentgenol* 2002;179(2):437–444.
26. Fang JF, Chan RJ, Wong YC, et al. Pooling of contrast material on computed tomography mandates aggressive management of blunt hepatic injury. *Am J Surg* 1998;176(4):315–319.
27. Santucci RA, McAninch JM. Grade IV renal injuries: evaluation, treatment, and outcome. *World J Surg* 2001;25(12):1565–1572.
28. Dinkel HP, Danuser H, Triller J. Blunt renal trauma: minimally invasive management with microcatheter embolization experience in nine patients. *Radiology* 2002;223(3):723–730.
29. Parker MS, Matheson TL, Rao AV, et al. Making the transition: the role of helical CT in the evaluation of potentially acute thoracic aortic injuries. *AJR Am J Roentgenol* 2001;176(5):1267–1272.
30. Cleverley JR, Barrie JR, Raymond GS, et al. Direct findings of aortic injury on contrast-enhanced CT in surgically proven traumatic aortic injury: a multi-centre review. *Clin Radiol* 2002;57(4):281–286.
31. Fishman JE, Nunez D Jr, Kane A, et al. Direct versus indirect signs of traumatic aortic injury revealed by helical CT: performance characteristics and interobserver agreement. *AJR Am J Roentgenol* 1999; 172(4):1027–1031.
32. Scaglione M, Pinto A, Pinto F, et al. Role of contrast-enhanced helical

CT in the evaluation of acute thoracic aortic injuries after blunt chest trauma. *Eur Radiol* 2001;11(12):2444–2448.

33. Wintermark M, Wicky S, Schnyder P. Imaging of acute traumatic injuries of the thoracic aorta. *Eur Radiol* 2002;12(2):431–442.

34. Beese RC, Allan R, Treasure T. Contrast-enhanced helical computerized tomography in the investigation of thoracic aortic injury. *Ann R Coll Surg Engl* 2001;83(1):10–13.

35. Exadaktylos AK, Sclabas G, Schmid SW, et al. Do we really need routine computed tomographic scanning in the primary evaluation of blunt chest trauma in patients with ''normal'' chest radiograph? *J Trauma* 2001;51(6):1173–1176.

36. Mirvis SE, Shanmuganathan K, Buell J, et al. Use of spiral computed tomography for the assessment of blunt trauma patients with potential aortic injury. *J Trauma* 1998;45(5):922–930.

37. Dyer DS, Moore EE, Ilke DN, et al. Thoracic aortic injury: how predictive is mechanism and is chest computed tomography a reliable screening tool? A prospective study of 1,561 patients. *J Trauma* 2000;48(4): 673–682; discussion 682–683.

38. Fishman JE, Nunez D Jr, Kane A, et al. Direct versus indirect signs of traumatic aortic injury revealed by helical CT: performance characteristics and interobserver agreement. *AJR Am J Roentgenol* 1999; 172(4):1027–1031.

39. Curry JD, Recine CA, Snavely E, et al. Periaortic hematoma on abdominal computed tomographic scanning as an indicator of thoracic aortic rupture in blunt trauma. *J Trauma* 2002;52(4):699–702.

40. Lane MJ, Mindelzun RE, Sandhu JS, et al. CT diagnosis of blunt pancreatic trauma: importance of detecting fluid between the pancreas and the splenic vein. *AJR Am J Roentgenol* 1994;163(4):833–835.

41. Lane MJ, Mindelzun RE, Jeffrey RB Jr. Diagnosis of pancreatic injury after blunt abdominal trauma. *Semin Ultrasound CT MR* 1996;17(2): 177–182.

42. Dondelinger RF, Boverie JH, Cornet O. Diagnosis of pancreatic injury: a need to improve performance. *JBR-BTR* 2000; 83(4):160–166.

43. Kim HS, Lee DK, Kim IW, et al. The role of endoscopic retrograde pancreatography in the treatment of traumatic pancreatic duct injury. *Gastrointest Endosc* 2001;54(1):49–55.

44. Canty TG Sr, Weinman D. Management of major pancreatic duct injuries in children. *J Trauma* 2001;50(6):1001–1007.

45. Nghiem HV, Jeffrey RB Jr, Mindelzun RE. CT of blunt trauma to the bowel and mesentery. *AJR Am J Roentgenol* 1993;160(1):53–58.

46. Rizzo MJ, Federle MP, Griffiths BG. Bowel and mesenteric injury following blunt abdominal trauma: evaluation with CT. *Radiology* 1989;173(1):143–148.

47. Killeen KL, Shanmuganathan K, Poletti PA, et al. Helical computed tomography of bowel and mesenteric injuries. *J Trauma* 2001;51(1): 26–36.

48. Hulka F, Mullins RJ, Leonardo V, et al. Significance of peritoneal fluid as an isolated finding on abdominal computed tomographic scans in pediatric trauma patients. *J Trauma* 1998;44(6):1069–1072.

49. Brody JM, Leighton DB, Murphy BL, et al. CT of blunt trauma bowel and mesenteric injury: typical findings and pitfalls in diagnosis. *Radiographics* 2000;20(6):1525–1536; discussion 1536–1537.

50. Killeen KL, Shanmuganathan K, Mirvis SE. Imaging of traumatic diaphragmatic injuries. *Semin Ultrasound CT MR* 2002;23(2):184–192.

51. Bergin D, Ennis R, Keogh C, et al. The ''dependent viscera'' sign in CT diagnosis of blunt traumatic diaphragmatic rupture. *AJR Am J Roentgenol* 2001;177(5):1137–1140.

CHAPTER 28

CT Screening: Principles and Controversies

Karen M. Horton, Leo P. Lawler, Elliot K. Fishman

INTRODUCTION

In the last decade, imaging technology has made impressive advances and now plays an invaluable role in the diagnosis, treatment, and follow up of disease. In particular, computed tomography (CT) has become the workhorse in radiology departments and is considered to be indispensable in the evaluation of a wide range of pathology. Computed-tomography advancements, including the introduction of multidetector CT (MDCT) and three-dimensional (3D) imaging, now offer unprecedented speed and resolution. Computed tomography has become so successful in imaging symptomatic patients that it now is being used to image healthy people as a means to screen for early disease. The concept of screening CT, however, has generated significant controversy.

This chapter will review the most common CT-screening examinations currently being performed throughout the country, including heart scans, lung-cancer screening, virtual colonoscopy, and whole-body scans. A discussion of the controversy and financial considerations surrounding CT screening also will be included.

CT-SCREENING STUDIES

Cardiac Scans for Coronary-artery Calcium Scoring

Cardiovascular disease remains the leading cause of death in the United States. Traditional cardiac risk factors (i.e., blood pressure, cholesterol, etc.) may not be adequate to identify patients at risk for future coronary events, as the first sign of heart disease may be a myocardial infarction. Computed-tomography scanning has been proposed as an imaging tool for early detection of coronary atherosclerosis even before symptoms occur. This early detection of coronary-artery disease using CT then could result in reduced mortality. Given the significance of preliminary studies, the CT calcium score is now being used clinically as a potential tool to identify people who are at risk for future "cardiac

events" so that the appropriate lifestyle or medical interventions can be made (1,2).

Preliminary findings suggest that the presence of coronary-artery calcification is indicative of a 4.2 overall relative risk of having a future cardiac event (3). A negative coronary-calcium score can rule out significant coronary-artery disease in symptomatic patients with atypical chest pain (4). The negative predictive value of a CT-screening examination for significant coronary-artery disease is estimated to be 90% to 95% (5).

Coronary-artery calcification is a marker for atherosclerosis, and the CT coronary-artery calcification score, established by Agatston, has been shown to be an accurate measure of coronary plaque burden and an accurate predictor of future cardiac events (1,6–8). The exact relationship, however, between coronary-artery calcium and the risk of future cardiac events is complex. Only calcified plaque is imaged with CT. Unstable noncalcified plaque cannot be detected. Thus, on rare occasions, patients who have low or negative calcium scores can have serious myocardial events, which often are catastrophic.

In addition, although the Agatston method for scoring coronary-artery calcium is currently the preferred method for CT evaluation of coronary calcium, some researchers question its reproducibility because its calculation involves multiplication of the area of a calcified plaque by an arbitrary coefficient based on peak plaque attenuation (9,10). Recent studies have shown that the use of the calcium-mass quantification in conjunction with scanner calibration (based on phantom calibration) may allow more accurate and more reproducible quantification of coronary calcium (11). In addition, this approach allows for changes in scanning protocols to reduce further radiation exposure and to adapt for new scanner generations (12). However, at this time, the Agatston score is the primary method of analysis (Figure 28-1).

In addition to dispute over the correct calcium-scoring method, there is persistent controversy regarding the use of

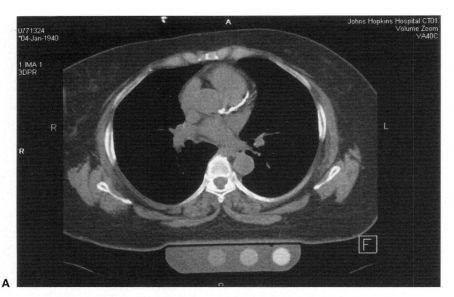

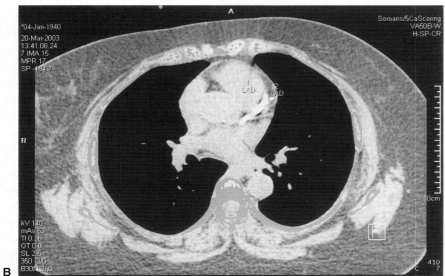

Artery	Number of Lesions (1)	Volume [mm²] (3)	Equiv. Mass [mg CaHA] (4)	Score (2)
LM	0	0.0	0.00	0.0
LAD	2	825.0	251.59	1015.6
CX	0	0.0	0.00	0.0
RCA	1	96.3	23.06	111.4
Total	3	921.4	274.65	1127.0

(1) Lesion is volume based
(2) Equivalent Agatston score
(3) Isotropic interpolated volume
(4) Calibration Factor: 0.833

Threshold = 130 HU

FIG. 28–1. Coronary-calcification scoring study. **A:** Coronary-artery calcification study demonstrates extensive calcification in the left anterior descending coronary artery on standard axial display. **B:** Computer-assisted highlighting program is used to help define the full extent of calcification on a semiautomated system approach. (See Color Fig. 28–1B) **C:** Calculation of Agatston score is 1127. Note software also provides the equivalent mass (mg CaHA) and volume score.

electron-beam CT (EBCT) versus MDCT for performing coronary-artery calcium-scoring examinations. The first reports in the early 1990s used EBCT. At that time, single-detector spiral scanners were not fast enough to image adequately the coronary arteries. However, by 1995, the first reported results of MDCT (2 detectors) appeared in the literature. A study comparing EBCT with 2-detector MDCT showed results to be comparable (13). Similarly, in a study by Becker and colleagues, there was excellent agreement between scores obtained on EBCT and MDCT (14). Four-detector row CT already has been proven to assess reliably and quantify coronary-artery calcification, especially when using retrospective electrocardiogram- (ECG) gated algorithms (14–16). The score obtained with EBCT correlates with the score obtained with gated MDCT studies; therefore, coronary-artery-calcium scoring can be done at CT-screening centers with either EBCT or MDCT scanners (14,17).

The technique for CT coronary-artery-calcium examinations depends on the type of scanner. On EBCT scanners, scans are obtained using a single breath hold and electrocardiogram (EKG) triggering. Patients are scanned in the supine position from the level of the pulmonary arteries through the base of the heart using a 350-mm field of view with a 512×512 reconstruction matrix. Three millimeter slices are obtained every 3.00 mm with an image-acquisition time of 100 milliseconds. Using an 8-detector row MDCT, prospective EKG gating is used in a sequential mode to obtain 2.00-mm to 5.00-mm slices through the heart at 2.50-mm intervals. One-hundred-forty kilovolts and 50 milliamperes (mAs) were used. This corresponds to an image acquisition of 360 milliseconds. Using new 16-detector row MDCT scanners, 3.00-mm reconstructions are obtained from data acquired using 1.50-mm collimation. Slice reconstruction with overlap (1.50 mm) has been shown to improve reproducibility of the calcium-quantity measurement (18). Three-millimeter slices at 300 mAs allow for images with high signal-to-noise ratio (SNR) that allows reliable detection of coronary calcium. The radiation exposure for this examination is in the range of 1 mSv. The faster MDCT scanners available also allow high-resolution CT angiography (CTA) to be performed of the coronary arteries (19).

In addition to the controversies surrounding the correct method of scoring the calcium and preferred scanning technology, there is some disagreement among physicians as to whether the radiologist, cardiologist, or technologist should be interpreting these examinations. The available software is easy to use and a trained technologist certainly can perform the scoring portion of the exam. However, should a cardiologist or radiologist, or both, review the study? Cardiologists may be more comfortable than the average radiologist in explaining the clinical significance of the examination results directly to a patient in the context of other potential risk factors (e.g., cholesterol, hypertension, smoking, family history). However, cardiologists are not trained in CT interpretation or qualified to review the entire exam, which includes portions of the lungs, bones, and upper abdo-men. Significant incidental findings are common on these examinations and include lung cancer, nodules, adenopathy, lung disease, etc. (20). A strong argument can be made for radiologist involvement in the interpretation of these examinations.

Lung-cancer Screening

Lung cancer is the number one cause of cancer deaths in the United States. The worldwide 5-year survival rate for lung cancer is only 8% to 15% (21). It is clear that if lung cancer is detected at an earlier stage and treated with aggressive surgical resection, the 5-year survival rate can be improved (22). For instance, when Stage-I cancer is resected, the 5-year survival rate is as high as 70% (22–25). Computed tomography is a powerful imaging modality that potentially could detect cancers in asymptomatic smokers.

Results of a landmark lung-cancer-screening study by Henschke and coworkers [Early Lung Cancer Action Project (ELCAP)], using CT and chest X-ray (CXR), demonstrated that low-dose CT is more sensitive than CXR for the detection of noncalcified nodules and for detection of lung cancer at an earlier stage (26). Low-dose CT detected more noncalcified nodules (23% versus 7%), as well as more cancers (2.3% versus 0.7%), than CXR (26). Therefore, in this series, 96% of the lung cancers detected were resectable. Similar studies comparing CT with CXR for lung-cancer detection were performed in Japan and also concluded that CT was more sensitive than CXR (27,28).

In addition to being more sensitive than CXR for the detection of lung cancer, CT also detects a high number of Stage-I cancers. In the Henscke trial, 85% of the cancers detected (23 of 27) were Stage I. In a similar study at the Mayo Clinic, 1520 patients were evaluated. Patients were at least 50 years old and had at least a 20-pack-per-year smoking history. After 3 years of scans, a total of 41 lung cancers were detected, 59% of which were Stage IA at the time of diagnosis. It is clear that CT can detect lung cancer at an early stage in high-risk smokers (29,30). In a large study of 1669 people in Japan who underwent biannual lung-cancer screening with CXR, low-dose spiral CT, and sputum cytology, 31 cases of lung cancer were detected on CT, 24 of which (77%) were not visible on CXR (31); 22 of the 24 were Stage IA (31).

Opponents to lung-cancer screening make several important points. First, when performing lung-cancer screening, many benign lesions are detected. For instance, in the study by Henschke and colleagues, 23% of patients had nodules requiring follow up (26). Similarly, in the study by Swensen and coworkers, 51% of the participants had at least one noncalcified nodule that needed to be followed (30). The vast majority of the small nodules detected will be benign, but will require serial follow-up scans to ensure stability. This adds significant cost to the healthcare system, as well as anxiety for patients. In addition, it has not been proven that detecting small cancers in asymptomatic patients will result in increased survival and decreased mortality, since even these small lesions may have spread already (32). A large multicenter prospective trial (National Lung Screening Trial) now is underway, sponsored by ACRIN and National Cancer Institute (NCI). This is a randomized trial comparing CXR and low-dose helical CT in 50,000 current or former smokers. The study is designed to have enough statistical power to determine if a 20% to 25% reduction in mortality from lung cancer is achievable with CT at 5 years. However, it will be many years before the results of these studies are available, as patients will need lengthy follow up in order to determine whether CT screening will improve long-term survival and mortality.

Because many studies are ongoing, the optimal CT protocol has yet to be determined. However, it is clear that scans should be performed with thin collimation (5 mm or less), single breath hold (to limit respiratory motion), and de-

creased mAs (to decrease radiation exposure). At John Hopkins Medical Insitutions, MDCT currently is used for lung-cancer screening using 2.50-mm collimation to create 3.00-mm slices. The kilovolt (kV) is 140 and the mAs is reduced to 80 to decrease the radiation dose. Due to the high contrast between the lung parenchyma and soft-tissue nodules, the technique can be adjusted in order to reduce significantly the radiation dose, so that it is equivalent to 2 or 3 chest X-rays (26,33) (Figure 28-2).

A promising new software technology is now in development that may aid in CT screening for lung cancer. Computer-aided diagnosis systems use sophisticated software programs to aid in lung-nodule detection (33,34). These systems can detect nodules and give accurate diameter and volume measurements and may come to play a role at CT-screening centers for the detection and follow up of lung nodules (Figure 28-3).

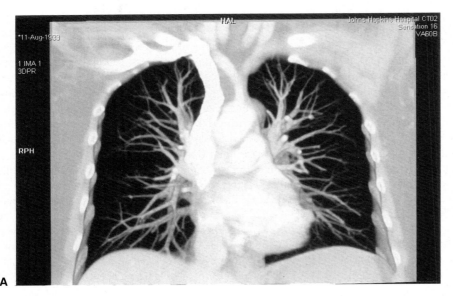

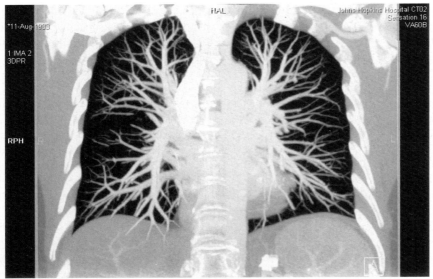

FIG. 28–2. Maximum-intensity-projection (MIP) technique used to enhance analysis of lung for detection of nodules. **A,B:** Use of 3D volume approach to analysis of the lung may help limit the number of false-positive diagnoses made.

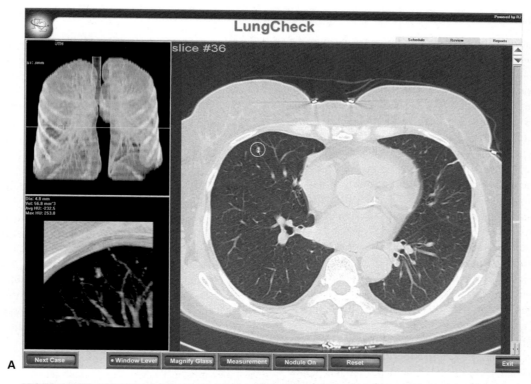

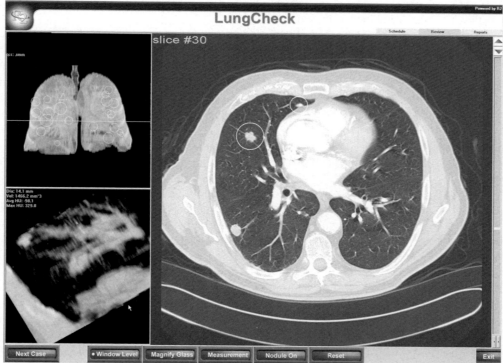

FIG. 28–3. Computer-assisted detection of lung nodules. **A,B:** Computer-assisted detection of lung nodules by prototype system from R2 Technologies (Sunnyvale, CA) may prove valuable for screening in the future.

Virtual Colonoscopy

Colon cancer is the third most common cancer in the United States and the second most common cause of cancer deaths (35). In the year 2002, more than 148,000 new cases of colorectal cancer were diagnosed in the United States. During that same time, nearly 57,000 people died from this disease (36). Given the prevalence of the disease, and the fact that almost all colon cancers arise from detectable precancerous polyps, an effective screening study would make a significant healthcare impact.

Among the colon-screening options available today, fiberoptic colonoscopy is considered the gold standard for colon-cancer screening, as well as for detection and removal of precancerous polyps. However, this examination is not ideal. It is expensive, invasive, and fails to identify some lesions. For example, in a recent study that included back-to-back colonoscopies, it was found that 27% of adenomas less than or equal to 5.00 mm were missed, 13% of adenomas 6.00 mm to 9 mm in size were missed, and 6% of adenomas greater than 1 cm were missed (37).

The concept of using CT for colon-cancer screening was introduced first in 1994. Since that time, the technique has made significant technical advancements and has gained widespread attention. The technique involves using the data acquired from a helical-CT scan combined with sophisticated computer software to generate both two-dimensional (2D) and 3D views of the colon in order to aid in detection of colon cancer and precancerous polyps.

First, the colon must be cleansed completely, as retained stool may obscure or simulate polyps. Various colonic cleansing agents are available. The Fleet prep kit #1 (Fleet Pharmaceuticals, Lynchburg, VA) was used in this study. This includes 45 cc of Phospho-soda, four 5-mg bisacodyl tablets, and one 10-mg bisacodyl suppository. This is considered to be a saline cathartic and is tolerated better by patients, resulting in less retained fluid. It should be avoided in patients with renal failure or congestive heart failure, however, as it may cause electrolyte problems.

Next, the colon must be distended maximally, as collapsed segments can obscure lesions. Colonic distention can be accomplished with either room air or carbon dioxide, and can be performed manually or via the use of a mechanical pump. At least 1.50 to 2.00 liters of air usually is necessary to distend the colon completely.

After the colon is distended, data are obtained in both the prone and supine positions, which has been found to increase the diagnostic accuracy of CT (38). While exact CT protocols vary, it is clear that thin collimation (less than 5 mm) should be performed with overlapping reconstruction, and an attempt should be made to limit the radiation dose by reducing the mA (35). The patient should be scanned in a single breath hold to reduce motion artifact. A 16-slice scanner at 0.75 collimation is used to create 1.00-mm slices every 1 mm. Typically, 120 kV and 200 mAs is adequate.

Images then are transferred to a workstation for interpretation. Initially, it is important to perform a comprehensive review of the axial scans, preferably with cine capabilities. Multiplanar reconstruction then can be performed to increase reader confidence and visualize the colon in multiple planes simultaneously. In addition to the axial scans and multiplanar reconstructions, volume-rendered and endoluminal views can be reviewed. There is some controversy as to whether the entire supine and prone dataset needs to be reviewed using endoluminal software. For instance, Dachman and associates evaluated 44 patients and found that interpretation times were shorter if routine endoluminal views were not performed (39). In another study by Macari coworkers, there was a significant decrease in interpretation times, from 40 minutes to 16 minutes, when only selected endoluminal views were reviewed (40). This did not result in a decreased sensitivity for polyp detection. Many different software manufacturers exist, which allow automated endoscopic "fly-through" imaging. However, even with the latest real-time software packages, CT colonoscopy still is a time-consuming examination requiring additional training for the technologists and radiologists. Even with skilled radiologists, the exam takes 20 minutes 30 minutes to interpret. If widespread CT screening is established, this could result in a significant time constraint for radiologists and is a strong argument for development of software to perform computer-assisted diagnosis.

Reviewing the diagnostic accuracy of CT colonoscopy is difficult given the variety of scanners, different scanning protocols and software packages used, and different methods of analysis over the last decade (per patient versus per polyp). However, it is clear that the sensitivity and specificity of CT colonoscopy have improved as scanner and computer technology has advanced. There has been one large trial evaluating single-detector CT and MDCT in 237 high-risk patients (41). The authors noted that the advantages of using MDCT included a shorter breath hold with less respiratory and motion artifact, as well as improved demonstration of colonic distention. The thinner collimation available with MDCT allows nearly isotropic images, resulting in high-resolution images in all imaging planes and improved endoluminal views (Figure 28-4).

Yee et al. utilized 3-mm collimation for CT colonoscopy in a large study of 300 patients (42). In the study, CT colonoscopy had a 100% sensitivity for detection of cancers (8 of 8) and an overall per-patient sensitivity and specificity of 90.1% (164 of 182) and 72% (85 of 118), respectively, for polyp detection. The per-patient sensitivity was 100% for polyps 1 cm or greater (49 of 49), 93% for polyps 5.00 mm to 9.90 mm (50 of 54), and 82% for polyps less than 5 mm (65 of 79) (42). The study also included a significant number of asymptomatic patients.

In addition to its use as a potential screening tool for colorectal cancer, CT colonoscopy has been found to play an important role in the evaluation of patients after failed

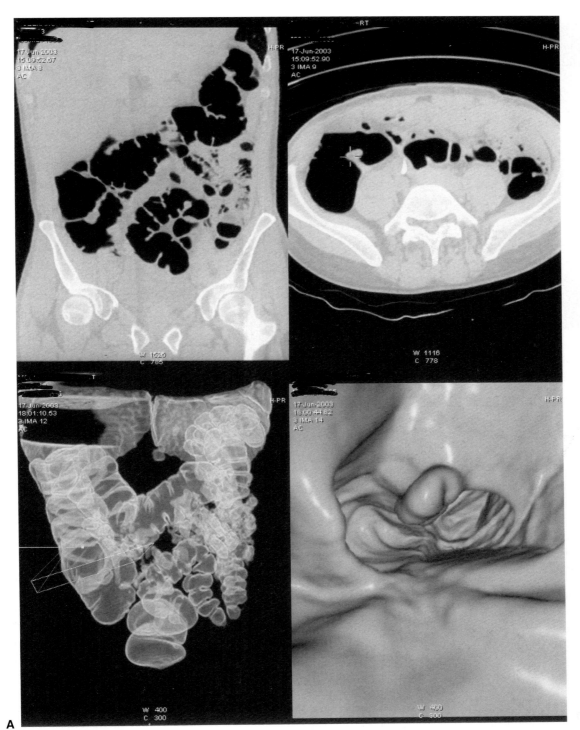

FIG. 28–4. Virtual colonoscopy. **A,B:** Computed tomography detects colonic polyp on this screening exam. The keys to a successful exam include adequate colonic distension, good patient prep, and good fly-through software. *(continued)*